Vera Pyle's Current Medical Terminology

Eighth Edition

by Health Professions Institute

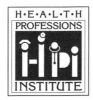

Health Professions Institute • Modesto, California • 2000

Vera Pyle's Current Medical Terminology
Eighth Edition
by Health Professions Institute

Published by:

Health Professions Institute
P. O. Box 801
Modesto, California 95353-0801
Phone (209) 551-2112
Fax (209) 551-0404
Web site: http://www.hpisum.com
E-mail: hpi@hpisum.com
Sally Crenshaw Pitman
Editor & Publisher

Printed by:
Parks Printing & Lithograph
Modesto, California

ISBN: 0-934385-33-5
Last digit is the print number: 9 8 7 6 5 4 3 2 1

ii

To those who have contributed to this book,
To those who read it and find it useful,
To all who love words.

and

To Dan Pae, who passed through life—
and made a difference.

"What is the use of a book," thought Alice, "without pictures or conversations?"

Lewis Carroll
Alice's Adventures in Wonderland

Contents

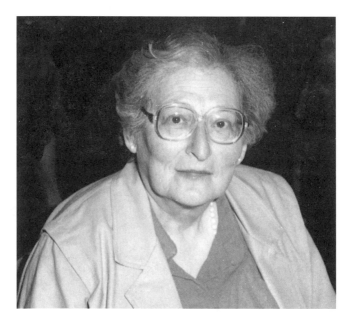

Vera Pyle, 1917-1998

Savoring Vera Pyle

One of the pivotal events in my life was meeting Vera Pyle in 1976. She taught medical transcription at City College of San Francisco and was supervisor of medical transcription at University of California Medical Center in San Francisco, and I owned a medical transcription business two hours away in Modesto, where medical transcriptionists formed a professional association. One of the inquiry letters sent to teaching hospitals in California reached Vera Pyle. She carried it back and forth from her office to her home for several weeks, planning to write an encouraging response. When her letter finally arrived, we were excited by her enthusiastic support and invited her to Modesto to speak at our November 1976 meeting. She visited my home, and that was the beginning of the beautiful friendship and mutually rewarding professional association that shaped our lives.

Vera Pyle and I worked together over the years to accomplish many things, some of them even great things. Helping to found the American Association for Medical Transcription (AAMT) in 1978, we served as national directors for two three-year terms (Vera's membership number is 12 and mine is 9). Each of us received the Distinguished Member Award, and our publishing company was the first corporate member. We have written and edited many publications and educational materials for medical transcription audiences, and we have worked together to set a professional tone and the highest professional standards for medical transcriptionists. Our leadership roles in the medical transcription profession were an essential part of the 23-year history we shared.

One of the important truths about history is that it doesn't deal just with the past, but with the present and the future. That's apparent when I think of the most valuable tangible result of our professional relationship—Vera Pyle's book, *Current Medical Terminology*. The past, the present, and the future are very much a part of this book and its importance to us as friends and professional colleagues

Life is to be savored—an important lesson we learned from Vera Pyle. She believed life is to be lived to the fullest and then remembered and shared with fondness and joy. It isn't that she had more treasured moments than the rest of us, but that she *savored* special times and experiences and shared them with friends and family with such obvious delight. She taught us to recognize the wonders of even ordinary life. Her generosity of spirit was reflected in her enjoyment of life, which she approached with keen insight and understanding, with hope and love and kindness.

A natural storyteller, Vera had the capacity to distill simple experiences into special moments to be re-created over and over and shared with friends. Perhaps a trivial example, but the "pat of butter" story comes to mind every time I think of the word *savor* in connection with her. A few years ago she was told by her doctor to reduce her fat intake to practically zilch, so she learned to spread only a tiny bit of butter on bread and then to gingerly place a bite of bread, butter side down, on her tongue and savor the taste. So even though she couldn't eat butter the way she liked, she made sure she received the maximum benefit of what she had. Who among us is so philosophical about our self-imposed culinary deprivations?

She went to a great deal of effort to provide special treats for her friends. For weeks before Christmas she baked persimmon puddings (little rich, moist individual cakes with walnuts), and carefully packed and mailed them to friends all over the world. She gave walking *sticks* (not *canes*, she emphasized) to elderly friends and silver spoons to newborns. She believed that every child deserves to be born with a silver spoon in its mouth, and she brought silver spoons from England for each of my six grandchildren (and for other friends as well). They were not ordinary spoons, but antique silver spoons purchased from an out-of-the-way antique dealer in London. She apologized that the one she bought most recently for my granddaughter was not as old as the others; it was made as recently as 1856. She took popcorn to friends in England, and a can of Spam to a friend who wondered if it would taste as good now as it did during World War II. And she brought me "worry beads" from Greece.

She savored friends and family. She never tried to impose her own desires or prejudices on anyone else, firmly believing that intelligent people should make their own choices, and she maintained that spirit of independence up until her death of cancer on July 24, 1998. What she said of her friend and mentor Dan Pae applies even more to her. "She passed through life—and made a difference." Her life has immeasurably enriched ours.

Sally Crenshaw Pitman

Adapted from editorial comments by Sally Pitman in *Perspectives on the Medical Transcription Profession*, "Our History" (Winter-Spring 1997-98), and "Savoring Life" (Summer 1998), published by Health Professions Institute.

Vera Pyle's Silver Book

I can see the handwriting on the wall—and it is misspelled.

One thing I have learned is that this is proving a bigger project than I had anticipated.

This is a continuing learning process, and one of the things I've learned is this: There is more than one right way.

How far should we go in trying to verify a word? One can spend hours researching a word, but in my book, that's artsy-craftsy, not professional.

What I am finding in medical word research is that nothing is gospel, nothing is graven on the tablet. It just depends on which tablet you check. This shakes your confidence, for how can you be as perfect as humanly possible when there are so many chances for error?

Medical transcriptionists don't dictate, physicians do.

Praise and credit rise to the highest person on the totem pole, criticism and blame fall on the lowest.

Collectively we could come up with many other quotable quotes from Vera Pyle. Her emphasis on quality medical transcription and the highest professional standards made her one of the most respected members of our profession. She provided an eloquent voice for medical transcriptionists. "Let me tell you a story" prefaced many of her favorite anecdotes, and they invariably ended with "Now you know all I know." And if you asked, "Are you sure?" she would inhale and launch another story.

Vera Pyle's love of *words* characterized her professional life. "How do you spell it and what is your source?" introduced her first column of new, difficult, and hard-to-find medical terms in November 1979, when she first began writing for medical transcriptionists. *Vera Pyle's Current Medical Terminology* is the first edition released since her death in 1998. It continues the professional traditions she established over twenty years ago.

Every book in its eighth edition has a history. What is apparent in the proud owners of the previous editions of *Current Medical Terminology* is that their fondness of the book is inextricably linked with their affection and respect for its author. For over twenty years Vera Pyle was associated with the best in medical transcription. To those who know and love this book and its author, it is often known as "the silver book," "my Vera," "Pyle," or "my bible."

Current Medical Terminology was written *by* medical transcriptionists especially *for* medical transcriptionists, although physicians and other health-care professionals find it useful as well. The unique qualities of the book are immediately apparent to anyone who gives more than a cursory glance at the words and phrases defined. First of all, the definitions are interesting, some even chatty, a few humorous or ironic, and many have quotations to show how the terms are used in medical dictation. Extensive cross-references help the reader on a word-search.

Vera Pyle always thought we are all word freaks. Long ago she wrote, "If I were cast away on a desert island, the book I would probably want to take with me is an *Unabridged Webster's* and I could be happy for years. Couldn't you? We get lost in a dictionary. We look up a word and we see something else that is exciting, and we look up another word, and so on. It's a common symptom among medical transcriptionists. I myself would rather have a dozen new medical words, researched and defined, than a five-pound box of candy. And I bet you would too."

As a lexicographer, Pyle never took her responsibility lightly, nor did she consider herself a self-appointed expert on medical language. Researching new medical terms and writing definitions proved to be a bigger challenge than she anticipated when she volunteered in 1979 to compile a list of new terms for bimonthly issues of *The AAMT Newsletter*. She spent hundreds of hours doing research in medical journals, dictionaries, equipment catalogs, and textbooks; corresponding with medical transcriptionists in all work settings; questioning physicians, nurses, pharmacists, surgical technicians, and lab technologists; and persuading friends in Central Supply to read her exactly how the name of an instrument was written on the package. That was many years before the Internet provided instant access to medical references.

Despite endless efforts to be correct in her findings, she admitted regret-fully, "There has been a time or two—or three—that I have rushed to press, triumphantly, with a word hot out of the operating room, newly born, nowhere else to be found, a real scoop—only to find it in print at a later date, and to learn that it had been given us—wrong."

Editing a word list for medical transcriptionists is not a job for the faint-hearted. Medical transcriptionists are necessarily perfectionists and can be ruth-less in their criticism of anyone who makes an *error* in spelling or defining a new medical term. Criticism, lots of it, is to be expected and borne with equa-nimity. Over the years Vera Pyle necessarily developed a thick skin.

When she first began writing, her task was to provide a *reliable* and *imme-diate* source of information to tens of thousands of medical transcriptionists. She recognized that medical transcriptionists need the words as soon as they are used in dictation; they cannot wait until they appear in dictionaries and reference books updated every five to ten years.

When she published spellings that were later proved incorrect, she was flooded with mail from irate readers. She was sure her mailman thought she was giving away gold bricks. One reader chastised her: "We need to 'know' when the dictator 'knows,' not after the fact. . . . If we knew the 'new' words by preview, the time and effort saved could be tremendous!" Pyle responded to the criticism with a marvelous fantasy of a modern-day Paul Revere who would ride through the countryside, shouting out the new terms that medical transcriptionists would need in the next day's dictation.

She tried to provide something for everybody. Deciding which words were worthy of inclusion in a word list was the first challenge. How could she be sure a word new to her was new to others in the field? She tried to determine if new terms will stand the test of time and not be merely faddish, trendy, highly personal, or regional among certain doctors. "My own criteria for using new words or slang would be (1) need for the word or term, (2) broad understanding of the term, and (3) potential for survival." Good judgment and a wealth of experience in medical transcription served her well.

Writing for a national audience of medical transcriptionists means that terms might be commonly used in certain regions of the country and not yet in circulation elsewhere. Doctors' in-language and jargon in one setting might not be accepted in other settings. Pyle often had to translate examples of abbreviations, acronyms, and brief forms that hospital residents and interns sprinkled in their dictation—a kind of medical "short-tongue" she thought made them feel professional. They often coined terms like *CABG* ("cabbage") and *COWS*, and she translated, defined, and illustrated how they are used in dictation.

> **COWS** (cold to the opposite, warm to the same)—a mnemonic device to help remember the Hallpike caloric stimulation response. "Caloric testing produced COWS." See *caloric testing*.

Understanding new procedures and explaining them to someone else in an interesting way, without being too technical, is always a challenge. Pyle's wonder and fascination with new techniques and her ability to describe them to a nontechnical audience are apparent in this definition:

> **subtraction films** (Radiol)—a method to visualize the arteries and veins on x-ray. A scout film is taken first, before the dye is injected. The scout negative is made into a positive (darkens it). Then the angiogram is taken

(this is a negative). Then a scout positive is taken and put under the dye-injected negative (the patient, not the film, has had the dye injection), which screens out the bone, so all that is then visible are the arteries and veins.

She believed that a picture was worth a thousand words, and she often used examples from dictation in order to provide a context and a word picture for an unusual phrase:

palmar beak ligament (Ortho)—"It has been suggested that instability result-ing from incompetence of the palmar beak ligament is responsible for initi-ating the progression of degenerative joint disease."

She made a special effort to explain terms used commonly in medical dictation but not defined elsewhere. Students and trainees in medical transcription found such definitions as the following particularly helpful:

pack-year smoking history—as "The patient has a 50-pack-year smoking his-tory." The patient has smoked a pack a day for 50 years, or two packs a day for 25 years, or five packs a day for ten years (or ten packs a day for five years!). It is the packs per day multiplied by the number of years of smoking; the cumulative result is the important factor.

One of Vera Pyle's most treasured compliments came from a physician who was chair of the medical record committee in the teaching hospital where she supervised the medical transcription department: "The medical transcrip-tionists make my residents appear to be better dictators than I know them to be." She always had enormous respect for physicians who were as conscien-tious in their dictation practices as in their medical practice. She taught us not to accept a doctor's spelling as definitive, but to appreciate the effort of a thoughtful physician giving a hint on the spelling of an unfamiliar new term or test.

She encouraged us to transcribe with accuracy and sensitivity what the dictators *mean*, not just what they *say*. Too medically sophisticated to insist on verbatim transcription, she nevertheless believed it's important not to tamper with a physician's dictating style, not to impose our own style and preferences on medical reports. The dictation is to represent their style, not ours. A physi-cian's style may need judicious editing, of course, but not *tampering*.

In the early years of producing word lists, somebody wrote to her, "Why don't you have *your staff* research the words more carefully?" "I am 'the staff'," she replied. But she enlisted the help of medical transcriptionists everywhere to contribute new terms they had encountered in dictation. "You're all medical word researchers on your own, on your jobs," she wrote. "New medical words tend to surface at university teaching hospitals, but a lot of you out there know things I don't know that haven't yet surfaced here. If you know enough to pick up on these things after we print them, why don't you tell me about them early on, before I fall on my face?"

Over the years Pyle's "staff" has grown to include many medical transcriptionists and others who have provided examples of new terms encountered in dictation. HPI staff and associates—Linda Campbell, Ellen Drake, Diane Heath, Georgia Green, Kathy Cameron, and John H. Dirckx, M.D.—have provided primary research, editing, and proofreading skills in production of each edition of the book.

In the early and mid-1980s, Bron Taylor of San Francisco contributed extensive lists of new AIDS terminology, when AIDS awareness was just beginning. Susan Turley provided scores of chemotherapy protocols and specialized nursing terms in the 1980s and early 1990s.

Of special help in this eighth edition were the many contributions of Arleen McGovern and Toni Mercandante from the popular Web site, *MT Desk.com*.

Now you know all I know. . . . I wish.

Sally Crenshaw Pitman
Editor & Publisher

Adapted from Sally Pitman, "Vera Pyle's Silver Book," *Perspectives on the Medical Transcription Profession* (Winter-Spring 1997-98, pp. 22-23), published by Health Professions Institute.

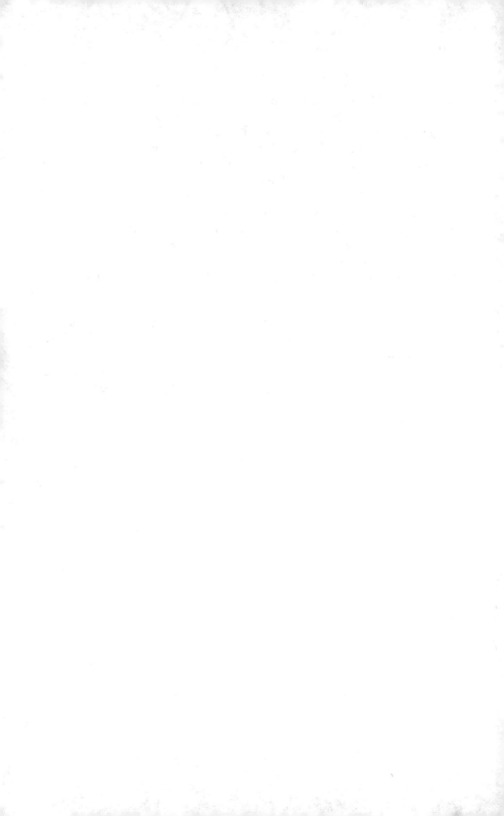

Preface

Words are a large part of the stock-in-trade of the medical transcriptionist, and we encounter new ones every day. There is the usual flurry of identifying the new word: "What do you hear? Yes, that's what I heard. What is it? What does it mean? How do you spell it? What's your source?"

Much has happened in medicine in the last ten years—monoclonal antibodies, magnetic resonance imaging (MRI), DNA recombinant method of producing biosynthetic hormones and other products, breakthroughs in our knowledge of cell function and reproduction, new methods of treatment without resorting to surgery, investigational drugs for treatment of AIDS and cancer. With all of these innovations, there are thousands of new words which, if you haven't yet heard, you soon will. In medicine, we can hardly say "current" for very long; thus, it is necessary to update *Current Medical Terminology* every two years.

New features include definitions of many specialized terms used in surgery and radiology. Under the entry *medication* is a quick-reference list of all the pharmaceuticals defined in main entries throughout the book, including drugs used in treating AIDS patients, chemicals, chemotherapy drugs and protocols, classes of drugs, contrast media, investigational drugs, natural substances, prescription and over-the-counter drugs, monoclonal antibodies, orphan drugs, radioisotopes, and solutions. In most cases we have listed both generic and brand name, the latter with capitalization where needed. Other lengthy quick-reference lists include those under main entries *device, disease, MRI terms, operation, pathogen, syndrome,* and *test.*

Extensive cross-referencing has been done. In most cases, the definition will appear with the form of the word most often used in dictation. That is, if the acronym, abbreviation, or brief form of the word is that most often dictated, then the definition will appear under that term, with a cross-reference to the other form. Sometimes a medical transcriptionist can hear or understand only one word of a phrase dictated by a physician; thus, cross-referencing under other important words of a phrase is provided.

I hope you will find this book even more useful than the earlier editions, which I know you all took to your hearts.

Vera Pyle, CMT
March 1998

xv

Introduction

This book is intended primarily for medical transcriptionists, but now I find that it is also being used by court reporters, health information management professionals, coders, legal secretaries, nurses, and students in the allied health professions. Also, with the continued importance of the patient's medical record in reimbursement systems, insurance claims examiners and Medicare evaluators refer to it as well. The recent increase in medicolegal cases has driven court reporters to expand their medical knowledge and reference libraries, and many have found this book to be a valuable tool. So it now becomes necessary to keep a diverse group of readers in mind.

Most medical transcriptionists are either hospital-based or work for off-site transcription services. They transcribe and edit the very detailed and highly technical medical and surgical reports that are used in the delivery of medical care. These written reports assure that everyone involved in that care knows the patient's medical history, what was found on physical examination and on laboratory examinations, the pathology discovered, the treatment given, the medications administered, and the response to therapy noted.

These reports are of importance medically and legally, and in research. They are valued by everyone who uses them (they are often the only legible documents in a patient's record), but the people who transcribe them are largely unknown, individually and as a profession.

New medical terms crop up daily—new medications, new operative procedures, new instruments, new equipment, new techniques, new research terms, new laboratory tests, new abbreviations—many of them—and with little documentation except for a physician's occasional attempt at spelling. It therefore becomes necessary to provide a reliable and immediate source of information to tens of thousands of medical transcriptionists.

References are made throughout the book to "the dictator." These definitions were originally written for an "in-group" of medical transcriptionists who know that "the dictator" refers to the physician or medical student or other healthcare professional who dictates the medical and surgical reports.

Perhaps an explanation is in order at this time to help familiarize new readers with how I research terms, and how I arrive at conclusions (or decisions) when research fails.

Many years ago when my younger daughter was five or six, I overheard an argument she was having with one of her playmates. I don't now recall what it was all about, but I do remember my daughter's clinching argument— "My mother says . . ." Her friend was not prepared to challenge Taffy's mother; end of argument.

No one since then has appointed me The Higher Authority, and the self-appointed are setting themselves up for being leaders with no followers. So I feel that ours must be a collaborative venture. We give our opinions, our reasons for them, and our sources. Our readers may evaluate our conclusions, discuss their differences of opinion, and decide to accept them or not. I hasten to add that we all have a strong instinct for self-preservation and try to make certain that our sources are generally respected and accepted and that our conclusions are those we can defend.

Where do we find entries for *Current Medical Terminology*? From words encountered in medical transcription, from questions from medical transcriptionists, from dozens of medical journals we read regularly. We consult medical textbooks, talk to physicians, and have friends in central supply. Over the years we have learned to be less trusting of the written, as well as the spoken, word.

Of all sources, dictionaries are perhaps my most trusted, although I have found errors in even the most respected. Next are books, although I am finding that they, too, often have errors; apparently proofreading is considered an expendable luxury. I should mention that books do have the disadvantage of being dated, even when newly published. Somewhere at the top of the list would be the trusted person in central supply who will read the label on the equipment, instrument, or medication container, although there are times when there may be more than one spelling, as in *Tycron* and *Ti-Cron*. Next are journals, in which I find the most current information available, but I do find errors in even the most prestigious.

A close tie for last place on my list of trusted sources would be catalogs of instrument manufacturers and the spelling given us by physicians. An old newspaperman once told me that typesetters were given instructions to "follow the copy, even if it goes out the window." There are a few physicians whose spelling is impeccable and whose dictation I *would* "follow out the window," but, unfortunately, they are all too few.

In researching words, sometimes hunches and the educated guess based on experience and the knowledge of analogous words or terms are all one has to go on and are useful. Here is an example: I came across the word *Versatex* as a cardiac pacemaker. I should tell you that it is fatal in this situation to trust; it is *essential* that one question—everything and always. At any rate I felt uncomfortable with that spelling (it was guilty until proven innocent), and I decided to pursue it further. Unable to document it, but finding analogous terms (Activitrax and Spectrax), I felt quite comfortable with the spelling *Versatrax*.

A reader inquired about *Angiocath PRN* and wanted to know the meaning of *PRN*. My first information about Angiocath PRN, trade name of a catheter manufactured by Siemens Medical Systems, came from the *Journal of Neurosurgery*. I can only hazard a more-or-less educated guess as to what is meant. As you know, *p.r.n.* (L. *pro re nata*) means "as circumstances may require." This catheter has many different uses and the PRN may *perhaps* make reference to that.

Medical equipment manufacturers and pharmaceutical companies are most imaginative in creating names for their products. They are so clever, and running these things to earth is so frustrating. Sometimes they provide clues, e.g., Cefobid is a third-generation cephalosporin medication (which accounts for the first syllable) and is to be taken twice a day (b.i.d.), which accounts for the last syllable.

Sometimes there is no clue; one has to know what the device or medication is used for to know what the abbreviation means, e.g., the EID percutaneous central venous large-bore catheter manufactured by Arrow International, Inc. The *EID* turns out to mean *e*mergency *i*nfusion *d*evice! Or how about the SRT vaginal speculum by Amko Manufacturing Company? The *SRT* is from *s*moke *r*emoval *t*ube; the device has a supplementary tube used when smoke evacuation is necessary in laser-induced tissue vaporization.

A few years ago I searched for the definitive spelling of a needle we've been spelling *Verres* for many years. I got a letter from a medical transcriptionist who said she had been told by a physician that that spelling was in error, that it should be *Veress*. She said that she had looked in a dozen different textbooks and the spelling she found was indeed *Veress*, and she also sent me a photocopy of an article about this needle, written by the physician who had developed it, a Dr. Veress. We must assume that Dr. Veress knows how to spell his name, so we have now changed our spelling of this instrument to *Veress*.

In the medical field we don't have to look far or wait long for new words, abbreviations, and acronyms to appear. Just stand still for a couple of hours and a dozen new ones will have been born!

Vera Pyle, CMT
July 1992

A Medical Transcriptionist's Fantasy

A letter from a reader came in yesterday's mail. I thought about it during a sleepless night and at 3 a.m. arose from my bed, sat down in front of the typewriter, and ventilated.

Prices on many things have gone through the roof; dinner out, a play, even a film, are now rare treats. But there is something we can still afford—fantasy.

First, let me quote from the letter:

> *I will again bring to your attention an item I mentioned in a previous survey, to which I have never received a response either directly or indirectly. That is—the providing of information, be it names of newly approved drugs, newly developed prostheses, etc. I recently noted a reprint in one of the local newsletters from another professional journal. It contained "new" items. Although our present Notebook is terrific, it is just too limited to provide us with the information we require; that is, we need to "know" when the dictator "knows," not after the fact. Every time a "new" word is dictated, it involves excessive time and effort not only on the part of the transcriptionists, but on the part of the people they ask for help in listening, only to determine in the end that the spelling is not available to them because it is a "new" item, at which point either the word is researched or left blank for fill-in. If we knew the "new" words by preview, the time and effort saved could be tremendous!*

Now, let us fantasize. Wouldn't it be marvelous if we had a modern-day Paul Revere who would ride through the countryside shouting, not "The British are coming!" but instead "lithotriptor!—a new extracorporeal stone-disintegrating machine! First used in Europe, now being brought to the United States! Generates shock that breaks up kidney stones! Lowercase 'L'!"—as he rides off into the cold, starry night. Or how about "Kim-Ray Greenfield filter—used in prevention of pulmonary emboli! Kim-Ray is capitalized and hyphenated!'' as he gallops, on his panting, snorting, sweating horse, to the next darkened village.

Let's fantasize further. Wouldn't it be wonderful if Dr. Andreas Grüntzig had called us and said: "Just wanted to let you know that I'm inventing a new balloon catheter; it will be a very nice thing to use in transluminal dilatation and in performing angioplasties. And, by the way, my name is spelled G-r-ün-t-z-i-g, in which case don't forget the umlaut over the *u*; or else, you can spell it *Gruentzig*, but in that case, don't use the umlaut. However, I will answer to either."

Or—if Dr. Richard Osgood had written, "You may be interested in being among the first to know that my colleague, Dr. Carl Schlatter (that's spelled S-c-h-l-a-t-t-e-r; don't forget the *c*, and remember there are two *t*'s), and I have just identified a new disease entity—osteochondrosis of the tuberosity of the tibia; also called apophysitis tibialis adolescentium, which we are going to call 'Osgood-Schlatter disease.' If he should call you and tell you about this and tells you it is 'Schlatter-Osgood' disease, remember you heard it from me first, and correctly!"

There has been the time or two—or three—that I have rushed to press, triumphantly, with a word hot out of the operating room, newly born, nowhere else to be found, a real scoop—only to find it in print at a later date, and to learn that it had been given us—wrong.

Paul Revere, where are you now that we need you?

Adapted from Vera Pyle, "A Medical Transcriptionist's Fantasy," *Journal of the American Association for Medical Transcription*, Winter 1983-84, p. 3.

In Defense of "Sterilely"

A question from a medical transcriptionist about the word *sterilely* prompted the following responses. They are quoted here to illustrate the dilemma medical transcriptionists face in striving for accuracy, and a warning about what might happen if they forget that *physicians dictate and medical transcriptionists transcribe.*

The question was how to spell the adverb form of the word *sterile*. The inquirer wrote:

> *I say that if you use this word as an adverb, you retain the original form of the word and add "-ly,"* making the spelling sterilely, *as it is in* futile, puerile, hostile, *etc. My colleagues see no point in dragging grammar into this and spell the word* sterilly, *as in "Sterilly we roll along."*

This is one of the questions to which I can say, with confidence, there is one and only one correct answer. The word is *sterilely*. I refer you to *Webster's Third International Dictionary, Unabridged* (1981), and to the *Random House Dictionary of the English Language, Unabridged*, 2nd ed. (1987); this is the only spelling given for this word.

I have just finished reading a book (in the nonmedical part of my life) about the people who colonized New England in the early 1600s, the Pilgrims and Puritans. Much of the journal written by Governor William Bradford of Plymouth was quoted, as well as letters written by many of the other men involved in the affairs of the Colony. Many of them were men of education, men who had studied at Cambridge. It was most interesting to see their spelling. In Elizabethan times there were no hard and fast spelling rules, and each person spelled as the spirit moved him, not even consistently with any individual. Shakespeare himself spelled his name a number of different ways. In those days this was not considered flouting of rules, since there were few if any rules. But that was then, and this is now.

Now there are dictionaries and rules. Sometimes there is more than one spelling of a word, and dictionaries will give preferred ones and acceptable ones. However, now, if one were to spell in a very personal manner, disregarding the rules, one would be open to criticism. And here I might give you Pyle's observation: Praise and credit rise to the highest person on the totem pole; criticism and blame fall on the lowest. So you see, we can ill afford to be cavalier about such things as correct spelling and grammar. Remember, we are judged and evaluated by people who know the rules and play by them, and they expect us to observe them as well.

A few months later I received the following comment, and apparently it struck a nerve; hence, the following response:

> *It was interesting to read the debate on the spelling of the word* sterilely. *Occasionally, due to progress in the English language, certain words or versions of certain words become outdated.* Sterilely *is one of them. I feel that proper grammar would dictate that we transcriptionists use the present-day terminology "in a sterile manner."*

Sterilely is not among my very favorite words. "I love you" and "I love your book" are higher on my list. Not too far behind comes ". . . the patient was taken to the recovery room in good condition." But I rise to the defense of *sterilely* for several reasons. First of all, there is nothing wrong with the word. Where has it been decreed that it is "outdated"? Words die when they are no longer viable and therefore no longer used. *Sterilely* is very much alive. If you don't believe it, transcribe operative reports in any hospital. If you don't want to believe it, just tell every surgeon in the country that it may no longer be used, that it is a forbidden word.

Imagine the unleashed fury of fifty thousand surgeons when they are told they may no longer say the WORD. I can see the backlash now—thousands of angry surgeons under the cover of night surging into the streets, chalking on fences and spray-painting on walls the naughty word—STERILELY, or possibly even (perish the thought) *sterilly*.

Carried to its logical conclusion, this stance puts us in the position of saying that physicians are permitted to use only those words that all transcriptionists can spell. Carried further there will then be no need for dictionaries, for drug books, for word books. Sounds like a dream, doesn't it? Now comes the alarm clock, shrilling the end of the dream. *Medical transcriptionists don't dictate, physicians do.*

I urge you—cease and desist. Don't type "The patient was draped in a sterile manner" when the surgeon dictates "The patient was sterilely draped," or the fence-chalking, spray-painting surgeons are likely to burn us in effigy.

Adapted from Vera Pyle, "A Question of Style," *Journal of the American Association for Medical Transcription*, Winter 1984-85, Fall 1985.

Medical Slang—Its Use and Abuse

The language of medicine is an ''in-language.'' It is the means of communication for a comparatively small, select group in a world divided into "us" and "them." Its use makes one feel part of that group of "us's." Medical abbreviations and medical slang are subspecies of this language (slanguage?) and are particularly dear to the hearts of the newest members of the in-group.

Its use makes medical students feel that they sound "professional." It has much the same effect as wearing a stethoscope. To only a slightly lesser degree, this applies also to the intern and resident. I once asked a resident in surgery the reason for this. He thought about it for a while, grinned, and replied, "Well, when you've just learned all these new long words, it's a pity not to use them, and you must admit that some of them *are* pretty impressive." Interestingly enough, the truly impressive people in medicine speak simply, almost in lay language.

Language changes. It is far from static. The English we speak now is far from the English of Chaucer or Shakespeare. The language of medicine also changes. Many of these changes fill a real need, in which case they are likely to last. Some of this change is frivolous, "trendy," highly personal, and likely to be understood by few. Much of this language is not yet found in dictionaries for these reasons. Dictionaries, after all, are *de*scriptive, not *pre*scriptive, and many of these words are too new, too ephemeral, too localized to make their way into dictionaries. And for these same reasons, we cannot be certain that we can use them safely in reports which are considered legal documents.

I think we must take a long look at what is now being dictated, and we may find it necessary to accept terms that have been frowned on in the past, that have not yet been accepted in dictionaries but are used constantly by physicians because they fill a need.

Some twenty years ago, we began hearing the word "bovied" but were told, "You can't make a verb of a noun." So we would type, "Bleeders were electrocoagulated with the Bovie unit." All these years later, I find "bovied" still used a great deal—a useful term, succinct, and universally understood. Another such word is "saucerize," which refers to creation of a saucer-shaped excavation surgically.

I believe 20/20 hindsight might well be the determining factor in knowing what is a needed term, likely to survive and ultimately enter the language, and what is for the moment "flip," likely to have only narrow, local application, and short survival. My own criteria for using new words or slang would be (1) need for the word or term, (2) broad understanding of the term, and (3) potential for survival.

A new slang expression I have encountered only occasionally is "romied" and it may or may not last. Although it may fill a need, it is not commonly understood. I am not prepared to use it. It is a verb coined from the acronym ROMI, *r*ule *o*ut *m*yocardial *i*nfarction, and used thus: "The patient was admitted with severe precordial pain and cardiac arrhythmias, and was romied." My guess is that it is one of those terms that will not have wide circulation and will not survive because too few will know the acronym from which it is derived. It is an example of a sub-subspecies of an in-language, and may be known to some cardiologists (probably the newest of them only) and hence will not be a viable means of communication to a broader spectrum of the medical population.

It should also be remembered that our spoken language differs from our written (more formal) language, and that terms used in the operating room or on the ward are not necessarily what should be written in a report.

The following are other examples of acronyms that have become words: CABG (coronary artery bypass graft) and pronounced "cabbage," as in "The patient was given a CABG," or even "The patient was CABG'd." These evoke rather interesting images. (We have the option of using the acronyms or writing out the terms in full.) You may be astonished to hear a physician dictate, "Caloric testing produced COWS." "COWS" stands for "cold to the opposite, warm to the same" and is a mnemonic device used in otolaryngology to help remember the Hallpike caloric stimulation response.

It may be interesting to enter the arcane world of the operating room and discover the slang peculiar to it. For example, a "peanut" is a small gauze sponge used in surgery. This word is in widespread use, but some operating room personnel have their own terms for it. Cotton pledgets are small cotton balls (sponges) which are rolled so that they have somewhat pointed ends. They are used to absorb blood or other fluids from the operative site. In some parts of the country they are known as "pollywogs." The term "stick-tie" means different things to different people in different operating rooms. In some operating rooms it refers to a suture ligature, or transfixion suture; in others it refers to a long strand of suture clamped on a hemostat. If a surgeon asks the scrub nurse for "Mets" (or "Metz"), Metzenbaum scissors are wanted. It is understandable that under the time pressures in surgery, "OR shorthand" would be used, but in a formal document the word should be transcribed "Metzenbaum scissors."

In the dim, distant past, some words originated as medical slang and are now firmly rooted in our language. "Gurney" is one such. I do not know its origin; it may well have been a trade name. It may also have been the brain-child of someone in one hospital and traveled with surgeons or nurses to others across the country. None of the references I have consulted gives a derivation. It is, however, such a commonly used word that it would be absurd now to say, "The patient was placed on a high wheeled cart for moving patients in a hospital and taken to the operating room."

So you see, we are dealing with not only the present but also the past and the future. We can, to some degree, judge from the kinds of words that have been accepted and have survived over the years which ones will have currency in the future. A surgical word we hear all the time is "prepped." Most attending surgeons with whose dictation I am familiar use "prepared." "Prepped" is, however, universally understood, and my inclination is to type whatever the dictator says; if residents feel that they are being "professional" by using it, I won't argue the point. It seems a lost cause anyhow. Perhaps I am getting too old to fight for lost causes; perhaps my sense of proportion tells me it's not worth it, or perhaps I am saving my ammunition for more important issues.

The purpose in dictating all this material, and the purpose in transcribing it, is communication—with other physicians, with nurses, with other healthcare professionals and paraprofessionals; with quality assurance, billing, risk management people; with insurance companies; with lawyers. If we are not successful in this communication, if we are "playing doctor" by being exclusionary with our in-language, if we are obfuscating rather than clarifying, what then is the point in all this effort?

Actually, I have more questions than I have answers. But these are questions that must be raised. I do want to be clear, to be understandable. It is *not*, I repeat, *not* our role to force doctors to do anything our way. This is not in any way a crusade. Doctors like us to be right, but they do resent our being righteous!

Adapted from Vera Pyle, "Medical Slang—Its Use and Abuse," *Journal of the American Association for Medical Transcription*, Fall 1983, pp. 38-39.

Notes

Sequence. Entries are alphabetized letter by letter, without regard to periods, spaces, and hyphens in main entries and subentries; the *'s* of possessive eponyms is ignored in alphabetizing. Initial numbers are alphabetized as if they were written out, although subscript and superscript numbers are ignored.

Medical specialties. To provide a context in which a term is likely to be encountered in medical transcription, one or more medical specialties may appear in parentheses in an entry. Medical specialties are not listed when they are obvious in context.

Anes	Anesthesiology
Cardio	Cardiology; Cardiac Surgery
Derm	Dermatology
ENT	Ear, Nose, and Throat
GI	Gastroenterology
Lab	Laboratory Medicine
Neonat	Neonatology
Nuclear Med	Nuclear Medicine
Neuro	Neurology; Neurosurgery
Ob-Gyn	Obstetrics-Gynecology
Oph	Ophthalmology
Oncol	Oncology
Oral Surg	Oral Surgery
Ortho	Orthopedics; Orthopedic Surgery
Path	Pathology
Peds	Pediatrics
Phys Ther	Physical Therapy
Plas Surg	Plastic Surgery
Pod	Podiatric Surgery
Psych	Psychiatry
Pulm	Pulmonary Medicine
Radiol	Radiology
Rad Oncol	Radiation Oncology
Rehab	Rehabilitation; Physical Medicine
Resp Ther	Respiratory Therapy
Thor Surg	Thoracic Surgery
Urol	Urology
Vasc Surg	Vascular Surgery

A, a

AA (acetabular anteversion).

AAA ("triple A")—medical slang for abdominal aortic aneurysm.

AAI (axial acetabular index).

AAMI (age-associated memory impairment).

AAMT (American Association for Medical Transcription)—a membership organization for medical transcriptionists. See *Certified Medical Transcriptionist*.

Aaron's sign—pain on pressure over McBurney's point in a patient with appendicitis.

Aarskog syndrome—characterized by shawl scrotum, long philtrum, short stature, downward eye slant, and thoracic deformity.

ab, AB (abortion or miscarriage) (Ob-Gyn)—common abbreviation used in dictation. *AB 2* (or *ab 2*) means that the patient has had two abortions or miscarriages.

abacavir—used in the treatment of AIDS. See *Ziagen*.

Abbe-McIndoe vaginal construction—uses split-thickness skin grafts.

ABBI (advanced breast biopsy instrumentation) **system**—a device used to perform breast biopsies, said to minimize the amount of pain, disfigurement, and scarring associated with open breast biopsy, allowing the surgeon to use local instead of general anesthesia, and reducing the time required for the procedure. In a one-step process, the ABBI device removes the entire specimen for biopsy. May also be referred to as the *ABBI procedure* or *system*.

Abbokinase (urokinase) thrombolytic drug.

Abbott-Rawson tube—a long gastrointestinal double-lumen tube.

Abbreviated Injury Scale (AIS).

ABC (airway, breathing, circulation).

ABC (argon beam coagulator).

ABCD (amphotericin B colloid dispersion)—a drug used to treat cryptococcal meningitis in AIDS patients.

ABCD rule of dermatoscopy—diagnostic method of identifying malignant melanoma with the use of a microscope. The parameters are

ABCD *(cont.)*
asymmetry, border, color, and differential structure. See *dermatoscope.*

abdominal compartment syndrome (ACS)—a sustained increase in intra-abdominal pressure due to alterations in respiratory mechanics, cardiovascular hemodynamics, and renal function. The syndrome may follow laparotomy for severe abdominal trauma, ruptured abdominal aortic aneurysm, and intra-abdominal infection. Only recently recognized, it carries a death rate of over 50%.

abdominal cutaneous nerve entrapment syndrome—a common source of unexplained severe abdominal pain. The cause is believed to be compression of the rectus muscle channel, creating ischemia of the ninth thoracolumbar nerve.

abdominal-sacral colpoperineopexy (Ob-Gyn)—a modified version of the abdominal-sacral colpopexy to correct posterior compartment defects and perineal descent associated with vaginal vault prolapse.

abduct—to draw away from a position parallel to the median axis. Cf. *adduct.*

"a-b-duction"—dictated by a physician to clarify that **ab**duction, not **ad**duction, is intended.

Abelcet (amphotericin B lipid complex) (formerly ABLC)—an antifungal agent used to treat candidiasis and severe systemic fungal infections in patients who have not responded to conventional amphotericin B therapy.

Aberdeen knot (Surg)—a crochet knot popularized by Cuschieri, used in laparoscopic suturing procedures. See *convertible slip knot.*

aberrant—wandering or deviating from the normal; abnormal. Cf. *apparent.*

aberrant ribonucleic acid—halts the production of the EAAT2 protein. A new test is being developed to detect this aberrant ribonucleic acid in the hopes of early detection of amyotrophic lateral sclerosis (Lou Gehrig's disease).

ab-externo laser sclerotomy.

ABGs (arterial blood gases)—refer to PO_2, PCO_2, and oxygen saturation. From these data and the serum pH, the bicarbonate (or base excess) can be calculated.

ab-interno laser sclerotomy.

abirritant—a soothing agent.

ABI Vest Airway Clearance System (the "Vest")—a portable device consisting of an inflatable vest connected by hose to an air-pulse generator which rapidly inflates and deflates the vest, compressing and releasing the chest wall, moving mucus toward the larger airways where it can be cleared by coughing or suctioning. Used by cystic fibrosis patients. Commonly referred to as *high frequency chest wall oscillation* (HFCWO). See also *ThAIRapy Vest.*

Ablatherm HIFU system—uses high-intensity focused ultrasound (HIFU) for endorectal treatment of localized prostate cancer. The procedure provides a nonsurgical alternative to surgical excision and radioactive seed implantation.

ablation—separation, eradication, extirpation, as in cryoablation, radiofrequency ablation.

ablative therapy with bone marrow rescue—an acceptable mode of therapy for many types of cancer.

ABLC (amphotericin B lipid complex) —a drug used to treat cryptococcal meningitis in AIDS patients.

ablepharon macrostomia syndrome (AMS)—inherited disorder in which the face, head, genitals, and abdomen do not develop normally. Children with AMS may experience delays in language development and, in some cases, mental retardation.

ABMT (autologous bone marrow transplantation).

abnormal uterine bleeding (AUB).

ABPA (allergic bronchopulmonary aspergillosis).

ABPM (ambulatory blood pressure monitoring).

ABPP (bropirimine)—a drug used to treat AIDS.

ABR (auditory brain stem response)— an audiometric technique to test for sensorineural hearing loss.

abreaction (Psych)—the reliving of an experience in such a way that previously repressed emotions associated with it are released.

abscess—circumscribed, localized collection of pus, usually caused by infection, and by the decomposition of tissue. Example: collar button abscess. See *Brodie's abscess*. Cf. *aphthous*.

Abscession—fluid drainage catheter.

absent bow-tie sign—used to identify bucket-handle tears of the knee menisci on MR imaging. Cf. *bow-tie sign of cervical fracture*.

Absolok—endoscopic clip applicator.

absolute neutrophil count (ANC).

absorbent—an agent or material that takes up or soaks up another material (usually a liquid). Cf. *adsorbent*.

ACA (anticentromere antibody).

ACAD (atherosclerotic carotid artery disease).

Acanthamoeba **keratitis**—an inflammation of the cornea caused by *Acanthamoeba*.

acanthosis—diffuse hyperplasia and thickening of the prickle-cell layer of the epidermis, as in psoriasis.

acarbose (Prandase)—for treatment of type II diabetes.

ACAT (automated computerized axial tomography).

accelerated idioventricular rhythm (AIVR).

Accellon Combi biopsampler—a cervical cytology collecting device that simplifies Pap smear process so that its fibers contact both exo- and endocervical mucosal surfaces.

Accel stopcock—used with high-flow percutaneous catheter introducer.

Ac'cents—permanent lash liner applied by plastic surgeon.

access—admittance, as "This gave easy access to the abdominal cavity." Cf. *axis, excess*.

Access MV system—a beating-heart bypass system which creates easier access and facilitates multiple vessel procedures.

Access Ostase—serum-based test for assessment of osteoporosis and Paget's disease of bone.

Accolate (zafirlukast)—used for prophylaxis and treatment of chronic asthma.

accommodation—adjustment, as of the eye for distance.

accordion sign—a finding indicative of pseudomembranous colitis on CT scans in patients who received oral contrast material. The accordion appearance depends on the degree of edema of the haustral folds and the amount of contrast material trapped between the folds.

Accu-Chek InstantPlus system—small monitor that uses a test strip and a fingerstick blood sample to provide a total cholesterol value in three minutes or a blood glucose value in 12 seconds.

Accu-Chek II Freedom—self-monitoring blood glucose system for visually impaired diabetics. It talks users through self-blood-testing with clearly spoken cues.

Accucore II—core biopsy needle with echo-enhanced tip for ultrasound guidance and precise depth markings.

accuDEXA—a bone mineral density assessment device. See *DEXAscan.*

AccuGuide injection monitor—a lightweight BMG monitor with auditory and BMG feedback to improve the efficiency of injecting small muscle groups.

AccuLase excimer laser—for use in transmyocardial revascularization procedures.

AccuLength arthroplasty measuring system—an intraoperative hip length measuring device for use during total hip arthroplasty.

Accu-Line knee instrumentation—to assist in total knee arthroplasty. Includes tibial resector, distal femoral resection instrument, dual pivot, chamfer resection guide, and patellar instruments.

Acculink self-expanding stent—for revascularization of stenotic carotid arteries secondary to atherosclerotic disease. The stent is advanced through a small incision in the femoral artery to the area of carotid occlusion. Once in place, the stent is deployed to maintain patency and prevent atherosclerotic plaque from becoming displaced. Carotid stenting offers a less invasive alternative to carotid endarterectomy procedures.

AccuPoint hCG Pregnancy Test Disc—for quick diagnosis.

Accupril (quinapril)—a once-a-day ACE inhibitor for hypertension.

Accurate Surgical and Scientific Instruments (ASSI)—a trade name, not a comment on quality.

Accuretic (quinapril hydrochloride/ hydrochlorothiazide)—an ACE inhibitor and diuretic combination tablet for once-daily administration in the treatment of essential hypertension.

AccuSharp instrument—used in carpal tunnel release.

AccuSite injectable gel—fluorouracil in a sustained-release formulation used for treatment of genital warts.

AccuSpan tissue expander. Also, *PMT AccuSpan.*

AccuSway balance measurement system—used to measure balance and sway in physical and rehabilitation therapy.

Accutane/Rezulin cocktail—combination of drugs being used together investigationally. The drug cocktail robs cancer cells of the protein they need to grow and programs them to age and die on schedule just as normal cells do.

Accutom—low-speed diamond saw.

Accuzyme—enzymatic debriding agent.

ACD (active compression-decompression) **resuscitator**—a suction device for cardiopulmonary resuscitation (CPR). The two researchers who developed it after hearing of a heart attack victim who had been resuscitated with a bathroom plunger (a.k.a. plumber's friend). It is easier

ACD resuscitator *(cont.)*
to use than standard CPR—a simple push-pull action—and studies have shown that the device pumps more blood through the heart and draws more air into the lungs.

ACD (allergic contact dermatitis).

ACE (Adriamycin, cyclophosphamide, etoposide)—chemotherapy protocol for small cell lung carcinoma.

ACE (angiotensin-converting enzyme) **inhibitor**—used to treat hypertension.

acecainide (Napa)—an antiarrhythmic drug which is actually a metabolite of procainamide (Procan SR). The chemical name for this drug, N-acetylprocainamide, is abbreviated *NAPA*. *Napa* is the trade name.

Acel-Imune—vaccine used prophylactically against diphtheria, tetanus, and pertussis in children up to 7 years of age.

Acel-P—vaccine used prophylactically against pertussis for adults.

acemannan (Carrisyn)—a drug used in AIDS treatment.

acetabular angle of Sharp.

acetabular anteversion (AA)—hip dysplasia measurement in children with cerebral palsy.

acetabular dysplasia—including maldirection, insufficiency, and incongruence.

acetabular head index (AHI).

acetabuloplasty—a variety of pelvic osteotomy procedures performed in children or young adults in whom hip pain or instability of the hip is present. The aim is to obtain concentric reduction of the hip joint and fashion a stable acetabular roof.

acetylator—an agent capable of metabolic acetylation.

acetylcholine receptor antibody (AChRab)—found in the sera of patients with myasthenia gravis.

ACG knee (Ortho)—for tricompartmental knee arthroplasty.

Achiever balloon dilatation catheter.

Achilles reflex—response to a tap on the heel of the foot. On percussion of the Achilles tendon just above the calcaneus, contraction of the muscles of the leg produces plantar flexion of the foot. Also, *gastrocnemius reflex, ankle jerk.*

Achilles tendon (English form), **tendo Achillis** (Latin form).

achondroplastic dwarfism—a disorder of connective tissue metabolism; the patient is normal except for bone growth and development.

Achromobacter lwoffi—see *Acinetobacter lwoffi.*

acidemia—see *isovaleric acidemia.*

acidic—having the characteristics of an acid. Cf. *ascitic.*

acid-related disorders (ARDs)—include dyspepsia, gastritis, GERD (gastroesophageal reflux disease), and PUD (peptic ulcer disease).

Acier stainless steel suture—nonabsorbable suture for use in abdominal wound closure, hernia repair, sternal closure, and certain orthopedic procedures including cerclage and tendon repair.

Acinetobacter lwoffi—normal flora of skin, mouth, and external genitalia, isolated from sputum and urine. Associated with conjunctivitis, keratitis, and chronic ear infections. Also, *Achromobacter lwoffi, Mima polymorpha, Moraxella lwoffi.*

AC-IOL (anterior chamber intraocular lens).

Aciphex (rabeprazole sodium)—proton pump inhibitor approved for healing of erosive gastroesophageal reflux disease (GERD), maintenance of healed erosive GERD, and healing of duodenal ulcers. Aciphex has also been approved for treatment of pathological hypersecretory conditions, including Zollinger-Ellison syndrome.

ACIS (Automated Cellular Imaging System)—immunohistochemical staining method used to diagnose or monitor numerous conditions, including cancer and infectious disease.

aCL (anticardiolipin antibody).

Acland-Banis arteriotomy set—used for end-to-side microvascular anastomosis.

Acland microvascular clamps—used in hand surgery.

ACL (anterior cruciate ligament) **drill guide**; **ACL repair**.

ACLS (advanced cardiac life support).

ACMI Martin endoscopy forceps.

ACM (automated cardiac flow measurement) **technology**—measures left ventricular outflow tract pressure ultrasonically and thus noninvasively.

acne rosacea—affects facial skin and may affect eyes (ocular rosacea), causing mild blepharoconjunctivitis or vision-impairing corneal involvement.

ACNM (American College of Nurse Midwives)—confers the credential CNM (Certified Nurse Midwife).

ACOP (Adriamycin, cyclophosphamide, Oncovin, prednisone)—chemotherapy protocol used in treatment of non-Hodgkin's lymphoma.

acoustical shadowing—a term used in ultrasonography. It refers to reflection of large amounts of ultrasonic waves from the surface of structures or materials that are physically incompressible (bone, gallstones), with blockage of further transmission.

acoustic stimulation test (AST) (Ob-Gyn)—an alternative to the standard nonstress test in managing high-risk pregnancies and identifying normal patterns of fetal activity and heart rate. The AST uses a sound-generating vibrator (also used by laryngectomy patients to generate a monotone quality of speech) which is applied to the abdomen over the position of the fetal head. Sound is produced for three one-second intervals. The test is considered normal if the fetal heart rate increases at least 15 beats per minute for at least 15 seconds.

acquired immunodeficiency syndrome (AIDS). See *AIDS*.

acquired von Willebrand's disease (AvWD)—a rare complication of an autoimmune or neoplastic disease, associated mostly with a lymphoid or plasma cell proliferative disorder.

acquisition time—MRI term.

Acra-Cut Spiral craniotome blade—a cranial blade with spiral geometric design.

acrivastine (Semprex-D).

acrocallosal syndrome, Schinzel type —rare disorder inherited as an autosomal recessive genetic trait and characterized by craniofacial abnormalities, absence or underdevelopment of the mass of white matter that unites the two halves of the brain, additional fingers and/or toes, loss of muscle tone, and mental retardation.

acrochordon (Derm)—a skin tag.

acrodysostosis—characterized by abnormally short and malformed

acrodysostosis *(cont.)*
bones of the hands and feet, nasal hypoplasia, and mental retardation. Some researchers believe acrodysostosis occurs randomly for no apparent reason; others believe it is a form of pseudohypoparathyroidism.

Acro-Flex artificial disk—flexible artificial disk intended as an alternative to spinal fusion.

acromesomelic dysplasia—a rare inherited progressive disorder characterized by premature fusion of metaphyses where the shafts of certain long bones meet their epiphyses. As a result, affected individuals exhibit unusually short forearms, abnormal shortening of bones of the lower legs, and short-limbed dwarfism.

AcryDerm border island dressing—a composite, or multilayered, dressing for the management of wound exudate moisture from acute and chronic wounds (not for use in third-degree burns). The island component is a highly absorbent hydrogel matrix placed on the adhesive side of a medical grade polyurethane transparent thin film.

AcryDerm hydrogel sheet.

AcryDerm Strands—absorbent wound dressing.

acrylic cement—very strong glue used to cement orthopedic joint replacements in place.

acrylic wafer TMJ (temporomandibular joint) **splint**—for TMJ pain and dysfunction. It is worn between the upper and lower teeth all the time until the patient's pain improves, and then only at night.

Acryl-X ultrasonic orthopedic cement removal system—for separation and simultaneous removal of acrylic bone cement, reducing risk of injury to bone.

AcrySof acrylic foldable intraocular lens—acrylic foldable lens allowing smaller incision in implant surgery.

ACS (abdominal compartment syndrome).

ACS (Advanced Cardiovascular System).

ACS Anchor Exchange device—used to exchange devices during interventional procedures such as PTCA, atherectomy, or stenting.

ACS Concorde—an over-the-wire catheter system for use in opening blocked coronary arteries. It allows for a minimal entry diameter and provides for easier advancement of catheter through tight or tortuous lesions.

ACS Endura—coronary dilation catheter used in heart-related operations.

ACS Hi-Torque Balance—middleweight guide wire.

ACS OTW (over-the-wire) **HP** (high pressure) **coronary stent**.

ACS OTW Lifestream coronary dilatation catheter—a perfusion catheter for treatment of blocked arteries in the heart.

ACS OTW (over-the-wire) **Photon**—coronary dilatation catheter.

ACS RX (rapid exchange) **Comet**—coronary dilatation catheter.

ACS RX Multi-Link stent—an expandable coronary stent with multiple linked rings that allows for flexibility and conformity.

ACS Tourguide II guiding catheter.

ACT (activated coagulation time).

ACT (adaptive cellular therapy)—see *RIGS/ACT*.

Actalyke—an activated clotting time (ACT) test performed at the bedside to monitor heparin anticoagulation

Actalyke *(cont.)*
therapy. It can provide test results within minutes.

ACTG (AIDS Clinical Trials Group).

ActHIB (*H. influenzae* type B vaccine).

Acticoat—silver-based antimicrobial burn barrier. Removes two of the greatest obstacles to wound healing: invasive infections and frequent dressing changes.

Acticon neosphincter—implantable prosthesis for the treatment of severe fecal incontinence. The device consists of a cuff (placed around the anal canal), a pressure-regulating balloon (placed in the abdomen), and a control pump (placed in the labium or scrotum).

ACTID (analgesic cell therapy implantable device)—cell-containing biocompatible pain-control implant.

Actigall (ursodiol)—given orally to dissolve small gallbladder stones without surgery. See also *MTBE, Chenix*.

Action-II (pimagedine)—a drug for diabetic patients with kidney disease.

Actiq (transmucosal fentanyl citrate)—an oral drug for chronic pain and cancer patients.

Actisite (tetracycline hydrochloride)—periodontal fiber used in scaling and root planing.

Actis venous flow controller (VFC)—placed in tourniquet fashion at the base of the penis to control erectile dysfunction caused by venous leak syndrome. It creates enough pressure to prevent venous drainage but does not interfere with arterial inflow or ejaculatory function.

Activa Parkinson's control therapy—utilizes bilateral brain stimulation to treat symptoms of advanced, levodopa-responsive Parkinson's disease.

Activase (alteplase, recombinant t-PA)—tissue plasminogen activator (tPA) commonly used to dissolve clots in the coronary arteries. This recombinant DNA drug is used to dissolve clots in the ventricles of the brain following intraventricular hemorrhage. Administered through a ventriculostomy drain, Activase dissolves the clots that cause ventricular dilatation and increased intracranial pressure.

activated charcoal—used as an antidote in some kinds of poisoning; it is an *adsorbent*, not an *absorbent*.

activated partial thromboplastin time (APTT).

Active Compression-Decompression (ACD) **Resuscitator.**

Activella (estradiol/norethindrone acetate)—hormone-replacement therapy for vasomotor symptoms associated with menopause, treatment of vulvar and vaginal atrophy, and prevention of postmenopausal osteoporosis.

Activent—antimicrobial ventilation tubes for myringotomy.

active phase arrest (Ob-Gyn) (*not* "of rest")—during labor, when the cervix stops dilating and no progress is being made toward delivery.

active specific immunotherapy (ASI).

activities of daily living (ADLs).

Activitrax pacemaker—specialized cardiac pacemaker containing a microphone that senses muscle activity during exercise. It can be programmed to increase the rate of a ventricle 5 to 10 beats per increment of sensed muscle tone.

ACT MicroCoil—delivery system for minimally invasive treatment of intracranial aneurysms.

actocardiotocograph—a fetal monitor that displays a tracing of the fetal heart rate and simultaneously records fetal movements and uterine contractions. Used to monitor pregnancies with multiple fetuses.

Actonel (risedronate)—bisphosphonate therapy used in prevention and treatment of osteoporosis.

Actos (pioglitazone HCl)—oral drug for treatment of type 2 diabetes mellitus. It belongs to the class of diabetic agents known as thiazolidinediones (TZDs).

Actron (ketoprofen)—a pain reliever.

Acucise (Urol)—retrograde procedure for incision of ureteral stricture and ureteropelvic junction obstruction.

Acu-Derm I.V./TPN dressing—provides a moisture- and vapor-permeable covering that reduces the risk of catheter movement.

Acufex (*not* Acuflex) **arthroscopic instruments**—rotary punch, straight and curved basket forceps.

Acufex bioabsorbable suture anchor —used in orthopedic surgery.

AcuFix anterior cervical plate system—multisegment plating system designed for fusing the anterior cervical spine.

Acular; Acular-PF (ketorolac tromethamine)—NSAID eye drops for allergic conjunctivitis or following cataract extraction.

AcuMatch A Series—acetabular component. Also, AcuMatch L and M series modular femoral hip prosthesis.

AcuNav—ultrasound catheter designed to capture images from inside the heart.

AcuPressor myotherapy tool—used in physical therapy.

acupressure without needles—stimulation of acupuncture points performed with fingers or an instrument with a hard, ball-shaped head. Another variation is reflexology, or zone therapy, where soles of feet and posteroinferior regions of the ankle joints are stimulated.

acupuncture lasers—helium-neon (He-Ne), gallium-arsenid (GaA).

Acuson computed sonography—for Doppler and color Doppler imaging.

Acuson V5M—multiplanar TEE (transesophageal echocardiographic) monitor.

Acusyst-Xcell—monoclonal antibody culturing system.

acute abdomen—an abdomen showing signs of acute inflammation.

acute cellular xenograft rejection— acute rejection reaction to transplantation of tissue of animal origin, addressed by the induction of T-cell tolerance.

acute compartment syndrome (Ortho) —found in tibial diaphyseal fractures. Delay in treatment can lead to contracture, infection, and occasionally amputation.

acute inflammatory demyelinating polyradiculoneuropathy (AIDP).

Acute Physiology and Chronic Health Evaluation (APACHE).

acute promyelocytic leukemia (APML).

acute repetitive seizure (ARS) **disorder**.

acute stroke team (AST)—staffed by specially trained physicians and/or nurses who respond immediately to cases of suspected stroke, either in patients already in the hospital or newly arrived in the emergency department.

ACUTENS—transcutaneous nerve stimulator that includes elements of acupuncture or acupressure, for control of pain. It is typed in all capital letters, as in TENS unit. See *TENS, PENS.*

acute zonal occult outer retinopathy (AZOOR).

Acutrainer—an electronic bladder retraining device for children and adults. It's a noninvasive option for voiding dysfunction and many types of urinary incontinence.

Acutrak fusion system—for fusion of interphalangeal and distal interphalangeal joints of hand and first toe. It is a small-bone fixation system using compression screw fixation with tapering variable pitch screw designs.

acylfulvenes—family of proprietary cancer therapy compounds.

A.D. (*auris dextra*)—right ear.

Adagen (pegademase bovine, PEG-ADA)—enzyme replacement for severe combined immunodeficiency disease.

Adalat CC (nifedipine)—used in treatment of hypertension.

Adamkiewicz artery—supplies blood to the thoracolumbar spinal cord. Injury to this artery may be a cause of cauda equina syndrome.

Adams test—a forward-bending test for scoliosis in which the observer is positioned posterior to the patient, who slowly bends forward, imitating a diver, to approximately 90° of lumbar flexion. The purpose is to detect rib asymmetry or prominence, which is indicative of scoliosis.

Adaptar—a "no-line" contact lens that can accommodate all stages of presbyopia.

adaptive cellular therapy (ACT)—see *RIGS/ACT.*

Adaptive Focusing Technology (AFT)—uses hyperthermia, or focused heat, to improve the results of both radiation and chemotherapy in cancer patients.

ADAS (Alzheimer Disease Assessment Scale)—evaluates memory, language, and praxis in Alzheimer patients. It notes changes in cognition and in activities of daily living.

ADCA (autosomal-dominant cerebellar ataxia) **type II**—a neurodegenerative disorder presenting with cerebellar ataxia and retinal degeneration.

ADC (analog-to-digital) **conversion quantization error**—MRI term.

Adcon-L—an antiadhesion barrier to prevent postoperative scarring and adhesions.

Adcon-P—a proprietary resorbable carbohydrate polymer liquid that is designed to inhibit scarring and adhesions in the peritoneal cavity.

ADD (attention-deficit disorder).

Adderall (formerly Obetrol)—for treatment of attention-deficit hyperactivity disorder.

Add-On Bucky digital x-ray image acquisition system.

adduct—to draw toward a position near or parallel to the median axis. Cf. *abduct.*

"a-d-duction"—dictated by a physician to clarify that **ad**duction, not **ab**duction, is intended.

Addvent atrioventricular pacemaker.

ADE (ara-C, daunorubicin, etoposide)—chemotherapy protocol for acute myeloid leukemia.

adenocarcinoma in situ (AIS) **of the cervix**—much less common than carcinoma in situ (CIS) but recently

adenocarcinoma in situ *(cont.)*
increasing in frequency. AIS is premalignant and highly curable.

Adenocard (adenosine)—slows conduction time through the AV node and
restores normal sinus rhythm in
patients with paroxysmal supraventricular tachycardia (PSVT), including SVT associated with Wolff-
Parkinson-White syndrome.

adenocyst—adenocystoma (adenoma in
which there is cyst formation). Cf.
adenosis.

adenoma—see *carcinoma ex pleomorphic adenoma*.

adenomatous hyperplasia (AH)—parenchymal nodule of the liver containing portal and biliary elements
and considered a regenerative, limited overgrowth. Some AH nodules
grow gradually and finally progress
to hepatocellular carcinoma (HCC),
suggesting that an AH nodule may
be premalignant. Distinguishing AH
from HCC is important.

adenomyomatosis—a proliferation of
epithelium with gland-like formations
and outpouchings of the mucosa into
or through the hypertrophied muscular layer. These hyperplastic mucosal
diverticula in the gallbladder are also
called *Rokitansky-Aschoff sinuses*.

Adenoscan—a cardiac diagnostic contrast medium used in nuclear perfusion imaging.

adenosine echocardiography—a study
in which the antiarrhythmic agent
adenosine (Adenocard) is given intravenously to assess patients with suspected coronary artery disease. It
causes the coronary arteries to constrict, thus producing ischemic symptoms without a stress test. Even if the
drug produces coronary artery constriction and exacerbates patient

symptoms, its effect is extremely
brief for it has a half-life of only
10 seconds.

adenosis—disease of the glands or abnormal development of glandular
tissue. Types: blunt duct, florid,
sclerosing. Cf. *adenocyst*.

adenovirus—a virus genetically engineered so that the virus is harmless
but able to carry desirable genes into
a variety of types of brain cells.
Though years away from use in
humans, scientists are working on
developing such viruses for potential
use in such debilitating conditions as
Alzheimer's, Huntington's, and Parkinson's diseases.

adenovirus test kit—for the detection
of adenovirus in stool samples. The
enzyme immunoassay uses a combination of antibodies to directly test
for the virus and reduces the time
required by traditional cell-culture
isolation.

Adept (icodextrin)—nonviscous solution for prevention of postoperative
adhesions.

AD/FHD (ratio of acetabular depth to
femoral head diameter).

adhesion preventative
Adcon-L
Adcon-P
Adept solution
Atrisol aerosol
Hylagel-Nuro
Hylasine
Incert sponge
Interceed Adhesion Barrier
Intergel solution
Parietex
Repel film
Sepracoat coating solution
Seprafilm
SprayGel adhesion barrier system

adhesive—see also *bandage, dressing*.
　Aron Alpha
　autologous fibrin tissue (AFTA)
　BA (bioactive) bone cement
　Biobrane
　Bioerodible Mucoadhesive (BEMA)
　BioGlue surgical
　bone cement
　CicaCare topical gel sheeting
　Coe-pak paste
　CoSeal resorbable synthetic sealant
　Coverlet
　Cover-Roll gauze
　cyanoacrylate
　Dermabond
　EMLA anesthetic disc
　fibrin glue
　fibrin sealant
　FloSeal matrix hemostatic sealant
　FocalSeal-S surgical sealant
　gelatin-resorcin-formalin tissue glue
　Hemaseel HMN biologial tissue glue
　Histoacryl tissue glue
　hydroxyapatite (HA)
　Implast bone cement
　Indermil topical tissue
　LPPS hydroxyapatite
　MCW cement
　methylmethacrylate cement
　Orthoset radiopaque bone cement
　Palacos cement
　Proceed hemostatic surgical sealant
　Simplex cement
　Soothe-N-Seal
　Superglue
　Surfit
　Surgical Simplex P radiopaque
　Tisseel surgical glue
　Vitex tissue
　Zimmer low viscosity
adiabatic fast passage—MRI term.
Adipex-P (phentermine HCl)—anorexiant for exogenous obesity.

adiposis dolorosa—rare disorder of fat metabolism of unknown cause; fat accumulates in painful lumps over the body. Also called *Dercum's disease.*
Adjustable Leg and Ankle Repositioning Mechanism (ALARM).
adjuvant therapy—auxiliary therapy.
Adkin's strut—used to retract the third rib to facilitate exposure to LIMA (left internal mammary artery) in MIDCAB (minimally invasive direct coronary artery bypass) procedures.
ADLs (activities of daily living) (Rehab). "Plan: Improve the patient's ADLs."
adnexa (Ob-Gyn)—the uterine appendages including the ovary and fallopian tube on each side. Adnexa is plural and always takes a plural verb: "The adnexa were unremarkable." Also, *ocular adnexa* (Oph).
Adolescent and Pediatric Pain Tool—see *APPT.*
adolescent idiopathic scoliosis (AIS).
adrenergic antagonist—a drug which blocks the action of naturally produced neurotransmitters on adrenergic receptors of sympathetic nervous system.
ADR-529—used to prevent cardiotoxicity in cancer patients receiving Adriamycin.
adRP (autosomal-dominant retinitis pigmentosa).
ADR Ultramark 4 ultrasound—portable microprocessor based on electrocardiography system.
AD7C—test that aids in diagnosis of Alzheimer's disease. Results are significantly elevated in patients with the disease and correlate with severity of dementia symptoms.

Adson maneuver—to rule in or rule out scalenus anticus syndrome.

adsorbent—an agent that attracts other molecules to, or maintains them on, a surface. Cf. *absorbent*.

ADTRA—composite external fixator ring (Ortho).

adult chronic immune thrombocytopenic purpura (ITP)—a disorder more commonly known as *idiopathic thrombocytopenic purpura*.

adult respiratory distress syndrome (ARDS).

advanced breast biopsy instrumentation (ABBI) **system**—permits sampling of a mammographic lesion while preserving the lesion's histologic architecture for complete pathologic analysis.

advanced cardiac life support (ACLS).

advanced cardiac mapping—multielectrode catheter is guided into the heart chamber, showing the heart's electrical activity, locating any points of arrhythmia, and targeting sites for curative catheter procedures.

Advanced Care cholesterol test—self-administered test for checking cholesterol. It measures total serum cholesterol levels in approximately 15 minutes.

advanced glycation end-products (AGE).

advanced real time motion analysis (ARTMA).

Advantage 24 (nonoxynol-9)—bioadhesive spermicidal female contraceptive.

AdvanTeq II TENS unit.

Advantim revision knee system—using Ortholoc instrumentation.

Advantx LC+—cardiovascular imaging system.

AED (automatic external defibrillator)—device used by emergency medical technicians in the field or by families trained in its use for patients at risk for sudden death.

AE (aryepiglottic) **fold**.

Ae-H interval (anterograde conduction)—a term used in electrophysiologic studies of supraventricular tachycardia.

aeroallergens—see *pathogen*.

AeroBid (flunisolide)—an oral inhaler used to treat asthma.

Aerochamber—a face mask which attaches to a bronchial inhaler device. The metered-dose aerosol can be breathed over several seconds by patients who have difficulty using inhaler devices.

aerogenous—descriptive term for bacteria which produce gas. Cf. *erogenous zones*.

Aeromonas sobria—a pathogen associated with left-sided segmental colitis. Chronic colitis frequently follows *Aeromonas* infection.

AeroTech II nebulizer—for administration of aerosolized drugs such as pentamidine.

AERx—pulmonary drug delivery system creating an aerosol from a liquid drug and delivering it locally to the lung or into the bloodstream via the lung. It allows people with diabetes to control meal-time glucose levels by inhaling insulin.

AERx electronic inhaler—believed to deliver morphine more quickly for breakthrough pain, providing rapid relief as the pain occurs.

Aescula left ventricular (LV) **lead**—cardiac lead for use with left-ventricle-based cardiac stimulation systems.

Aesop 2000—a surgical robot capable of maneuvering and positioning a laparoscope in response to a surgeon's voice commands. Aesop (or AESOP) is an acronym for Automated Endoscopic System for Optimal Positioning.

aesthetic—artistic or beautiful in appearance. Cf. *asthenic.*

A-FAIR (arrhythmia-insensitive flow-sensitive alternating inversion recovery) imaging.

AFBG (aortofemoral bypass graft).

affect—(verb) to change; to produce an effect, as "This should not affect the outcome"; (noun) outward appearance of an inner emotion (Neuro, Psych), as "The patient demonstrated a flat affect" (or "flattened affect"). Cf. *effect.*

afferent—moving towards the center, as in an afferent defect in ophthalmology. Cf. *efferent.*

affinity chromatography.

Affirm—a one-step pregnancy test that detects chorionic gonadotropin in human urine. The test is said to be 99% accurate and effective as early as the first day of a missed period and may be taken at any time of the day, giving visual results in one to two minutes.

Affymetrix GeneChip system—for lab analysis of genes associated with cancer. It provides rapid genetic analysis using miniaturized, high-density arrays of DNA probes and proprietary software to analyze and manage genetic information.

AFIP (Armed Forces Institute of Pathology). Pathologists often send specimens to AFIP for consultation.

Afipia felis—a bacterium found in the lymph nodes of a patient with cat-scratch disease. First identified by AFIP (Armed Forces Institute of Pathology). Not currently regarded as a cause of cat-scratch disease. See *Bartonella henselae.*

Aflexa (glucosamine)—an OTC product intended to help promote healthy joints.

AFM (Adriamycin, fluorouracil, methotrexate [with leucovorin rescue])—chemotherapy protocol for metastatic breast carcinoma.

AFM (atomic force microscopy).

AFO (ankle-foot orthosis).

AFP (alpha-fetoprotein) **lab test**.

AFT (Adaptive Focusing Technology).

after-depolarizations (Cardiol)—used in study of cardiac arrhythmias by electrophysiology.

afterloading—see *RAB* (remote afterloading brachytherapy).

Agar-IF (immunofixation in agar) of blood serum.

agarose gel electrophoresis (AGE).

Agatston score—quantifies calcium in coronary arteries as a risk factor for coronary artery disease.

AGC (anatomic graduated components).

AGE (advanced glycation end-products)—used in ophthalmology.

AGE (agarose gel electrophoresis).

age-associated memory impairment (AAMI)—used in the context of senile dementia and Alzheimer's disease workup. Alzheimer's disease is not an age-associated memory impairment, while senile dementia is.

Agee carpal tunnel release system—a one-portal system used in endoscopic carpal tunnel release.

Agee endoscope—used to perform endoscopic carpal tunnel release surgery.

Agee-WristJack fracture reduction system—multiplanar ligamentotaxis to restore palmar tilt in distal radial fractures.

Agenerase (amprenavir)—protease inhibitor with antiviral activity, used for treatment of HIV.

age-related macular degeneration (AMD or ARMD). See *"dry" age-related macular degeneration* and *"wet" age-related macular degeneration*.

AGF (angle of greatest flexion).

AGF (autologous growth factors).

Aggrastat (tirofiban HCl)—antiplatelet drug for unstable angina.

aggregate—a mass or cluster of material, as aggregate measurements.

aggregated human IgG (AHuG).

Aggrenox (extended-release dipyridamole/aspirin)—capsules to be taken twice daily to reduce the combined risk of death and nonfatal stroke in patients who have experienced a transient ischemic attack or completed ischemic stroke.

aggressive angiomyxoma—a rare variant of myxoid tumor with a vascular component. It is a slow-growing soft-tissue tumor that occurs mostly in the female pelvis and perineum, primarily in young premenopausal women. These tumors tend to infiltrate surrounding tissue, are locally aggressive, and have recurrence rates of up to 70%. No metastases have been reported. The tumor can resemble a Bartholin gland abscess or can be misdiagnosed as angiomyofibroblastoma.

agonist—a drug that stimulates activity of a receptor in the way it would be stimulated by naturally produced substances. Cf. *antagonist*.

Agrelin (anagrelide)—used for its antiplatelet properties in treating thrombocytosis (a blood disorder) with high platelet counts and blood clotting causing cardiovascular events, such as a heart attack or stroke.

Agris-Dingman submammary dissector —used for a transaxillary approach to breast augmentation.

AGUS (atypical glandular cells of undetermined significance).

AH (adenomatous hyperplasia).

ahaustral—without haustra, the bands running circumferentially around the large bowel.

AHG (antihemophilic globulin)—can be administered via AV fistula for intravenous infusion control of intermittent bleeding in hemophilia.

AHI (acetabular head index).

AHI (apnea/hypopnea index).

AHIMA (American Health Information Management Association)—a professional association for health information management professionals who have credentials of the Registered Health Information Administrator (RHIA), Registered Health Information Technician (RHIT), Certified Coding Specialist (CCS), and Certified Coding Specialist–Physician-based (CCS-P).

Ahn thrombectomy catheter—for the treatment of thromboemboli. Named for Samuel Ahn, M.D., the catheter incorporates a distal dual balloon design to more effectively remove thromboemboli, as well as a proximal-indicator safety balloon that allows the surgeon to visually determine inflation volume. The distal dual balloon traps blood clots more effectively and prevents contamination caused by blood spurting into the operator's face and eyes.

AHR (airway hyperreactivity).

AHuG (aggregated human IgG).

AI (acetabular index)—hip dysplasia measurement in children with cerebral palsy.

AICA (pronounced "i'-ka") (anterior inferior communicating artery).

AICD (automatic implantable cardioverter-defibrillator).

AID (artificial insemination-donor).

AIDP (acute inflammatory demyelinating polyradicular) neuropathy.

AIDS (acquired immunodeficiency syndrome)—a disease that attacks the immune system, leaving the body susceptible to such opportunistic infections as *Pneumocystis carinii* pneumonia, candidiasis, and cancers like Kaposi's sarcoma. These may also be accompanied by neurological manifestations. AIDS is caused by a retrovirus and transmitted by sexual contact or by contaminated hypodermic needles, blood or blood products (contaminated blood in blood transfusions, and occasionally contamination by blood through an open wound in the skin), or by contact with the virus in semen. See related entries: *AIDS drugs, AIDS virus, ARV, cytokines, HIV, HTLV/III,* and *Kaposi's sarcoma.*

AIDS-associated ophthalmic pneumocystis (Oph).

AIDS dementia complex—a progressive primary encephalopathy caused by HIV type 1 infection involving principally the subcortical white matter and deep gray nuclei, manifested by a variety of cognitive, motor, and behavior abnormalities. Also called *AIDS encephalopathy, HIV dementia complex,* and *HIV encephalitis.*

AIDS drugs—in alphabetic entries throughout the book, as well as in the main entries *cytokine, protein,* and *medication.*

AIDS encephalopathy—see *AIDS dementia complex.*

AIDS-KS (AIDS-related Kaposi's sarcoma).

AIDS-related complex (ARC)—a term used to describe a variety of symptoms and signs found in some persons infected with HIV, including decrease in CD4 cells, recurrent fevers, unexplained weight loss, swollen lymph nodes, and/or fungus infections of mouth and throat. Most clinical findings formerly denoted as ARC are now in groups 3 or 4 of the CDC AIDS classification system, although the term *ARC* is still used to describe these symptoms and diagnoses. ARC is also commonly described as symptomatic HIV infection.

AIDS vaccine—not yet available after years of research due to the rapid rate of mutation of the HIV virus. A number of designs are under study with the common factor being that they each use specific parts of HIV (genes or proteins) to activate the body's immune defenses. Methods undergoing clinical trials include those involving recombinant subunit vaccines (e.g., gp120, which has made it to Phase III trials), DNA vaccines, live recombinant viral or bacterial vector vaccines, synthetic peptide vaccines, and combination vaccines using two or more of these methods.

AIDSVAX B/B—a genetically engineered, aluminum adjuvanted sub-

AIDSVAX B/B *(cont.)* unit investigational vaccine based on gp120. It is the first AIDS vaccine to enter Phase III clinical trials in North America.

AIDS virus—a retrovirus of the cytopathic lentivirus group that invades and inactivates helper/T-cells of the immune system. See *helper cell; HIV; pathogen.*

AIH (artificial insemination–husband).

AILD (angioimmunoblastic lymphadenopathy with dysproteinemia).

Ailee sutures and needles.

AIM CPM (continuous passive motion) **for hand.**

AIMS (Abnormal Involuntary Movement Scale)—a scale for rating tardive dyskinesia.

AIOD (aortoiliac obstructive disease).

AIP (acute intermittent porphyria).

air-bone gap—in audiology testing. (*Not* "ear-bone gap" or "air-borne gap.")

Aircast Swivel-Strap—ankle brace to treat ankle instability.

AirCom—compression-molded polyethylene used in modular components.

air conduction (*not* ear conduction)—refers to the transmission of sound through the ear canal, tympanic membrane, and ossicular chain to the cochlea and auditory nerve. Air conduction is tested by holding a vibrating tuning fork near the external auditory meatus. Cf. *bone conduction, Rinne test, Weber test.*

air contrast barium enema—radiology procedure.

AirFlex carpal tunnel splint.

air-fluid level (Radiol)—a line representing the level of a collection of fluid seen in profile, with air or gas above it. Cf. *free air.*

air hunger—in patients with chronic extreme anemia, uremia, and diabetic acidosis who have great difficulty struggling to breathe; long, deep, or panting breathing.

Airlift balloon retractor—used in Laparolift system for gasless laparoscopy.

Air-Limb—designed to provide protection and edema control for a patient's leg following amputation.

AirMax—external nasal dilator designed to improve breathing capacity during exercise.

Airprene hinged knee prosthesis—with breathable lining support, reportedly offers more comfort than ordinary material, superior compression and muscle stability, and hinged stainless steel side bars to provide increased support.

air-space disease (Radiol)—disease or abnormality of lung tissue that encroaches on space normally filled by air, as seen on chest x-ray.

air splint (also *inflatable splint*)—blown up like a balloon and usually used to immobilize the foot and ankle. There are other such splints used for the arm or the whole leg. Usage: "This is an acute ankle sprain, so she will be placed in an air splint and should keep her foot elevated."

Air Supply—a wearable air purifier to reduce exposure to a variety of germs, pollen, dust, and other airborne hazards, so that patients can breathe cleaner, healthier air.

air trousers—medical (or military) antishock trousers. See *MAST trousers.*

airway, breathing, circulation (ABC)—must be assessed immediately on trauma patients before anything else is done.

airway hyperreactivity (AHR)—found on helical CT scan following methacholine bronchoprovocation in asthmatics.

AIS (Abbreviated Injury Scale)—a system of scoring trauma injuries to each anatomic system.

AIS (adenocarcinoma in situ).

AIS (adolescent idiopathic scoliosis).

AIVR (accelerated idioventricular rhythm).

AJ (ankle jerk) (Neuro)—Usage: "He has preserved reflexes throughout, evaluated at 2+ AJs, 3+ KJs, trace brachioradialis, and 1+ biceps." (Note: *KJ* is *knee jerk*.)

akathisia—motor restlessness often localized in the muscles, resulting in inability to sit or lie quietly; a side effect of some antipsychotic drugs. Example: "A protracted akathisia-like dystonic-type reaction to this medication is very remote." Cf. *extrapyramidal signs, pyramidal signs, tardive dyskinesia*.

A-K diamond knife—precalibrated.

akinesia—see *Nadbath*.

Akne-mycin (erythromycin)—prescription ointment for acne vulgaris, indicated as acne therapy for sensitive skin.

Akros extended care mattress—for pressure relief.

Alamast (pemirolast potassium)—ophthalmic solution for prevention of itchy eyes due to allergic conjunctivitis.

alanine aminotransaminase (ALT) (formerly *SGPT*)—a liver function test. See *ALT*.

alar flaring—flaring (dilatation) of the nostrils on inspiration, sometimes the only sign of dyspnea in a small child. Also called *nasal flaring*.

ALARM (Adjustable Leg and Ankle Repositioning Mechanism)—used in orthopedic surgery.

AlaSTAT latex allergy test—measures IgE antibodies specific to latex in blood samples. According to the FDA, at least 15 deaths and 1,000 reactions due to latex allergy have been reported. The American Academy of Allergy and Immunology recommends testing healthcare and latex industry workers, spina bifida children, and people who have such risk factors as multiple surgeries, unexplained anaphylaxis, or oral itching after eating avocados, bananas, kiwi, or chestnuts.

Alatest Latex-specific IgE allergen test kit—used to measure the circulating levels of immunoglobulin E (IgE) specific to latex. Although only about 1% of the general population is thought to have type I latex allergy, in healthcare workers and others in occupations exposing them to latex, this allergy may affect more than 14%.

Albarran deflecting level (Urol)—attached to a cystoscope, allowing slow water irrigation during prostate resection for benign prostatic hypertrophy.

Alberts' Famous Faces Test—neurological test.

albumen—the white of the egg; it contains protein and not cholesterol. Cf. *albumin*.

albumin—the major plasma protein present in human serum. Cf. *albumen*.

albuminocytologic dissociation—cerebrospinal fluid protein elevation.

Albunex—ultrasound contrast medium for cardiac studies.

albuterol (Proventil, Volmax)—a bronchodilator given orally or administered through inhalers.

albuterol sulfate inhalation solution —for use in patients with reversible obstructive airway disease and acute attacks of bronchospasm.

ALCAPA (anomalous origin of left coronary artery from the pulmonary artery) **syndrome**—a condition resulting in infarction with myocardial necrosis in affected neonates with almost entirely collateral circulation-dependent perfusion of the left ventricle and poor global left ventricular function. In the past infants rarely survived because of severe left heart failure, but revascularization with good functional recovery is improving the clinical outcomes for these infants. Also called *Bland-Garland-White syndrome*.

Alcian blue—a stain used in testing for mucopolysaccharides.

alcohol ablation—surgical technique to treat cardiomyopathy. A catheter is threaded into the heart and pure alcohol is injected to induce a controlled heart attack, killing part of the overgrown heart muscle that blocks the flow of blood.

alcohol, ethanol, EtOH—used interchangeably when referring to the consumption of alcohol.

alcoholic blackout—anterograde amnesia experienced by alcoholics during episodes of drinking, even when not fully intoxicated. Indicative of early but still reversible brain damage.

Alcon crescent blade (Oph).

Alcon pocket blade (Oph).

Aldara cream 5%—a self-administered cream for treatment of external genital and perianal warts.

aldesleukin (Proleukin)—a recombinant interleukin-2 product used as an antineoplastic and biological response modifier in the treatment of metastatic renal cell carcinoma. Administered intravenously.

aldosterone-producing adenoma (APA).

Aldurazyme—a once-weekly enzyme replacement therapy for treatment of patients with mucopolysaccharidosis I (MPS I), which includes Hurler, Hurler-Scheie, and Scheie syndromes.

alendronate (Fosamax)—the first non-hormonal drug to treat osteoporosis.

Alesse—an oral contraceptive drug.

Aleve (naproxyn sodium)—a nonsteroid anti-inflammatory drug.

Alexagram—breast lesion diagnostic test. See *Alexa 1000 system*.

alexandrite (solid-state) **laser.**

Alexa 1000 system—noninvasive diagnostic system for determining whether a breast lesion is malignant or benign (reportedly 95% accurate), as an alternative to more invasive surgical breast biopsy procedures. Immediate diagnostic results are provided by the Alexagram test.

AlexLAZR—an alexandrite laser used for the removal of tattoo pigments and pigmented lesions, with reduced risk of scarring and tissue damage.

alfa—international spelling for *alpha*. The pharmaceutical nomenclature committees in several countries are moving toward a common spelling of new generic drugs. Since many languages that use the Roman alphabet have replaced the digraph *ph* with *f*, the United States Adopted Name (USAN) council has agreed to use this spelling in newly approved

alfa *(cont.)*
generic names. This change does not retroactively affect current drug names, however. Thus, "alpha" becomes "alfa" in *interferon alfa* and *dornase alfa*, but not in *alpha tocopherol* or *alpha amylase*.

alfacalcidol—used in treating hypocalcemia and osteopenia resistant to vitamin D therapy.

Alferon LDO—see *interferon alfa-n3*.

Alferon N—see *interferon alfa-n3*.

AlgiDERM—alginate wound dressing.

alginate wound dressing—made from soft, nonwoven fiber derived from seaweed and usually produced in pad, rope, or ribbon form. It absorbs wound exudate and forms a gel-like covering over the wound. Most alginate dressings absorb many times their own weight. See *dressing*.

AlgiSite—alginate wound dressing.

alglucerase (Ceredase)—treatment for Gaucher's disease, a rare hereditary metabolic disease. It is an enzyme which acts in the place of a deficient enzyme. The drug increases red blood cell and platelet counts, improves splenomegaly, and diminishes cachexia from Gaucher's disease.

algorithm—a problem-solving procedure, step-by-step, as with a computer; e.g., "We discussed the following: Should he not improve, there would be two more stools for ova and parasites and for culture. If these are normal, and should he still have symptomatology, he would have a barium enema. If this is normal and symptomatology still persists, he would have flexible sigmoidoscopy, and finally, if his symptomatology still persists, then an upper GI with small bowel series. I told him that there is no urgency in approaching this algorithm." See *DRC (dynamic range control) algorithm*.

Algosteril—alginate wound dressing.

ALHE (angiolymphoid hyperplasia with eosinophilia).

ALI (acute lung injury).

aliasing artifact (wrap-around ghosting)—MRI term.

Alibra (alprostadil/prazosin HCl)—a two-drug combination therapy for the treatment of erectile dysfunction. It is formulated into a microsuppository and delivered to the urethra via a single-use plastic applicator.

alien hand sign (Neuro)—sequela of an extensive stroke in the medial frontal cortex. The hand opposite the affected side of the brain (the alien hand) instinctively grasps and does other purposeful behaviors that cannot be controlled by the patient. Often the patient must use the unaffected hand to hold and restrain the "alien hand."

aliquot ("al´-e-kwat")—an equal part of a whole, as in a solution. Used thus: "The patient was then given 5 mg of Valium in 2.5 mg aliquots to minimize the artifact in this EEG."

AlitraQ—a nutritionally complete formula for patients with impaired GI function.

alkaline phosphatase antialkaline phosphatase (APAAP) **antibody test**—venous blood test technique for determining CD4, CD3, CD8, CD22, and other factors.

Alkeran (melphalan).

alkylating (*not* alkalating) **agent**.

ALL (acute lymphoblastic leukemia)—seen primarily in children.

ALL (acute lymphocytic leukemia).

Allegra-D—nonsedating antihistamine drug containing fexofenadine, a chemical entity derived from terfenadine, with decongestant.

Allen-Brown shunt—a vascular access shunt, used in performing dialysis.

Allen picture test (Oph)—used to test visual acuity, especially in young children who can identify pictures better than they can read Snellen letters.

Allen's test—for diagnosing occlusion of the ulnar and radial arteries.

allergic bronchopulmonary aspergillosis (ABPA)—characterized by asthma, recurrent lung infiltration, recurrent episodes of purulent cough with or without fever, sputum plugs containing *Aspergillus fumigatus*, wheezing, peripheral blood eosinophilia, and immunologic evidence of hypersensitivity to *A. fumigatus.*

allergic contact dermatitis (ACD).

allergic salute—repeated rubbing of the nose upward to scratch an itchy nose and open the obstructed airway (seen in patients with allergies).

allergic shiners—darkening of the skin around the eyes, resembling periorbital hematomas, as a symptom of allergic rhinitis.

Allevyn dressing—nonadherent dressing material that is absorbent even under pressure.

alligator grasper/forceps.

Allis sign—a sign of fracture of the femoral neck, when the fascia between the crest of the ilium and the greater trochanter relaxes.

Alliston procedure—used in the correction of gastroesophageal reflux.

AlloDerm—cadaveric dermal matrix from which all cellular components have been removed. It is used in plastic surgery for facial contouring.

AlloDerm processed tissue graft—patented by LifeCell.

allodynia—pain resulting from a nonnoxious stimulus to normal skin.

AlloMatrix injectable putty—bone graft substitute that combines bioassayed demineralized bone matrix, surgical-grade calcium sulfate, and a biocompatible plasticizing agent, creating a moldable putty with osteoconductive and osteoinductive properties.

Allon system—enables physicians to maintain normal body temperature in patients undergoing surgery. In addition to preventing hypothermia, it allows a physician to lower brain temperature in order to improve patient outcome.

allopurinol (Zyloprim)—commonly used as a treatment for gout. A solution of this drug is also used to preserve kidneys taken from cadavers prior to being transplanted.

Allovectin-7—a DNA/lipid complex containing the human gene encoding the HLA-B7 antigen. It is injected directly into a tumor, where it is absorbed by the malignant cells and the HLA-B7 antigen expressed, alerting the immune system to the presence of foreign tissue. This induces the type of powerful immune response seen in organ transplant rejection.

all-trans retinoic acid (ATRA; tretinoin; Vesanoid). See also *Retin-A.*

allusion—an indirect reference to something, as "He made allusion to a history of some kind of tropical disease." Cf. *elusion, illusion.*

allylamines—class of antifungal drugs. Example: naftifine (Naftin).

Alm self-retaining retractor.

Alocril (nedocromil sodium ophthalmic solution)—for treatment of itch associated with allergic conjunctivitis in patients age 3 and over.

Aloe Vesta antifungal ointment.

Aloka color Doppler system—provides real-time, two-dimensional blood flow imaging with Cine Memory. Also, *Aloka 650.*

Aloka SSD—ultrasound system and probes.

alopecia androgenetica—male pattern baldness.

Aloprim (allopurinol sodium)—an intravenous formulation for treatment of leukemia, lymphoma, and solid tumor malignancies in cancer therapy patients who cannot tolerate oral drugs.

Alora (estradiol)—a patch for moderate to severe vasomotor symptoms of menopause.

alosetron—drug shown to reduce abdominal pain and discomfort of irritable bowel syndrome.

alpha-BSM (bone substitute material)—a calcium phosphate bone substitute material used to repair or replace autologous bone.

alpha-fetoprotein (AFP)—a globulin produced by the liver and other tissues of the fetus and newborn. Its level normally declines after one year of age. Normal value in amniotic fluid, less than 20; an elevated value (over 100,000) indicates the presence of an embryonal tumor, spina bifida, or Down syndrome.

alpha Gal antibody—anti-pig antibody, the source of hyperacute rejection of a porcine xenograft.

Alphagan (brimondine tartrate)—ophthalmic solution to lower intraocular pressure in patients with open-angle glaucoma or ocular hypertension.

alpha interferon—see *alfa.*

Alpha Leukoferon—used for the treatment of HIV/AIDS in hemophiliacs.

AlphaNine—factor IX clotting agent, given by injection to patients with hemophilia B.

alpha$_1$-proteinase inhibitor—an intravenous drug for patients with emphysema due to alpha$_1$-antitrypsin deficiency.

AlphaStar—a flexible, modular, lightweight operating room table.

Alphatec mini lag-screw system (MLS) for forefoot surgery.

Alphatec small fragment system (SFS) for extremity fractures.

alpha-TGI (alpha-triglycidyl isocyanurate)—see *teroxirone.*

alpha-2 antiplasmin functional assay—blood test to diagnose dysantiplasminemia, a rare inherited cause of a bleeding disorder.

alprostadil (Caverject, Edex, prostaglandin E1).

Alprox-TD (alprostadil)—a vasodilator combined with skin penetration enhancers, resulting in a topical treatment for male impotence.

ALPS (anterior locking plate system).

ALPS (autologous leukapheresis, processing, and storage)—collection and cryogenic storage of a patient's own peripheral (circulating) blood stem cells, increasing disease management options available to cancer patients and oncologists.

Alredase (tolrestat)—a drug used to treat diabetic retinopathy.

Alrex (loteprednol etabonate)—treatment for seasonal allergic conjunctivitis.

ALS Functional Rating Scale (ALS-FRS)—an instrument for evaluation of functional status and functional change in patients with ALS (amyotrophic lateral sclerosis). May be used as a screening measure in situations where muscle strength cannot be measured directly, or as an adjunct to myometry.

Alström's disease—a symptom complex including pigmentary retinopathy, diabetes, renal disease, and obesity, with sensorineural deafness and with severe visual loss in the first decade after diagnosis.

ALSVs (arm and lesser saphenous veins).

ALT (alanine aminotransferase) (newer name for *SGPT*)—an enzyme whose level in the serum is elevated in hepatitis, cirrhosis, and other liver diseases.

ALT (argon laser trabeculoplasty).

Altace (ramipril)—an ACE inhibitor used to treat congestive heart failure following myocardial infarction.

Alta reconstruction rod—for complex cervical or femoral fractures.

Alta tibial/humeral rod—a titanium alloy rod used to provide rotational stability and reduce interference with endosteal revascularization to promote fracture healing.

ALTE (apparent life-threatening event).

Altemeier's procedure—perineal rectosigmoidectomy for rectal prolapse.

alteplase—see *Activase*.

alternans test—noninvasive cardiac diagnostic test designed to identify certain patients at risk for sudden life-threatening arrhythmias (cardiac arrest) and sudden cardiac death. The test works like a "super stress test," measuring extremely subtle beat-to-beat fluctuations in the heartbeat called *T-wave alternans*.

Alternaria—an inhalant antigen.

Alteromonas putrefaciens—gram-negative organism.

Altmann classification of congenital aural atresia.

ALT-RCC (autolymphocyte-based treatment for renal cell carcinoma)—a treatment in which a small number of the patient's WBCs are removed, activated in the laboratory, and then returned to the patient to combat the cancer cells. This procedure, done on an outpatient basis (two visits per month for six months), has been shown to increase survival time.

altretamine (Hexalen, Hexastat)—chemotherapy drug used to treat ovarian carcinoma.

Altropane—^{123}I-based radioimaging agent for the early diagnosis of Parkinson's disease. May also be used in the early diagnosis of attention-deficit/hyperactivity disorder.

alumina-alumina (this is *not* a stutter)—total hip replacement prosthesis.

alumina bioceramic joint replacement material.

ALVAD (abdominal left ventricular assist device).

alveolar ridge—upper flattened surface of the mandible and lower flattened surface of the maxilla, in the sockets of which the teeth are rooted.

Alzate catheter.

ALZ-50—a protein found in the central nervous system of patients with Alzheimer's disease. This may prove to be a good clinical marker in the diagnosis of this disease. Cf. *A68*.

Alzheimer's disease—presenile dementia characterized by cortical atrophy and ventricular dilatation.

Alzheimer's Disease Assessment Scale (ADAS)—notes changes in cognition and in activities of daily living.

Amadeus microkeratome—combines computer monitoring unit, one-handed operation, vacuum system, and integrated blade-loading system.

Amaryl (glimepiride)—used to lower blood glucose in patients with non-insulin-dependent (type 2) diabetes mellitus whose hyperglycemia cannot be controlled by diet and exercise alone.

Amazr catheter—used to perform radiofrequency ablation of the inner atrial wall in treatment of refractory atrial fibrillation.

Ambien (zolpidem tartrate)—a non-benzodiazepine sleep agent. Patients are said to fall asleep within 30 minutes and sleep 7-8 hours without awakening, and feel better the following day.

AmBisome—an amphotericin B antifungal agent used intravenously, particularly for fungal infections in febrile neutropenic patients as well as for the treatment of visceral leishmaniasis.

amblyopia—dimness of vision not due to refractive error or organic lesion in the eye.

Ambu bag—a low-tech resuscitation tool in the emergency room.

Ambulator shoe—used in management of hyperkeratotic lesions of the foot.

ambulatory blood pressure monitoring (ABPM).

AMD or **ARMD** (age-related macular degeneration).

Amdray (valspodar)—a multidrug resistance modulator used in treating certain patients with acute myelogenous leukemia (AML) in combination with chemotherapy.

AME bone growth stimulators—noninvasive; can be used over casted or noncasted fracture sites for treatment of nonunion secondary to trauma. See *PEMF*.

Amelogen—composite dental restorative.

Amen (medroxyprogesterone).

AME PinSite Shields—for protection of the site (soft skin) into which are inserted halo pins, external fixation pins, Ilizarov fixation, and traction pins. Made by AME (American Medical Electronics).

Amerge (naratriptan HCl)—for treatment or reduction of menstrually associated migraines.

American Association for Medical Transcription—see *AAMT*.

American College of Nurse Midwives (ACNM).

American Health Information Management Association—see *AHIMA*.

American Liver Foundation (ALF)—offers free hepatitis B and C screening in 100 cities in the U.S. Intron (interferon alfa-2b) is now available as a treatment.

American Thoracic Society classification of dyspnea:

grade I—can keep pace walking on level ground with a normal person of similar age and body build, but not on hills or stairs.

grade II—can walk a mile at own pace without dyspnea but cannot keep pace with a normal person.

grade III—becomes breathless after walking about 100 yards or for a few minutes on level ground.

grade IV—becomes breathless while dressing or talking.

AMI (acute myocardial infarction).

Amicus separator—a blood collection device that separates and removes the white blood cells to provide a

Amicus *(cont.)*
"leuko-reduced" platelet product for transfusion. White blood cells have been associated with a variety of transfusion reactions.

amifostine (Ethyol, gammaphos)—used to treat advanced ovarian carcinoma. It acts as a protective agent when cisplatin is used for chemotherapy.

amiloride (Midamor)—commonly prescribed potassium-sparing diuretic. Administered via inhalation to treat cystic fibrosis.

Amin-Aid—a special formula dietary supplement usually used by patients with chronic renal failure.

amine precursor uptake and decarboxylation (APUD) **cells**—neural crest cells which are derived from gut endoderm and give rise to carcinoid tumors, usually in the GI tract.

aminobiphosphonates—a class of drugs used for treatment of postmenopausal syndrome.

aminoglutethimide (Cytadren).

aminoglycoside ototoxicity—toxicity of the ear attributed to the use of aminoglycosides (neomycin, streptomycin, and kanamycin), affecting mainly the inner and outer hair cells.

aminopyridine—see *4-aminopyridine.*

aminosalicylic acid (Paser).

aminosterols—a class of naturally occurring pharmacologically active small molecules with potential to treat a number of diseases.

Amiscan—a technetium-99m-labeled agent for imaging of acute myocardial infarction.

Amis 2000 respiratory mass spectrometer.

AMK (Anatomic Modular Knee) **total knee system**.

AML (acute myeloblastic leukemia)—seen at any age, but mostly in adults.

AML (Anatomic Medullary Locking) **total hip system**.

AML (angiomyolipoma)—solid renal tumor.

amlodipine besylate (Lotrel, Norvasc)—calcium channel blocking drug to treat hypertension and angina.

AMMOL (acute myelomonoblastic leukemia)—seen at all ages but somewhat more often in adults.

amnioinfusion (Ob-Gyn)—a treatment that replenishes depleted amniotic fluid via an intrauterine infusion of saline solution. Used in post-term pregnancies to decrease the incidence of cord compression, variable heart rate decelerations, meconium aspiration, and resultant morbidities.

amniotic fluid index (AFI) (Ob-Gyn)—a means of estimating amniotic fluid volume by using ultrasound and taking measurements of the largest pocket of fluid in each of the four quadrants of the uterus. Abnormally low AFI values correlate with the development of fetal distress, intrauterine passage of meconium, and the need for cesarean section.

AMO Array—foldable intraocular lens that can be implanted through small-incision cataract surgery.

AMOL (acute monoblastic leukemia)—seen at all ages, but a higher proportion of patients are adults.

amorphous silicon filmless digital x-ray detection technology—used in the fields of appendicular bone mass measurement and computer-assisted arthritis detection.

ampakine CX-516—drug that looks promising for improving memory, particularly in Alzheimer's patients.

Amphotec (amphotericin B cholesteryl sulfate)—used for treating invasive aspergillosis.

amphotericin B colloid dispersion (ABCD)—for cryptococcal meningitis.

amphotericin B lipid complex (Abelcet, ABLC)—reformulation of the antifungal drug, amphotericin B. It is said to be more effective in treating cryptococcal meningitis in AIDS patients.

Amplicor Chlamydia Assay—a highly sensitive lab test for *Chlamydia* that can detect the infection in four hours, even in difficult samples such as male urine, compared to the cell culture method that takes several days to a week. It uses polymerase chain reaction technology. See *polymerase chain reaction*.

Amplicor CT/NG test—screening test for chlamydia and gonorrhea that uses polymerase chain reaction technology to check for both diseases simultaneously.

Amplicor *Mycobacterium tuberculosis* test—a PCR (polymerase chain reaction) assay for the direct detection of *Mycobacterium tuberculosis*.

Amplified *Mycobacterium Tuberculosis* Direct (MTD) **test**—a saliva test for tuberculosis that provides results in four to five hours instead of days, with 95.5% accuracy.

amplified perversity—epidemiological term referring to the tendency for harmful trends such as improvement in treating drug-sensitive disease leading to increase in severity of an epidemic, i.e., even more intractable drug-resistant strains.

Ampligen—mismatched double-stranded RNA used to treat AIDS patients. Also called *polyribonucleotide*.

AMPPE ("amp-pee") (acute multifocal placoid pigment epitheliopathy) (Oph)—an acute disease involving rapid loss of vision and multifocal off-white, plaque-like spots of the retinal pigment epithelium of uncertain etiology but believed to be associated with a viral infection. Eventually resolves with restoration of vision. May be treated with topical or systemic steroids and, if associated with infection, an antibiotic. May be accompanied by vitreous floaters.

amprenavir—HIV protease inhibitor that achieves significant concentrations in the cerebrospinal fluid, suggesting that it crosses the blood-brain barrier and may provide potent antiviral activity in the brain, a key viral reservoir.

amrinone—a cardiotonic medication that was changed to *inamrinone*, due to medication errors that occurred because of name similarity to *amiodarone*.

AMS (ablepharon macrostomia syndrome).

AMS (American Medical Systems) **700 CX** inflatable penile prosthesis.

AMS (automatic mode switching)—used in cardiac pacemakers.

amsacrine (AMSA, Amsidyl)—chemotherapy drug used to treat adult acute leukemia.

Amset ALPS (anterior locking plate system)—provides anterior decompression and stabilization of the thoracolumbar and lumbar spine.

AMS 700 CXM penile prosthesis.

Amsidyl (amsacrine).

Amsler grid—a grid with a small dot in the middle; it tests for irregularities in the central 20° of the visual field.

AMT-25-enhanced MR images—MRI term.

amygdala—general term for an almond-shaped structure; specifically a nucleus of the basal ganglia.

ANA (antinuclear antibody)—detected by immunofluorescence in patients with rheumatoid arthritis, lupus erythematosus, and other autoimmune diseases.

anabaseine—an ant pheromone considered a possible drug candidate to slow deterioration of memory function in Alzheimer patients.

anabolic steroids—used illegally as street drugs and by body builders and other athletes to build muscle mass, but they are useful in AIDS treatment for patients with wasting syndrome.

Anadrol-50 (oxymetholone).

anagen—the phase in which hair grows. See *telogen*.

anagrelide (Agrelin).

anakmesis—arrest of maturation of leukocytes, resulting in smaller proportions of mature granular cells in the bone marrow, as observed in agranulocytosis. Also, leukanakmesis—arrest of maturation of white cell series.

anal EMG PerryMeter sensor—used for biofeedback in incontinence training.

analog-to-digital (ADC) **conversion quantization error**—MRI term.

analog-to-digital converter—MRI.

anal wink (or *anal reflex*)—contraction of the anal sphincter when the area around the anus is stroked. Loss of this response is indicative of a neurologic problem.

Anandron (nilutamide)—used to relieve bone pain of advanced prostatic carcinoma.

Anaprox (naproxen)—nonsteroidal anti-inflammatory drug.

Ana-Sal—saliva-based HIV test.

Anastaflo intravascular shunt—inserted into both ends of a severed coronary artery, preventing excessive blood loss. An interior channel within the Anastaflo conveys blood to the heart muscles beyond the grafting site while the replacement artery is sutured.

anastomoser—a coined word for an anastomosis stapler.

anatomical snuffbox—shallow depression between two tendons in the wrist, just proximal to the base of the thumb.

anatomic graduated components (AGC)—used in joint replacements.

ANCA (antineutrophil cytoplasmic antibodies)—associated with cases of the syndrome of lung hemorrhage and nephritis.

ancestral organs—five organs identified in acupuncture (brain/spinal cord, liver/gallbladder, bone marrow, uterus, and blood system).

Anchorlok soft-tissue anchor.

anchovy—a term used in microsurgery and hand surgery and refers to a rolled-up piece of fascia lata (that looks like an anchovy) and is used thus: "Operation: Carpal/metacarpal joint arthroplasty, with tensor fasciae latae anchovy." Also: "The fascia lata was initially rolled into an anchovy and tied together with corner chromic sutures. This anchovy would not adequately fill the irregular joint cavity. The anchovy was then unraveled and the fascia lata divided into three strips. These were carefully inserted into the joint space with the joint opened and distracted."

ancrod—see *Viprinex.*

Ancure system—minimally invasive endovascular repair of abdominal aortic aneurysm.

Andes virus—variation of hantavirus pulmonary syndrome found in Argentina and Chile.

Andractim (dihydrotestosterone gel)—used to treat male hormone deficiency in men, a condition also known as geriatric hypogonadism, or "male menopause." May also be used to treat benign prostatic hypertrophy.

Andrews spinal frame/table (Neuro)—frame attaches to an operating table and is used like the Hastings frame to keep the patient in a flexed knee-chest position. With the patient in the prone kneeling position for spinal surgery, the abdomen is kept from contact with the table, reducing vena caval pressure and bleeding intraoperatively. It distributes the patient's weight and relieves pressure on the knees. Also, *Andrews SST-3000.* See also *Hastings table.*

Androderm testosterone transdermal patch—mimics the natural diurnal testosterone cycle. Patches are placed on the upper arms, thighs, back, or abdomen to improve male libido, erectile function, energy, and mood.

Androgel (testosterone)—a topical testosterone gel used to treat impotence.

Androsorb—topical testosterone cream for the treatment of testosterone deficiency in males.

anechoic—in echocardiography, an area not generating echoes.

AneuRx stent graft system—for treatment of abdominal aortic aneurysm.

AngeCool RF (radiofrequency)—a catheter ablation system used in the treatment of atrial arrhythmias.

AngeFlex leads—used with Sentinel implantable cardioverter-defibrillator.

Angelchik antireflux prosthesis—used in repair of sliding hiatal hernia and gastroesophageal reflux. The abdomen is entered and the stomach and a small portion of the esophagus pulled down below the diaphragm. The small C-shaped silicone prosthesis is placed around the esophagus and tied and the abdomen closed. The prosthesis then lies around the esophagus, below the diaphragm, and above the stomach, reinforcing the esophageal sphincter.

Angiocath PRN—a flexible catheter.

Angiocidin—soluble protein that is a potent inhibitor of new blood vessel formation (angiogenesis).

Angiocol—used to inhibit capillary development and tumor growth. May be used to treat metastatic cancers, including malignant melanoma and colorectal cancer.

angiographically occult intracranial vascular malformation (AOIVM).

angiography, arteriography—the radiographic study of arteries into which radiopaque medium has been injected. Still pictures may be taken immediately after injection, or motion pictures may be made showing the flow of blood and contrast medium through vessels. See *digital subtraction angiography; fluorescein angiography; indocyanine green angiography.*

angioimmunoblastic lymphadenopathy with dysproteinemia (AILD).

AngioJet Rheolytic thrombectomy system—a device to treat peripheral

AngioJet *(cont.)*
blood clots. It is a minimally invasive catheter system which allows rapid and safe removal of intravascular blood clots from leg and arm arteries and bypass grafts and would be an alternative to current methods, drug or surgery therapy.

angiolymphoid hyperplasia with eosinophilia—uncommon smooth-surfaced nodules, consisting of lymphocytes and eosinophils involving dermis and subcutaneous tissue.

angioma—see *cherry angioma.*

AngioMark—MRI contrast agent for noninvasive breast imaging.

Angiomax (bivalirudin)—anticoagulant for patients with unstable angina undergoing PTCA.

angiomyolipoma (AML).

angioplasty, laser—used to ablate obstructing tissue. Causes less subintimal hemorrhage than balloon dilatation.

AngioOptic microcatheter—used for angiographic diagnosis of the peripheral vascular system.

Angio-Seal—a hemostatic puncture closure device. See *HPCD.*

AngioStent—balloon-expandable stent and delivery system for the treatment of malignant strictures in the biliary tree.

angiotensin-converting enzyme (ACE) **inhibitor**. See *ACE inhibitor.*

angiotensin II—a vasoconstrictor associated with primary aldosteronism and secretion of large amounts of renin in the blood in some hypertensive patients.

angle
antegonial
Baumann's
Boehler's (Böhler's)

angle *(cont.)*
center-edge angle (CE) of Wiberg
central collodiaphyseal (CCD)
cerebellopontile
cerebellopontine
Cobb
costosternal
gonial
Lovibond's

Angle's class III malocclusion.

Angstrom MD—an implantable single-lead cardioverter-defibrillator.

angular frequency; **angular momentum**—MRI terms.

anhedonia (Psych)—loss of feelings of pleasure in things that usually give pleasure. Example: "The patient describes anhedonia and low energy."

animal-assisted therapy (AAT)—used in treating autistic children, stroke victims, nursing home patients, and others who respond to animals, when it is difficult for human therapists to make contact.

anion gap ("an-eye-on")—referring to electrolytes.

aniseikonia—inequality in size and shape of an object, as seen by each eye.

anisocoria—inequality of diameter of the pupils. Cf. *anisophoria.*

anisophoria—condition in which the visual lines of the pupils are not on the same horizontal plane; caused by unequal pull on the muscles of the eyes. Cf. *anisocoria.*

anisoylated plasminogen streptokinase activator complex (APSAC)—see *anistreplase.*

anistreplase (Eminase)—also known as *APSAC* (anisoylated plasminogen streptokinase activator complex). Used to break up thrombi obstructing the coronary arteries after a patient has a myocardial infarction.

ankle air stirrup.

AnkleCiser exerciser (Phys Ther).

ankle jerk—see *Achilles reflex.*

ankle mortise—the normal articulation between the talus and the distal tibia and fibula. See *mortise.*

anlage (pl., anlagen)—a primordial structure in the developing embryo.

ANLL (acute nonlymphoid leukemia).

Annamycin—liposomal anthracycline used in treatment of refractory breast cancers with overexpression of P-glycoprotein in the tumor cell, which promotes drug resistance.

ANNs (artificial neural networks).

AnnuloFlex—a flexible annuloplasty ring for mitral valve repair.

AnnuloFlo—annuloplasty ring system.

annulus of Zinn. Also *anulus.*

anomaly
cervical aortic arch
cervical rib
cor triatriatum dexter
DiGeorge (DGA)
Ebstein's cardiac
Pelger-Huët
Taussig-Bing

anorexia—see *reversed anorexia syndrome.*

anorexia nervosa—severe caloric restriction due to distortion of body image, with dangerous nutritional deficiency. See *bulimorexia.*

anserine bursitis syndrome—associated with pes anserine bursitis.

Anspach—neurosurgical and orthopedic surgery instruments, including craniotomes, cranial perforators, and diamond dissecting cutters.

Antabuse (disulfiram)—given to recovering alcoholics to thwart their consumption of alcohol. This drug is often misspelled "Antiabuse" because it is "anti-alcohol."

Antagon (ganirelix acetate injection)—inhibits premature luteinizing hormone surges in women undergoing controlled ovarian hyperstimulation.

antagonist—a drug that inhibits or counteracts the action of naturally produced substances on a receptor. Examples: *adrenergic antagonist, beta antagonist.* Cf. *agonist.*

antecolic—in front of the colon, e.g., antecolic anastomosis and antecolic gastrojejunostomy.

antegonial angle or notch—just in front of the gonion (the most inferior, posterior, and lateral point of the external angle of the mandible). An anatomical landmark in oral and plastic surgery.

antegrade scrotal sclerotherapy—treatment for varicocele consisting of puncture of dilated vein of the pampiniform plexus by scrotal access and injection of a sclerosing agent under fluoroscopy after control of venous drainage. This is an alternative to the traditional methods of choice, which include high vasal ligation and retrograde sclerotherapy, and the newer methods of microsurgical and laparoscopic ligation.

anterior chamber acrylic implants (Oph).

anterior chamber maintainer (ACM) —an instrument used in intracapsular cataract extraction when the lens is subluxated.

anterior cruciate ligament (ACL).

anterior inferior communicating artery (AICA).

anterolisthesis—spondylolisthesis with anterior displacement of a vertebral body on the one below it.

antestrogen drug—a drug that counteracts the effects of estrogen. Also, antiestrogen.

anthelix, antihelix—of the ear.
anthracenediones—a class of chemotherapy drugs, e.g., *mitoxantrone.*
**Anthron heparinized antithromboge-
nic catheter**—used in angiography.
anthropometry—measurement of the
human body in order to assess general nutritional status of an individual or population group.
anti-aliasing techniques (MRI)—mathematical methods for eliminating
wrap-around and zebra artifacts. The
artifacts appear because of the nature
of the processing of the raw data that
produce the image (two-dimensional
Fourier transform, 2DFT). Doubling the size of the field of view
(FOV), called oversampling, can be
helpful, and newer imaging protocols include a "no phase wrap"
function to eliminate aliasing artifacts.
antibody
acetylcholine receptor (AChRab)
Acusyst-Xcell monoclonal
ANA (antinuclear antibody)
anticardiolipin (aCL)
anti-CD11a humanized monoclonal
anti-CD18 humanized
anticentromere (ACA)
anticytoplasmic (ACPA)
anti-D (WinRho)
anti-EA
anti-EGF-receptor antibody
    for cancer
antifibrin
anti-HA
anti-HAV
anti-IgE humanized monoclonal
anti-IL-8
anti-La
antimitochondrial
antineutrophilic cytoplasmic
    (ANCA)

antibody *(cont.)*
antiphospholipid
anti-Ro
anti-Sm
anti-VEGF
Bexxar radiolabeled monoclonal
BR96-doxorubicin monoclonal
C100-3 hepatitis C virus (anti-HIV)
CC49 monoclonal
CD5+
CD18
cryptosporidiosis
CytoTAb polyclonal
dacliximab monoclonal
Diffistat-G polyclonal
Duffy blood antibody type
E5 monoclonal
Ha-1A monoclonal
HB_cAb
HB_eAb
HB_sAb
I-B1 radiolabeled
IgM-RF (rheumatoid factor)
ImmuRAIT-LL2 (IgG 2A
    monoclonal)
infliximab monoclonal
islet cell (ICA)
Kell blood antibody type
Kidd blood antibody type
LDP-02 humanized monoclonal
LeuTech radiolabeled
Lewis blood antibody type
LymphoCide
MAb-170 monoclonal
MabThera (rituximab) monoclonal
monoclonal
Oncolym radiolabeled monoclonal
opsonizing
OvaRex MAb (monoclonal)
PM 81 monoclonal
ProstaScint (CYT-356 radiolabeled
    with 111 indium chloride)
    monoclonal
ReoPro (abciximab) monoclonal

antibody *(cont.)*
   Rituxan (rituximab) monoclonal
   7E3 monoclonal antiplatelet
   thyroperoxidase
   TI-23 cytomegalovirus monoclonal
   2C3 anti-VEGF (vascular
      endothelial growth factor)
   WinRho SD (anti-D)
   XMMEN-OE5 monoclonal
antibody molecules (immune globulins)
   —have heavy and light chains. There
   are five classes of heavy chains (G,
   A, M, D, and E), IgG, IgA, IgM,
   etc., and two classes of light chains
   (kappa and lambda).
anticardiolipin antibody (aCL).
**anti-CD11a humanized monoclonal
   antibody**—designed to specifically
   block the T-cells that are overactive
   in psoriasis.
anti-CD18 humanized antibody—used
   for the prevention or alleviation of
   reperfusion injuries and mortality
   following treatment of shock.
anticentromere antibody (ACA)—appears in the majority of patients with
   CREST syndrome. See *CREST syndrome.*
**anticonvulsant hypersensitivity syn-
   drome**—a potentially fatal drug reaction with cutaneous and systemic
   reactions. The hallmark features of
   fever, rash, and lymphadenopathy
   are accompanied by multiorgan system abnormalities.
Anticort—inhibits adrenal cortisol
   synthesis, thus lowering circulating
   cortisol levels in the blood and
   modulating the immune response of
   infected individuals, leading to a
   more effective response to HIV and
   other autoimmune diseases.
anticytoplasmic antibody (ACPA) **test**
   —detects autoantibodies to components of neutrophilic cytoplasm by

immunofluorescence. Useful in diagnosing Wegener's granulomatosis
and gauging its extent and severity.
anti-D antibody (WinRho SD)—used
   in intermittent doses for treatment of
   childhood idiopathic thrombocytopenic purpura (also referred to as
   immunothrombocytopenic purpura).
anti-EA antibody—*EA* stands for *early
   antigen* of Epstein-Barr virus. Patients with chronic mononucleosis
   syndrome are thought to test positive
   to the antibody.
anti-EGF-receptor antibody—used
   in cancer treatment.
antiendomysial antibody test—blood
   test to detect celiac disease, a condition in which the gluten in wheat,
   oats, barley, and rye damages the
   small intestine.
antifibrin antibody imaging—a method to diagnose deep vein thrombosis; it is thought to be a safer, faster,
   and more accurate way to detect
   blood clots than venography. In the
   procedure, a radiolabeled antifibrin
   antibody is injected into the patient.
   It then attaches itself to the fibrin in
   the clot; within an hour, imaging
   reveals the clot.
antigen
   CA1-18 tumor marker
   CA 15-3
   CA 19-9
   CA 72-4
   CEA (carcinoembryonic)
   common acute lymphoblastic
      leukemia (CALLA)
   ENA (extractable nuclear)
   epithelial membrane (EMA)
   Goa (Gonzales blood)
   HbAg (or HBAg) (hepatitis B)
   HB_eAg (hepatitis B "e")
   HB_sAg (hepatitis B surface)
   Histoplasma capsulatum (HPA)

antigen *(cont.)*
HLA (human lymphocyte)
inhalant
PHA (phytohemagglutinin)
PLA-I (platelet)
PSA (prostate-specific antigen)
PSA-ACT
PSMA (prostate-specific membrane)
Rh (Rhesus) factor
SD
Sm
vWF (von Willebrand's factor)
Anti-Gliadin IgG, Anti-Gliadin IgA —
ELISA autoimmune tests trademarked by Great Smokies.
anti-HA, anti-HAV (antibody to hepatitis A virus).
antihelix, anthelix—of the ear.
antihemophilic globulin (AHG).
Antihist-1 (clemastine fumarate)—over-the-counter antihistamine.
anti-IgE humanized monoclonal antibody—used to block or interfere with the process that leads to allergy symptoms in allergic rhinitis.
anti-IL-8 antibody for inflammation.
anti-La antibody—an unusual antibody found in patients with Sjögren's disease. Cf. *anti-Ro*.
antimesenteric border of ileum—a surgical landmark; the side of the small bowel opposite the insertion of the mesentery.
antimicrobial catheter cuff—placed subcutaneously where a central venous catheter exits from the skin. It slowly releases silver ions which prevent infection from microorganisms along the catheter exit site.
antimitochondrial antibody.
antineutrophilic cytoplasmic antibody (ANCA)—indicative of an acute necrotizing vasculitis.
antinuclear antibody (ANA).

antiphospholipid antibodies—found in the serum of women who experience recurrent spontaneous abortions. These antibodies inhibit the normal formation of syncytiotrophoblasts in the placenta and jeopardize the pregnancy.
antiphospholipid syndrome (APS)—characterized by arterial and venous thrombosis, thrombocytopenia, and antiphospholipid or anticardiolipin antibodies, which can lead to stroke or transient ischemic attack. Frequently seen in young individuals and often associated with transient ischemic attacks or strokes. Clinically similar to multiple sclerosis. See *antiphospholipid antibodies*.
antipsychotic drug side effects—akathisia, extrapyramidal and pyramidal signs, and tardive dyskinesia.
anti-RHO-D titer (Lab).
anti-Ro antibody—an unusual antibody found in patients with Sjögren's disease. Cf. *anti-La*.
antisense oligodeoxynucleotides (also known as ODNs)—proposed as a new therapy for patients with cancer, including malignant brain tumors. Antisense ODNs have been used successfully to block glioblastoma gene expression in vitro and expression of multiple genes with the central nervous system of experimental animals.
antisense technology—zeros in on a cancer gene to halt malignancy at its roots.
Anti-Sept bactericidal scrub solution.
anti-Sm antibody—found in lupus erythematosus. The *Sm* is for *Smith*.
antistreptolysin titer (AST).
anti-Tamm-Horsfall protein—found in interstitial cystitis.
antiteichoic acid titer (Lab).

antithrombin III (ATnativ)—used to inhibit blood coagulation in patients with an antithrombin III deficiency. It is given intravenously prior to surgery or obstetrical procedures to prevent the formation of thrombi and emboli. Note the unique spelling of *ATnativ*, with two initial capital letters.

antithymocyte globulin (ATG).

anti-TNF drugs (antitumor necrosis factor)—the investigational N-acetyl-L-cysteine (NAC), Procysteine, and pentoxifylline (Trental). Tumor necrosis factor has been linked to wasting syndrome and HIV activation in AIDS.

antitussives—a class of drugs used as cough suppressants.

anti-VEGF antibody—an inhibitor of angiogenesis (blood-vessel growth) that may hinder the growth of cancer tumors by starving their blood supply.

Antizol (fomepizole)—injectable antidote administered for ingestion, or suspected ingestion, of ethylene glycol (antifreeze).

Antopol-Goldman lesion—subepithelial hematoma of the renal pelvis.

anuresis—inability of the kidneys to produce or excrete urine. Cf. *enuresis*.

anxiolytics—antianxiety drugs; minor tranquilizers.

Anzemet (dolasetron mesylate)—used for the treatment and prevention of nausea and vomiting in postoperative patients and patients receiving chemotherapy.

AoBP (aortic blood pressure).

AO (American Optical) **indirect ophthalmoscope**.

AOIVM (angiographically occult intracranial vascular malformation).

A-OK ShortCut knife—an ophthalmic knife with a unique rounded tip and short length for intraocular incisions. Also called *ShortCut knife.*

AOPA (ara-C, Oncovin, prednisone, asparaginase)—chemotherapy protocol.

AOPE (Adriamycin, Oncovin, prednisone, etoposide)—chemotherapy protocol.

Aortic Connector System—for performance of sutureless anastomoses during coronary artery bypass graft procedures.

aortic root (*not* route)—"The patient underwent an aortic root reconstruction procedure with aortic valve replacement."

aortobifemoral reconstruction.

aortofemoral bypass graft (AFBG).

aortoiliac obstructive (or occlusive) **disease** (AIOD).

AOVM (angiographically occult vascular malformations).

APA (aldosterone-producing adenoma).

APAAP (alkaline phosphatase antialkaline phosphatase).

APACHE CV Risk Predictor—Internet-based product that can help physicians anywhere predict a patient's risk of death or serious complications before the patient elects to undergo an invasive heart procedure.

APACHE III (Acute Physiology and Chronic Health Evaluation) **score**—originally designed as a predictor of death on admission to the ICU. It is now used to predict length of stay for long-term hospitalizations.

apallic syndrome—parasomniac conscious state.

A-pattern strabismus.

APC (adenopolyposis coli) **gene**—implicated in the development of colorectal carcinoma.

APE (ara-C, Platinol, etoposide)—chemotherapy protocol for children with advanced Hodgkin's disease.

Apex irrigation system (ENT).

Apex Plus excimer laser—used in the treatment of myopia, hyperopia, and astigmatism. It combines an erodible mask with an Axicon prismatic lens system for ablation of hyperopia.

Apex universal drive (ENT).

Apgar score (named for Dr. Virginia Apgar, an anesthesiologist)—rating of the condition of the newborn infant, performed at one and five minutes after birth. The criteria are color, heart rate, respiration, reflex response to nose catheter, and muscle tone. "The infant's Apgars were 8 and 9 at one and five minutes."

1. Color: If the infant is pale or blue, the score for color is 0; if the body is pink and the extremities are blue, the score is 1; if the body and extremities are pink, the score is 2.

2. Heart rate: If the heart rate cannot be elicited, the score for heart rate is 0; if it is less than 100, the score is 1; if more than 100, the score is 2.

3. Respiration: If respirations can not be elicited, the score for respiration is 0; if irregular or slow, the score is 1; if respirations are good, crying, the score for this is 2.

4. Reflex response: If there is no reflex response to the nose catheter, the score is 0; if the infant grimaces, the score is 1; if the infant sneezes or coughs, the score is 2.

5. Muscle tone: If the infant is limp, the score for muscle tone is 0; if there is some flexion of the extremities, the score is 1; if the infant is active, the score is 2. All the subscore totals are added together for the total score on a scale of 1 to 10 at one and five minutes.

APGAR—in Family APGAR Questionnaire, the acronym formed from the initial letters of adaptability, partnership, growth, affection, and resolve. Sometimes abbreviated FAPGAR. See *Apgar score.*

apheresis (from Greek *aphairesis*, taking away)—removal of a component of the blood from the intravascular circulation. This process is used now as apheresis of plasma, erythrocytes, leukocyte fractions, platelets, and cold precipitable serum proteins in blood banking. It is used in treating babies who are Rh incompatible and is likely to be used in the future for selective aphcresis of autoantibodies in the treatment of rheumatoid arthritis, systemic lupus erythematosus, and other autoimmune diseases. See *lymphapheresis, plasmapheresis.* Cf. *electrophoresis.*

aphtha (pl., aphthae), adj., aphthous ("af-thus")—the small ulcers of the oral mucosa known colloquially as "canker sores." Cf. *abscess.*

Aphthasol (amlexanox oral paste 5%) —prescription medication used specifically for treatment of canker sores, in patients with normal immune systems.

apical impulse—a thrust noted over the apex of the heart. May be referred to as *PMI, point of maximal impulse.*

APL (abductor pollicis longus).

APL (acute promyelocytic leukemia).

APLD (automated percutaneous lumbar diskectomy).

Apley sign.

Apligraf (graftskin)—living skin product that looks and feels like human skin, indicated for treatment of lower extremity venous ulcers. It has two primary layers, including an outer epidermal layer made of living human keratinocytes and a dermal layer consisting of human fibroblasts. The keratinocytes and fibroblasts are derived from donor tissue that is thoroughly screened for a wide range of infectious pathogens.

APML (acute promyelocytic leukemia).

apnea—see *obstructive sleep apnea* (OSA).

apnea/hypopnea index (AHI).

APO (Adriamycin, prednisone, Oncovin)—chemotherapy protocol used to treat non-Hodgkin's lymphoma.

apocrine metaplasia—a change in the cells lining a breast duct so they appear similar to a lactating breast, often associated with mammary dysplasia.

Apo E-4 (apolipoprotein E-4)—thought to increase the risk for Alzheimer's disease. It also appears to be associated with poor recovery from traumatic brain injury.

Apo-Etodolac (etodolac)—NSAID for osteoarthritis.

apolipoprotein E—the E4 allele of this gene may become a predictor of coronary heart disease mortality.

Apollo hip prosthesis.

Apollo knee prosthesis.

Apollo triple lumen papillotome.

apomorphine—oral medication for erectile dysfunction.

apophysis—a projecting part of a bone; a bony outgrowth, such as a tubercle, process, or tuberosity, not separated from the main portion of the bone. Cf. *epiphysis, hypophysis.*

apoptosis (pronounced "a-puh-toe-sis") —a naturally occurring process of programmed cell death that researchers hope to use for treatment of cancer and other disorders. It can be induced by ischemia, reperfusion, and pressure-overload-induced hypertrophy.

Apo-Zidovudine (azidothymidine, AZT) —drug used to treat AIDS. The proprietary name is used in the U.S.; in Canada it is both apozidovudine and apo-zidovudine.

apparent—visible, obvious, evident. Cf. *aberrant.*

appendectomy, inversion-ligation.

appendicovesicotomy—technique for continent urinary diversion. Also, *Mitrofanoff procedure.*

appendicular ataxia—muscular incoordination of the extremities.

appendicular bone mass measurement—see *amorphous silicon filmless digital x-ray detection arm artery, LIMA (left internal mammary artery).*

applanation—flattening of the cornea by pressure.

applanation tonometry—measures intraocular pressure. See *Schiötz tonometry.*

applanometer—an instrument used to determine the intraocular pressure in testing for glaucoma. See *tonometry.*

apple peel syndrome—jejunal atresia, caused by the distal small bowel coming straight off the cecum and twisting around the marginal artery like an apple peel.

apposition—the placing or bringing together of two adjacent parts, e.g., drawing together the cut edges of an incision on closure of a wound: "The wound edges were placed in apposition and sutured in place." Cf. *opposition*.

Appraise—diabetes monitoring system that allows patients to collect their own specimens for hemoglobin $A1_c$ and microalbumin.

apprehension test—refers to the apprehensive appearance of a patient in testing for a subluxed or dislocated shoulder. The arm is held abducted and extended while it is in external rotation, and the test is considered to be positive if the patient appears to be apprehensive. "There is a positive mild to moderate apprehension test."

approach—see *operation*.

APPT (Adolescent and Pediatric Pain Tool)—a scale used to measure pain experienced by patients undergoing Ilizarov limb-lengthening procedures. It is a measurement of current pain, including a visual analogue scale, a listing of 42 words that describe the qualitative aspects of pain, and two body diagrams. Cf. *HSC Scale*.

Apri (desogestrel and ethinyl estradiol) **tablets**—brand name generic oral contraceptive.

apron—excessive subcutaneous fat that hangs from the abdominal wall like an apron; also called *hanging panniculus*.

aprosody (Psych)—lack of variation in voice features like pitch, loudness, tempo, and intonation, such as encountered in Parkinson's disease.

aprotinin (Trasylol)—a protease inhibitor that reduces blood loss during heart bypass surgery.

APR total hip system—porous, coated cement fixation.

APS (antiphospholipid antibody syndrome).

APSAC (anisoylated plasminogen streptokinase activator complex). See *anistreplase*.

APSGN (acute poststreptococcal glomerulonephritis).

Apt-Downey alkali denaturation test —performed to rule out maternal source of bleeding in newborn.

Aptosyn (exisulind)—a drug used to treat adenomatous polyposis coli. May also be used to treat prostate cancer.

APTT (activated partial thromboplastin time).

APUD (amine precursor uptake and decarboxylation).

apudoma—tumor composed of APUD cells; potentially malignant or overtly malignant gastrin-secreting tumor; the most frequent cause of the Zollinger-Ellison syndrome. See *APUD, Zollinger-Ellison syndrome*.

Aquacel hydrofiber wound packing and dressing.

"aquacise"—a coined word denoting buoyant exercise in water.

Aqua-Flow collagen glaucoma drainage device—permanently implanted under the sclera (without entering the interior of the eye) for immediate reduction of eye pressure associated with open-angle glaucoma.

Aquaphor gauze—non-adhering dressing.

aquaporin 1—protein identified as enabling the kidneys to form concentrated urine, a process that is critical for preventing severe dehydration during times of water deprivation. The discovery of this protein has potential implications for treat-

aquaporin 1 *(cont.)*
ment of diseases associated with fluid retention or refractory edema, including congestive heart failure and cirrhosis.

AquaShield—reusable, one-piece, completely waterproof orthopedic cast cover.

Aquasil Smart Wetting dental impression material.

Aquasorb transparent hydrogel dressing—a conformable gel dressing that promotes healing by maintaining a moist environment. Healing can be monitored because the dressing is transparent. Cf. *Curasorb, ClearSite,* and *Ventex.*

Aquaspirillum itersonii—a gram-negative organism.

Aquatab C, Aquatab D, and **Aquatab DM**—products for a persistent, nonproductive cough, nasal congestion, and bronchial secretions.

aqueous flare (Oph)—scattering of slit-lamp light beam when the light is directed into the anterior chamber. This is found with increased protein in the aqueous and is an indication of iritis. See *cell and flare.*

arachidonic acid—an unsaturated fatty acid that occurs in certain fats and in animal phosphatides.

arachnoid (Greek *arachne,* spider)—the membrane between dura and pia mater; the weblike strands between it and the pia give rise to the name.

araldehyde-tanned bovine carotid artery graft (heterograft or xenograft).

Arava (leflunomide)—for treating active rheumatoid arthritis in adults. It works by inhibiting an enzyme (DHODH) involved in the autoimmune process that leads to rheumatoid arthritis.

arbovirus (arthropod-borne virus)—any one of a group of viruses carried by mosquitoes and ticks. Arboviruses are the cause of some febrile diseases, such as yellow fever, and of types of viral meningitis. See *togavirus.*

arbutamine—a cardiac stimulant. Cf. *GenESA System.*

ARC (AIDS-related complex).

arcade of Frohse—see *Frohse.*

Arcanobacterium haemolyticum—a bacterial throat infection seen in adolescents and young adults, and may mimic a viral exanthem, toxic erythema, or drug eruption.

arch bar—a wire or bar support, shaped to fit the arch of the teeth, used to splint a fractured jaw or loosened teeth. See *Winters arch bar.*

Arcometer—an instrument to measure kyphosis.

ARDs (acid-related disorders).

ARDS (adult respiratory distress syndrome).

Aredia (pamidronate disodium)—used for treatment of osteolytic bone lesions in multiple myeloma patients.

Arenberg-Denver implant—a pressure-sensitive unidirectional inner-ear valve implant. For use in patients with Mondini's dysplasia, and to control endolymphatic hypertension and hydrops in Ménière's disease, congenital hydrops, and large vestibular aqueduct syndrome.

AREx inhaler—a noninvasive device that delivers a drug through an inhaler rather than intravenously, thus allowing more flexibility for outpatients.

AREZ (anterior root exit zone).

ARF (acute renal failure)—a critical condition characterized by oliguria

ARF *(cont.)*
and rapid deterioration in renal function.

ARF (acute respiratory failure).

ArF excimer laser—used for tissue ablation.

argatroban (Novastan).

argentaffin carcinoma.

arginine tolerance test (ATT)—for growth hormone.

argon beam coagulator (ABC)—used for hemostasis in minimally invasive surgery instead of electrocautery, and for treating highly vascular pleural malignancies.

argon/krypton laser—a vitreoretinal laser used for iridotomies and trabeculoplasties, for management of glaucoma, and in macular procedures. May be used for other kinds of surgery.

argon laser—is used for photocoagulation in diabetic retinopathy and detached retina. May be used for other kinds of surgery. Cf. *laser, CO_2 laser, Nd:YAG laser*.

argon laser trabeculoplasty (ALT)—a procedure used in treating glaucoma and ocular hypertension which do not respond to medical management, before resorting to filtering surgery.

Argosy Cameo CIC (completely-in-the-canal) **hearing aid** with digital magnetic sensing and remote adjustment of volume for various listening situations.

Argyle CPAP nasal cannula.

Argyle Turkel safety thoracentesis system.

Aria—coronary artery bypass graft which incorporates the proprietary biomaterial Thoralon in patients with few or no suitable native vessels.

Arias-Stella phenomenon.

ariboflavinosis—a vitamin deficiency state, indicated by flattening of the papillae of the tongue.

Aricept (donepezil HCl)—used in the treatment of Alzheimer's disease.

Aries-Pitanguy correction of mammary ptosis.

Arimidex (anastrozole)—for treatment of advanced breast cancer in postmenopausal women whose disease has progressed despite tamoxifen therapy.

aripiprazole—a drug used for treatment of schizophrenia.

ARM (age-related maculopathy).

arm and **lesser saphenous veins** (ALSVs)—an alternative for infrapopliteal arterial bypass grafts when the greater saphenous vein (GSV) is not available.

arm board or **armboard**.

ARMD (age-related macular degeneration). See *"dry" age-related macular degeneration; "wet" age-related macular degeneration*.

Arneth's grouping of polymorphonuclear neutrophils—according to the number of lobes in their nuclei, e.g., one lobe, class I; two lobes, class II; three lobes, class III, etc.

Arnett-TMP (trimandibular plate) **system** (Plas Surg)—a fixation device for orthognathic, craniofacial, midface, and mandibular applications.

Arnold's nerve—the auricular branch of the vagus nerve.

Aromapatch nasal inhaler—OTC single-use patch indicated for aroma inhalation of essential oils.

AromaScan—aroma analysis device developed for use in beverage, food, and perfume industries, now being used to check breath samples for evidence of infection, producing a

AromaScan *(cont.)*
kind of "fingerprint" of the air. If the device produces a suspicion for lung infection, physicians can prescribe antibiotics while they await lab results.

Aromasin (exemestane)—oral aromatase inactivator for treatment of postmenopausal women with advanced breast cancer whose tumors no longer respond to tamoxifen.

AR-177—an oligonucleotide inhibitor for treatment of HIV.

Arrequi laparoscopic knot pusher ligator.

arrest of labor—stopping of progress in labor (*not* "a rest of labor").

arrhythmia mapping system—a catheter-based system to aid in the diagnosis of complex ventricular tachyarrhythmias.

Arrowgard Blue Line catheter—a central venous catheter that contains chlorhexidine and silver sulfadiazine antiseptics bonded onto the outer surface to reduce the risk of catheter-induced bacteremia.

Arrow-Howes multilumen catheter—provides multiple apertures with the use of only one venipuncture site, thus permitting hyperalimentation, central venous pressure monitoring, intravenous administration of medications, and blood sampling without the necessity of multiple needle punctures.

Arrow PICC—a radiology device for insertion of central venous lines.

Arrow pneumothorax kit—for nonsurgical treatment of pneumothorax, using percutaneous catheter-over-needle technique.

Arrowsmith corneal marker (Oph).

Arrow Twin Cath—multilumen peripheral catheter.

ARS (acute repetitive seizure) **disorder**.

ArtAssist—compression dressing or wrap.

arterial—referring to an artery. Cf. *arteriole*.

arterial blood gases (ABGs).

arterial line (A-line).

arterial obstruction, signs and symptoms of (also known as the classic five P's): pain, pallor, pulselessness, paresthesia, and paralysis.

arterial oxygen saturation (SaO_2).

arterial switch procedure—for correcting transposition of the great vessels.

arteriole—a tiny arterial branch. Cf. *arterial*.

arteriovenous oxygen difference (AVD O_2, AV DO_2, $AVDO_2$).

arteritis—inflammation of an artery or arteries. Examples: giant cell arteritis; Takayasu's arteritis. Cf. *arthritis*.

artery of Adamkiewicz—the great anterior radicular artery.

Arthro-BST—arthroscopic probe for diagnosis of arthritis. Provides objective diagnosis of cartilage disease and evaluation of cartilage repair after therapy.

Arthopor acetabular cup (*not* Arthropor, although it is often pronounced that way). The acetabular component attached to the femoral stem constitutes the prosthesis used in hip arthroplasty. These sintered (calcareous) porous-coated hemispherical cups are made with holes in various shapes and sizes on the top to accommodate screws and locking pins. They come in three depths: low profile, deep profile, and extra deep

Arthopor *(cont.)*
profile. The cups are designated Arthopor I, II, and III.

arthritides ("ar-thrit-ih-dees")—plural form of *arthritis.*

arthritis—inflammation of a joint. Cf. *arteritis.*

ArthroCare Coblation-based cosmetic surgery system—used for skin resurfacing for treatment of wrinkles.

ArthroCare System—for rapid tissue removal, resection, and hemostasis in the knee and shoulder as well as for soft tissue sculpting of meniscus and articular cartilage, using Coblation technology.

Arthro-Flo system—provides powered irrigation for arthroscopy.

Arthro-Lok system—Beaver blades for arthroscopic surgery and all types of meniscal tears. Blades include banana, rosette, retrograde.

ArthroProbe laser system—a laser system for arthroscopic surgery, which provides both resection and hemostasis. Used through an arthroscopic cannula.

ArthroSew—arthroscopic suturing device.

Arthrotec (diclofenac sodium/misoprostol)—used for relieving the signs and symptoms of osteoarthritis and rheumatoid arthritis in patients at high risk for ulcers and their complications induced by nonsteroidal anti-inflammatory drugs.

ArthroWand—used to apply radiofrequency in procedures using Coblation technology. See *CAPS ArthroWand.*

Arthus reaction—immune complex deposition in dermal walls; it can cause gangrene at the site of injection of an allergen. Named for a French bacteriologist (d. 1945).

artifact (Radiol)—a finding which mimics but is not a disease process, e.g., a nipple shadow resembling a lesion seen on a chest x-ray, a wrinkled film, or movement. Misleading images in radiology may be due to a variety of sources, such as patient movement, software or hardware failure, or human error. Examples:
aliasing (wrap-around ghosting)
analog-to-digital (ADC) conversion quantization error
barium
beam hardening
"black comets"
braces
broadband noise detection error
calibration failure
chemical shift phenomena
coin
construction
corduroy
crescent
crinkle
cross-talk effect
crown
data-clipping detection error
data spike detection error
DC (direct current) offset
developer
distortion of limitations of image reconstruction algorithm
double exposure drift
eddy current
edge ringing
equipment
faulty RF (radiofrequency) shielding in MRI scanner room permitting coherent RF noise which distorts image
flow effect (MRI)

artifact *(cont.)*
 fog
 foreign material (within the patient,
  within the MRI scanner room,
  within the MRI magnet bore)
 geophagia
 Gibbs phenomenon
 glass eye
 half-moon
 image post-processing errors
 imbalance of phase or gain
 intensifying screen
 kink
 kissing-type
 large clothing
 lettering
 "magic angle"
 magnetic susceptibility
 main magnetic field inhomogeneity
 mercury
 mitral regurgitation
 moiré
 movement
 paramagnetic
 patient motion
 pellet
 pica
 "pseudofracture"
 quadrature phase detector (QPD)
 radiofrequency (RF) spatial distribution problem reconstruction
 reticulation
 screen craze
 skin fold (skin crease)
 skin lesion
 slice profile
 stimulated echo
 subcutaneous injection of contrast
 summation shadow
 superimposition
 swamp-static
 temporal instability
 tree
 truncation band

artifact *(cont.)*
 wheelchair
 wrap-around ghost (aliasing)
 wrinkle
 zebra
artificial blood
 Fluosol plasma expander
 Hemolink
 Hextend blood plasma volume
  expander
 pyridoxylated stroma-free
  hemoglobin (SFHb)
 recombinant hemoglobin (rHb1.1)
artificial heart
 Symbion J-7-70-mL-ventricle
 University of Akron
artificial insemination–donor (AID).
artificial insemination–husband (AIH).
artificial lung—see *IVOX* (intravascular
 oxygenator).
artificial neural networks (ANNs)—
 the task-oriented computer algo-
 rithms modeled on the human brain.
 This is a diagnostic tool to predict
 the presence of pulmonary embolism by using findings from ventila-
 tion-perfusion lung scans and from
 clinical examination.
artificial skin—see *Integra*.
ARTMA (advanced real time motion
 analysis) **virtual patient technology**
 —used in endoscopic navigation system and telesurgery.
ARUM pin—for fixation of Colles'
 fractures as an alternative to the
 usual intrafocal pinning procedure. It
 consists of a pin and a special nut.
 The pin is cut close to the nut, and
 the nut is designed so that it slides
 between the tendons very precisely.
ARV (AIDS-related virus)—the term
 given to the AIDS virus by the
 group of scientists working at U.C.
 San Francisco under Dr. Jay Levy.

ARV *(cont.)*
The virus is now officially known as *HIV*. See *HIV*.

Arvin (ancrod)—a drug used to dissolve blood clots following a stroke. Obtained from snake venom.

aryepiglottic fold (AE fold).

arylcyclohexylamines—a category of drugs including phencyclidine (PCP), a street drug of abuse.

A.S. *(auris sinistra)*—left ear.

ASA (acetylsalicylic acid, aspirin). The trade name of the drug marketed by Lilly is *A.S.A.* (with periods).

Asacol (mesalamine)—used to treat ulcerative colitis.

ASAP solution—mineral supplement solution that acts as a broad-spectrum antimicrobial agent.

A-scan—an ultrasound device used to differentiate abnormal from normal tissues in the eye.

Ascent guiding catheter—directs balloon catheters rapidly into coronary arteries or other sites where obstructions are treated.

Aschoff-Tawara node—atrioventricular node.

ascitic—characterized by ascites or an accumulation of fluid in the peritoneal cavity. Cf. *acidic*.

ascribe—to attribute; e.g., "The patient ascribes occasional shortness of breath to the fact that she has put on a great deal of weight in the past four months, although she still smokes more than a pack a day." Cf. *describe*.

ASCUS (atypical squamous cells of undetermined significance).

AS-800—artificial sphincter for surgically treating urinary incontinence in women.

aseptic loosening—seen in some cemented custom-made prosthetic replacements for bone tumors of the limbs.

ASF (anterior spine fusion).

ASH (asymmetric septal hypertrophy) —the newer term for what was formerly called *IHSS* (idiopathic hypertrophic subaortic stenosis).

A-SHAP (Adriamycin, Solu-Medrol, high-dose ara-C, Platinol)—chemotherapy protocol for advanced lymphoma.

ash leaf spots in the eye—seen in cases of tuberous sclerosis.

ASI (active specific immunotherapy)— using the patient's own tumor to elicit an immune response.

ASIA impairment scale—classification of spinal cord injury established by the American Spinal Injury Association.

A No motor or sensory function preserved in sacral segments.

B Sensory but not motor function preserved in at least sacral segments.

C Motor function preserved below the neurologic level; majority of key muscles have motor score < 3.

D Motor function preserved below the neurologic level; majority of key muscles have motor score of 3 or >.

E Motor and sensory function normal.

ASIF plates. (ASIF, Association for the Study of Internal Fixation.)

ASIS (anterior superior iliac spine).

AS-101—a drug used in treating AIDS patients.

A68 (Path)—a protein found in the brains of patients with Alzheimer's disease. Cf. *ALZ-50*.

Asnis 2 guided screw system—for treatment of hip fractures.

aspartate transaminase (AST) (formerly *SGOT*)—a liver function test.

Aspen electrocautery—used in arthroscopic procedures.

Aspen laparoscopy electrode—electrosurgical device used in laparoscopic surgical procedures.

Aspen ultrasound system—a maneuverable digital ultrasound system that utilizes high-frequency transducers, and enables the imaging of small body parts, such as breast, testicle, and thyroid.

Aspergillus—the fungus causing aspergillosis, which is seen in disseminated form in AIDS. See *Penicillium*.

aspheric—refers to the reflecting surface of a lens.

aspiration biopsy cytology (ABC).

aspiration-tulip device—used for in vitro percutaneous removal of rigid clots, such as a platelet-rich arterial plug.

aspartate aminotransferase (AST) (formerly called *SGOT*)—see *AST*.

ASPS (alveolar soft-part sarcoma)—soft tissue tumors as opposed to bone tumors.

assay—see *test*.

ASSI—bipolar coagulating forceps and disposable cranio blades (no hyphen and no period after *cranio*) and wire pass drills for use in neurosurgery and other surgical specialties. (ASSI, Accurate Surgical and Scientific Instruments Corporation.)

Assistant Free calibrated femoral-tibial spreader (Ortho).

assisted same-day microsurgical arthroscopic lateral-approach laser-assisted (SMALL) fluoroscopic diskectomy.

AST (acute stroke team).

AST (antistreptolysin titer).

AST (aspartate transaminase) (newer name for *SGOT*)—an enzyme whose level in the serum is elevated in myocardial infarction, liver disease, and other conditions.

astasia–abasia—inability to stand or to walk, although the legs are otherwise under control.

Astelin (azelastine) **nasal spray**—for treatment of seasonal allergic rhinitis.

asthenic—lacking in strength and energy, or pertaining to an individual with an ectomorphic body build. Cf. *aesthetic*.

asthenopia—eye discomfort that feels like eyestrain and may also be accompanied by headache.

asthenospermic—poor motility of sperm.

asthma—synonym for reversible obstructive airway disease.

astigmatic keratotomy—surgical incision of the cornea to correct astigmatism.

astigmatism—an eye condition in which there is unequal curvature of one of the refractive surfaces of the eye, causing lack of sharpness in focus of a ray of light on the retina.

astigmatism with the rule—has the greater curvature along the vertical meridian of the eye. *Astigmatism against the rule* has the greater curvature in the horizontal meridian.

Astler-Coller modification of Dukes' C classification of carcinoma—provides a subscript for the C (C_1, C_2).

Aston cartilage reduction system—includes cartilage rasps and nasal scissors for nasal reconstruction.

Astra profiles (Lab)—blood chemistry analyzers.

Astringedent topical hemostatic solution used by dentists. Does not contain epinephrine and can be infused using a Dento-Infuser.

asymmetric septal hypertrophy (ASH) —newer term for *IHSS* (idiopathic hypertrophic subaortic stenosis).

Atacand (candesartan cilexetil)—for once-daily treatment of hypertension. Atacand belongs to a group of antihypertensive medications called angiotensin II receptor blockers.

ataxia
appendicular
equilibratory
Marie's
telangiectasia

atevirdine—for HIV-positive patients.

ATFL (anterior talofibular ligament).

ATG (antithymocyte globulin)—used to prevent rejection of transplanted kidney.

atherectomy—the removal of atherosclerotic plaque from an artery by means of a rotary cutter introduced into the artery through a special catheter under radiographic guidance. Atherectomy methods include directional, extraction, and rotational.

atherectomy catheter—a catheter (such as AtheroCath and Simpson) used to retrieve cholesterol plaque from diseased arteries. See *Simpson atherectomy catheter*.

AtheroCath Bantam coronary atherectomy catheter—for performance of nonsurgical directional coronary atherectomy, a procedure for shaving obstructing plaque from coronary vessels.

atheroma—see *protruding atheromas*.

Athlete coronary guidewire—said to have optimal steering characteristics and unique stiffness, kink resistance, and pushability of the 3 cm radiopaque tip segment because of improved jointless spring technology (one-piece core wire). Used for recanalization of total coronary occlusion when conventional wires fail to cross.

Atkinson endoprosthesis—a silicone rubber tube with a preformed distal shoulder. Also, *Atkinson tube*.

Atkinson tube stent—used over Nottingham introducer.

Atkinson-type lid block—local eye anesthesia.

ATL duplex scanner—uses B-mode imaging and pulsed Doppler ultrasound in noninvasive evaluation of the extracranial carotid artery system.

ATL real-time Neurosector scanner —used in ultrasonography. (ATL, Advanced Technology Laboratories.)

ATL (acute tumor lysis) **syndrome**.

ATLS (advanced trauma life support) **examination**.

ATM (acute transverse myelitis).

ATN (acute tubular necrosis).

ATnativ (antithrombin III).

ATNR (asymmetric tonic neck reflex).

ATO (Arsenic TriOxide)—drug used in treatment of multiple myeloma.

atomic force microscopy (AFM)— used by dental researchers to test strength and stiffness of dentin by pushing the atoms and molecules apart to observe how they respond. The goal is to create a tighter, more permanent bond between teeth and plastic-based fillings now used to repair most cavities.

atorvastatin—an HMG-CoA reductase inhibitor with a lipid-lowering effect on triglycerides and other lipoprotein fractions in patients with primary hypertriglyceridemia.

atovaquone (Mepron)—a drug used to treat refractory *Pneumocystis carinii*, especially for AIDS patients who have severe side effects from Bactrim or Septra.

ATRA (all-trans retinoic acid).

atracurium besylate—a skeletal muscle relaxant. "The patient was given 50 mg of thiopental sodium and a total of 12 mg of atracurium besylate, after which she was intubated with a 3.5 mm endotracheal tube."

Atragen—used for treatment of acute promyelocytic leukemia (APL) and Kaposi's sarcoma.

Atraloc needle—double-pointed needle used for blood vessel anastomoses; the double point allows the needle to be passed in either direction without reversing it on the needle holder, thus saving time.

Atrauclip hemostatic clip.

atresia, bilateral congenital aural—see *stereolithography*.

Atrial View Ventak AV implantable cardioverter-defibrillator.

Atridox—a drug delivery system used for treatment of periodontal disease. Said to be faster, less painful, and less costly than scaling and root planing, the Atridox product is applied to the infected periodontal pocket as a fluid, where it molds to the shape of the problem area and quickly solidifies, releasing doxycycline for a period of seven days as it is bioabsorbed.

Atrigel drug delivery system to administer leuprolide acetate over a 120-day period to treat patients with advanced prostate cancer.

atrio-His (pronounced "hiss") **tract or pathway in the heart**, as in *bundle of His*.

atrioventricular nodal reentry tachycardia (AVNRT).

Atrisol aerosol—thin polymeric barrier sprayed over surgical sites to prevent formation of adhesions.

Atrovent (ipratropium bromide)—inhalation solution for relief of bronchospasm in COPD.

Atrioverter—a very small implantable defibrillator device, specifically used to treat patients who do not respond to medical control of atrial fibrillation.

ATT (arginine tolerance test)—a test for growth hormone.

attention-deficit disorder (ADD) (newer name for *minimal brain dysfunction* in children)—a group of developmentally inappropriate symptoms in children, such as moderate to severe distractibility, short attention span, hyperactivity, emotional lability, and impulsivity. Also called *hyperkinetic child syndrome, minimal brain damage, minimal cerebral dysfunction, minor cerebral dysfunction*.

atypical glandular cells of undetermined significance (AGUS).

atypical squamous cells of undetermined significance (ASCUS)—cells in a Pap smear that show cellular atypia (structural abnormalities) but no clear evidence of premalignant change. About 20% of women with ASCUS will eventually develop squamous intraepithelial lesions or invasive carcinoma.

AUA Symptom Index (Urol)—a seven-item patient questionnaire about benign prostatic hypertrophy, developed by the American Urological Association. Each item is rated on a scale of 1 to 5 and then totaled for the AUA Symptom Score.

AUB (abnormal uterine bleeding).

AuBMT (autologous bone marrow transplantation).

Auchincloss modified radical mastectomy.

AudioScope, Welch Allyn—an instrument for screening hearing loss in children; it is combined with an otoscope in a single device.

auditory brain stem response (ABR).

Auer body; rod—found only in myelogenous and monocytic leukemia.

Aufrecht's sign of tracheal stenosis—faint breath sounds heard about the jugular notch.

augmentative communication device (also known as *alternative communication device*)—used by individuals with speech disorders such as cerebral palsy and autism as an alternative or adjunct to verbalizations. This can range from a simple picture board to a computerized system using a wireless connection to a computer.

Augmentin (amoxicillin/clavulanate)—a stronger adult dose to be given every 12 hours for treatment of more severe infections as well as respiratory tract infections.

Augustine guide and **scope**—for oral blind intubation of the trachea of patients presenting with difficult airways.

Aura desktop laser for ENT surgery.

aural—pertaining to the ear, or to the sense of hearing, as aural acuity or aural surgery. Cf. *oral*.

Aura Laser system—used in outpatient surgical and dermatologic procedures.

auramine-rhodamine stain (Path).

auramine-stained buffy coat smear—a rapid diagnostic test for mycobacteremia, with moderate sensitivity and high specificity.

auricular acupuncture—performed on the ear for treatment of various parts and organs of the body. The ear has many acupuncture points that correspond to parts and organs of the body.

auricular perichondritis—occurs as a result of ear piercing so high that it perforates the auricular cartilage, implanting infecting organisms, usually either *Pseudomonas aeruginosa* or *Staphylococcus*, and resulting in complications such as the need for incision and drainage, antibiotic irrigation, placement of drains, necrosis, liquefying chondritis, and cosmetic deformity.

auris dextra (A.D.)—right ear.

auris sinistra (A.S.)—left ear.

Aurora diode-based dental laser system—used for gingival surgery as well as recontouring, dental implant, and the removal of diseased soft tissue.

Aurora MR breast imaging system—a dedicated MRI system to detect lesions in patients with dense breasts for whom x-ray mammography may be unrevealing.

Ausculscope—detects carotid bruits.

Austin Flint murmur of relative mitral stenosis—differs from the murmur of true mitral stenosis by having no audible opening snap.

Austin Moore hip prosthesis—named for Dr. Thomas Austin Moore. (No hyphen.)

Auth atherectomy catheter.

AUTI (asymptomatic urinary tract infection) (pronounced "ah-dee").

**Autima II dual chamber cardiac pacemaker.

autoaugmentation (Urol)—a means of establishing a low-pressure, adequate capacity bladder. A large wide-mouthed mucosal diverticulum is fashioned to augment bladder storage capacity.

AutoCat—automatic intra-aortic balloon pump.

Autoclix—fingerstick device for blood glucose testing.

autoclot—a preformed clot of the patient's blood, reinjected to stop bleeding.

autocrine motility factor (AMF)—a protein secreted by cancerous cells which can be detected in the urine. The test for AMF aids in early detection of bladder cancer.

Autoflex II—continuous passive motion (CPM) unit.

autogenous—a synonym for *autologous*, which is most often used to refer to blood transfusions of the patient's own blood (see *autologous transfusion*). *Autogenous* usually refers to a patient's own bone or bone marrow used for graft material (autograft).

Autolet—a fingerstick device for blood glucose testing.

AuTolo Cure Process—for treatment of chronic nonhealing wounds.

autologous bone marrow transplant (AuBMT).

autologous clot—used for control of hemorrhage. Some of the patient's blood is mixed with epsilon aminocaproic acid, and clot forms. This is then cut in small fragments. Gelatin sponge is then soaked in 50% diatrizoate sodium, and the clot alternated with strips of the gelatin sponge is injected into the bleeding vessels until hemorrhage stops.

autologous fat graft—use of the patient's own fat (to fill a cavity, such as that left by removal of a tumor or cyst).

autologous fibrin glue—used in surgery for acoustic neuromas, with blood for the glue taken at the time of routine blood draw. Used routinely to seal the ear and internal auditory canal in order to reduce the incidence of cerebrospinal fluid leak.

autologous fibrin tissue adhesive (AFTA)—uses a combination of ethanol and freezing to precipitate fibrinogen.

autologous growth factors (AGF)—properties in a patient's own blood that enable the orthopedic surgeon to speed healing and growth process of human bone.

autologous leukapheresis, processing, and storage (ALPS).

autologous transfusion—transfusion of one's own blood or blood components, thereby eliminating risks (e.g., hepatitis and alloimmunization) associated with homologous blood transfusion. Also called *autogenous*.

autolymphocyte-based treatment for renal cell carcinoma (ALT-RCC) — used in the treatment of stage IV metastatic renal cell carcinoma.

automated cardiac flow measurement technology—see *ACM*.

Automated Cellular Imaging System (ACIS)—HER2 protein expression system for the guidance of breast cancer therapy. (About 30% of breast cancer patients have a particularly aggressive cancer identified by the elevated expression of the HER2 protein. This protein is important for normal cell division; however, if

Automated *(cont.)*

patients overexpress this protein, their cancer can spread very rapidly.)

automated external defibrillator (AED)—used to provide a quick response and early defibrillation to victims of sudden cardiac arrest. This device is used by fire departments, corporations, and businesses that train employees in its use.

automated lamellar keratoplasty (Oph).

automated percutaneous lumbar diskectomy (APLD)—technique for treating a herniated lumbar disk. The procedure is performed under local anesthesia, and the herniated disk is extracted through a cannula inserted into the disk by using either pituitary forceps or a Nucleotome aspiration probe. The Nucleotome uses suction to aspirate nucleus pulposus into a side port and then a sleeve is pneumatically pushed across the portal opening, making a clean cut through the disk material.

Automator—a computerized device that attaches to the telescopic rods used in the Ilizarov leg lengthening procedure. Programmed to automatically adjust the hardware four times per day to increase bone distraction. Before this development, the adjustment was done manually by the patient.

AutoPap—automated screening device to analyze Pap smear slides for signs of cervical cancer prior to examination by trained personnel.

AutoPap 300 QC automatic Pap screener—a system used in labs to recheck Pap smear slides initially classified as normal.

Autoplex—Factor VIII inhibitor bypass product (anti-anti Factor VIII) (yes, anti-anti).

autosomal-dominant cerebellar ataxia (ADCA) **type II**. See *ADCA*.

autosomal-dominant retinitis pigmentosa (adRP).

Auto Suture Multifire Endo GIA 30 stapler—for laparoscopic use in appendectomy, bowel resection, blebectomies, and wedge resections.

Auto Suture Premium CEEA stapler —used for circular anastomosis requiring double and triple stapling technique in intestinal procedures.

autotransfusion system—see *Cell Saver Haemolite.*

auxiliary transplant—a procedure in which the donor organ (or part of an organ, such as the liver) is placed alongside the patient's own damaged organ, sharing the same blood supply. Then it's a case of "survival of the fittest," and the stronger of the two organs takes over. The liver is the only organ that can regenerate, so only a portion of a liver can function until it grows to be normal size.

AV (atrioventricular) **bundle in heart** —a term used in electrophysiologic studies of supraventricular tachycardia. See *Kent bundle*.

Avakine—now *Remicade.*

Avandia (rosiglitazone maleate)—an oral medication that increases insulin sensitivity in type 2 diabetic patients. Can be used in combination with metformin.

Avanta metacarpophalangeal and proximal interphalangeal joint soft skeletal implants, made of Silflex II, a silicone elastomer (Hand Surg).

Avapro (irbesartan)—an angiotensin II receptor blocker used to treat hypertension.

AVA 3Xi—advanced venous access device that is flexible enough for routine cardiac care and surgery,

AVA 3Xi *(cont.)*
designed specifically for high-risk cardiovascular, trauma, and organ transplant surgeries.

Avelox (moxifloxacin)—a second-generation quinolone antibiotic.

aversion therapy (Psych)—a type of therapy used to change behavior patterns by associating them with unpleasant stimuli.

avian influenza A (H5N1) **virus**—isolated in human patients in Hong Kong in 1997. Previously known to infect only birds.

Avicidin—an anticancer drug.

Avicine—essentially nontoxic investigational therapeutic cancer vaccine which elicits a highly specific immune response to the human hormone and growth factor hCG, a cancer-associated oncofetal protein. The vaccine blocks hCG's facilitation of tumor growth, angiogenesis, invasion, and immunosuppression.

Avita—a prescription acne cream.

Avitene—microfibrillar collagen hemostatic material; used like Gelfoam; applied topically for hemostasis in localized oozing, in areas inaccessible for suturing, and in procedures involving friable organs or vessels.

Avitene Ultrafoam collagen hemostat—collagen sponge used to obtain hemostasis in surgical procedures.

AVM (arteriovenous malformation).

AVM (atrioventricular malformation).

AVNRT (atrioventricular nodal reentry tachycardia).

AvocetPT—a rapid prothrombin time (PT) meter.

Avonex (interferon beta-1a)—used for the treatment of relapsing-remitting forms of multiple sclerosis.

AvWD (acquired von Willebrand's disease).

Aware AccuMeter rapid HIV test.

Aware breast self-examination pad—consists of two 10-inch polyurethane circles with silicone lubricant sealed between them. Provides increased sensitivity on palpation that may help detect an abnormality.

axial acetabular index (AAI)—hip dysplasia measurement in children with cerebral palsy.

axial images—MRI term.

axial proton-density-weighted image (MRI). Also, *axial T2-weighted image.*

axillofemoral bypass—used only in high risk patients.

axis—a real or imaginary straight line going through a structure, around which it revolves, or would revolve if it could. For example, HPA (hypothalamic-pituitary-adrenal) axis. Cf. *access, excess.*

Axokine—for the treatment of Huntington's disease; it is infused via an implantable pump in the brain.

Axostim nerve stimulator.

AxyaWeld bone anchor system—uses suture material and bone anchors to secure soft tissue structures in surgical procedures, utilizing ultrasonic energy to weld polymeric materials, thereby eliminating knot-tying by the surgeon.

ayw1, ayw2, ayw3, ayw4, ayr—these are hepatitis B surface antigen (HB$_s$Ag) subdeterminants.

azacitidine (5-AZA; 5-AZC).

azalides—a class of antibiotics. The first drug in this group is azithromycin (Zithromax), which is similar to erythromycin.

azathioprine (Imuran)—drug now used to treat juvenile diabetics, although its more common use has been as an antirejection drug after organ trans-

azathioprine *(cont.)*
plant. It appears to suppress the immune system and stop its attack on the beta cells of the pancreas that produce insulin. It is administered in pill form rather than in an injection like insulin.

AzdU (azidouridine)—a drug reported to be much less toxic than AZT to human bone marrow cells in in vitro studies. Used to treat patients who are HIV-positive or have AIDS.

Azelex (azelaic acid)—used in the topical treatment of mild to moderate inflammatory acne vulgaris.

azidothymidine (now zidovudine).

azidouridine (AzdU).

azithromycin (Zithromax)—antibiotic for treating AIDS patients with MAC infection; also for strep pharyngitis, chlamydial infections, urethritis, toxoplasmosis, and cryptosporidiosis.

Azmacort (triamcinolone acetonide) —a drug used to treat asthma. Easy to misspell as it does not follow the spelling of *asthma*.

azodicarbonamide—a drug that inhibits HIV and may also help prevent rejection of transplanted organs.

AZOOR (acute zonal occult outer retinopathy).

AZT (azidothymidine, Retrovir)—now *zidovudine*.

Aztec (zidovudine).

Azulfidine En-Tabs (sulfasalazine delayed-release tablets)—for treatment of rheumatoid arthritis in patients who have responded inadequately to, or are intolerant of, analgesics or other nonsteroidal anti-inflammatory drugs. They are enteric-coated to reduce stomach absorption and minimize gastrointestinal irritation.

azygos lobe, **azygos vein**—unpaired. (*Not* azygous or azygus.)

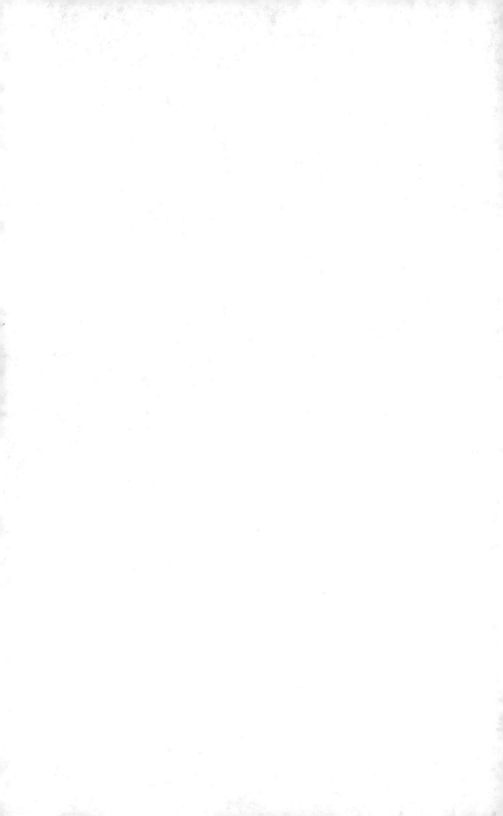

B, b

Baastrupi's syndrome—intervertebral disk collapse after severe lordosis, leading to "kissing spines."

babesiosis—infection with the tickborne parasite *Babesia.*

Babinski sign—upward deviation of the great toe on stroking the sole of the foot, an indication of brain stem injury. A positive Babinski is an extensor plantar response: "The toes are upgoing." A negative Babinski is a flexor plantar response: "The toes are downgoing."

BA (bioactive) **bone cement**—consisting of Bis-GMA resin and bioactive-lasting fixation of implants to bone under weightbearing conditions.

BABYbird respirator (BABY, all caps)—a time-cycled infant ventilator. Also, *Bird respirator.*

BabyFace—3-D surface rendering accessory for diagnostic ultrasound systems that makes it possible for a physician to view a fetus in three full dimensions.

Babytherm IC—a thermostatically controlled gel mattress for warming newborns.

Bachman, anterior internodal tract of—in the heart.

bacillary angiomatosis (BA)—a condition in which nodular tumors made up of densely proliferating blood vessels appear in the skin, bone, brain, spleen, and other tissues. Caused by *Bartonella henselae* and detected by a serum immunofluorescent antibody test.

bacillus—see *pathogen.*

bacillus Calmette-Guérin (BCG)—an attenuated strain of tubercle bacillus, once used as a vaccine and still used in parts of the Third World, so it may turn up in past histories, especially now with drug-resistant TB becoming a problem. Variations include cell-free fractions, Glaxo, Montreal, Pasteur, Phipps, and Tice.

Bacillus circulans—a pathogen causing endophthalmitis, a complication of cataract extraction.

Bacillus coagulans (Lab).

BackBiter—grooved orthopedic instrument which cuts from the rear to allow easier access to the anterior horn of the meniscus.

BackTracker—assesses on-the-job low-back stress in flexion/extension, lateral flexion, and rotation.

backward failure—a phenomenon that occurs when all the blood returned to the heart cannot be pumped out. Venous pressure rises and the lungs and viscera congest.

Bacon-Babcock—operation for correction of rectovaginal fistula.

BacT/Alert—an automated blood culture system.

BACTEC—an automated blood culture system.

bacteria—see *pathogen.*

bacterial endophthalmitis—a serious postoperative complication of intraocular or cataract surgery.

bactericidal—see *cidal.*

Bacteroides corrodens—a genus of anaerobic gram-negative rods, found normally in the oropharynx. Has been isolated from infected tonsils, in pharyngitis, pneumonia, and postoperative wound infections. Also called *Eikenella corrodens.*

Bactrim (sulfamethoxazole and trimethoprim; Septra)—a combination antibiotic which is one of the drugs of choice for treating *Pneumocystis carinii* pneumonia in AIDS patients. Physicians may dictate either Bactrim or Septra or the generic abbreviations, *TMP-SMZ* or *SMZ-TMP.*

Bactroban Cream (mupirocin calcium 2%)—topical antibiotic for treatment of impetigo and secondary infection of traumatic skin lesions.

baculovirus—an insect virus which is being used in research to develop an AIDS vaccine. See *AIDS vaccine.*

Baculovirus Expression Vector System (BEVS)—a process in which genetically engineered baculoviruses are injected into bioreactors containing proprietary insect cells. The engineered baculoviruses infect the cells and "program" them to manufacture a desired protein. After being supplied with nutrients and oxygen, the cells are harvested and the protein extracted.

BAEP (brain stem auditory evoked potential).

BAER (brain stem auditory evoked response) (pronounced "bear").

Baerveldt glaucoma implant—implantable intraocular device for treatment of glaucoma.

Baffe's anastomosis—between the inferior vena cava and the left atrium.

bagassosis—extrinsic allergic alveolitis caused by exposure to moldy sugar cane.

BagEasy—disposable manual respirator.

BAGF (brachioaxillary bridge graft fistula).

bagged—ventilated by hand using an Ambu bag, as "The patient was being bagged via endotracheal tube in the emergency room."

Baggish hysteroscope—an operative sheath used in both Nd:YAG laser and conventional surgery in the uterine cavity as well as aspiration from the uterine cavity. Also, *Baggish contact panoramic hysteroscope.*

Bagolini lens—used in testing and assessing retinal correspondence in eye deviations.

bagpipe sign—a continuous wheeze at the end of expiration.

Baim-Turi cardiac device.

Bair Hugger—a plastic warming body cover.

Bakanjian flap (ENT)—a deltopectoral flap turned in a radical neck dissection.

Bakelite—strong, lightweight material used to make cystoscopy sheaths.

Bakes dilator (no apostrophe)—a common duct dilator.

BAK interbody fusion system—a system of spinal implants, surgical instruments, and procedures that aid minimally invasive surgical placement of implants between the vertebrae to stabilize the spine and facilitate fusion. Also, *BAK/C* (cervical) and *BAK/T* (thoracic).

BAK surgical procedure—uses the BAK interbody fusion system to stabilize and fuse spinal vertebrae in patients with chronic back pain as a result of degenerative disk disease.

BAL (bronchoalveolar lavage).

Baladi Inverter—a medical device that provides better access to the aorta in cardiac procedures than other clamps. The Inverter preserves the cylindrical shape of the aorta in beating- and still-heart procedures and thus provides less traumatic access than with a side-biting clamp.

balanced electrolyte solution (BES).

balanced salt solution (BSS) (Oph).

BalAsa (balsalazide disodium)—anti-inflammatory drug for oral administration. Used for treatment of acute ulcerative colitis in adults.

bald gastric fundus (Radiol)—absence of rugal folds when the gastric fundus is distended by gas or by the presence of barium from an (immediately previous) upper GI study.

Baldy-Webster operation—for correction of uterine retrodisplacement.

Balke protocol—for cardiac exercise stress testing.

Ballard gestational assessment (Ob-Gyn).

Baller-Gerold syndrome—craniosynostosis.

ballism—intense and violent flailing movements. Also, *ballismus, hemiballism, hemiballismus.*

balloon catheterization—used to stop bleeding following childbirth in order to avoid emergency hysterectomy postpartum. An interventional radiologist performs the dual procedure of embolization of the bleeding blood vessel and balloon catheterization to stop bleeding.

balloon dissector—used as an alternative to blunt dissection. The dissector is inserted with the balloon uninflated through a small incision and between the tissue layers. The balloon is then filled with air or saline to cause the desired dissection of the tissue planes.

Balloon-on-a-Wire—cardiac device.

balloon tuboplasty—opens blocked fallopian tubes without surgery. Technique is similar to that used in the Grüntzig balloon catheter angioplasty. In the tuboplasty, a guide wire is passed up through the uterus and eased through the fallopian tube to the point of blockage, which is then perforated. The balloon catheter is inserted and inflated to further enlarge the opening.

Ball operation—for treatment of pruritus ani.

ball therapy—see *Swiss ball therapy.*

Baltic myoclonus—the benign form of Unverricht-Lundborg syndrome, a progressive myoclonus epilepsy associated with progressive dementia. See *Unverricht-Lundborg syndrome.*

banana blade—a Beaver blade used in arthroscopic surgery.

banana sign—shape of the fetal cerebellum secondary to small size of the posterior fossa, seen in spina bifida.

bandage—see also *dressing*.
Ace
butterfly
Champ elastic
Comperm tubular elastic
E Cotton
Elastic Foam
Elastomull
Esmarch
Flexilite conforming elastic
Fractura Flex
Hydron Burn Bandage
Kerlix
Liquiderm liquid healing
POP (plaster of Paris)
Profore four-layer
spica
Tricodur Epi (elbow) compression support
Tricodur Omos (shoulder) compression support
Tricodur Talus (ankle) compression support
Velpeau

bandeau (Plas Surg)—a narrow band or fillet; bandlike. A type of defect.

band-ligator device—used to obtain large particle biopsies in the GI tract. It was originally designed for esophageal variceal ligation.

bands—immature neutrophils. More than 10% band cells indicates inflammation or infection.

band-snare technique (GI)—provides a large sample of mucosa and submucosa and can be used for either large particle biopsy or for endoscopic mucosal resection.

Bang's horseshoe-crab blood test—see *LAL test*.

banjo-string adhesion.

Bankart procedure—operation on the shoulder girdle to treat recurrent shoulder dislocation.

BAR (biofragmentable anastomotic ring). Example: *Valtrac BAR*.

Bárány's symptom (ENT)—see *caloric testing*.

barbotage ("bar-bow-tahzh")—alternate injection and withdrawal of fluid.

Barcat technique, modified—treats distal hypospadias utilizing apposing, fully mobilized, meatal-based skin flaps.

Bardach's modification (Plas Surg)—Obwegeser's mandibular osteotomy.

Bard biopty gun—see *Biopty gun*.

Bard BTA test—used for the detection of recurrent bladder cancer. Cf. *BTA stat test*.

Bard cardiopulmonary support system—a portable heart-lung machine that does not require opening the patient's chest. The patient's blood is shunted to an external machine via a narrow catheter inserted into the femoral vein up to the heart. The blood is oxygenated, warmed, and pumped back into the body via a second catheter threaded through the femoral artery.

Bard Clamshell Septal Umbrella—a device for closure of atrial and ventricular septal defects, similar to the Bard PDA Umbrella.

Bard Composix mesh graft material.

Bard endoscopic suturing system—used in treatment of gastroesophageal reflux disease.

Bardenheuer's bifurcation procedure, modified—a procedure for correction of radial ray defect, or club hand. See *pouce flottant*.

Bard Memotherm—colorectal stent used for treatment of malignant obstructions arising from colon cancer.

Bard PDA (patent ductus arteriosus) **Umbrella**—device used to close patent ductus arteriosus defects in infants. The device is inserted via a catheter, positioning a balloon on each side of the orifice. When the balloons are expanded, slight pulling causes the arms or ribs of the umbrella to expand further and come flush to the orifice. Slight pushing then causes the arms of the other balloon to expand and come flush on the opposite side of the orifice, thus closing the patent ductus.

Bard's sign—on cardiac palpation, a prominent and broad thrust sustained throughout ventricular systole in left ventricular hypertrophy.

Bard Sperma-Tex preshaped mesh.

Bard TransAct intra-aortic balloon pump—a device to assist the heart before and after open heart surgery and complex balloon angioplasty procedures.

Bard Visilex mesh—graft material for laparoscopic hernia repair.

Bard XT coronary stent—a one-piece Y-shaped stent implanted in a patient. It is described as a modular zigzag design or a true bifurcated stent with a dedicated "trouser" balloon delivery system.

bare lymphocyte syndrome—a condition in which the lymphocytes do not express MHC class I and/or II antigens on their surface, resulting in severe combined immunodeficiency disease.

barium artifact (Radiol)—overlooked dried barium on table tops, intensifying screens, or on patient gowns appearing to be within the patient and misleading the radiologist.

Barlow test—for dysplasia of the hip.

barotrauma—tissue injury caused by abnormally high or low atmospheric pressure, e.g., in flying, scuba diving; also, from high respirator pressures.

Barouk button space—used with conventional Keller arthroplasty technique for reconstruction of hallux valgus deformities.

Barouk microscrew—used with a shortening osteotomy for correction of hallux valgus.

Barouk microstaple—used with a closing wedge osteotomy for solid fixation using only a single implant.

Barraquer forceps and scissors—used in ophthalmology procedures.

Barr body—see *buccal smear.*

barrel-stave osteotomy (Ortho).

Barrett's esophagus (BE)—one or more zones of metaplasia (cell transformation) in the distal esophagus, by which the normal squamous epithelium is replaced by columnar epithelium resembling that of the gastric mucosa. This change occurs chiefly in persons with hiatal hernia or gastroesophageal reflux disease, in whom the distal esophagus is repeatedly exposed to acid gastric juice. The condition is associated with an increased risk of esophageal carcinoma. Various procedures may reduce the risk of malignant change. After an IV injection of a photosensitizing agent, which concentrates in zones of abnormal tissue, argon dye laser treatment of the lower esophagus selectively destroys sensitized metaplastic cells.

Barron disposable trephine (Oph).

Barron donor corneal punch—steel blade with vacuum base to immobilize the cornea for cutting the button for transplantation.

Barron pump—four-speed pump used to control delivery of chemotherapeutic agents through an arterial line.

Barron radial vacuum trephine—corneal trephine made of solid steel.

Bartonella bacilliformis—a bacterial pathogen causing Carrión's disease, a tropical infection.

Bartonella elizabethae—a bacterial pathogen isolated from a patient with endocarditis involving an artificial aortic valve.

Bartonella henselae—a bacterial pathogen causing bacillary angiomatosis and associated with cat-scratch disease. *B. henselae* is transmitted among cats by the cat flea and from cats to humans by means of a cat scratch.

Bartonella quintana—bacterial pathogen causing bacillary angiomatosis-peliosis. It was formerly called *Rochalimaea quintana* or *Rickettsia quintana* and was the cause of trench fever in World War I. *B. quintana* infection is transmitted by the human body louse.

Bartter's syndrome—hypokalemic alkalosis, hyperaldosteronism secondary to adrenal cortical hyperplasia, hypertrophy and hyperplasia of the juxtaglomerular apparatus of the kidneys, and normal blood pressures associated with subnormal reactivity of blood pressures to angiotensin II.

basal ganglia—gray masses in the cerebrum involved in motor coordination.

baseball stitch—"A baseball stitch of 00 chromic was used to complete the uterine repair."

base excess—one of the measurements on a blood gas study related to bicarbonate. "The arterial blood gases showed pH 7.35, PO_2 110, PCO_2 40 with a base excess of -3 and saturation of 95%."

bas-fond ("bah-fawn")—bladder fundus.

basic fibroblast growth factor (bFGF)—one of several compounds the body uses to stimulate growth of blood vessels.

basidiobolomycosis—fungal disease caused by *Basidiobolus ranarum*, most often found in tropical regions of Africa. The fungus, usually limited to the skin, has also been found to invade the gastrointestinal and urinary tracts of some patients, producing nonspecific peptic ulcer-like symptoms such as fever, nausea, vomiting, anorexia, weight loss, and gastrointestinal bleeding.

Basidiomycetes—class of smut and rust fungi causing problems in allergic individuals who work around wheat and granaries.

basis pontis—the ventral portion of the pons; part of the brain stem.

Bassen-Kornzweig abetalipoproteinemia.

Batchelor technique—a modified procedure to correct hindfoot valgus deformity, achieving immediate stability.

Bateman UPF II bipolar endoprosthesis (Universal proximal femur)—hip replacement system made by Kirschner.

Batista procedure (left ventriculectomy)—radical surgical procedure for treatment of end-stage heart failure by removing a piece of the left ventricle, surgically reducing the size of the chamber, ultimately allowing the heart to beat more effi-

Batista *(cont.)*
ciently, as a possible alternative to heart transplantation.

Baton laser pointer—device used in minimally invasive surgery, allowing a surgeon to point out anatomical details on a video screen without having to physically point or use verbal descriptions. It is mounted on a lightweight headset and is activated by a small mouthpiece switch.

Batten disease—a form of cerebral macular degeneration.

batten graft—see *spreader graft*.

Battey-avium complex—see *MAC infection*.

Battle's sign—discoloration (ecchymosis) over the mastoid process, a sign of basilar skull fracture.

Bauhin, valve of—ileocecal valve.

Baumann, angle of.

Baycol (cerivastatin sodium)—cholesterol-lowering HMG-CoA reductase inhibitor for treatment of patients with primary hypercholesterolemia and mixed dyslipidemia who have not responded to dietary control.

Bayley Scales of Infant Development—from manual by Nancy Bayley.

Baylor bleeding score—identifies patients at increased risk for rebleeding following endoscopy.

bayonet bipolar forceps.

bayonet-type incision—a rectilinear incision with a jog near the middle, giving it a configuration like that of a rifle with a bayonet attached.

Bayou virus—a hantavirus pulmonary syndrome identified in the blood of patients from Louisiana and eastern Texas. The carrier is believed to be the rice rat (*Oryzomys palustris*).

Baypress (nitrendipine).

Bazex syndrome—palmoplantar keratoderma with features similar to psoriasis on the hands, associated with carcinoma of the upper respiratory tract; this is a cutaneous marker to an internal malignancy.

BB shot—small, 0.46 cm in diameter round pellet used in air rifles or BB guns. "There was a small BB-sized cystic lesion on the lateral thigh."

BBVP-M (BCNU, bleomycin, VePesid, prednisone, methotrexate)—protocol for advanced non-Hodgkin's lymphoma resistant to CHOP chemotherapy protocol.

B-cell (also called *B-lymphocyte*)—part of the immune system; some mature B-cells become plasma cells, which secrete antibodies, but not without help from T-cells, one variety of which is attacked by the AIDS virus. See *T-4 cell, helper cell*.

Bcl-2—see *BRCA*.

BCT (breast-conserving therapy).

BCX-34—used to treat cutaneous T-cell lymphoma.

BDD (body dysmorphic disorder)—obsession and distress with physical appearance.

Bdellovibrio ("del´-o-vib´-re-o")—a genus of parasitic gram-negative organisms that live on certain other gram-negative bacteria.

BDNF (brain-derived neurotrophic factor)—used to treat ALS (amyotrophic lateral sclerosis).

BDProbeTec ET system—for direct qualitative detection of *Chlamydia trachomatis* and *Neisseria gonorrhoeae*.

B–D (Becton-Dickinson) **spinal needle**.

BE (Barrett's esophagus).

BEAC (BCNU, etoposide, ara-C, Cytoxan)—chemotherapy protocol for advanced non-Hodgkin's lymphoma.

Beacon minimally invasive incontinence surgical line from UroMed.

beads of methylmethacrylate—see *methylmethacrylate, beads of.*

BEAM (brain electrical activity map, or mapping)—a computerized EEG that maps different areas of the brain.

Beamer injection stent system—a Percuflex stent that provides for contrast injection during ureteral stent placement. Can convert to drainage stent.

beam-hardening artifact (on CT scans)—streaks seen when the beam passes through tissues of vastly different densities (e.g., in petrous bone next to the brain, the parenchyma will be streaked).

beam splitter—used with an operating microscope to permit use of attachments that will enable a second person to look through the microscope with the surgeon; makes it possible to take photographs and videotape what is seen through the microscope.

beaten silver appearance—increase in convolutional markings on x-rays of the skull.

Beau's line—a transverse groove in the nail seen in fingernails. Can result from severe emotional or physical shock. Cf. *Mees' line.*

beat-knee syndrome—alternative term for prepatellar bursitis, carpet layer's knee, coal miner's knee, housemaid's knee.

Beaver blade—see also *blade.*
arachnoid shape
banana
cataract knife
discission knife
keratome
retrograde
rosette
sickle-shape

Beaver DeBakey blades—for hip surgery.

beaver fever—the hikers' and canoeists' "affectionate" term for giardiasis.

BEB (blind esophageal brushing).

becaplermin (Regranex).

Bechert lens-holding forceps.

Beck Depression Inventory (Psych).

Becker accelerator cannula—a liposuction cannula.

Becker tissue expander/breast prosthesis—an inflatable tissue expander used to reconstruct the breast following mastectomy. Also serves as a permanent breast implant. Only the access port and tubing have to be removed in a brief outpatient procedure under local anesthesia with intravenous sedation.

Beckwith-Wiedemann syndrome—a congenital syndrome characterized by the presence of macroglossia, omphalocele, gigantism, and sometimes other associated anomalies.

becquerel (Bq)—the unit of measurement in the International System of Measurement (SI) that is the absorbed dose equivalent in radioactivity. See *International System.*

bedewing of cornea ("bee-doing")—swelling and superficial clouding of the cornea, caused by increased intraocular pressure for an extended period of time. The surface of the cornea becomes "grainy" in appearance, thus interfering with the transmission of light rays. May also be referred to as *Sattler veil.*

Bedge antireflux mattress—egg-crate foam wedge used to elevate the upper body to prevent gastroesophageal reflux.

beef-lung heparin—used in heparinized saline solution to dilate the vein and determine its patency in forming an arteriovenous fistula for a long-term access route for hemodialysis, and at the end of the procedure to check the patency of the radial artery-to-cephalic vein anastomosis.

behavioral mapping (Rehab).

Behavioral Pathology in Alzheimer's Disease Rating Scale—rates behavioral symptoms in seven categories: delusional ideation, hallucinations, activity disturbance, sleep disturbance, depressive symptoms, anxiety, and aggressive behavior.

Behçet's ("bay-shets") **syndrome**—severe uveitis and retinal vasculitis, optic atrophy.

Bellini's duct carcinoma—a rare variant of renal cell carcinoma.

Bell's phenomenon—the eye rolls upward and outward on attempting to close the eye.

Bellucci scissors (ENT).

belly of muscle—the center of the muscle where its area of greatest mass lies. The site where an intramuscular injection may be given in certain large muscles in the arms, legs, and buttocks.

Belos compression pin.

Belzer's solution—a solution that preserves organs until transplantation. Contains lactobionate and raffinose (to prevent cellular swelling) and some other ingredients (gluthathione and allopurinol) that prevent oxidative damage, and still other ingredients that will help to restore adenosine triphosphate levels to normal after re-perfusion.

BEMA (Bioerodible Mucoadhesive)—pre-formed film designed for both systemic and local drug delivery across oral mucosal membranes.

BEMP (bleomycin, Eldisine, mitomycin, Platinol)—chemotherapy protocol for squamous cell carcinoma of the uterine cervix.

benazepril (Lotensin)—ACE inhibitor used to treat hypertension.

bench method—refers to manual performance of a laboratory test (at a workbench, hence the name) rather than automated machinery. "Calcium determinations were 10.3 and 9.7 on the SMA, and 9.7 by bench method."

Bender Gestalt test (Neuro)—mental status examination.

Benecol margarine—contains a plant-derived substance (stanol esters), shown to help lower cholesterol. It is sold as a nonprescription food product.

Benedikt's ipsilateral oculomotor paralysis (Neuro).

BeneFix—hemophilia B blood clotting factor.

BeneJoint—a topical cream for temporary relief of arthritis pain.

Benelli mastopexy (also, pursestring mastopexy; modified Benelli round block mastopexy)—a procedure used for true ptosis of breasts or tubular breast deformity.

benign—normal, not showing evidence of disease or abnormality; a benign tumor is one that is not malignant.

benign intracranial hypertension (BIH).

benign necrotizing otitis externa (BNOE).

benign paroxysmal positional vertigo (BPPV)—a common form of vertigo that is precipitated by certain specific movements, such as bending over, looking upward, or even rolling over in bed.

benign prostatic hypertrophy or **hyperplasia** (BPH)—treated by a variety of surgical procedures and medications which are increasingly replacing the traditional treatment, TURP (transurethral resection of the prostate). Surgical procedures include laser resection, microwave thermotherapy, intraurethral coils and springs, balloon dilatation, cryotherapy, and focused extracorporeal ultrasound. Medical treatments include 5-alpha reductase inhibitors, alpha-adrenergic blockade, and antiandrogens.

Benjamin binocular slimline laryngoscope (ENT).

Benjamin-Havas fiberoptic light clip —used as light source in laryngoscopes.

Benjamin pediatric laryngoscope.

Benjamin proverbs (Psych).

Bennett bone retractor.

Bennett's fracture—alternative name for carpometacarpal thumb ray fracture, thumb fracture-dislocation, stave of thumb.

Bennett PR-2 ventilator—a time-cycled ventilator, used mainly in treating children.

Bennett's quadriceps plastic procedure—for traction contractures of the knee.

Bennett self-retaining retractor blade.

Bentley Duraflo II—extracorporeal perfusion circuit with universal biocompatibility protection to prevent blood reactions.

bent malleable retractor.

bentonite flocculation test—to diagnose trichinosis.

Bentson guide wire (Radiol).

benzalkonium chloride patch test— for allergies.

benzodiazepines—a class of drugs that includes antianxiety agents and sedatives.

BEP (bleomycin, etoposide, Platinol)— a standard chemotherapy protocol used to treat testicular carcinoma, ovarian carcinoma, and chronic myelogenous leukemia.

bepridil (Vascor)—a calcium channel blocker that relaxes the smooth muscle of the coronary arteries and relieves angina. Because it can cause arrhythmia and blood disorders, it is reserved for use in patients who have not responded to other antianginal medications.

BER (benign early repolarization).

beractant (Survanta).

Berens 3-character test—eye test used in small children who do not know the letters of the alphabet.

Berger's disease—appears to be a variant of Henoch-Schönlein nephritis, but without the rash. Cf. *Buerger's disease.*

Berkeley-Bonney retractor—a self-retaining three-blade abdominal retractor. See *Goligher modification.*

Berkeley optic zone marker (Oph).

Berkow formula—a method of assessing the percentage of body surface that has been burned. This is an adaptation of the Rule of Nines, but makes allowance for the age of the patient. In a one-year-old child, for example, the head is larger in proportion to body size; therefore, the head is rated at 19, while the head of an adult would be rated at 7. See *Rule of Nines.*

Berkson-Gage calculation—for determining breast cancer survival rates.

Berman locator—a magnetic device used in locating intraocular foreign bodies.

Berotec (fenoterol)—drug used to prevent bronchial asthma attacks.

berry aneurysm—abnormal berry-like dilatation of an artery.

Bertel's position—used to visualize the floor of the orbits and the orbital fissures on x-rays.

Berwick's dye (Gyn).

BES (balanced electrolyte solution).

besipirdine hydrochloride—investigational drug for treatment of mild or moderate Alzheimer's disease. It is reported to have improved memory and enhanced cognitive functioning in Alzheimer's patients.

Bessey-Lowry units—measure alkaline phosphatase. See also *Bodansky unit, King-Armstrong unit.*

Best right-angle colon clamp.

BeStent—a balloon-expandable stent for use in arteries measuring 2.5 mm to 5.5 mm in diameter.

BeStent2—Medtronic laser-cut stent for use after coronary arteries have been opened with balloon catheters in PTCA.

best spectacle-corrected visual acuity (BSCVA)—a term ophthalmologists use in referring to vision correction.

beta antagonist—see *antagonist*. Also known as *beta blocker.*

Beta-Cath system—an intracoronary catheter for use with beta irradiation, to prevent recurrence of stenosis after vascularization procedure.

beta-endorphin—an opiate-like peptide that acts on the central nervous system; it is of anterior pituitary origin. See *endorphins.*

beta interferon—see *interferon beta, Betaseron.*

BetaKine (TGF-beta-2)—used for treatment of ophthalmic diseases, cancer-related disorders, multiple sclerosis, and dermal wounds. (TGF stands for transforming growth factor.)

beta-lactamase—an enzyme produced by certain bacteria which is able to split the beta-lactam chemical ring structure of penicillins and cephalosporins. Beta-lactamase-positive bacteria are resistant to the antibiotic effect of penicillins and cephalosporins.

betamethasone mousse—used topically for treatment of scalp psoriasis and other scalp dermatoses.

Betapace (sotalol).

Betaseron (interferon beta-1b, recombinant human)—drug approved to treat the symptoms of multiple sclerosis. It alters cell response to surface antigens and enhances immune cell production. While not a cure, it helps relieve the debilitating symptoms. Also used to treat CMV retinitis in AIDS patients.

Betaseron needle-free delivery system —for use by multiple sclerosis patients to self-administer Betaseron (interferon beta-lb) for subcutaneous injection. It uses a burst of carbon dioxide to propel a stream of medication through the skin.

Betaxon (levobetaxolol HCl ophthalmic suspension 0.5%) **eye drops**—used for lowering intraocular pressure in patients with chronic open-angle glaucoma or ocular hypertension.

bethanidine—used to treat ventricular fibrillation.

Bethesda rating scale—assigns a category for Pap smears in which the cells have abnormal features that quantitatively or qualitatively fall short of dysplasia, termed ASCUS (atypical squamous cells of uncertain significance).

Betoptic S (betaxolol HCl)—used to lower intraocular pressure in glaucoma patients.

Betz cells—large pyramidal cells forming layer of the gray matter of the brain. Vladimir Betz, Russian anatomist.

Bevan incision—vertical elliptical skin incision in the abdomen.

BEVS (Baculovirus Expression Vector System).

Bexxar (iodine ^{131}I tositumomab)—combines monoclonal antibody technology with the power of radiation to treat cancer in non-Hodgkin lymphoma patients who are refractory to chemotherapy.

bFGF (basic fibroblast growth factor).

BFNC (benign familial neonatal convulsions).

BFU-E (burst-forming unit—erythroid).

bG (blood glucose).

BHT (breath hydrogen test).

Biad SPECT imaging system.

Biafine RE (radiodermatitis emulsion)—used for protection against skin reactions induced by radiation therapy.

Biafine WDE (wound dressing emulsion)—used to manage dermal wounds, ulcers, and burns.

Biaxin (clarithromycin).

bibasally—at the bases of both lungs (on chest x-ray).

Bible printer's lung—extrinsic allergic alveolitis caused by exposure to moldy paper.

bicalutamide (Casodex)—an oral medication used to treat advanced cancer of the prostate. It is used in conjunction with a luteinizing-hormone-releasing hormone analog, e.g., goserelin (Zoladex) or leuprolide (Lupron), reducing the body's production of testosterone. (Testosterone activates growth of the cancer cells.)

Bicarbolyte—a bacteriostatic solution, premixed liquid bicarbonate dialysate. Used for hemodialysis.

biceps jerk (BJ) (Neuro).

Bielschowsky's head tilt—a test of oblique ocular muscle paralysis.

biennial—occurring every two years. Not to be confused with "biannual" (occurring twice a year).

Bier ("beer") **block anesthesia**—used in surgery of the extremities.

Bierman needle—used for bone marrow biopsy and aspiration.

BIFC (benign infantile familial convulsions).

biferious pulse (or bisferious)—see *bisferious pulse* (pulsus bisferiens, or biferiens).

bifidity—used to describe an iatrogenic deformity following rhinoplasty in which a retrograde cartilage-splitting or intracartilaginous incision was inappropriately performed in a patient with thick cartilages, resulting in a wide interdomal distance.

bifoil balloon catheter—see *percutaneous transvenous mitral commisurotomy*.

BIH (benign intracranial hypertension).

Bihrle dorsal clamp and T-C needle holder—for fixation and suturing of the dorsal vein complex in urologic surgery.

BiLAP—bipolar cautery unit with cutting and coagulation functions.

bilateral juxtafoveal telangiectasis (BJT)—characterized by leaking parafoveal retinal capillaries resulting in retinal edema. It affects middle-aged and elderly patients and is treated with laser photocoagulation for macular edema.

bilateral PC-IOL (posterior chamber intraocular lens) **implantation**—used to correct pediatric aphakia.

bilateral ureteral obstruction (BUO).

bi-level positive airway pressure (BiPAP).

bilharziasis—another name for schistosomiasis. Infection with flukes of the genus *Schistosoma*.

biliary decompression (internal biliary drainage)—promotes Kupffer cell recovery in obstructive jaundice.

biliary reconstruction—a procedure using side-to-side anastomosis choledochocholedochostomy in liver transplant patients.

Bilibed—phototherapy system in which the infant, placed inside a special garment on a plastic film support, lies over the light source. The baby is exposed to light via a special section in the rear of the garment, eliminating the need for eye shielding.

Biliblanket Phototherapy System—an alternative to phototherapy light used to treat jaundice in newborn babies. This device consists of a small jacket that gives off high-intensity fiberoptic light.

BiliBottoms—light-permeable disposable phototherapy diaper for newborns with jaundice.

BiliCheck—handheld battery-powered system that measures bilirubin levels without needing a blood sample.

bili lights—slang for the fluorescent lights (bilirubin lights) used as phototherapy for infants with hyperbilirubinemia.

Bili mask—an eye shield used on infants undergoing phototherapy for bilirubinemia.

bilirubinometer—see *Colormate TLc BiliTest System*.

Billroth gastroenterostomy. Billroth I is a partial resection of the stomach (65-75%), and anastomosis of the end of the stomach to the duodenum. (The stomach is first tapered to the size, or caliber, of the duodenum.) The Billroth II is used for duodenal ulcer; a gastrojejunostomy is performed, bringing the jejunal loop up to the remnant of the stomach posteriorly through a hole in the transverse mesocolon, or anterior to the transverse colon. The antecolic anastomosis is used more frequently because it is a simpler procedure.

biloma—encapsulated collection of bile due to biliary tract injury.

Bing auditory acuity test. A vibrating tuning fork is placed at the mastoid process and the acoustic meatus is closed off and opened. If the patient hears a decrease and increase in sound (a positive Bing), hearing is normal or the hearing loss is sensorineural. If the patient does not notice any difference in sound (a negative Bing), there is a deficit in conductive hearing.

binge, bingeing—overindulging in excessive amounts of food (as in bulimia) or alcohol.

binocular infrared oculographic (BIRO) **system**—allows binocular recordings with simultaneous measurements of horizontal and vertical eye movements.

bioabsorbable closure device—bovine collagen plug and anchor used after angioplasty to stop bleeding.

bioactive (BA) **bone cement**.

Biobrane adhesive—a biosynthetic skin substitute. The adhesive is used to protect clean superficial abrasions and burns. It maintains a clean

Biobrane *(cont.)*
   wound until healing takes place, or is removed when autografting is necessary and possible. See *Biobrane glove, Biobrane/HF.*

Biobrane glove—a glove-like wrapping made of a biosynthetic skin substitute. It is used to protect clean excised burn wounds of the hand until healing occurs, or is removed when autografting is possible.

Biobrane/HF—experimental skin substitute made from human neonatal fibroblasts cultured in a mesh of Biobrane, which is a dressing made of a thin layer of silicone bonded to nylon mesh. Researchers believe this graft could replace cadaveric allograft skin for temporary wound closure after burn wound excision.

BioBypass—gene-based angiogenic therapy designed to stimulate new blood vessel formation in the heart and other tissues affected by inadequate blood flow.

biocavity laser—a semiconductor laser scalpel with a blood analysis system built into the handle to give a surgeon immediate feedback on whether cells being removed are cancerous.

Biocell RTV implant—saline-filled breast implant used as an alternative to, or replacement of, gel-filled or silicone implants.

Bioceram two-stage series II, or **type S** —endosteal dental implants.

Bio-Chromatic hand prosthesis.

Bioclot protein S assay—a test for the anticoagulant protein S, which is considered an important naturally occurring anticoagulant in human blood. Measuring deficiency in protein S can identify patients at risk for clotting disorders such as deep venous thrombosis and pulmonary embolism.

Bioclusive transparent dressing—a clear, waterproof sterile dressing that protects the wound, permits continuous wound monitoring, is vapor permeable (thus preventing skin maceration), and prevents dehydration of the wound.

Biocoral (Neuro)—processed madreporic coral. See *madreporic coral.*

Biocor porcine stented aortic and mitral valves and stentless porcine aortic valve.

Biocor 200—a high performance oxygenator device that replaces the function of the lungs during open-heart surgery.

Biodel—a biodegradable polymer formed into wafers or beads impregnated with a chemotherapy drug or antibiotic. Used to treat osteomyelitis and malignant gliomas. See *Gliadel, Septacin.*

Biodex System—for multijoint testing and rehabilitation.

Bioerodible Mucoadhesive (BEMA).

Bio-eye—hydroxyapatite ocular implant that allows motility and fibrovascular ingrowth. It can be coupled directly to an artificial eye.

biofeedback therapy—used in occupational therapy: *electromyographic feedback*—used to increase or decrease muscle function; *goniometric biofeedback*—used to study range of motion; and *thermal biofeedback*—used to treat vascular problems like Raynaud's syndrome and reflex sympathetic dystrophy.

Biofilter hemoconcentrator—used in open heart surgery to prevent fluid overload.

BioFIT Herbgels—a line of "natural" remedies, nutrients, and food products.

Biofix system—bioabsorbable fixation rod made of Dexon sutures by Acufex.

biofragmentable anastomotic ring (BAR).

Biofreeze with Ilex—topical analgesic ointment, may be used to enhance benefits of ultrasound, electrical stimulation, and massage therapy.

BioGlue—surgical adhesive used for repair of aortic dissections.

BioHy—high-molecular-weight sodium hyaluronate product for treatment of pain associated with osteoarthritis of the knee.

bio-interference screw (Ortho).

Biojector 2000—jet injection systems for needle-free drug delivery.

Biolex wound cleanser.

Biologically Quiet Screw—trade name for a screw used in anterior cruciate ligament reconstruction. The biodegradable screw does not have to be removed. About six weeks postoperatively it begins to metabolize, and by six months the space that had been occupied by the screw has been replaced by new cancellous bone marrow.

Biologically Quiet suture anchor—a mini-screw implant for soft tissue repair in the shoulder.

BioLogic-DT system—a blood detoxification system used for treating acute hepatic coma.

BioLogic-HT system—used for whole-body extracorporeal hyperthermia treatment for AIDS patients.

Biolox ball head—ceramic head for total hip replacement and hemiarthroplasty.

Biomatrix ocular implant—an implant made of hydroxyapatite and used in patients who have had enucleation or evisceration of an eye. About six to eight weeks after surgery, the blood vessels and tissues have grown into the implant, and the artificial eye is then attached to the implant. This lets the artificial eye move naturally with the other eye, for very good cosmetic effect. See *enucleation, evisceration, hydroxyapatite.*

BioMend—type 1 collagen membrane made from bovine Achilles tendon and utilized in dental implants.

biomicroscope—a microscope used to visualize living tissue in the body. Used synonymously with slit lamp in ophthalmology. It permits study of the structures of the eye, with the intense beam of light permitting visualization through the tissues of these structures. See *slit-lamp biomicroscopy.*

Bionicare 1000—a stimulator system used to reduce pain and symptoms of osteoarthritis of the knee.

Bionx SmartNail bioresorbable implant—used to maintain fixation and accurate alignment of small bone fractures, osteochondral fragments, or osteochondritis dissecans lesions.

BIO-OSS (all caps)—a bone filler used in oral and maxillofacial surgery. This is a bovine-derived natural bone matrix with all protein removed. Once implanted, it will be invaded by lamellar bone and is osteoconductive, which means it becomes vascularized just as normal bone.

Biopatch—foam wound dressing.

Bioplus dispersive electrode (Cardio).

BioPolyMeric graft for femoropopliteal bypass.

Bioport collection and transport system—a sterile, self-contained device to preserve the viability of aerobic microbial specimens.

biopsy—see *operation*.

Biopty (*not* biopsy) **cut needle**—a needle used in breast biopsy and prostate biopsy.

Biopty (*not* biopsy) **gun**; **Bard Biopty gun**—a device used in needle core breast biopsy and prostate biopsy.

BioRCI screw—orthopedic screw used for fixation of bone-tendon-bone or soft-tissue grafts during anterior cruciate ligament and/or posterior cruciate ligament reconstruction.

bioresorbable implants—experimental implants for repair of facial fractures and osteotomies. Most common polymers used are polyglycolic acid (PGA), polylactic acid (PLA), and levo-PLA.

Biosafe PSA4—can measure prostate-specific antigen on even a small blood sample collected by the patient.

BioScrew bio-absorbable interference screws—used in knee arthroscopy.

BioSorb resorbable urology stent products.

BioStar strep A 01A test—accurate, rapid strep test which can be used to assist in selection of appropriate antibiotic treatment.

Biostent—an agent to prevent restenosis following balloon angioplasty.

BioStinger—low-profile fixation device developed for the performance of BioStinger meniscal fixation surgical technique.

biosurgery—a rapidly growing field in which surgeons use solutions or gels to enhance or replace traditional invasive surgery. Used in areas such as wound care, burn care, cosmetic augmentation, orthopedics, and reduction of tissue adhesions in surgery.

Biosyn suture—synthetic monofilament suture with similar features to a braided suture, without promotion of bacterial growth.

Biot's breathing—an irregular breathing commonly found in meningitis.

Bio-Tense—a relaxation tool that looks much like the sunglasses given to patients following cataract surgery. It combines specific audio frequencies delivered through stereo headphones with continuous flashing *flicker phenomena* to relax patients with hypertension, depression, insomnia, chronic pain, headaches, and arthritis.

Biotrack coagulation monitor—a monitor which, with only one drop of blood, can calculate the APTT value to assess heparin levels while a cardiac catheterization is being performed.

Bio-Tract—proprietary strain of *Lactobacillus salivarius* which inhibits *Helicobacter pylori* bacteria in vitro.

Biotropin—human growth hormone used to treat HIV-positive patients.

BioZ system—a digital noninvasive cardiac function monitoring system used as an alternative to the invasive right heart catheter for monitoring critically ill patients.

BIP (bleomycin, ifosfamide [with mesna rescue], Platinol)—chemotherapy protocol for cervical carcinoma.

BiPAP (bi-level positive airway pressure).

biplane sector probe—used with Bard Biopty gun to perform transrectal prostatic ultrasonographic biopsy.

biphasic helical CT scan—computed tomographic study in which an imaging agent is injected, scans are taken (the arterial phase), and delayed scans (the delayed phase) are additionally performed.

bipolar affective illness (also *manic-depressive*; *bipolar disorder*)—alternating attacks of mania and depression.

bipolar coagulation—electrosurgery using a pair of electrodes. Tissue between them is coagulated by flow of current from one to the other. Also, *bipolar forceps*.

bipolar disorder—see *bipolar affective illness*.

bipolar esophageal recording.

bipolar urological loop—a device used in endoscopic surgical procedures such as resection of prostate tissue and nonmalignant tumors of the bladder wall. It is said to offer the benefit of tissue resection in a saline environment physiologically compatible with the human body.

BIPP (bismuth-iodoform-paraffin paste) —ribbon gauze used to pack the ear canal after surgery.

BI-RADS—Breast Imaging and Reporting Data System of the American College of Radiology. Mammographic findings may be characterized by the term *BI-RAD* followed by an arabic numeral, e.g., BI-RAD 3.
Category 0: Need additional imaging evidence
Category 1: Negative
Category 2: Benign finding
Category 3: Probably benign finding
Category 4: Suspicious abnormality
Category 5: Highly suspicious for malignancy

Birbeck granule—identification of this part of a Langerhans' cell is diagnostic of histiocytosis X. Also called *X-body*.

birdcage splint—descriptive term for a splint used on a digit with a crush injury: "The wound was dressed and a birdcage splint was applied to the index finger."

Bird cup (Ob-Gyn)—attached to a vacuum source to facilitate vacuum-assisted vaginal deliveries. Also, *Bird OP cup*, for posterior presentations.

birdlike facies (Neuro)—refers to a "pinched" facial expression in which eyes are squinting and lips are slightly pursed.

bird's nest filter (BNF)—temporarily placed caval filter to treat a patient for phlegmasia cerulea dolens and limb-threatening ischemia due to sudden complete occlusion of thigh and iliac veins. Suitable and effective for short-term use during caval thrombolysis. See *Gianturco-Roehm bird's nest vena cava filter*.

Bird respirator—see also *BABYbird respirator*.

birdshot chorioretinopathy—autoimmune ophthalmologic disease of unknown cause, diagnosed by positive HLA-A29 titer.

Birkhauser eye testing chart.

birthing ball—a physical therapy ball that can support up to 300 pounds. A woman in labor sits on the ball in a natural, comfortable, squatting-type position, which opens the pelvic outlet, supports pressure points, and helps gravity work with the woman's body to speed labor.

bisferious pulse (or biferious) (pulsus bisferiens, or biferiens)—a pulse

bisferious pulse *(cont.)* with two beats, sometimes palpable in combined aortic stenosis and aortic regurgitation.

Bishop-Koop ileostomy—a procedure to decompress an intestinal graft, such as might be performed during complete intestinal transplantation.

bishop's nod—rhythmic nodding of the head, synchronous with the pulse, in aortic regurgitation. Cf. *de Musset's sign.*

Bishop's score of cervical ripening (Ob-Gyn)—a score for estimating the prospects for induction of labor in a primigravida. A score of less than or equal to 4 would be considered an unfavorable cervix. See *dinoprostone.*

bisoprolol (Zebeta)—a beta blocker, given once a day, to treat hypertension.

BIS (bispectral index) **Sensor**—a one-piece sensor used to acquire the signals necessary to produce the bispectral index. A noninvasive, direct, quantitative measurement of the effects of anesthetics on the brain.

bite line—a horizontal line of whitened, thickened buccal mucosa caused by habitual biting or chewing of the surface.

biventricular pacing—a therapy in which wires are implanted in both of the two lower chambers of the heart so that both sides of the heart are paced at the same time. This therapy is being evaluated for its use in the treatment of congestive heart failure. It affects more than 3 million people in the U.S.

Bivona TTS (tight-to-shaft) **tracheostomy tube**.

BJ (biceps jerk) (Neuro).

Bjerrum's scotoma—further development of Seidel's scotoma.

BJT (bilateral juxtafoveal telangiectasis).

BKS-1000 refractive set (Barraquer-Krumeich-Swinger)—used to section and reshape the cornea.

"black comets" (Radiol)—characteristic streaks resulting from dirty automatic film processor.

Black Creek Canal virus—identified in a single case of hantavirus pulmonary syndrome in southern Florida. The carrier is believed to be the cotton rat (*Sigmodon hispidus*).

Blackfan-Diamond syndrome—a rare hypoplastic anemia seen in infants and young children; caused by defective erythropoiesis and lack of adequate nucleated erythrocytes in the bone marrow, but with normal platelet and leukocyte counts. Also known as *Josephs-Diamond-Blackfan syndrome.*

black hairy tongue—discoloration and alteration of the surface texture of the tongue by fungal infection.

blackout—loss of consciousness; syncope.

black-patch delirium—hallucinations caused in some patients with both eyes patched.

bladder carcinoma classification—see *Jewett's classification.*

bladder neck support prosthesis—for control of urinary incontinence. The device is an elastic vaginal pessary with two prongs on one side of the ring that elevate the bladder neck against the pubic bone and facilitate pressure transmission around the bladder neck.

BladderScan—measures postvoid residuals and bladder distention by ultrasound to avoid catheterization.

Bladder Tumor Assay—a method of monitoring urinary specimens. The test is said to be more sensitive than cytology in detecting low-grade carcinomas that may have insufficient cellular activity for cytologic identification.

blade or **knife**
Acra-Cut Spiral craniotome
Alcon crescent
Alcon pocket
arachnoid-shape
ASSI disposable cranio blade
banana
Bard-Parker
Beaver cataract knife
Beaver DeBakey
Beaver discission knife
Beaver keratome
Bennett self-retaining retractor
Curdy
Dyonics disposable arthroscope
5-prong rake
Franceschetti-type freeblade
Hebra
K-Blade
LaserSonics EndoBlade
LaserSonics Nd-YAG Laser Blade
    scalpels
Merlin bendable
MVR
Paufique
RAD40 sinus
sickle-shape
Superblade
Swann-Morton surgical
3-prong rake
Typhoon microdebrider

Blaivas classification of urinary incontinence.

Blake drains—flat, round, and hubless silicone nonclogging wound drains.

Blakemore-Sengstaken tube—a triple-lumen tube. It is useful in stopping hemorrhage from gastric and esophageal varices, to suction gastric contents, and in differentiating between bleeding from esophageal varices and other causes of upper gastrointestinal bleeding. This tube has a gastric balloon (always inflated), an esophageal balloon, and a gastric tip that permits suction.

Blalock-Taussig procedure (Cardio)—for "blue baby" syndrome.

Bland-Garland-White syndrome—see *ALCAPA syndrome.*

bleb, filtering (Oph).

Bledsoe brace—for knee and lower extremity fractures.

bleed (noun)—a hemorrhage, usually gastrointestinal. Intracranial bleeds are common in very premature infants.

bleeding time—see *Duke; Ivy.*

Blenoxane (bleomycin sulfate)—used to treat malignant pleural effusion and prevent recurrent pleural effusion.

blepharitis—inflammation of the eyelid margin.

bLES (bovine lavage extract surfactant)—see *surfactant, heterologous.*

Blessed Information Memory Concentration (IMC) **Test**—a cognitive screening test used to evaluate patients with dementia and Alzheimer's disease. Scores are given as the number of errors out of a possible 34. Also called *Blessed IMC Test.*

blind esophageal brushing (BEB)—a method of diagnosing infectious esophageal disease in patients with AIDS. This technique protects the endoscopist from exposure to HIV better than the standard procedure of esophagogastroduodenoscopy.

blind headache—the old lay name for any headache preceded by ocular

blind headache *(cont.)*
phenomena. May still appear in past histories, in the patient's words.

BlisterFilm—transparent dressing.

Bloch, clear cells of.

Bloch equation—MRI term.

Block cardiac device.

Blom-Singer indwelling low pressure voice prosthesis—a prosthetic device used to improve esophageal speech in patients after laryngectomy. See also *Panje voice button.*

blood, artificial—see *artificial blood.*

blood-brain barrier—barrier by which many substances that pass easily through vessel walls in other parts of the body are chemically prevented from passing through blood vessel walls into central nervous system tissue.

blood coagulation factors—see *coagulation factors, blood.*

blood flow, superior mesenteric artery.

blood glucose (bG).

Bloodgood's syndrome—see *fibrocystic breast syndrome.*

blood patch—a method of stopping postspinal tap headaches. The patient's own blood is injected into the epidural space and seals the hole in the dura made by the spinal tap needle. This prevents leakage of cerebrospinal fluid, the cause of the headache pain, also called *postspinal headache.*

blood perfusion monitor (BPM)—incorporates laser and fiberoptic technology to provide continuous tissue perfusion data. See *Laserflo.*

blood pool—the circulating blood, into which radionuclides are injected for various types of circulatory scans.

Blood Shield—a device that attaches easily to the tip of a conventional suction catheter to limit the degree of splash which occurs during vascular graft flushing, and to increase the efficiency of a standard suction tip in collecting shed blood for autotransfusion.

Bloom syndrome—a genetically transmitted syndrome whose manifestations are short stature, sun-sensitive facial erythematous lesions, and susceptibility to diarrhea and respiratory infections with a compromised immune system. Individuals with this condition have a striking predisposition to develop various neoplasms at an early age.

blot test—see *Western blot electrotransfer test.*

blow-by oxygen—a tube with humidified flowing oxygen is positioned near the patient's nose and allowed to blow by. FiO_2 (forced inspiratory oxygen) is not precise.

blow-in fracture.

blown pupil—slang for a dilated pupil unresponsive to light in a brain-damaged patient.

blow-out fracture—a result of blunt impact to the orbit. It usually involves the floor of the orbit.

Blue Angel syndrome—a pathological infatuation in which partners in a relationship sacrifice themselves and their own best interests.

blue bloater—a patient with severe respiratory failure, showing dyspnea, cyanosis, and peripheral edema due to right ventricular failure. Cf. *pink puffer.*

blue diaper syndrome—tryptophan malabsorption.

blue-dot sign—when, in testicular torsion, the infarcted appendix epididymidis can be seen through the scrotal skin.

Blue FlexTip catheter—a cardiac catheter with a special blue flexible tip to decrease the risk of vessel perforation.

blue rubber-bleb nevus syndrome.

blue toe syndrome—multiple emboli of atheromatous material in small arteries, causing cyanosis and pain in the toes.

blue velvet syndrome—feelings of euphoria, excitement, or depression, following repeated intravenous injections of strong analgesics with talcum filler. Signs include apical thrust, tachycardia, systolic murmur, pulmonary rales, hepatomegaly, ankle edema.

Blumberg's sign—rebound tenderness over the site of a suspected abdominal lesion, a sign of possible peritonitis.

Blumenthal irrigating cystitome—used during cataract surgery.

Blumer's shelf—in anorectum.

Blumgart technique—for hepaticojejunostomy.

blunt dissection (also, *blunt finger dissection* and *finger dissection*)—separating tissues with the fingers or a sponge.

blunted costophrenic angle—on chest x-ray, a costophrenic angle that is flattened or distorted by scarring or pleural fluid.

Bluntport disposable trocar—used in minimally invasive surgeries, such as laparoscopy.

B-lymphocyte—see *B-cell*.

Blythe uvulopalatoplasty—performed with standard electrocautery.

BM (bone marrow).

BMD (bone mineral density).

B-mode—see *B-scan*.

BMP (bone morphogenic protein).

BMP cable system—used for trochanteric reattachment, fracture fixation, and cerclage cabling.

BMT (bone marrow transplantation).

BNCT (boron neutron capture therapy).

BNF (Bird's Nest filter).

BNOE (benign necrotizing otitis externa).

Boas sign (also point, test)—tender area to the left of the twelfth thoracic vertebra. May be mentioned in workups for gallbladder disease and is indicative not of cholecystitis or cholelithiasis but gastric ulcer. Do not confuse with *psoas*.

boat hook—a combination of a Sinskey hook and an iris hook. The boat hook is used to manipulate an intraocular lens. It is so named because it is similar in shape (a C curve going in one direction with a straight short tip going in the opposite direction) to boating hooks used by sailors.

Bochdalek's hernia—congenital hernia through a hiatus in the posterolateral part of the diaphragm because of the persistence of the pleuroperitoneal canal in an infant.

Bodansky unit—unit of measurement of alkaline phosphatase. Very high levels (over 100 Bodansky units) are seen in primary biliary cirrhosis. Alcoholic liver disease, cholestatic hepatitis, and drug-induced cholestasis also produce high alkaline phosphatase levels. Also, *King-Armstrong* and *Bessey-Lowry* measurements of alkaline phosphatase.

body

Auer

Barr

Councilman

creola

cytomegalic inclusion

body *(cont.)*
    cytoplasmic inclusion
    Gamna-Gandy
    Heinz
    Hirano
    inclusion
    Lafora inclusion
    Lewy inclusion
    lyssa inclusion
    Negri inclusion
    Pick inclusion
    psammoma
    vitreous
    X-body
body dysmorphic disorder (BDD).
body mass indices (BMI)—used to identify and monitor obesity in children. Also used in monitoring parenteral nutrition for metabolic support.
body of Luys (subthalamic nucleus)— an important "way-station" in the extrapyramidal system. Also called *corpus Luysii* and *nucleus of Luys.*
body surface Laplacian mapping (BSLM)—noninvasive way to map out the heart's electrical activity in patients with arrhythmias. This technique utilizes Laplacian electrodes to translate the three-dimensional heart into a two-dimensional picture.
Boehler's angle (or Böhler's)—radiologic view of the two superior surfaces of the calcaneus.
Boerema hernia repair—used to repair type 2 paraesophageal hernia, often followed by gastropexy to prevent volvulus following the repair.
Boerhaave's syndrome—a spontaneous rupture of the esophagus.
boggy uterus—undesirable soft, spongy uterus felt on abdominal palpation following delivery, rather than firm uterus which is needed to stop hemorrhaging.

Böhler's angle—see *Boehler's angle.*
Bohlman triple-wire technique—posterior cervical fusion for stabilization of cervical spine fracture.
Boltzmann distribution—MRI term.
bolus—a single dose of a drug given intravenously over a few minutes, usually by the I.V. push method. A bolus produces immediate therapeutic levels of the drug and is used in emergency situations. See also *I.V. push.*
bombé—curved or swelling outward.
Bonaccolto utility and splinter forceps —for ophthalmology use.
Bondek absorbable sutures.
bone age according to Greulich and Pyle (Radiol).
bone and limb growth velocity ratios (Ortho, Ped).
Bone Bullet suture anchor—used to attach soft tissue to bone in hallux valgus repair, midfoot reconstruction, scapholunate ligament reconstruction, ulnar or radial collateral ligament reconstruction, PIP joint ligament reconstruction, and profundus tendon reattachment.
bone cement—see *adhesive.*
bone conduction (ENT)—refers to the transmission of sound through the bones of the skull to the cochlea and auditory nerve. Bone conduction is tested by holding an activated tuning fork against the mastoid bone. Normally the sound is heard twice as long by air conduction as by bone conduction. See *Weber test, air conduction, Rinne test.*
bone-cutting forceps.
bone density measurements—a study performed with amorphous silicon filmless x-ray technology.

Bonefos (disodium clodronate tetrahydrate)—a drug used to treat increased bone resorption (loss of bony substance) in patients with carcinoma.

bone marrow edema pattern on MR imaging—seen in an epiphysis and may indicate posttraumatic or stress fractures, osteonecrosis, transient osteoporosis, reactive changes underlying degenerative articular disease, and a self-resolving condition referred to as *transient bone marrow edema syndrome.*

bone marrow transplantation (BMT).

bone mineral density (BMD).

bone morphogenic proteins—induce bone growth at a site of injury.

bone paste (skeletal repair system)—injectable biomaterial that may soon replace the painful pins and screws and casts used to hold fractures in place while healing. The material hardens in 15 minutes. As the fracture heals, the hardened biomaterial is replaced by living bone.

BonePlast—bone void filler; biocompatible plaster-of-paris-based material that resorbs and is replaced with bone during the healing process.

bone replacement material—see *graft.*

bone scan—see *TSPP rectilinear bone scan.*

bone surface lesions—may be endosteal, intracortical, paracortical, parosteal (juxtacortical), periosteal, or subperiosteal.

bone wax—a sticky material prepared from beeswax and used to control bleeding on bony surfaces.

bone window—CT setting which optimizes the visualization of osseous structures. See *brain window, pulmonary parenchymal window, soft tissue window, subdural window.*

Bonney test—used for diagnosis of stress incontinence. It produces continence by restoring the anterior vaginal wall hammock. See *Miyazaki-Bonney test.*

bony island (Radiol)—benign developmental abnormality consisting of a localized zone of increased density in a long bone.

Bookler swivel-ball laparoscopic instrument holder—features a clamp tip for holding instruments such as trocars and graspers.

Bookwalter retractor system—a metal circular frame on a post to which many retractors are clamped to expose the surgical field from all directions. Used in colorectal, vaginal, and small-incision surgery. Note on spelling: There is no *Buckwalter* or *Buchwalter retractor.*

BOOP (bronchiolitis obliterans with organizing pneumonia).

Boorman gastric cancer typing system (types 1-4):
1   polypoid carcinoma
2   ulcerocancer
3   ulcerating and infiltrating carcinoma
4   diffusely infiltrating carcinoma

Booth wire osteotomy.

BOP (bleomycin, Oncovin, Platinol)—chemotherapy protocol for metastatic testicular carcinoma, malignant germ cell tumor of ovary, and teratoma of the ovary.

Bordetella—genus of small gram-negative coccobacilli, or rods, of the family *Brucellaceae,* formerly *Haemophilus.* The organism causing whooping cough is *B. pertussis* (formerly *Haemophilus pertussis).*

Bores radial marker—used in refractive eye surgery.

Bornholm disease (also called "devil's grip")—caused by coxsackievirus.

boron neutron capture therapy (BNCT)—for treatment of brain tumors. Patients are injected with a nontoxic boron compound that accumulates in the brain. A beam of low-energy neutrons is then fired at the tumor area, reacting with the compound to produce cancer-killing nuclear particles. It is reportedly far less traumatic than current treatments and has fewer side effects. Currently the treatment is only available at nuclear reactor sites, where the beams can be safely generated.

Borrelia burgdorferi—tick-borne spirochete which causes Lyme disease.

Bosker TMI System—a transmandibular implant (TMI) for cosmetic reconstruction of the mandible or to treat fractures caused by accident or radiation therapy. Mandibular fixation device using an osseointegrated rigid box-frame structure which can induce bone growth in the mandible.

Bosker transmandibular reconstructive surgical system—a procedure named for a reconstructive maxillofacial surgeon who utilizes a transmandibular approach.

boss (noun), **bosselated** (adj.)—a rounded eminence, as on the surface of a bone or tumor; for example, bosselated surface.

Bosworth procedure—repair of acromioclavicular separation, using screw fixation of the clavicle to the coracoid.

"bother" score—see *International Prostate Symptom Score.*

Botox (botulinum toxin, type A)—used in treatment of postlaryngectomy tracheoesophageal speech failure after placement of a tracheoesophageal voice prosthesis.

botulinum toxin, type A—used for treatment of blepharospasm and strabismus of dystonia. Type A is used investigationally for treatment of pediatric cerebral palsy and cervical dystonia; type B (for cervical dystonia); and type F (for cervical dystonia and essential blepharospasm). See *Botox; Clostridium botulinum toxin, type A; Oculinum.*

bouche de tapir ("boosh duh tahpeer") (Fr., tapir's mouth)—elongation of the face, so that it resembles that of a tapir, caused by extreme weakness of the muscles about the mouth.

Bouin's solution—a fixative for gastrointestinal biopsy specimens (and other tissue specimens).

Bourns-Bear ventilator—volume-cycled ventilator that delivers a pre-set volume of air.

Boutin thoracoscope.

boutonnière deformity of the finger.

bovied (lowercase)—verb form denoting the use of the Bovie electrocautery.

Bovie ultrasound aspirator.

bovine heterograft—see *graft.*

bovine lavage extract surfactant—see *surfactant, heterologous.*

bovine pericardium strips—used to seal air leaks during surgical stapling of emphysematous lung tissue in lung volume reduction surgery. See *Peri-Strips.*

bovine spongiform encephalopathy (BSE)—also known as "mad cow disease." This malady causes progressive degeneration of brain tissue and produces symptoms of agitation, clumsiness, and eventual death in cows. It is believed that this disease

bovine *(cont.)*
can be spread to humans by ingesting meat from infected animals. BSE causes symptoms strikingly similar to the human brain infection called Creutzfeldt-Jakob disease.

bovine superoxide (Orgotein).

Bowen Hutterite syndrome—a very rare disorder inherited as an autosomal recessive genetic trait. Major symptoms may include low birth weight, microcephaly, a prominent nose, an underdeveloped jaw, "rocker-bottom feet," and failure to thrive.

Bowen wire tightener—tightens stainless steel wires and breaks them at precisely the proper length. Also, Bowen wire cutters and wire holders.

Bowman's layer of the cornea (Oph).

bow-tie sign—an abnormality seen on x-ray which is associated with a cervical facet fracture. The body and facet of the cervical vertebra rotate and overlap, causing a shadow in the shape of a bow tie to appear.

boxcarring (Oph)—segmentation of blood in retinal vessels; a sign of death.

boxer's fracture—caused by striking close-fisted hand on hard object, as in boxing. "Preliminary interpretation of x-rays of the left hand is of a boxer's-type fracture of the distal aspect of the second metacarpal."

boxer's nose—a nasal deformity (usually from a fracture) that looks like that which boxers often acquire in their occupation.

Boyle uterine elevator—used to retract the uterus during hysterectomy. Replaces standard self-retaining retractors and bowel packing. Consists of a long rod with a cervical cup on one end. Advantages are that a small abdominal incision can be used, and less manipulation of abdominal contents helps to avoid postoperative catheterization and decreases total hospital length of stay.

Boynton needle holder.

BPA (burst-promoting activity).

BPD (biparietal diameter) (Ob-Gyn).

BPD (bronchopulmonary dysplasia).

BPI (bactericidal/permeability-increasing) **protein**—a human host-defense protein that kills bacteria, neutralizes endotoxins, and inhibits neovascularization. Used to develop new antifungal agents.

BPM (blood perfusion monitor).

BPPV (benign paroxysmal positional vertigo).

BPTI (brachial plexus traction injury) **syndrome**.

Bq (becquerel).

BRACAnalysis—comprehensive gene test used to detect hereditary breast and ovarian cancer. The BRCA1 and BRCA2 gene mutations are believed to be responsible for 90 percent of early-onset hereditary breast and ovarian cancers.

brace—see also *braces for children* and *orthosis.*
Aircast Swivel-Strap
Bledsoe
Cast Boot hip abduction
chair-back
clamshell
CRS (Counter Rotation System)
Cruiser hip abduction
C.Ti.
DonJoy Goldpoint knee
49er knee
Friedman Splint
gait lock splint (GLS)
Galveston metacarpal

brace *(cont.)*
Jewett
Kicker Pavlik harness
Liberty CMC thumb
KS 5 ACL brace
Kydex
Lenox Hill
LSU reciprocation-gait orthosis
Moon Boot
Newport MC hip orthosis
Nextep knee
OS-5/Plus 2 knee
Palumbo knee
PMT halo system
postoperative flexor tendon traction
Rhino Triangle
Rolyan tibial fracture
Seton hip
SmartBrace
SmartWrap elbow
Swede-O-Universal
Swivel-Strap
TLSO (thoracolumbosacral)
Townsend knee
UBC (Univ. of British Columbia)
Ultrabrace
Wheaton Pavlik harness

braces artifact (Radiol)—orthodontic hardware degrading image quality on CT and MRI studies of the neck and posterior fossa structures.

braces for children—polypropylene hip abduction brace for treating hip dysplasia in toddlers up to $2^1/2$ years of age. The following are trademarks:
Cast Boot
Cruiser hip abduction
Friedman Splint
Kicker Pavlik harness
Rhino Triangle

brachial—refers to the arm, as in brachial plexus, a network of nerves located partly in the neck and partly in the axilla. Cf. *branchial, bronchial.*

brachioaxillary bridge graft fistula (BAGF)—used for patients on chronic hemodialysis when sites for direct arteriovenous anastomosis are no longer usable.

brachioradialis transfer—Ober-Barr procedure for weakness of the triceps muscle.

brachiosubclavian bridge graft fistula (BSGF)—used for patients on chronic hemodialysis when sites for direct arteriovenous anastomosis are no longer usable.

BrachySeed—iodine ^{125}I for treatment of prostate cancer.

brachytherapy—interstitial implantation of radioactive isotopes, permitting the localized delivery of high doses of radiation to a tumor mass. See separate entries:
afterloading brachytherapy
episcleral plaque brachytherapy
intraluminal brachytherapy
IOHDR (intraoperative high dose rate) brachytherapy
I-Plant brachytherapy seeds
permanent brachytherapy
remote afterloading brachytherapy (RAB)
Symmetra I-125 brachytherapy seeds
Ultraseed brachytherapy
vascular brachytherapy

Brackmann facial nerve monitor.

Brackmann II EMG system—used in complex cranial motor nerve monitoring.

Braden score—measures potential for alteration of skin integrity in bedridden patients.

bradyarrhythmia—a disturbance in the heart rhythm, resulting in a slow, irregular heartbeat.

Bradycor—drug that may improve functional outcome in patients with severe traumatic brain injury.

bradykinin—endogenous peptide that causes vasodilation, induces contraction of smooth muscle, and induces hypotension.

bradyphemic (Neuro)—afflicted with slow speech.

Bragg peak (Radiol, Neuro)—photon beam therapy.

Brailler—see *Perkins Brailler*.

"brain attack"—a concept developed to educate the public on the warning signs of stroke, transient ischemic attacks, and amaurosis fugax.

brain death—irreversible coma.

brain death syndrome—state in which brain function, including autonomic control, is totally and permanently absent. See *Harvard Criteria for Brain Death*.

brain-derived neurotrophic factor (BDNF).

brain electrical activity map (BEAM).

brain or **intraventricular temperature monitoring**—difficult to monitor as there are no commercially available devices yet for measuring brain temperature.

brain plasticity—the phenomenon that allows remodeling of detailed connections in the brain during learning and underlies the progressive development of behavioral skills and abilities. Researchers are investigating the use of electrical stimulation of the nucleus basalis to magnify and accelerate plasticity changes involved in stroke recovery.

brain stem—two words, as a noun and an adjective.

brain stem auditory evoked potential (BAEP).

brain stem auditory evoked response (BAER).

brain tests, noninvasive
BAEP—brain stem auditory evoked potential
BAER—brain stem auditory evoked response
EP—evoked potential
ER—evoked response
MEP—multimodality evoked potential (a combination of visual, somatosensory, and brain stem auditory evoked potential)
SEP—somatosensory evoked potential
SER—somatosensory evoked response
VEP—visual evoked potential
VER—visual evoked response

brain window—CT setting which optimizes radiologic visualization of intracranial anatomy. See *bone window, pulmonary parenchymal window, soft tissue window, subdural window*.

branched calculus (Radiol)—staghorn calculus.

branched chain DNA assay—uses a series of DNA probes to capture, target, and amplify viral RNA in a specimen. Cf. *polymerase chain reaction*.

branchial arches, cleft—pertaining to gill-like structures in embryo that become modified into structures in the ear and neck. Cf. *brachial, bronchial*.

branchio-oto-renal (BOR) **syndrome**—a rare, autosomal dominant genetic disorder involving branchial cleft and renal anomalies, hearing loss, and other otologic manifestations.

branch retinal vein occlusion—said to be second only to diabetic reti-

branch *(cont.)*
nopathy as the most common form of retinal vascular disease.

Brandt cytology balloon—used for esophageal brushing to diagnose fungal esophagitis and esophageal cytomegalovirus in AIDS patients.

Brandt-Daroff exercises—a method of treating benign paroxysmal positional vertigo.

Branemark endosteal implants (ENT).

Branham's sign—compression over an arteriovenous fistula causing slowing of the pulse, which gives a positive sign. Also called *Nicoladoni-Branham's sign.*

Branhamella catarrhalis (new genus—formerly *Neisseria).*

brash—burning sensation in the stomach. Cf. *water brash.*

BRAT diet—for children who, after having been on intravenous fluids, are started on *bananas, rice cereal, applesauce,* and *toast.*

brawny edema or **brawny induration.**

Braxton Hicks contractions—sometimes called *false labor.* Light, irregular contractions, usually painless; may become more intense, frequent, and regular later in pregnancy.

BRCA1, BRCA2 (breast cancer one and two)—genes thought to act as a tumor suppressor in breast cancer. An estimated 85% of women who inherit a defective copy of BRCA2 will develop breast cancer during their lifetime, as compared to 10% of women in the general population.

BreakAway absorptive wound dressing.

BreastAlert—differential temperature sensor (DTS) screening device for early detection of breast disease.

breast bolster—device that helps to increase tissue depth of the breast during fine needle biopsy. It is most effective in moderately large breasts that are flaccid and easily compress to a thin tissue depth.

BreastCheck—a handheld electronic device for breast self-examination. It uses miniature pressure sensors which are glided over the breast, gently "palpating" in a manner similar to the human hand.

breast-conserving therapy (BCT)—breast cancer treatment limited to lumpectomy, axillary dissection, and radiation therapy.

BreastExam—used by physicians for breast cancer detection. See *Breast-Check.*

breast fibrocystic disease, stages of:
mazoplasia—in patients in late teens and early 20s
adenosis—early 30s and 40s
cystic disease—late 30s through 40s and early 50s

Breast Imaging and Reporting Data System of the American College of Radiology (BI-RADS).

breast reconstruction donor sites for autogenous tissue—transverse rectus abdominis myocutaneous flap, latissimus dorsi, gluteal free flap, lateral transverse thigh flap or "saddle bags," and Rubens flap, a modification of the deep circumflex iliac artery iliac crest flap. See *Rubens flap.*

breast reconstruction pattern—see *fleur de lis pattern.*

breast reduction technique—a short-scar procedure that uses the inferior pedicle (tissue situated on the bottom part of the breast) to give consistent, controllable results over

breast *(cont.)*

breast shape. By retaining fat and parenchyma (the main tissue of the breast) centrally beneath the nipple and areola, direct contouring of the breast with consistent control over shape becomes possible. Very little reliance is placed on postoperative settling, with essentially no bottoming out.

Breathe Right nasal strips—temporary treatment for nasal congestion, including a version with Vicks mentholated vapors.

breath excretion test

breath hydrogen excretion

breath pentane

C-cholyl-glycine breath excretion

C-urea breath excretion

Helicobacter pylori breath excretion

breath-hold MR cholangiography in adults and children vs. **non-breath-hold** studies in infants.

breath hydrogen excretion test—serves two functions: (1) a screening test in premature infants to detect necrotizing enterocolitis; (2) a reliable indicator of lactose intolerance at high levels of concentration; not reliable at lower concentration levels. See also *breath excretion test* entries.

breath pentane—an indicator of heart transplant rejection. Measurement of breath pentane via gas chromatography is considered a marker for cardiac transplant (allograft) rejection. Previously found to correlate closely with the severity of an inflammatory process, breath pentane may replace expensive and hazardous fluoroscopic or echocardiograph-guided bioptome biopsies of the transplanted heart. See also *breath excretion test* entries.

Brecher and Cronkite technique—for platelet counting.

Breisky-Navratil retractor (Ob-Gyn) —used in sacrospinous ligament fixation. Also, Navratil retractor.

Bremer AirFlo Vest—for thoracic stabilization. Can be used in CT and MRI scanning, where movement causes artifact.

Bremer Halo Crown system—for cervical traction and stabilization. Can be used in CT and MRI scanning.

Brent pressure earring—used for treating earlobe keloids.

Brescia-Cimino AV fistula—arteriovenous fistula, used as hemodialysis access.

Breslow classification system—pathologic classification of melanoma.

Bretschneider-HTK cardioplegic solution.

Brett's syndrome (also *Janus syndrome*)—used to indicate an occasional radiologic finding of a clear lung on one side and opaque shadow on the other side. This aspect is observed in Fallot's tetralogy with atresia of a branch of pulmonary artery or in truncus arteriosus with solitary pulmonary artery.

Breuerton view—a special x-ray view of the hand, to permit visualization of early changes of the joints from rheumatoid arthritis.

Brevibacterium linens.

Brevibloc (esmolol HCl).

Brevi-Kath epidural catheter—spring-guide catheter used for the administration of local anesthetics into the epidural space for pain management.

Bricanyl (terbutaline sulfate)—for use in children age 6 and older for relief of reversible bronchospasm.

Bricker ureteroileostomy.

bridging osteophytes—osteophytes on adjacent vertebrae that meet and fuse, forming a "bridge" across the joint space.

bridle suture *(not* bridal)—used in eye surgery.

Brief Neuropsychological Mental Status Examination (BNMSE).

bright signal—MRI term.

brimonidine tartrate—an alpha$_2$ agonist used to reduce intraocular pressure spikes following argon laser trabeculoplasty. See *argon laser trabeculoplasty.*

brim sign (Radiol)—in Paget's disease, a thickened pelvic brim.

bris—the Jewish circumcision rite, from the Hebrew *berith.* Also, *briss.*

Bristow coracoid process transfer—for recurrent anterior dislocation of the shoulder. The procedure stabilizes the shoulder.

brittle bone disease (osteogenesis imperfecta)—marked by a china-blue discoloration of the sclerae.

BR96-doxorubicin—monoclonal antibody (BR, Bristol Myers).

broach—an elongated, tapered, and serrated cutting tool for shaping and enlarging holes.

broad beta disease—hyperlipoproteinemia type 3, one of a group of inherited disorders of fat metabolism.

Broca's motor speech area of the brain (Neuro).

Brockenbrough–Braunwald sign—spike-and-dome configuration of pressure gradient at cardiac catheterization in which the pulse pressure is unchanged or actually reduced following an extrasystolic beat. It is believed to reflect worsening of obstruction of the left ventricular outflow tract during the potentiated beat, with diminished stroke volume and aortic pulse pressure.

Brockenbrough cardiac device.

Brockenbrough needle—used in diagnostic cardiovascular procedures, such as with a Mullins sheath in transseptal catheterization.

Broders' index (devised by A. C. Broders, an American pathologist)—a classification of the malignancy of tumors, based on the degree of differentiation, and therefore the aggressiveness, of the tumor; graded from 1 to 4, grade 1 representing the most differentiation and the best prognosis, and grade 4 the least differentiation and the poorest prognosis.

Brodie's abscess—centrally placed radiographic lucency in the metaphysis adjacent to the growth plate, usually in adolescents and associated with subacute or chronic hematogenous osteomyelitis. Named for Benjamin Brodie in 1832.

bromocriptine-dopamine agonist—has been found to help stave off craving for alcohol in men who inherited the minor allele (A1) of the gene for the D2 dopamine receptor (DRD2). While no studies have included women, researchers believe this drug may help the 69% of alcoholics who have the A1 allele. More studies and easier identification tests are needed before widespread clinical use, but physicians may give alcoholics a trial of the drug without determining whether the patient has the inherited gene. Its effectiveness (or lack thereof) would be considered diagnostic.

bromodeoxyuridine (BUdR, broxuridine). See *BUdR.*

bromontan—a drug widely used in Russia by armed forces personnel, cosmonauts, and athletes. It reportedly increases powers of concentration and stimulates physical activity.

Brompton solution (from the Brompton Hospital in London), used for analgesia in terminal cancer patients. Contains cocaine, morphine sulfate, Compazine, ethyl alcohol, and syrup. Also, *Brompton mixture*.

bronchial—refers to the bronchi and bronchial tubes. Cf. *bronchiole, brachial, branchial.*

bronchial artery embolization—for treatment of bronchial bleeding and life-threatening hemoptysis.

bronchial dehiscence—disruption of the anastomosis secondary to airway ischemia in the watershed area in lung transplantation. These areas may heal spontaneously, require stenting or dilatation, or go on to bronchial stricture or rejection. See *watershed region.*

bronchial sleeve resection—procedure to treat centrally located lung cancer, while sparing distal parenchyma. It requires full mobilization of the hilum and dissection of the bronchi and vessels. Successful reconstruction involves frozen section analysis of regional lymph nodes and confirmation of free margins prior to bronchial anastomosis.

bronchial washings cytology.

bronchiole—one of the smaller branches into which the segmental bronchi divide. Cf. *bronchial.*

bronchiolitis obliterans—a term for signs of chronic rejection of a transplanted lung. Also called *progressive parenchymal restriction.* As the process continues, the radiologist sees the lungs decrease in size, the vascular markings decrease, and the interstitial markings increase.

bronchiolitis obliterans with organizing pneumonia (BOOP)—cryptogenic organizing pneumonia or proliferative bronchiolitis. Forms of this disease may be referred to as *idiopathic BOOP* and *BOOP reactions.* Cf. *obliterative bronchiolitis.*

bronchiolocentric—used in radiologic reports, as in "abnormalities are bronchiolocentric."

Bronchitrac L catheter—a flexible suction catheter designed specifically to reach the left lobe of the lung without having to twist the catheter or reposition the patient.

bronchoalveolar lavage (BAL).

Broncho-Cath—a double-lumen endobronchial tube.

bronchogram, tantalum—using powdered tantalum.

bronchoprovocation testing—administration of an agent known to induce or aggravate bronchoconstriction.

Bronkosol (isoetharine HCl)—used to treat bronchial asthma. Easy to misspell because it does not follow the spelling of *bronchial.*

Brontex (codeine phosphate and guaifenesin)—antitussive/expectorant.

bronze diabetes—diabetes with accompanying pancreatic damage. Also called *iron storage disease.*

bronze disease—Addison's disease; called "bronze" because one of the symptoms of this hypofunction of the adrenal glands is a bronze or brownish color of the skin.

Brooke Army Hospital splint—used in tendon repair.

Brooke ileostomy.

Brooker classification—a system of classifying periarticular heterotopic ossification following total hip arthroplasty. It consists of grades 1 through 4, with grade 1 showing islands of bone in the periarticular soft tissues and grade 4 showing osseous ankylosis (complete bony fusion) of the hip.

bropirimine (ABPP)—a drug used to treat AIDS.

Broselow tape or **chart**—used to determine a child's weight. It is part of trauma cart equipment.

Brostrom procedure—repair of ankle ligament injuries using direct suturing to reconstruct a ligament with available tissue and reimplant into the bone.

Browlift BoneBridge system—an instrument allowing browlift suture fixation without implant.

Brown-Adson tissue forceps.

Brown dermatome—oscillating blade-type dermatome.

Browne—see *Denis Browne clubfoot splint*.

Brown-McHardy pneumatic dilator—used in treatment of dysphagia associated with achalasia. The unit of measure used in procedures with this dilator is p.s.i. ("sigh"), pounds per square inch.

Brown-Roberts-Wells (BRW) **stereotactic system**—consisting of an arc system, frame, stereotactic adapter used in performing stereotactic procedures on the brain.

Brown's tendon sheath syndrome—the superior oblique tendon is short, causing strabismus.

Brown two-portal technique—for endoscopic carpal tunnel release.

Broxine (broxuridine)—radiosensitizer for breast and brain tumors.

Bruce protocol—staging on cardiac treadmill test. Scored in mets—1 met equals 3.5 ml O_2/kg/min. There are six stages, I through VI.

Bruch's membrane—glassy-appearing membrane of the choroid of the eye. (K.W.L. Bruch, Swiss anatomist.) Usage: "Vascularization was found of the inner part of Bruch's membrane in the enucleated eye."

Brudzinski's sign—a positive sign in meningitis. Bending a patient's neck (pressing the chin toward the sternum) produces flexion of the knees and hips.

Brueghel's syndrome—see *Meige's syndrome*.

Bruel-Kjaer transvaginal ultrasound probe.

Bruel-Kjaer ultrasound scanner—used in intracavitary prostate ultrasonography. "Incremental multiplane scanning of the prostate and seminal vesicles in real-time mode was performed using the Bruel-Kjaer ultrasound scanner, type 1846, and a 7 MHz 112° rectal multiplane transducer, type 8551."

Bruening syringe—for Teflon insertion into vocal cords.

Bruhat maneuver—CO_2 laser surgery neosalpingostomy.

Bruininks-Oseretsky Test of Motor Proficiency (Phys Ther).

bruit ("broo′ee") (pl., bruits)—a sound or murmur heard on vascular auscultation, especially an abnormal one. Example: aneurysmal bruit.

brunescent—dark brown, as in brunescent cataract.

Bruno-Helfand physical therapy—combines whirlpool, electrical stimu-

Bruno-Helfand *(cont.)*
lation, foot and toe exercises, to improve circulation.

Bruns bone curette.

Bruser's skin incision—in knee surgery.

Brushfield spots—frequently found on the iris of patients with Down syndrome.

brush marks (Oph)—lid margin vascular dilation.

brux, bruxism—to grind the teeth spasmodically. "She complained of a weak chin and malocclusion, and desired a normal bite and profile. She bruxes and clenches, but denied any TMJ (temporomandibular joint) pain or dysfunction."

BRW (Brown-Roberts-Wells) **CT stereotaxic guide**—may also be used with MRI and PET scan techniques.

Bryant's traction—used on small children for the correction of congenital hip dislocation, or for stabilization of femur fractures. Overhead suspension is used, so that the hips are flexed to 90°.

B-scan (also called *B-mode*)—an ultrasound technique which permits visualization of structures by delineating echoes from these structures in various shades of gray. It can differentiate between the lumen of an artery and the arterial wall, to determine the thickness of the wall.

BSCVA (best spectacle-corrected visual acuity).

BSD-2000—uses hyperthermia to treat tumors deep in the body and precisely heat surface tumors by directing radiofrequency/microwave energy.

BSE—see *bovine spongiform encephalopathy.*

BSGF (brachiosubclavian bridge graft fistula).

BSS (balanced salt solution) (Oph).

BSS Plus—balanced salt solution with added bicarbonate, dextrose, and glutathione, used as a sterile intraocular irrigating solution. It is better than plain BSS in preserving the integrity of the corneal epithelium following surgery.

BTA stat test—rapid, single-step immunoassay of the urine to detect recurrent bladder cancer. The disposable test device contains two monoclonal antibodies that detect the presence of a newly identified human complement factor H-related protein (hCFHrp). The BTA stat test is said to be simpler and faster than urine cytology and is simpler than the original Bard BTA test.

bubble boy disease—see *pegademase bovine.*

bubble ventriculography—used in diagnosing hydrocephalus.

buccal mucosa *(not* buckle)—the mucosa lining the inside of the cheek.

buccal smear—test used in X-chromosome determinations; made from cells scraped from the buccal mucosa, placed on a slide, and stained; demonstrates the Barr bodies (sex chromatin) seen in normal females.

Buchwalter—see *Bookwalter retractor.*

Buckwalter—see *Bookwalter retractor.*

bucindolol—used for treatment of congestive heart failure.

bucket-handle pattern of fracture—seen in a metaphyseal lesion of the distal femur in abused infants.

bucket-handle tear of the knee meniscus.

Buck-Gramcko retractor.

Buck restrictor (Ortho).

Buck's traction—used on the leg and in knee injuries. Also used as a temporary measure to help reduce muscle spasm, while the patient is awaiting surgical repair for fracture of the hip.

bucrylate—a liquid acrylic monomer which polymerizes on contact with blood, forming a plug for a vessel. Used to stop bleeding in life-threatening situations.

Budd-Chiari syndrome—acute parenchymatous jaundice. Related terms:
Budd's disease
Budd's jaundice
Chiari's disease
Rokitansky's disease
von Rokitansky's disease

Budde halo retractor system (Neuro).

buddy splint—used in dislocation of fingers or toes; the dislocated digit is taped to an adjacent digit (its "buddy"), which acts as a splint.

budesonide (Rhinocort)—a topical corticosteroid spray administered intranasally to treat allergic rhinitis.

Budin toe splint—treats overlapping toes and hammertoes.

BUdR (bromodeoxyuridine, broxuridine)—clinical radiosensitizer, used in tumors that are poorly radioresponsive to enhance radiotherapy response. Used concurrently with irradiation. Cf. *FUdR, IUdR.*

Buechel-Pappas total ankle prosthesis—a 3-piece titanium and ultra-high-molecular-weight polyethylene prosthesis that can be used to restore a functioning ankle joint even in a patient with previous fusion.

Buerger Allen exercise (Phys Ther)—used to increase circulation.

Buerger's disease—an inflammatory disease of the blood vessels which can lead to ischemia and gangrene. Cf. *Berger's disease.*

buffalo hump—a zone of focal edema over the upper mid back, seen especially in Cushing's syndrome and in prolonged adrenal steroid therapy.

buffy coat—layer of white blood cells found on centrifugation of anticoagulated blood between the plasma and the red cells. You may hear of a test being "buffy coat positive." See *buffy coat smear.*

buffy coat smear—used in diagnosis of lupus erythematosus, in determining the presence of certain protozoa and fungi in the peripheral blood, and for some bone marrow exams.

Bugbee electrode.

bulbosity—the condition of being bulbous; used in describing a nasal tip in plastic surgery procedures.

bulimia nervosa—binge eating followed by self-induced vomiting or purging.

bulimorexia—an eating disorder including features of both *anorexia nervosa* (severe caloric restriction due to distortion of body image, with dangerous nutritional deficiency) and *bulimia nervosa* (binge eating followed by self-induced vomiting or purging).

Bullard intubating laryngoscope.

bull's eye lesion—a skin lesion consisting of concentric rings of erythema.

Bumex (bumetanide)—a loop diuretic for use in treatment of acute edema associated with congestive heart failure, hepatic and renal disease, including nephrotic syndrome.

bunching suture.

bundle-nailing method of treating bone shaft fractures—a two-step method. It lacks the stability of Küntscher's

bundle-nailing *(cont.)*
method but has the advantage that no bone-damaging boring of the medullary canal is needed.

bunionectomy
Joplin
Keller
Kreuscher
scarf osteotomy
tricorrectional
Wu

bunion last—used in management of hyperkeratotic lesions of the foot. See *last*.

Bunnell
active hand and finger splints
finger extension splint
knuckle bender
tendon transfer

Bunny boot—orthopedic brace.

BUO (bilateral ureteral obstruction).

bupropion—antidepressant found to be significantly useful in smoking cessation.

Burch colposuspension—for stress incontinence.

Burch iliopectineal ligament urethrovesical suspension.

Burch laparoscopic procedure.

Burhenne steerable catheter with basket inserted.

buried bumper syndrome—a complication of gastrostomy tube placement whereby the tube migrates anteriorly to lie partially or completely outside the gastric wall, where it becomes embedded in the abdominal wall as the gastric site heals and reepithelializes behind it. The internal "bumper" of the gastrostomy tube burrows into the gastric mucosa and becomes permanently embedded. It must be freed surgically and a new gastrostomy tube inserted.

buried penis—an infrequent congenital penile deformity in which the penile shaft is buried below the surface of the prepubic skin because of an abnormally prominent suprapubic fat pad and dense fascial bands retracting and tethering the penis.

buried vaginal island—see *vaginal wall sling procedure.*

Bürker chamber for macrophage counting.

Burkitt's lymphoma—one of the cancers to which AIDS patients are particularly susceptible.

burn diagram—see *Lund Browder.*

burning mouth syndrome (BMS)—characterized by chronic orofacial pain usually unaccompanied by mucosal lesions or other clinical signs. Several oral sites are usually affected (lips, palate, tongue). Symptoms include oral burning, dry mouth, thirst, dysgeusia, change in eating habits, irritability, and depression. Most commonly seen in postmenopausal women of Asian-American or American Indian heritage, and most often found in the western United States.

burning vulvar syndrome—see *vulvar vestibulitis syndrome.*

burns classification
first degree—erythema, involving only epidermis. Only superficial destruction of tissue and no blistering.
second degree—entire epidermis and some of the dermis involved. There are blisters, mottling of the surface, and pain. In deeper burns, hair follicles and sebaceous glands may be destroyed.
third degree—full thickness of skin injury.

burns classification *(cont.)*
> fourth degree—extends to subcutaneous tissue, muscle, or bone. There may be charring.

Burow's solution *(not* Burrow's, but pronounced the same).

burst-forming unit-erythroid (BFU-E).

burst fracture—a type of spiral column injury, commonly caused by motorcycle or automobile accidents or falls from great heights, causing the vertebral body to explode or "burst."

burst-promoting activity (BPA).

BUS (Bartholin's, urethral, Skene's) **glands**.

Buselmeier shunt—a vascular access shunt, used in performing dialysis.

Busulfex (busulfan)—injection used in combination with cyclophosphamide as a conditioning regimen prior to allogeneic hematopoietic progenitor cell transplantation for chronic myelogenous leukemia.

butenafine—the first of a class of antifungal agents.

butorphanol tartrate—see *Stadol NS.*

butterfly bandage.

butterfly drain—a soft tissue drain consisting of a butterfly needle connected to a Vacutainer; used after surgery.

butterfly flap—technique used in hand surgery for treatment of incomplete syndactyly.

butterfly needle—a fine-gauge needle with color-coded plastic tabs on each side (like wings of a butterfly) for gripping while inserting. Useful for drawing blood from a hand vein or used for scalp vein I.V. in premature infants.

butterfly rash—a rash that has a shape roughly like that of a butterfly; it is seen over the malar area and bridge of the nose in systemic lupus erythematosus.

butterfly shadow—on x-ray.

Button and **Button-One Step gastrostomy devices**—skin-level, nonrefluxing feeding devices available in sizes for both children and adults.

buttonpexy fixation—internal fixation procedure for stomal prolapse in pediatric patients.

butyl-DNJ (deoxynojirmycin).

butyrylcholesterinase—used to reduce the levels of cocaine in the blood.

butyrylcholinesterase inhibitors—for treatment of Alzheimer's disease.

B-VAT (Baylor Visual Acuity Test). Mentor BVAT is a computer screen chart used in testing visual acuity.

BVM device (bag-valve-mask)—a resuscitating device consisting of a ventilating bag with a valve, attached to a mask.

bypass circuit (Cardio).

C, c

CA (cardiac-apnea)—see *CA monitor*.

"CA"—slang for carcinoma.

CAB (combined androgen blockade)—significantly increases survival in patients with advanced prostate cancer.

cabergoline (Dostinex)—for treatment of hyperprolactinemic disorders. The tablets are taken just twice weekly.

CABG ("cab-bage")—coronary artery bypass graft. "The patient underwent a CABG," or "The patient was given a CABG."

CAC (cisplatin, ara-C, caffeine)—chemotherapy protocol.

CAD (computer-aided diagnosis).

CAD (coronary artery disease).

CAD (cyclophosphamide, Adriamycin, dacarbazine)—chemotherapy protocol for metastatic sarcoma.

CADD-Prizm pain control system (PCS)—drug delivery system that provides measured therapy for management of pain.

Cadence AICD (automatic implantable cardioverter-defibrillator).

Cadet cardioverter-defibrillator.

CAE (cyclophosphamide, Adriamycin, etoposide)—chemotherapy protocol for refractory non-Hodgkin's lymphoma.

CAF (cyclophosphamide, Adriamycin, fluorouracil)—chemotherapy protocol for advanced breast cancer.

Cafcit (caffeine citrate)—oral solution for short-term treatment of apnea of prematurity in infants between 28 and 33 weeks' gestational age.

café au lait macules (CALMs)—may be treated with the frequency-doubled Q-switched neodymium:YAG laser and the Q-switched ruby laser.

caffeine—given to premature infants to prevent episodes of apnea.

Caffinière prosthesis—cemented prosthesis used in replacement of the trapeziometacarpal joint.

CA15-3 RIA—a radioimmunoassay for monitoring breast cancer, based on two monoclonal antibodies which react with circulating antigen expressed by human breast carcinoma cells. This monitors a breast cancer patient's response to therapy. Used in

CA15-3 RIA *(cont.)*
the manner of carcinoembryonic antigen.

CAFTH (cyclophosphamide, Adriamycin, fluorouracil, tamoxifen, Halotestin)—chemotherapy protocol for hormone-sensitive metastatic breast carcinoma.

CAGE (cutting, annoyance, guilt, eye-opener)—an acronym for questions about cutting down on drinking, annoyance at others' concern about drinking, feeling guilty about drinking, and using alcohol as an eye-opener in the morning. Referred to as the CAGE test, its brevity gives it an advantage in a busy medical office.

CAGEIN (catheter-guided endoscopic intubation)—used at the start of endoscopy as a method to intubate the esophagus in patients who have constricted anatomy, such as from Zenker's diverticulum.

caisson disease—decompression sickness (called "the bends"), seen in workers and divers who work for long periods of time under water, breathing air at higher than atmospheric pressure, and then come up too quickly. The name is from the watertight structures in which underwater construction is performed, as in building bridges or tunnels.

"cake mix" kit—for hematopoietic progenitor assay.

calamus scriptorius—the lowest portion of the floor of the fourth ventricle, shaped like a writing pen (hence its name). Used in surgical correction of syringomyelia.

Calandruccio triangular compression fixation device—used for fixation of the distal tibia.

calcarine fissure—sulcus on medial surface of the occipital lobe; the visual cortex is around this fissure.

calcar reamer (Ortho).

Calcijex—injectable calcitriol for treatment of bone-loss disease in dialysis patients.

calciphylaxis—an untreatable, rare, generally fatal, necrotizing cutaneous syndrome.

calcipotriene (Dovonex)—topical cream for the treatment of psoriasis. This vitamin D_3 derivative is an alternative to steroid-based creams.

Calcitek drill system—for use in oral and maxillofacial surgery.

Calcitek spline dental implant system.

Calcitite—alloplastic material used as bone replacement. It is a solid hydroxyapatite, similar to cortical bone. See *hydroxyapatite*.

calcium acetate (PhosLo)—buffering agent for hyperphosphatemia of end-stage renal failure.

calcium and magnesium-free Hanks' balanced salt solution (CMF-HBSS).

calcium channel blockers—a class of drugs commonly used to treat angina, hypertension, and arrhythmias, and now a part of some chemotherapy protocols. Certain types of cancer are resistant to the effects of chemotherapy agents, but this resistance can be overcome with the use of calcium channel blockers such as nifedipine and verapamil. See also *P-glycoprotein*.

calcium entry blockers—alternative name for calcium channel blockers.

calcium pyrophosphate deposition (CPPD) **of the spine**—a relatively uncommon arthropathy characterized by clinical features of pseudogout,

calcium *(cont.)*
radiographic manifestations of chondrocalcinosis, and the pathological deposition of calcium pyrophosphate crystals in hyaline and fibrocartilage. It is sometimes the cause of mechanical low back pain or nerve root compression syndrome. Also called *CPPD disease.*

calculi—see *cat's-eye calculi.*

Calcutript—a lithotripter used for stone disintegration in the ureter.

Caldwell view—occipitofrontal view for x-raying the ethmoid and frontal sinuses.

CALF (cyclophosphamide, Adriamycin, leucovorin [rescue], fluorouracil)—chemotherapy protocol.

CALF-E (cyclophosphamide, Adriamycin, leucovorin [rescue], fluorouracil, ethinyl estradiol)—chemotherapy protocol for breast carcinoma.

caliber—the internal diameter of a needle; also known as the *bore.* Cf. *caliper.*

calibration failure—MRI term.

Caligamed—an ankle orthosis that can be worn in a shoe to offer full immobilization of the ankle joint. It is used to treat chronic ankle instability, immediate post-injury immobilization, protection postoperatively after ligament restructuring, or as a conservative treatment for torn ligaments.

caliper (often plural)—instrument with two curved legs used to measure a width or thickness indirectly—for example, the thickness of a skin fold. Examples: Jameson, Lange skin-fold, Machemer, Oscher, Stahl, Tenzel, Vernier. Cf. *caliber.*

CALLA (common acute lymphoblastic leukemia antigen).

Callaway formula—used to calculate a person's optimal daily calorie intake: Multiply your weight by 4.3 and your height in inches by 4.7. Add these results together plus 655 calories. From this resulting number subtract your age multiplied by 4.7. That number represents the number of calories you burn at rest. Multiply that by 1.3 and you get the number of calories you burn with moderate activity. If you keep within that calorie count, you will lose weight; if you go below the lower number, your metabolism will slow down.

Calleja exercises (Ortho).

callous (adjective)—hard, as "There is a callous area on the heel of the left foot." Cf. *callus.*

callus (noun)—localized growth of a hard, horny epidermal material, as "There is a callus on the palm of the hand, near the ring he is wearing on his ring finger." Cf. *callous.*

callus distraction—a technique that corrects limb shortening by callus formation and induces bony union of nonunited fractures.

Calmette-Guérin—see *bacillus Calmette-Guérin.*

CALMs (café au lait macules).

Calnan-Nicolle synthetic joint prosthesis—used to lengthen a shortened metatarsal.

caloric testing of vestibular function—stimulates the labyrinth by instilling fluid into the ear (either above or below body temperature). Resulting nystagmus lasting more than two minutes indicates hyperirritability of the labyrinth. Absence of response indicates eighth nerve damage. Also called *cold water calorics.* See *Bárány's symptom.*

calorimeter—a device to measure an individual's caloric burn.

Caluso PEG tube—a percutaneous endoscopic gastrostomy tube.

calusterone—an androgen used experimentally in treatment of carcinoma.

Calypso Rely catheter—rapid-exchange PTCA balloon angioplasty catheter.

CAM (cystic adenomatoid malformation).

cameral fistula—a very rare condition of the coronary arteries, with an arteriovenous fistula between the artery and one of the cardiac chambers. Also called *coronary artery cameral fistula.*

Camey ileocystoplasty—see *LeDuc-Camey ileocystoplasty.*

Camey reservoir—a continent supravesical bowel urinary diversion, performed for bladder reconstruction to treat invasive bladder cancer. Also, *Camey ileocystoplasty.*

Camino intracranial catheter—inserted into the lateral ventricle, subarachnoid space, or subdural space, this catheter uses a transducer to monitor intracranial pressure.

Camino microventricular bolt—a catheter with a transducer on the end. Used to monitor intracranial pressure and facilitate draining of cerebrospinal fluid through a ventriculostomy.

CAMIS (computer-assisted minimally invasive surgery).

Camitz palmaris longus abductorplasty—for severe thenar atrophy secondary to carpal tunnel syndrome.

CA (cardiac-apnea) monitor—for newborns.

cAMP (cyclic adenosine monophosphate)—a second-messenger neurotransmitter.

Campath—a humanized monoclonal antibody to the leukocyte antigen CD52. It is used for the treatment of chronic lymphocytic leukemia refractory to standard therapies (alkylating agents, fludarabine).

Campbell de Morgan spots—see *cherry angioma.*

Camptosar (irinotecan)—antineoplastic for metastatic cervical, colon, and rectal carcinoma.

Campylobacter fetus—a gram-negative organism causing enteritis in AIDS patients.

Campylobacter jejuni—enteric pathogen in humans, probably transmitted by infected animals, or from consumption of contaminated water or foods of animal origin.

CAM tent (Peds).

Cam (controlled ankle motion) walker—an air-filled ankle-support device, looking something like a padded boot with a rocker foot. (Note: Only the initial letter in *Cam* is capitalized.)

Canal Finder System—for use in endodontic applications, and specialized biomaterials for dentistry and other medical specialties.

canaliculus—a small canal; generally refers to the one that leads from the lacrimal punctum to the lacrimal sac of the eye. Cf. *colliculus.*

canalith repositioning maneuver—used to resolve or decrease intensity of symptoms in patients with disorders of the vestibular system with a component of benign postural vertigo.

canals (or canaliculi) of Sondermann—blind outpouchings from the canal of Schlemm.

Cancell—a biologic remedy, especially popular in the Midwest and Florida. Proponents claim it returns cancer cells to a "primitive state" from which they can be digested and rendered inert. The FDA has found no basis for the claims.

cancellous (adj.)—descriptive term for a reticular, spongy, or lattice-like structure, mainly of bony tissue.

cancellus (noun)—any structure arranged like a lattice.

cancer classifications—see *classification and staging.*

cancer marker—see *tumor marker.*

Candela 405-nm pulsed dye laser.

Candida albicans—a fungus which can disseminate in AIDS, but is also an exceedingly common cause of dermatitis, vaginitis, and thrush in persons with intact immune systems. Also, esophageal candidiasis is seen in AIDS patients.

Candida glabrata—a pathogen causing vaginitis.

C&S, C and S—culture and sensitivity. Do not confuse with CNS (central nervous system).

CA 19-9—tumor marker which is a sialylated Lewis A antigen expressed by many adenocarcinomas of the digestive tract.

Cannon waves—a phenomenon in which the two chambers of the heart may contract at the same time, when the heart loses coordination of the atria and ventricles. Blood then flows upward across the mitral and tricuspid valves, and a venous wave is seen in the neck. Named for a physician named Cannon, who first observed this phenomenon.

Cannulated Plus screw system.

canstatin—a collagen fragment that inhibits angiogenesis. It has a variety of anticancer applications.

Cantlie line—the plane separating the right and middle hepatic vein territories, not marked by any anatomical feature but usually running along or to the right of the line joining the gallbladder fossa with the inferior vena cava.

Cantor tube—see *mercury artifact.*

CA1-18 tumor marker—a tumor-associated antigen used in diagnosis and management of GI and lung cancer patients.

CAP (cyclophosphamide, Adriamycin, Platinol)—chemotherapy protocol for ovarian carcinoma.

CAPD (continuous ambulatory peritoneal dialysis).

Capetown aortic prosthetic valve.

capillary blood sugar (CBS).

capillary leak syndrome—extravasation of plasma fluid and proteins into the extravascular space, sometimes resulting in fatal hypotension and reduced organ perfusion; an adverse effect of aldesleukin (interleukin-2) therapy.

Capio CL transvaginal suture-capturing device—for suturing a sling to Cooper's ligament through a transvaginal approach without the need for an abdominal incision.

Capiox SX—gas and heat exchange oxygenation system.

capnograph (*capno-* pertains to carbon dioxide)—a graph displaying the results from an infrared spectrometer. The capnograph shows the results as CO_2 wave forms, and as numbers denoting value for $ETCO_2$ (end-tidal carbon dioxide concentration).

capnography—used in anesthesiology to record measurement of end-tidal carbon dioxide.

CaPPi (calcium pyrophosphate)—one of the salts of which bone is composed.

CAPPr (cyclophosphamide, Adriamycin, Platinol, prednisone)—chemotherapy protocol.

capravirine (formerly AG 1549)—an antiretroviral agent for HIV-infected patients.

Caprogel (aminocaproic acid)—topical gel for bleeding in the eyes, usually as a result of trauma.

CAPS ArthroWand—collagen shrinkage wand used in arthroscopic surgery.

Capset (calcium sulfate) **bone graft barrier**—applied following bone graft procedure to keep grafted bone or bone substitute from migrating and to prevent unwanted tissue formation before the grafted material has had time to integrate and heal.

CAPS-free diet:
C caffeine
A alcohol
P pepper
S spicy foods

capsulorrhexis (also capsulorhexis)—circular anterior capsulotomy; rupture of a structure enveloping an organ, vessel, or joint. See *continuous circular capsulorrhexis technique, posterior capsulorrhexis with optic capture,* and *two-stage capsulorrhexis for endocapsular phacoemulsification.*

CAPSure ArthroWand—applies radiofrequency to achieve capsular shrinkage.

Capsure steroid-eluting electrode.

CAPS X—thermal ArthroWand for capsular shrinkage.

captopril (Capoten)—a common antihypertensive drug now also used to treat diabetic nephropathy and prevent diabetic renal disease in patients with type 1 diabetes mellitus.

caput—the head; also used in reference to the expanded part of an organ or muscle. Cf. *caput medusae.*

caput medusae—dilated veins around the umbilicus. So named because of the resemblance to the snakes which formed the hair of Medusa in Greek mythology. Seen in patients with cirrhosis of the liver, and in some newborns. Cf. *caput.*

Carabello sign—a rise in arterial blood pressure during left heart catheter pull-back in patients with severe aortic stenosis.

carbacephems—a class of antibiotics similar to cephalosporins. Example: loracarbef (Lorabid).

Carbatrol (carbamazepine sustained-release)—primary therapy for control of partial and some types of generalized seizures. It is also used as an antipsychotic and an analgesic for trigeminal neuralgia.

Carbex (selegiline)—used for treating Parkinson's disease.

Carbomedics prosthetic heart valve (CPHV).

Carbo-Seal—zero-porosity cardiovascular composite graft.

carbolfuchsin stain—Tilden's method, to study mouth organisms.

carbon dioxide laser—see *laser.*

carbon fiber—synthetic ligament material.

carbonaceous material—smoke inhalation debris deposited in the nose and upper respiratory tract.

carbonate-apatite (Lab).

carbovir—a drug used to treat AIDS.

carboxyhemoglobin—levels measured in patients exposed to fires and in attempted suicides using automobile exhaust. Carbon monoxide binds competitively with hemoglobin molecules, excluding oxygen.

carcinoembryonic antigen (CEA)—present in many cases of carcinoma, particularly of the lung, digestive tract, and pancreas. It is valuable in testing treated cancer patients for recurrence of metastases.

carcinoma ex pleomorphic adenoma—a type of malignant pleomorphic adenoma (appearing as two or more distinct forms of tumor) that usually occurs in the salivary glands of older adults. An epithelial malignancy arises in a preexisting mixed tumor, with metastasis only of the malignant epithelial component. Also called *malignant mixed tumor.*

carcinoma in situ (CIS).

carcinoma of bladder classification—see *Jewett's classification.*

cardiac allograft vascular disease (CAVD)—cardiac disease occurring after heart transplantation.

Cardiac Assist intra-aortic balloon catheter—a device to assist the heart before and after open-heart surgery and complex balloon angioplasty procedures.

cardiac device—see *device* and specific categories, such as *catheter.*

cardiac hybrid revascularization procedure—in which minimally invasive surgery is first used to treat the principal coronary artery, while interventional therapies such as balloon angioplasty and coronary stenting are then used to treat other blocked vessels.

cardiac retraction clip—used to retract the fatty layer over the heart during coronary artery anastomosis.

cardiac risk factors—elevated blood lipids, obesity, habitual dietary excesses, lack of exercise, hypertension, cigarette smoking, and stress.

cardiac shock wave therapy (CSWT).

cardiac sling—used to support the heart and expose the circumflex branch of the coronary artery during surgery.

Cardiac T Rapid Assay—a rapid bedside assay to diagnose myocardial infarction. Uses cardiac troponin T, which is found inside the cardiac muscle and released into the blood only when cells are damaged.

cardiac troponin T—used to test for myocardial infarction. The protein troponin T is elevated in myocardial infarction and is cardiac-specific, unlike CK-MB which may indicate other muscle injury. Also, the diagnostic window for troponin T is from one hour (before CK-MB shows up) to 14 days (long after CK-MB has returned to normal).

Cardia Salt Alternative—a salt substitute used by hypertensive patients.

Cardima Pathfinder microcatheter for diagnosis of cardiac tachyarrhythmia.

CardioBeeper CB-12L—cardiac monitoring device that allows for transmission of a complete 12-lead ECG, utilizing prefitted reusable electrodes, over a standard telephone line.

Cardiocap 5—a patient monitor designed for use in the operating room, ambulatory surgery unit, induction area, or PACU.

CardioCard—stores digital electrocardiogram records on an optical memory card.

CardioCoil coronary stent—a self-expanding stent used for prevention of re-stenosis following PTCA.

CardioFix Pericardium—patch for intracardiac repair and pericardial closure.

Cardiofreezer cryosurgical system.

cardiokymography (CKG)—for measuring interference in pacemaker function. Cardiokymography is used clinically at some institutions for detecting segmental wall motion abnormalities of the heart. It may interfere with cardiac pacemaker function and can cause the pacemaker to operate at its upper rate limit.

Cardiolite scan—a cardiac scan showing areas of myocardial infarction, using the radioactive imaging agent ^{99m}Tc sestamibi (Cardiolite).

Cardiomed Bodysoft epidural catheter—thermosensitive material of catheter softens when warmed to body temperature, minimizing patient trauma.

Cardiomed endotracheal ventilation catheter.

Cardiomed thermodilution catheter.

cardiomyoplasty—a surgical treatment for weakened heart muscle leading to congestive heart failure. In cardiomyoplasty, the latissimus dorsi muscle is surgically excised except for a pedicle that contains its blood and nerve supply. It is then inserted into the chest cavity through an opening created by excision of the second rib on the anterior chest. Two pacing electrode leads are placed in the muscle flap, and two sensing leads are placed on the heart itself. These leads are connected to a programmable pulse pacemaker which is placed surgically beneath the rectus abdominis muscle. The pacemaker synchronizes the contraction of the muscle flap to the R wave of the heart's own electrical rhythm. The number of bursts from the pacemaker is gradually increased after surgery until, after a few months, the skeletal muscle contracts with every heartbeat or every other heartbeat. After exposure to burst stimulation from the pacemaker, the skeletal muscle gradually changes its muscle fibers at the cellular level until they resemble those of heart muscle, which can contract repeatedly without fatigue.

cardioplegic solution—an iced solution injected into the coronary arteries during open-heart surgery to produce cardiac arrest. Composed of calcium, magnesium, potassium, chloride, and sodium bicarbonate in solution, it produces cardiac standstill, and protects the myocardium from damage due to intracellular ion imbalance and acidosis. Types:
ECS—extracellular-like, calcium-free solution
ICS—intracellular-like, calcium-bearing, crystalloid solution

Cardiopoint—cardiac surgery needles.

cardiopulmonary support system (CPS).

CardioSEAL septal occluder—a cardiac implant used in a minimally invasive, catheter-based procedure to close heart defects.

Cardiosol—a patented human organ preservation solution designed for use during heart transplantation and open-heart surgery. Also, *HK-Cardiosol* and *CP-Cardiosol*.

Cardio Tactilaze peripheral angioplasty laser catheter—contains an Nd:YAG laser to vaporize atheromatous plaques.

CardioTec scan—a cardiac scan showing areas of myocardial infarction, using the radioactive imaging agent ^{99m}Tc teboroxime (CardioTec). Used for emergency scans, it clears rapidly from the blood to allow subsequent scans, if necessary.

cardiothoracic ratio (CTR).

cardiotocography—method of fetal monitoring.

Cardizem Lyo-Ject—an injectable form of Cardizem, given in 25 mg doses.

Cardizem Monovial—advanced infusion delivery system for the injectable form of Cardizem, prescribed for certain heartbeat irregularities.

Cardura (doxazosin mesylate).

CARES (Cancer Rehabilitation Evaluation System)—cancer-specific health-related quality-of-life assessment.

Carlesta—an over-the-counter topical preparation for the prevention and treatment of skin irritation associated with adult incontinence.

Carmeda BioActive Surface—extracorporeal circuit whose surface reduces thrombogenesis and preserves platelet function.

C-arm fluoroscopy—image intensifier, portable x-ray unit used in the operating room.

carmine dye (also called *cochineal extract*)—color additive extracted from dried female cochineal insects and commonly used in fruit drinks, candy, yogurt, and other foods. It can cause anaphylactic shock in some people.

carmustine wafer—biodegradable wafer impregnated with carmustine, inserted into the cavity after surgical removal of recurrent glioblastoma multiforme, delivering medication directly to brain tumor site.

Caroli disease—one of the reasons for liver transplant in children.

Carolina rocker—a wheelchair on a rocker platform, used in physical therapy for patients with stroke, and also for tardive dyskinesia.

carotene—the yellow or red coloring found in egg yolk, carrots, and sweet potatoes. Cf. *creatine, creatinine, keratin.*

carotid angioplasty with stenting—noninvasive alternative to carotid endarterectomy. A balloon catheter is threaded from groin to neck and pushed into the clogged section under fluoroscopic guidance. After flattening of plaque and removal of the balloon, another catheter deposits the metal stent to keep the artery open.

CarotidCoil stent—designed to resist compression after placement in the neck arteries to maintain blood flow to the brain.

carotid sinus massage—used as the provocative test for the detection of sinus node disease, which is the most common indication for pacemaker implantation.

carpal compression test—performed by applying direct pressure on the carpal tunnel, and considered by many to be more sensitive and specific than the Tinel or Phalen tests.

Carpal Lock cock-up splint (Phys Ther).

carpal tunnel syndrome (CTS)—caused by repetitive hand motions, such as prolonged keyboard use, or hammering, filing, or writing, resulting in compression of the soft

carpal tunnel *(cont.)*
median nerve against the volar carpal ligament by the nine comparatively harder tendons that are in the tunnel with it. Depending on the degree of pressure, symptoms range from aching and numbness over the median nerve distribution (but sparing the little finger), to constant hypesthesia and paralysis of the abductor pollicis brevis. Also, *repetitive strain injury.*

Carpentier-Edwards Perimount RSR pericardial bioprosthesis—a tissue heart valve designed for patients with small heart valves. It is implanted in a position that improves blood flow and decreases the need for anticoagulant drugs.

Carpentier-Edwards Physio annuloplasty ring.

carphology—purposeless plucking at clothing or bedclothes; sometimes seen in dementia or terminal illness.

carprofen (Rimadyl)—a nonsteroidal anti-inflammatory drug.

CarraFilm—transparent film dressings used as wound coverings for wounds with light exudate.

CarraSmart foam—a self-adhesive foam dressing with water-attracting properties used for skin ulcers, pressure sores, burns, abrasions, and lacerations. This "smart" foam manages the moisture balance of a wound with its absorption and evaporative properties.

Carra Sorb H—a calcium alginate wound dressing used in the management of heavily exuding wounds.

Carra Sorb M—a freeze-dried gel with aloe vera gel extract, containing acemannan, used for the medium exudating wound.

Carrasyn Hydrogel—wound dressing.

Carrión's disease—a tropical infection caused by *Bartonella bacilliformis.*

Carr-Purcell-Meiboom-Gill sequence—MRI term.

Carr-Purcell sequence—MRI term.

Carswell's grapes—clusters of tubercles around the smaller bronchioles, looking like a bunch of grapes; seen in pulmonary tuberculosis.

Carter pillow—a foam cushion which immobilizes and elevates simultaneously; often used in replantation procedures.

Carter-Thomason suture passer—for ligation of bleeding vessels in the abdominal wall as well as other laparoscopic surgical applications.

Carticel autologous cultured chondrocytes—a tissue repair product used to grow a patient's own cartilage cells to repair knee damage.

Cartilade—shark cartilage that presently has a use patent for inhibition of angiogenesis.

carvedilol (Coreg)—antihypertensive medication.

CAS (contralateral acoustic stimulation).

CAS (coronary artery scan).

caseation—necrosed tissue resembling cheesy material.

CA 72-4—a cancer antigen serum tumor marker to monitor metastatic gastric cancer.

CASH (classic abdominal Semm hysterectomy).

Casodex (bicalutamide)—an antiandrogen for the treatment of advanced prostate cancer.

CAST (Cardiac Arrhythmic Suppression Trial)—a cardiac protocol. May be followed by a roman numeral.

cast, casting material
Cotton Loader position
Fractura Flex
Gypsona
Hexcelite
hip spica
MaxCast
Minerva-type
Risser localizer
Sarmiento
spica
Castanares face-lift scissors.
Castaneda anastomosis clamp.
Castaneda bottle—used in the culture of certain organisms from blood.
Cast Boot (trademark)—polypropylene hip abduction brace for treating hip dysplasia in toddlers up to $2^1/2$ years of age.
Castleman's disease—a rare B-cell lymphoproliferation disorder that occurs in two forms. The more common localized Castleman's disease often presents as an asymptomatic mediastinal mass and usually is cured by surgical removal of the mediastinal mass. The rarer form, multicentric Castleman's disease, often presents as multisystem illness with widespread lymphadenopathy. It has a poor prognosis but may respond to prednisone, chemotherapy or surgical removal of affected nodes and spleen.
Castroviejo-Colibri forceps.
cast syndrome—a rare but sometimes fatal condition in which a body cast occludes the blood supply to the duodenum.
CAT ("cat") (computerized, or computed, axial tomography). Also called *ACAT, CT,* and *CAT scan.* See *computed tomography scan.*

Cataflam (diclofenac potassium)—immediate release tablets for acute and chronic treatment of rheumatoid arthritis, osteoarthritis, and ankylosing spondylitis. Also for management of pain and primary dysmenorrhea. Not for patients hypersensitive to aspirin, other nonsteroidal anti-inflammatory drugs, or diclofenac.
Catapres (clonidine).
cataract—opacity of the lens of the eye, or its capsule, or both. Types include *brunescent, mature, posterior subcapsular, senile,* and *traumatic.*
Catarex—surgical device for cataract removal through a 1 to 2 mm hole created in the lens capsule. It uses a mechanical energy source, with the procedure taking less than 10 minutes.
Catatrol (viloxazine)—bicyclic antidepressant.
catch—term for a sharp, localized pain, usually in the chest, and provoked or aggravated by drawing a breath (inspiration).
CATCH 22—acronym for the major features of microdeletion of chromosome 22q11:
C cardiac defect
A abnormal face
T thymic hypoplasia
C cleft palate
H hypocalcemia
cat cry syndrome—a chromosome abnormality including multiple heart and eye abnormalities, mental retardation, microcephaly, and a mewing cry, thus its name. Also called *cri du chat syndrome.*
cat's eye calculi (Radiol)—gallstones in the common bile duct resulting from metallic surgical clips from previous

cat's eye calculi *(cont.)*
surgical procedure, so-called because of radiographic appearance of stones.

cat's eye pupil (also, *cat's eye reflex*) — unusual appearance of the pupil resembling that of a light shining into a cat's eye. It is seen in retinoblastoma.

cat's eye reflex—sign of retinoblastoma.

catgut—see *surgical gut.*

cathepsin D—lysozomal enzyme used to label fibroblasts, macrophages, sweat ducts and glands, smooth muscle, and stratum granulosum in normal tissue, and now being used as a prognostic marker in breast tumors.

catheter
Abscession fluid drainage
Achiever balloon dilatation
ACS Concorde
ACS Endura coronary dilation
ACS OTW (over-the-wire)
    Lifestream coronary dilatation
ACS OTW (over-the-wire) Photon
ACS RX Comet coronary dilatation
ACS Tourguide II guiding
AcuNav ultrasound
Ahn thrombectomy
Alzate
Amazr
Angiocath PRN
AngioOptic microcatheter
Anthron heparinized
arrhythmia mapping system
Arrowgard Blue Line
Arrow-Howes multilumen
Arrow Twin Cath
Ascent guiding
atherectomy
AtheroCath
AtheroCath Bantam coronary
    atherectomy

catheter *(cont.)*
Auth atherectomy
balloon biliary
Beta-Cath system
bifoil balloon
Blue FlexTip
Brevi-Kath epidural
Bronchitrac L
Burhenne steerable
Calypso Rely
Camino intracranial
Camino microventricular bolt
Cardiac Assist intra-aortic balloon
Cardima Pathfinder microcatheter
Cardiomed Bodysoft epidural
Cardiomed endotracheal ventilation
Cardiomed thermodilution
Cardio Tactilaze peripheral
    angioplasty laser
Cath-Finder
CCOmbo
central venous (CVC)
Cheetah angioplasty
Chemo-Port
Chilli cooled ablation
CliniCath peripherally inserted
Closure System by VNUS
Comfort Cath I or II
Conceptus Soft Seal cervical
Conceptus Soft Torque uterine
Conceptus VS (variable softness)
Constellation mapping
Cook TPN
Cool Tip
Cordis Predator PTCA balloon
Cordis Trakstar PTCA balloon
coudé
CrossSail coronary dilatation
cutdown
Cutting Balloon microsurgical
    dilatation
Dale Foley
Datascope
Dorros infusion/probing

catheter *(cont.)*

Double J indwelling
Double J ureteral
Du Pen long-term epidural
DURAglide3 stone balloon
EAC (expandable access catheter)
EchoMark
EndoCPB (endovascular cardio-
pulmonary bypass)
Endosound endoscopic ultrasound
Endotak C lead
EnSite cardiac
Erythroflex
e-TRAIN 110 AngioJet
Evert-O-Cath
eXamine cholangiography
Express PTCA
FACT (Focal Angioplasty Catheter
Technology)
Falcon coronary
Fast-Cath introducer
Flexguard Tip
Flexxicon Blue dialysis
Fogarty adherent clot
Fogarty balloon biliary
Fogarty graft thrombectomy
Force balloon dilatation
Freezor cryocatheter
Gold Probe bipolar hemostasis
Grollman
Groshong
Grüntzig balloon (Gruentzig)
Hartzler ACX-II or RX-014 balloon
HealthShield mediastinal wound
drainage
Hickman
Hieshima coaxial
Hohn central venous
Hurwitz dialysis
Hydrolyser microcatheter
ICP (intracranial pressure)
Illumen-8 guiding
ILUS (intraluminal ultrasound)
Infiniti

catheter *(cont.)*

InfusaSleeve II
Intracath
Intran disposable intrauterine
pressure measurement
intravascular ultrasound (IVUS)
intrepid PTCA angioplasty
ITC balloon
IVUS (intravascular ultrasound)
Jackman orthogonal
Jelco intravenous
JL4 (Judkins left 4 cm curve)
JL5 (Judkins left 5 cm curve)
Judkins 4 diagnostic
Kaye tamponade balloon
KDF-2.3
Kifa
Kinsey atherectomy
Kish urethral illuminated
KISS (Kidney Internal Splint/Stent)
Koala intrauterine pressure
Konton
L-Cath peripherally inserted
neonatal
Lifestream coronary dilatation
Livewire TC ablation
MammoSite RTS (radiation therapy
system)
Marathon guiding
Mark IV Moss decompression-
feeding
Max Force
Mercator atrial high-density array
MicroMewi multiple sidehole
infusion
Millar MPC-500
Millenia balloon
Moss decompression feeding
MS Classique balloon dilatation
multiflanged Portnoy (for hydro-
cephalus shunts)
Multipurpose-SM
Naviport deflectable tip guiding
Neo-Sert umbilical vessel

catheter *(cont.)*
  nephrostomy-type
  NeuroVasx (Sub-Microinfusion)
  Nexus 2 linear ablation
  NoProfile balloon
  NovaCath multi-lumen infusion
  Nutricath
  OmniCath atherectomy
  On-Command (male and female)
  Oracle Focus
  Oracle Megasonics
  Oracle Micro
  Oracle Micro Plus
  Oreopoulos-Zellerman
  Pace bipolar pacing
  P.A.S. Port
  P.A.S. Port Fluoro-Free
  Pathfinder
  Periflow peripheral balloon
  PermCath double-lumen ventricular
    access
  Phantom V Plus
  PIC (peripherally inserted)
  PICC (peripherally inserted central)
  Pico-ST II
  pigtail
  Pipelle endometrial suction
  Polystan
  ProCross Rely over-the-wire
    balloon
  Pro-Flo XT
  Quinton Mahurkar dual lumen
  Ranfac cholangiographic
  Reddick cystic duct cholangiogram
  Reddick-Saye screw
  Redifurl TaperSeal IAB
  Reliance urinary control insert
  remote access perfusion (RAP)
    cannula
  Response electrophysiology
  Rigiflex TTS balloon
  Rivas vascular
  Rsch-Uchida transjugular liver
    access needle-catheter

catheter *(cont.)*
  Sable
  SCA-EX ShortCutter
  SCOOP 1; SCOOP 2
  Seroma-Cath
  SET three-lumen thrombectomy
  Shaldon
  Sherpa guiding
  SPI-Argent II peritoneal dialysis
  Simpson atherectomy
  Simpson peripheral AtheroCath
  Skinny dilatation
  Slinky
  soaker
  Soft Torque uterine
  Soft-Vu Omni flush
  Solo catheter with Pro/Pel coating
  SoloPass
  Sones woven Dacron
  Speedy balloon
  SPI-Argent II peritoneal dialysis
  split sheath
  Spyglass angiography
  Stamey-Malecot
  St. Jude 4F Supreme electro-
    physiology
  Sub-Microinfusion
  Suction Buster
  Supreme electrophysiology
  SureCuff
  surgically implanted hemodialysis
    (SIHC)
  Swan-Ganz
  swan-neck
  Swartz SL Series Fast-Cath
    introducer
  Syntel latex-free embolectomy
  Tactilaze angioplasty laser
  Targis microwave catheter-based
    system
  Taut cystic duct
  Tenckhoff peritoneal dialysis
  Tennis Racquet
  thermodilution

catheter *(cont.)*
  Tis-u-trap endometrial suction
  Torcon NB selective angiographic
  Tourguide guiding
  Tracker-18 Soft Stream
  transluminal extraction (TEC)
  transtracheal oxygen
  T-TAC (transcervical tubal access)
  TTS (through the scope)
  twist drill
  Uldall (*not* Udall) subclavian
    hemodialysis
  Ultra 8 balloon
  UltraLite flow-directed
    microcatheter
  umbilical artery (UAC)
  Ureflex
  UroMax II
  vanSonnenberg-Wittich
  Vas-Cath
  Vector and VectorX large-lumen
    guiding
  Ventra
  Ventureyra ventricular
  Verbatim balloon
  Veripath peripheral guiding
  vessel-sizing
  Visa II PTCA
  Vision PTCA
  Vitesse Cos laser
  Vitesse E-II
  VNUS Restore
  Von Andel
  Was-Cath
  whistletip ureteral
  Witzel enterostomy
  Workhorse percutaneous trans-
    luminal angioplasty balloon
  Wurd
  XL-11
  Xpeedior 60
  X-trode electrode
  Z-Med
  Zuma guiding

catheter balloon valvuloplasty—performed for severe calcific aortic stenosis.

catheter-directed thrombolysis and endovascular stent placement—treatment for SVC (superior vena cava) syndrome.

catheter vitrector—Verbatim balloon probe.

Cath-Finder—catheter tracking system, part of the P.A.S. Port system that tracks the catheter tip during placement, without fluoroscopy.

CathLink implantable vascular access device.

Cath-Secure—a hypoallergenic tape with an attached fastener to hold a triple-lumen central catheter in place.

CathTrack catheter locator system—handheld device used to determine catheter tip placement.

cat-scratch disease (CSD)—a *Bartonella henselae* infection acquired through the bite or scratch of a cat.

Cattell Infant Intelligence Scale.

cauda—tail, or structure resembling a tail. See *tail.*

caudate, adj., having a tail, as in "caudate lobe." Cf. *chordate, cordate.*

cauliflower ear—slang term for an external ear deformed by repeated or severe trauma, as in boxers and wrestlers.

cautery (electrocautery)
  BiLAP bipolar
  bipolar
  Concept handheld
  Mira
  NeoKnife
  Op-Temp
  Scheie ophthalmic
  wet field

CAV (cyclophosphamide, Adriamycin, vincristine)—chemotherapy protocol for neuroblastoma.

CAVD (cardiac allograft vascular disease).

Caverject (prostaglandin E1, PGE1, alprostadil)—intracavernous injection as treatment for erectile failure. Produces penile rigidity and an erection with satisfactory vaginal intercourse.

CaverMap surgical device—assists in sparing vital nerves typically damaged during prostate cancer surgery.

cavernous hemangioma—one of the most common benign intraorbital tumors, found typically within the cone of the extraocular muscles. Removal of cavernomas located in the basal, inferomedial, and lateral aspect of the orbit may be done by a microneurosurgical transconjunctival approach. Other surgical approaches include transcranial and direct orbital.

Cavilon barrier ointment—forms an occlusive barrier to block transepidermal water loss.

Cavitron ultrasonic surgical aspirator (CUSA)—used in the resection of lung tumors. It can fragment and aspirate tissue at a selected margin from a tumor, leaving airways and vessels intact to be ligated. This operation can be performed in a bloodless fashion with direct visualization of adequate margins. It can also be used to resect large masses of residual germ cell tumor following chemotherapy by insertion directly through the tumor pseudocapsule, fragmenting the giant mass and collapsing the pseudocapsule, facilitat-ing exposure of mediastinal vessels and nerves. The collapsed pseudocapsule can then be excised, allowing the underlying lung to expand normally.

CAVP16 (cyclophosphamide, Adriamycin, VP-16)—chemotherapy protocol.

cavum conchal cartilage graft—a graft harvested from the lower cavernous portion of the concha of the auricle, used in rhinoplasty. See also *cymba conchal cartilage graft*.

C-bar web-spacer—a device used to prevent burn contractures. It is a plastic appliance that fits around the wrist and has a protrusion that supports the thumb and stretches the web space so that the configuration of the thumb and the rest of the fingers is much like a letter *C*.

CBF (cochlear blood flow) (ENT).

CBFV (cerebral blood flow velocity).

CBP (chronic bacterial prostatitis)—may be treated with the antiobiotic Maxaquin.

CBP-1011—drug used in treatment of idiopathic thrombocytopenic purpura.

CBS (capillary blood sugar)—a test for hypoglycemia. It enables a patient to take a blood sugar reading by a fingerstick.

CBWO (closing base wedge osteotomy).

C Cap (compliance cap)—a device on containers of medications for glaucoma, to help patients track medication compliance.

CCB (calcium channel blocker).

CCD (central collodiaphyseal angle) in the shaft and neck of long bones.

CCE (clubbing, cyanosis, and edema).

CCE (counterflow centrifugation elutriation).

CC49 monoclonal antibody—labeled with 177 lutetium. Given intravenously to patients with advanced adenocarcinoma.

CCH (circumscribed choroidal hemangioma).

C-cholyl-glycine breath excretion test —highly sensitive test indicating bacterial overgrowth in small intestine or ileal disease. See *C-urea breath test.*

CCO (continuous cardiac output).

CCOmbo catheter—measures pressures inside the heart with continuous cardiac output (CCO).

CCPD (continuous cyclical peritoneal dialysis)—method of maintenance dialysis in patients with end-stage renal disease.

CCS (Certified Coding Specialist).

CCS-P (Certified Coding Specialist–Physician-based).

CCUP (colpocystourethropexy).

CD (color Doppler) (Rad).

CDA (chenodeoxycholic acid)—used to dissolve gallstones in patients at higher surgical risk, who are slender, who have noncalcium gallstones, and who tend to have higher serum cholesterol levels. Cf. *2-CdA.*

CDAD (*Clostridium difficile*-associated diarrhea).

CDC—the Centers (*not* Center) for Disease Control and Prevention in Atlanta, Georgia, federal clearinghouse for information on epidemic diseases. In addition to being a pool of information for researchers and practicing physicians, the CDC sometimes has investigational drugs available.

CDCR (conjunctivodacryocystorhinostomy).

CDE (cyclophosphamide, doxorubicin, etoposide)—chemotherapy protocol for small cell lung carcinoma.

CD4-IgG—a drug used to treat HIV-positive mothers and babies.

CD4, recombinant soluble human (Receptin, rCD4)—a drug used in the treatment of AIDS.

CD5+ monoclonal antibody—used in treating graft-versus-host disease.

CD5-T lymphocyte immunotoxin— see *XomaZyme-H65.*

CD8 AIS CELLector—a device used in treatment for Kaposi's sarcoma, a rare form of skin cancer that affects HIV-positive patients. The CD8 AIS CELLector isolates the patient's CD8 cells, which serve to separate and multiply the patient's own cancer-killing cells. Additional applications include the processing of stem cells for transfusion or bone marrow transplantation, and the treatment of cancer and AIDS.

CD18 antibodies—may, in the future, help reduce some kinds of heart damage after a heart attack. In research trials, the antibodies prevent the attachment to the artery walls of polymorphonuclear leukocytes which form as a result of heart injury, usually attaching first to arterial walls and then squeezing through them into the heart tissue. With CD18 antibodies, the PMNs continue to circulate harmlessly through the body.

CD26—a protease. This HIV co-receptor acts as a door for cell penetration. Scientists hope to use this new target to develop a vaccine for all HIV strains.

CDH (congenital dysplasia of the hip). Also, dislocation.

CDI (Cotrel-Dubousset instrumentation).

CDI 2000 blood gas monitoring system—bedside (point of care) monitoring system that measures arterial pH, PCO_2, and PO_2. The system decreases therapeutic decision time and is advantageous for patients needing frequent blood gas monitoring. Lack of blood loss and reduced infection risk to patient and operator are major advantages.

cDNA (complementary DNA).

CDP (computerized dynamic posturography).

CDR (computed dental radiography).

Cd-texaphyrin—photosensitizing agent used in laser surgery.

CE (capillary electrophoresis)—a technique for rapid separation and analysis of peptides and proteins.

CEA (carcinoembryonic antigen).

CEA (carotid endarterectomy).

CEAker—an anti-CEA monoclonal antibody labeled with indium 111; used to detect recurrent colorectal carcinoma.

CEAP classification—used in diagnosis of chronic venous disease of the lower extremities: assesses **c**linical manifestations, **e**tiologic factors, **a**natomic involvement, and **p**athophysiologic features.

CEA-Scan—a diagnostic imaging product for screening of colorectal cancer. The technique uses radiolabeled antibodies in conjunction with technetium 99m to detect tumors within hours, using conventional gamma cameras. The use of a small fragment of antibody will reduce immune reactions by patients to the foreign protein.

CEA-Tc 99m—carcinoembryonic antigen (a monoclonal antibody) plus ^{99m}Tc (a technetium isotope) imaging agent. See *RAID, ImmuRAID*.

CEB (carboplatin, etoposide, bleomycin)—chemotherapy protocol for metastatic testicular carcinoma.

Cebotome—orthopedic tool by Zimmer. Also, *Neurairtome, Surgairtome*.

CECA (cisplatin, etoposide, cyclophosphamide, Adriamycin)—chemotherapy protocol.

CECT (contrast enhancement of computed tomographic) head and body imaging.

Cedax (ceftibuten)—oral, broad-spectrum cephalosporin antibiotic, used in the treatment of pharyngitis, tonsillitis, acute bacterial otitis media, and acute bacterial exacerbation of chronic bronchitis.

Cedell fracture—fracture of posterior process of the talus which may result in tarsal tunnel syndrome.

CeeOn heparinized intraocular lens.

CEF (cyclophosphamide, epirubicin, fluorouracil)—chemotherapy protocol for breast carcinoma.

cefmetazole (Zefazone)—a second-generation cephalosporin similar in action to that of cefoxitin (Mefoxin). Used for treating infections by susceptible gram-positive and gram-negative bacteria; given prophylactically in abdominal surgery.

cefpodoxime proxetil (Vantin)—second-generation cephalosporin antibiotic used to treat respiratory, urinary, and skin infections as well as gonorrhea.

cefprozil (Cefzil)—a cephalosporin antibiotic used to treat ENT, pulmonary, and skin infections.

ceftibuten (Cedax)—a third-generation cephalosporin that is similar to Ceclor in its action.

Cefzil (cefprozil).

Celebrex (celecoxib)—modified nonsteroidal anti-inflammatory drug that does not cause GI bleeding. It is used to relieve the signs and symptoms of osteoarthritis and adult rheumatoid arthritis. A COX-2 inhibitor.

Celestin latex rubber tube—used in dilation of the esophagus in treatment for peptic stricture.

Celexa (citalopram HBr)—SSRI (selective serotonin reuptake inhibitor) in an oral solution for treatment of depression. May also be useful in treating Alzheimer's disease.

celiac dimple—the anatomic area of slight depression in the abdomen.

celiacography—used to diagnose hemangiomata.

celiprolol (Selecor)—a cardioselective beta blocker drug for hypertension and angina. Other possible uses include post myocardial infarction prophylaxis, migraine, and arrhythmias.

cell
Betz
Bloch
clue
Deiters'
eating (phagocyte)
eukaryotic
foam
gelbe
glitter
ground-glass
HeLa
helle
helper
hybridoma
inducer
islet

cell *(cont.)*
koilocytotic
Kulchitsky
Kupffer
LAK (lymphokine-activated killer)
Leydig
LUCs (large undifferentiated cells)
macrophage colon-forming (M-CFC)
mast
NK (natural killer)
null
oxyphil
peripheral blood progenitor (PBPC)
Pelger-Huët
phagocyte
prickle-cell layer
Sézary
stem
suppressor
Tart
T-cell (thymus)
T-8 suppressor
T-4
theca
thymus dependent
TRC
umbrella
universal donor
zymogen

cell and flare (*not* flair) (Oph)—an accumulation of white blood cells and an increase of protein in the aqueous which can be seen on slit-lamp examination of the anterior chamber of the eye. A sign of iritis or ciliary body inflammation.

Cellano phenotype (Kell blood group) —see *McLeod blood phenotype.*

cell assay test—see *Raji cell assay test.*

CellCept (mycophenolate mofetil)—a drug shown to decrease the incidence of transplant rejection by half.

cell-mediated immunity (CMI).

Cellolite—a form of patty material (see *cottonoid patty*) produced as an alternative to cottonoid; made of polyvinyl alcohol foam cross-linked with formaldehyde, and impregnated with particles of barium sulfate.

Cellpatch—an investigational drug delivery system that enables both the formation of a standardized small epidermal bleb and exposure of the circular base of the bleb to drug. The epidermis is split off by suctioning without bleeding or discomfort in a layer superficial to dermal capillaries and nociceptor nerves. Transdermal invasion is thus avoided.

cell ratio—see *helper/suppressor*.

Cell Recovery System (CRS)—an automated medical device used to brush and retrieve cells from surfaces of internal organs, such as the bladder. The endoscopic procedure is minimally invasive and can be performed in a physician's office.

Cell Saver Haemolite—a washed red cell autotransfusion system for use in low-volume blood loss procedures. Can be used intraoperatively and postoperatively.

celltrifuge—a coined word for a device to remove white blood cells from blood of patients with leukemia.

Cellugel ophthalmic viscosurgical device (OVD)—viscoelastic solution for use in the anterior segment of the eye. It is used to create and maintain space, to protect the corneal endothelium and other intraocular tissues, and to manipulate tissues during surgery.

cellular xenograft rejection—rejection reaction involving the transplantation of cells or tissue of animal origin, thought to be T-cell mediated as in an allograft rejection response.

cellular xenotransplantation—transplantation of tissue or cells of animal origin, more successful than solid organ xenotransplantation.

Celsior—an organ preservation solution used to preserve the heart prior to cardiac transplantation and to promote graft function in the initial 48 hours after cardiac transplant.

CEM (cytosine arabinoside, etoposide, methotrexate)—chemotherapy protocol.

cement—see *adhesive*.

Cementless Sportorno (CLS) hip arthroplasty stem.

cementophyte—an excrescence of cement (such as methylmethacrylate), the result of a previous arthrotomy, in contrast to osteophyte, which is a bony excrescence or osseous outgrowth.

Cemex system (Ortho)—an integrated system that contains, prepares, and extrudes bone cement.

Cenestin (synthetic conjugated estrogen)—used for treatment of vasomotor symptoms due to menopause.

Cenflex central monitoring system.

Centauri Er:YAG laser system—for tooth procedures, including decay removal, cavity preparation for restorations, and related applications. It works by vaporizing the bacteria along with the decay to provide a virtually sterile area for restoration. Reportedly eliminates the need for traditional dental anesthesia and the drill.

center-edge (CE) **angle of Wiberg**.

Centers for Disease Control and Prevention (CDC).

centigray (cGy)—an SI unit of absorbed radiation dose equal to 1 rad. See *gray*.

centimeter (cm)—often pronounced "sonameter."

centistoke—a unit of measurement of plasma viscosity and serum viscosity.

Centovir—a drug used to treat cytomegalovirus infection. Also known as *monoclonal antibody C-58*.

Centoxin (nebacumab)—the Ha-1A monoclonal antibody which acts as an immunostimulant. See *Ha-1A monoclonal antibody*.

central venous catheter (CVC)—an intravenous catheter inserted into the subclavian vein (occasionally into the internal jugular vein) and advanced so that the tip is just above the right atrium. Used to administer fluids, drugs, or total parenteral nutrition on a long-term basis.

Centralign Precoat Hip prosthesis—precoat cemented hip replacement components by Zimmer.

centric relation-centric occlusion (CR/CO).

CEP (CCNU, etoposide, prednimustine)—chemotherapy protocol.

cephalopelvic disproportion (CPD)—a condition in which the head of the fetus is too large to enter the pelvic outlet; used in ultrasound and x-ray pelvimetry reports.

cephalosporins—a group of antibiotics with a broad spectrum of antibacterial activity, divided into first-, second-, and third-generation cephalosporins. This designation has nothing to do with when these antibiotics were discovered or first marketed, but instead divides them by their therapeutic antibiotic properties. First generation, such as cefazolin (Ancef) and cephalexin (Keflex), are generally inactivated by bacteria that produce penicillinase. Third genera-tion, such as cefixime (Suprax) and ceftazidime (Fortaz, Tazidime), show the greatest activity against gram-negative bacteria and resistant strains of bacteria.

Cephulac (lactulose)—used to prevent and treat portal-systemic encephalopathy.

Ceptaz (ceftazidime pentahydrate)—cephalosporin antibiotic.

c-erb B-2 oncogene—a factor predicting treatment response and prognosis in node-negative breast cancer patients.

cerclage—encircling, hooping, banding. Also *cervical cerclage*, used for incompetent cervix in pregnancy. See *Dall-Miles cable grip*.

cerebellopontile angle tumor—a brain tumor located between the cerebellum and the pons. It involves cranial nerves V through VIII. Spasms of eyelid muscles, oscillating eye movements, loss of corneal sensation, and impaired hearing are characteristic symptoms.

cerebral blood flow velocity (CBFV).

cerebral perfusion pressure (CPP).

cerebrolysin (FPF 1070)—drug that appears to improve cognitive function, noncognitive psychiatric symptoms, and behavior in Alzheimer's disease patients.

cerebrovascular accident (CVA)—a stroke.

Cerebyx (fosphenytoin)—intravenous antiepileptic drug for acute treatment of status epilepticus (nonstop uncontrolled seizures). Cerebyx will gradually replace I.V. Dilantin (phenytoin).

Ceredase (alglucerase)—replacement enzyme used for treatment of Gaucher's disease.

Ceresine—a pyruvate dehydrogenase stimulator for use in treatment of traumatic brain injury, including bleeding into the brain.

Ceretec—technetium 99m (Tc-99m) contrast imaging agent commonly used with SPECT imaging to detect cerebrovascular accidents. It may also be used to help diagnose Alzheimer's disease.

Cerezyme—replacement enzyme for treatment of Gaucher's disease.

Cernevit-12 (multivitamin for infusion) —lyophilized sterile powder containing water-soluble and fat-soluble vitamins. It is used as a maintenance dosage for patients receiving parenteral nutrition.

ceroid-like histiocytic granuloma—see *xanthogranulomatous cholecystitis*.

Certified Coding Specialist (CCS).

Certified Coding Specialist–Physician-based (CCS-P).

Certified Medical Transcriptionist (CMT)—an individual who has satisfied the requirements for voluntary certification through the American Association for Medical Transcription (AAMT).

Certified Nurse Midwife (CNM).

Cervex-Brush—used to simultaneously obtain ectocervical and endocervical cells for cytologic exam.

cervical aortic arch—an anomaly in which the aortic arch retains a cervical position. (The heart and aortic arches begin as cervical structures and migrate to the thorax during fetal development.) It is of no clinical significance in terms of symptomatology, but important in the differential diagnosis of pulsatile masses in the neck.

cervical intraepithelial neoplasia—see *CIN*.

cervical rib—a congenital anomaly in which an extra rib arises from a cervical vertebra. There is controversy over whether this is a normal variant or a condition requiring surgery.

cervical collar or support
 AOA halo traction
 Bremer Halo Crown
 Georgiade visor
 Houston Halo traction
 Miami Acute Collar
 Miami J collar
 Philadelphia collar
 Plastizote
 PMT halo system

cervicography, cervigram (Ob-Gyn)— a noninvasive technique for photographing the cervix. It is similar to colposcopy but less expensive. Colposcopy requires extensive expertise to perform and to read, but cervicography, in combination with a Pap smear, appears more reliable in detecting malignant and premalignant lesions than either procedure alone.

Cervidil (dinoprostone) **vaginal insert** —used to ripen the cervix for vaginal deliveries.

CES (cranial electrical stimulation).

cesium chloride—used in myocardial scanning.

cetiedil citrate—a drug used to treat sickle cell crisis.

cetirizine (Reactine, Zyrtec))—a nonsedating, long-acting antihistamine.

Cetrotide (cetrorelix for injection)—a luteinizing hormone-releasing hormone antagonist. It is used for the prevention of premature ovulation in patients undergoing controlled ovarian stimulation.

Cetus trial—a trial of tumor necrosis factor in conjunction with interleukin-2 in the treatment of cancers that have been unresponsive to other therapy. Cetus is the corporation that manufactures tumor necrosis factor. See *tumor necrosis factor*.

cf. (L., *confer*, compare).

CF (counting fingers) (Oph).

C_3F_8 gas (perfluoropropane)—used in pneumatic retinopexy, for correcting detached retina.

C-fiber—small unmyelinated nerve fiber.

CFIDS (chronic fatigue immune dysfunction syndrome).

CFL (calcaneofibular ligament).

CF-200Z Olympus colonoscope—a colonoscopic instrument which enables high-power magnified observation of the surface of colorectal neoplasms.

CFU (colony-forming unit).

CFU-E (colony-forming unit—erythroid).

CFU-GM (colony-forming unit—granulocyte, monocyte).

CFU-meg or **CFU-MK** (colony-forming unit—megakaryocyte).

CF-UM3 echocolonoscope.

CGL (chronic granulocytic leukemia).

cGy (centigray).

CHAG (coralline hydroxyapatite Goniopora)—a bone graft substitute material made by conversion of the calcium carbonate structure of reef-building sea corals into pure hydroxyapatite.

Chadwick's sign—purplish or bluish discoloration of the cervix and vaginal mucosa, a normal finding in pregnancy early in gestation. Also, *Jacquemier's sign*.

chair—see *wheelchairs* for list of chairs used in Rehabilitation reports.

chair-back brace (Ortho).

chalazion—chronic inflammatory granulomatous process of a meibomian gland. See *meibomian cyst, tarsal cyst*.

chamfer reamer (lowercase *c*).

Champ cardiac device.

Champion Trauma Score (CTS)—a scoring system used to evaluate multiple trauma injuries.

Chan wrist rest—a device used by ophthalmic surgeons to stabilize their hands, particularly when performing vitrectomies.

Chance fracture—a fracture of the lumbar vertebrae caused by extreme forward flexion of the spine above and below a seat belt during an automobile accident. Dr. C. Q. Chance first described this type of traumatic spinal fracture in 1948. Also known as a *seat belt fracture* and a *fulcrum fracture* because the seat belt acts as the point of a fulcrum which separates the upper and lower segments of the spinal column.

chandelier sign—extreme tenderness of the uterine adnexa, elicited on pelvic examination. (The term fancifully implies that the pain causes the patient to leap into the air and cling to the chandelier.)

charcoal—see *activated charcoal*.

CharcoCaps homeopathic formula for relief of intestinal gas.

Charcot-Bouchard aneurysm—aneurysmal formation in small arteries within the neural parenchyma.

Charcot-Leyden crystals—found in sputa of patients with bronchial asthma. Also, in aspiration of visceral larva migrans lesions. See *visceral larva migrans*.

Charles Bonnet syndrome—condition wherein elderly patients see strange figures or objects during hallucinations.

Charles flute needle (Oph).

charley horse—a painful spasm in a lower extremity, generally due to injury or strain.

Charnley Howorth Exflow system—a sterile air system for operating rooms to reduce infection rate, particularly used during arthroplasties.

Charnley reamer—used in hip replacement.

Charnley wire tightener—used in total hip arthroplasty.

CHART (continuous hyperfractionated accelerated radiotherapy).

Chattanooga Balance System—a computer system attached to two foot pads. Used to document postural sway and instability in patients with strokes, head injuries, and neuromuscular disorders.

Cheatle slit—for takedown of colostomy.

Cheatle's syndrome—see *fibrocystic breast syndrome.*

Check-Flo introducer—used to introduce balloon, electrode, closed-end, and other catheters; the seal on this prevents blood reflux and air aspiration.

checking—fine control of voluntary movement; the act of stopping a motion when its goal or purpose has been attained.

cheese worker's lung disease—extrinsic allergic alveolitis caused by exposure to moldy cheese.

Cheetah angioplasty catheter.

cheilectomy ("ky-lék-to-me")—(1) excision of a lip; (2) an operative procedure in which bone edges that impede joint motion are removed, e.g., in hallux rigidus.

chelation therapy—the oral or intravenous administration of medications such as ethylenediaminetetraacetic acid (EDTA) to remove metals such as lead, iron, and calcium from the body. It is used in alternative medicine, although its efficacy as a treatment for atherosclerosis has not yet been established in mainstream medicine.

Chemet (succimer)—heavy metal chelating agent for lead poisoning; treatment of cystine kidney stones and mercury poisoning.

chemical shift imaging (CSI) (Rad).

chemical shift phenomena (MRI term)—spatially mismapped signals occurring at the interface of tissues with different chemical shifts. Fat suppression technique is helpful.

chemoembolization—the use of DSM (degradable starch microspheres) administered simultaneously with a chemotherapy drug. These microspheres temporarily block the blood flow at the capillary level. The chemotherapy drug is then concentrated in the region of the cancer and achieves high tissue uptake. See *DSM.*

Chemo-Port catheter—for administration of chemotherapeutic agents or for the delivery of nutritional fluids.

chemoprevention—administration of a natural or man-made agent to retard or prevent development or progression of cancer.

chemosis—edema of the conjunctiva of the eye.

chemotherapy code for evaluating progress:
-2 definitely worse
-1 probably worse

chemotherapy code *(cont.)*
   0 no change since last scan
   +1 probably better
   +2 definitely better
chemotherapy drugs—see *medication.*
chemotherapy protocol—see individual main entries alphabetically throughout the book. Also listed under *medication.*
Chemstrip bG—a plastic strip used in checking blood glucose. Cf. *Dextrostix*, used in a similar manner. The blood spot on the treated strip is wiped off and rinsed with water, and then the resulting color is compared with a color chart, which gives the blood glucose value.
Chemstrip MatchMaker blood glucose meter—for self-testing by diabetics.
ChemTrak AccuMeter—screens for *H. pylori* bacteria commonly associated with stomach ulcers.
ChemTrak *Helicobacter pylori* test—a one-step test that can detect the presence of *H. pylori* within minutes during an office visit.
Chenix (chenodiol)—oral drug given to dissolve small gallbladder stones in patients without surgery. See *Actigall, MTBE.*
chenodiol (Chenix).
Cherf leg holder—supports lower extremity during knee and hip surgery.
Cherney incision—lower transverse abdominal incision.
cherry angiomas—benign hemangiomas that are round, cherry-red, dome-shaped papules; usually seen in the elderly. Called *Campbell de Morgan spots,* or *De Morgan's spots.*
Cherry-Crandall test—of serum lipase.
cherry red endobronchial lesions of Kaposi's sarcoma—a finding on bronchoscopy.

Chester-Erdheim disease—a rare lipid storage disorder characterized by hardening of the growth areas of the long bones of the body. Lipid cell deposits (histiocytes) are found in various vital organs of the body such as heart, lungs, peritoneum, kidneys, and other tissues. Severity of the disease differs with each patient, but the outcome is generally fatal.
chest, flail—see *flail chest.*
chest PT—the use of positioning (postural drainage) and clapping with a cupped hand over the patient's chest and back (frappage) to loosen pulmonary secretions. The patient may cough up the secretions, or they may be suctioned out. Also, *percussion.*
chest shell—used for noninvasive extrathoracic ventilation (NEV) during transport.
chevron incision—the name derives from the V shape of the incision.
C'H$_{50}$—total hemolytic complement.
CHF (congestive heart failure).
Chiari I malformation (Peds).
Chiba needle (also, *Skinny needle*)—used in percutaneous transhepatic cholangiography.
Chibroxin (norfloxacin)—topical ophthalmic antibiotic.
Chick CLT—operating table and frame for orthopedic surgery.
Chilaiditi's ("ky-la-dee-tees") **syndrome**—interposition of the colon (sometimes the small intestine) between the liver and the diaphragm. This is a result of a congenital anomaly of the diaphragm or the falciform ligament, which is a fold of peritoneum from the diaphragm to the surface of the liver.
Child's class (A, B, and C)—a classification system for esophageal varices.

Child's classification of hepatic risk criteria—class A, class B, and class C. Relates to operative risk.

Child-Pugh class A, B, or **C**—used in hepatic disease.

Child-Turcotte classification—used in hepatic surgery.

Chilli—cooled ablation catheters incorporating real-time position management (RPM) navigation technology.

Chirocaine (levobupivacaine)—local anesthetic used in a wide range of surgical procedures, including pain relief during childbirth.

Chlamydia pneumoniae—linked to brain samples from late-onset Alzheimer's patients. This finding could lead to new diagnostic and treatment regimens.

Chlamydia trachomatis—a gram-negative organism.

chloracetate esterase (Leder stain).

chlorotrianisene (Tace)—estrogen.

ChlVPP (chlorambucil, vinblastine, procarbazine, prednisone)—chemotherapy protocol for Hodgkin's disease.

chocolate agar—a culture medium.

CHOD (cyclophosphamide, hydroxydaunomycin, Oncovin, dexamethasone)—chemotherapy protocol used to treat CNS lymphoma.

Cho/Dyonics two-portal endoscopic system (Hand Surg).

choked disk—edema and hyperemia of the optic disk, usually associated with increased intracranial pressure. Also called *papilledema*.

Cholestagel (colesevelam hydrochloride)—renamed Welchol in May 2000. It is used for treatment of hypercholesterolemia. It is said to be four to five times more potent than cholestyramine.

cholecystectomy—see *endoscopic laser, laparoscopic laser, video-laseroscopy*.

cholecystitis—see *xanthogranulomatous cholecystitis*.

cholecystocholedocholithiasis—gallstones in gallbladder and common duct.

cholecystokinin (CCK)—thought to be one of the important hormones regulating gallbladder contraction. See *noncholecystokinin substance*.

choledochofiberscope—Olympus URF-P2 translaparoscopic.

cholescintography—radionuclide test; ^{99m}Tc PIPIDA is injected intravenously, giving prompt visualization of the liver, bile ducts, and gallbladder. Absence of dye in the gastrointestinal tract indicates obstruction of the common duct. If the gallbladder is not visualized, this is an indication of acute cholecystitis or of obstruction of the cystic duct or hepatic duct. See *PIPIDA*.

Cholestech LDX system with the TC (total cholesterol) and **Glucose Panel**—used to measure cholesterol and glucose levels at the same time from a single drop of blood and receive the results within five minutes. The system consists of a portable blood analyzer and disposable test cassettes and measures total cholesterol, HDL cholesterol, triglycerides, and glucose levels, and provides a calculated LDL cholesterol.

CholesTrak home cholesterol test—used by patients with high cholesterol who are trying to achieve better cholesterol levels through diet and exercise.

Choletec (^{99m}Tc mebrofenin)—radionuclide imaging agent.

chondromalacia patellae (*not* patella, even though only one knee is involved); *patellae* is (Latin) genitive case, meaning *of the patella*.

Chonstruct chondral repair system—used for repair of chondral defects of the articular cartilage. A paste consisting of a mixture of the patient's cancellous bone and articular cartilage is used as an anatomic patch for repair of the defect with a supportive matrix to promote new cartilage formation.

CHOP (cyclophosphamide, hydroxydaunomycin, Oncovin, prednisone)—chemotherapy protocol used to treat non-Hodgkin's lymphoma and CNS lymphoma.

Chopart ankle dislocation of navicula and cuboid across talus and calcaneus.

CHOP-BLEO (cyclophosphamide, hydroxydaunomycin, Oncovin, prednisone, bleomycin)—chemotherapy protocol used to treat non-Hodgkin's lymphoma.

CHOPE (cyclophosphamide, Halotestin, Oncovin, prednisone, etoposide)—chemotherapy protocol used to treat Hodgkin's and other lymphomas.

chordate—having a notochord (primitive backbone). See *caudate, cordate*.

chordae—plural of *chorda*; e.g., chordae tympani. Do not confuse with *chordee*.

chordee—a congenital defect that involves stricture of the fibrous tissue of the penis and that causes the penis to bow. This condition is often associated with a hypospadias. Do not confuse with *chordae*.

chordoma (*not* cordoma)—a malignant tumor arising from the embryonic remains of the notochord (primitive backbone).

chordotomy—see *cordotomy*.

chorionic villi biopsy (CVB).

chorioretinopathy, birdshot (Oph).

choristoma—a benign tumor containing tissues foreign to the tissue in which the tumor is found, e.g., bone found in muscle tissue.

choroidal hemangioma—benign vascular hamartoma.

choroidal neovascularization (CNV).

choroidal neovascular membrane.

Chow technique—a modified technique for performance of endoscopic carpal ligament release through an open slotted cannula, performed under local anesthesia without a tourniquet; developed by Dr. James Chow.

Chrisman and Snook procedure—modification of the Elmslie procedure using half of the peroneus brevis tendon to correct lateral ankle instability.

Christmas disease—factor IX deficiency (hemophilia B). See *hemophilia A*. Named for the child in whom it was first identified.

Christmas tree appearance of pancreas (Radiol).

Christmas tree pattern—seen in the skin eruption of pityriasis rosea.

Christoudias fascial closure device—for closing wounds.

chromatography
    affinity
    gas

ChromaVision digital analyzer—an automated intelligent microscopy system used for prenatal screening

ChromaVision *(cont.)*
for Down syndrome and for HIV and cancer detection.

chromohydrotubation—a test used in the evaluation of infertility. Dye is injected into the cervix through the vagina; a laparoscopic incision permits visualization of where the dye goes, to determine if the fallopian tubes are patent. Also called *chromopertubation.*

chromosomally mediated-resistant *Neisseria gonorrhoeae*—a penicillin-resistant gonococcus.

chromosome 14q—a tumor marker for patients with nonpapillary renal cell carcinoma (RCC). Patients with 14q deletion are found to have higher stages and grades of nonpapillary RCC.

chronic—persistent or prolonged, as in chronic bronchitis, chronic steroid therapy.

chronic bacterial prostatitis (CBP).

chronic fatigue immune dysfunction syndrome (CFIDS)—newer name by the Centers for Disease Control for what is usually called *chronic fatigue syndrome.*

chronic fatigue syndrome (CFS) (also known as *chronic fatigue immune dysfunction syndrome, myalgic encephalomyelitis, postviral fatigue syndrome,* and *yuppie flu*)—characterized by fatigue, irritability, sleep loss, forgetfulness, and muscle pain. Many of the patients are also depressed, and whether this is one of the symptoms of the disease or relates to the isolation, exhaustion, pain, and the fact that many physicians do not recognize this as a disease entity is not known. Symptoms last for months or even years, and

seem to affect more women than men. See also *chronic fatigue immune dysfunction syndrome.*

chronic intestinal pseudo-obstruction —syndrome manifested by signs and symptoms of obstruction but without true mechanical obstruction. See *familial visceral neuropathy.*

Chronicle implantable hemodynamic monitor from Medtronics.

chronic "lunger"—a pejorative term not used in the patient's presence. "The patient is a chronic lunger who no longer smokes." It refers to a patient who has had chronic long-term lung disease, particularly tuberculosis or chronic obstructive pulmonary disease.

chronic myeloid leukemia (CML).

chronic myelomonocytic leukemia (CMML).

chronic pulmonary emphysema (CPE).

chronotherapy—a technique for administering chemotherapy drugs that follows the body's biorhythms; it shows increased effectiveness in shrinking tumor size when compared to standard administration schedules.

Chronulac—lactulose solution used as a laxative.

Chrysalin—synthetic peptide used to accelerate healing of chronic wounds.

CHRYS CO$_2$ laser—a portable carbon dioxide laser as small as a desktop computer. Intended for use in physician offices and outpatient surgery centers.

chrysiasis—a rare blue-gray skin discoloration that occurs in sun-exposed sites of some patients who receive gold salts for treatment of psoriatic arthritis.

CHUK (conserved helix-loop-helix ubiquitous kinase)—protein that is believed to play a key role in inflammatory response. Identification of this protein may help treat a number of inflammatory diseases, including rheumatoid arthritis, inflammatory bowel disease, septic shock, and asthma.

chymonucleolysis—use of chymopapain to break down nucleus pulposus of herniated disk. Rarely used but will continue to appear in dictation as patients return with continued back problems.

Ciaglia percutaneous tracheostomy introducer—allows for bedside placement of tracheal tube for fewer complications than traditional open surgical technique.

cibenzoline succinate—a generic name officially changed to *cifenline succinate* in 1993.

Cibis ski needle—a flat needle used as an aid in placing an encircling band in retinal surgery.

CicaCare topical gel sheeting—adhesive topical gel sheeting used for the management of hypertrophic and keloid scars and to lessen the overall effect of scarring following surgery.

CIC (completely-in-the-[ear] canal) **hearing aid**. See *Argosy Cameo* and *Unitron Esteem*.

cidal level (serumcidal; bactericidal): the amount of an antibiotic needed in the blood to kill an organism.

cidofovir (HPMPC, Vistide)—an antiviral drug taken every two weeks for AIDS-related cytomegalovirus-related eye disorders. Previously, foscarnet and ganciclovir had to be taken daily.

cidofovir topical gel (Forvade)—used in the treatment of refractory herpes simplex virus (HSV) lesions in patients with AIDS.

CIE (countercurrent immunoelectrophoresis)—test for amebic antigen.

cifenline succinate (Cipralan)—twice-daily antiarrhythmic unrelated to any other currently available. It is effective in suppressing a variety of ventricular arrhythmias.

CIF-4 needle (Oph).

cilazapril—a once-daily, long-acting, potent ACE inhibitor for hypertension. For morbid hypertension, it may be combined with HCTZ for a more effective regimen. See *HCTZ*.

Cilco Slant lens—a single-piece intraocular lens with a design that incorporates slanted haptics and a low profile for easy insertion through the longer scleral tunnel and more acute angle of entry now used in intraocular lens surgery. *Slant* is a trade name. Also called *Slant lens*.

Ciloxan (ciprofloxacin)—an antimicrobial drug for topical ophthalmic use.

CIN (cervical intraepithelial neoplasia)—a designation to describe preinvasive lesions of the cervix. The degree of abnormal cytology is expressed in grades 1-3. CIN-2 is severe dysplasia.

cinchonism ("sin-koh-nism") (from cinchona, the plant from which quinine is obtained)—the manifestations of quinine toxicity: tinnitus, blurred vision, nausea, headache, and possibly thrombocytopenia.

cinctured—encircled.

cineangiography—studies of the cardiac vasculature performed by teams including cardiologists and radiologists.

cineangiography *(cont.)*
The cine (motion picture) films can be studied later by many physicians.

cine CT (computed tomography) **scanner**—provides a movie of the contractions of the heart wall and the blood flow in the brain. It can evaluate coronary artery bypass graft function, detect regional thickening of the myocardium or abnormalities in wall motion, and estimate cardiac output. Also, *ultrafast CT.*

cine view in MUGA (cinematograph in multiple gated acquisition) **scan**—a moving picture of the cardiac cycle, constructed from individual frames, of which each is a composite image of one point in the cardiac cycle obtained by cardiac gating.

cingulate gyrus ("sing-gyu-late")—an elevation of the brain surface, just above the corpus callosum.

CIP (chronic intestinal pseudo-obstruction).

Cipralan—see *cifenline succinate.*

Cipro (ciprofloxacin).

ciprofloxacin (Ciloxan, Cipro)— fluoroquinolone antibiotic.

Cipro HC Otic suspension (ciprofloxacin hydrochloride/hydrocortisone)—a combination product used to treat bacterial infection of acute otitis externa, as well as the severe localized pain that accompanies such an infection.

circinate ("sur-sin-ate")—ringlike or circular.

circinate-pattern interstitial keratopathy—occurs in soft contact lens wearers.

circinate retinopathy—condition marked by white spots encircling the macular area, which results in complete foveal blindness.

circle of death—attributed to an aberrant obturator artery that can bleed from both sides of an injury because of existing anastomosis. In laparoscopic herniorrhaphies, there is the danger of not identifying the aberrant artery because of the limited visibility of abdominal and pelvic anatomy. If inadvertently cut, it may bleed profusely, resulting in the death of the patient. It is, therefore, important that physicians performing laparoscopic procedures be able to identify internal anatomy "with their eyes closed," so to speak, and that they anticipate such anomalies.

Circon video camera—used for arthroscopy. The camera is connected to the arthroscope and provides color reproduction reported to be almost identical to that perceived by the human eye. Also, *Saticon and Newvicon, Vidicon vacuum chamber pickup tube for camera.*

Circon videohydrothoracoscope—an instrument that allows for viewing and irrigation through the same port during thoracoscopy, a minimally invasive surgical procedure.

Circon-ACMI electrohydraulic lithotriptor probe (Urol).

CircPlus—compression dressing or wrap.

circulation—see *extracorporeal circulation.*

circulator boot therapy—an external compression device attached to the lower extremity and timed to the cardiac cycle. As the heart pumps and the pressure head of the blood reaches the extremity, the boot gives the blood an extra push to force it through diseased vessels. The device also helps stimulate alternative blood

circulator *(cont.)* vessels to bring oxygenated blood to diseased parts of the extremity.

Circulon dressing or wrap.

circumduction ("sur-kum-duk-shun") —the rotational movement, active or passive, of an eye, or of an extremity. Cf. *sursumduction.*

circumduction-adduction shoulder maneuver—see *Clancy test.*

circumferential fracture—extends completely around the skull, leaving the skull essentially in two pieces.

circumscribed choroidal hemangioma (CCH).

circus-movement tachycardia (CMT).

circus senilis (often used interchangeably with *arcus senilis)*—a hazy gray ring around the periphery of the cornea, composed of lipid droplets.

CIRF (cocaine-induced respiratory failure).

CirKuit-Guard—device for cardiovascular and vascular surgery.

cirsodesis ("sur-sod-ee-sis")—ligation of varicose veins.

CIS (carcinoma in situ).

cisapride—see *Propulsid.*

cisatracurium besylate (Nimbex).

CISCA (cisplatin, cyclophosphamide, Adriamycin)—chemotherapy protocol.

cisplatin (cis-platinum, Platinol)—an antineoplastic drug. When cisplatin first appeared, it was called *cis-platinum*, although this term is rarely used today. *Cisplatin* (lowercase *c*) is the current approved name in all nomenclature systems. If a doctor dictates cis-platinum, it would be better to type the internationally recognized name, cisplatin.

cisternogram—see *metrizamide CT.*

cisternography—see *oxygen cisternography.*

cis-retinoic acid—see *isotretinoin.*

cite—to bring forward, as for illustration; to quote, as proof or by way of authority; to summon to appear. "It may be necessary to cite an example." Cf. *site.*

citicoline—used for the treatment of strokes.

citrate phosphate dextrose (CPD).

Citrobacter amalonaticus (formerly *C. freundii)*—associated with enteritis, septicemia, urinary tract infections, pneumonia, and burn and wound infections.

citrovorum rescue (Oncol)—see *leucovorin rescue.*

Citscope—a disposable arthroscope.

citta ("sit'-ah")—the craving for unusual foods during pregnancy (strawberries, pickles, etc.).

CIWA-A scale—see *Clinical Institute Withdrawal Assessment-Alcohol.*

CK (creatine kinase).

CK$_1$, CK$_2$, CK$_3$—isoenzymes of creatine kinase.

CK/AST (creatine kinase/aspartate aminotransferase) **ratio.**

CKC (cold knife cone) **biopsy.**

CKPT (combined kidney and pancreas transplant).

Cladosporium—an inhalant antigen.

cladribine (Leustatin)—a chemotherapy drug used to treat hairy cell and lymphocytic leukemia. Unlike other leukemia treatments which attack the cancer cells as they are dividing, this attacks the cells at rest. Since 90% of cancer cells are dormant at any given time, other treatments must be given continuously for many weeks. Cladribine is given in a single 7-day

cladribine *(cont.)*
course. It is also studied for use against other types of leukemias, lymphomas, and autoimmune diseases such as multiple sclerosis and rheumatoid arthritis.

Clagett-Barrett esophagogastrostomy.

clamp or **clip**
Acland microvascular clamp
Atrauclip hemostatic clip
Benjamin-Havas fiberoptic light clip
Best right-angle colon clamp
Bihrle dorsal clamp
cardiac retraction clip
Castaneda anastomosis clamp
Cope crushing clamp
Cope modification of Martel intestinal clamp
Cunningham clamp
Dardik clamp
Duvall lung-grasping clamp
Filshie female sterilization clip
Fukushima C-clamp
Glassman clamp
Goldstein Microspike approximator
Gregory clamp
Gusberg hysterectomy clamp
Hemoclip
Hem-o-lok
Jahnke anastomosis clamp
Klintmalm clamp
Lane bone-holding clamp
Ligaclip
Locke clamp
Masters intestinal
Mayfield three-pin skull clamp
mosquito clamp
Multiclip
Neuromeet nerve approximator
Olsen cholangiogram clamp
Omed bulldog vascular clamp
Parker-Kerr intestinal clamp
Perneczky aneurysm clamp
Raney clip

clamp *(cont.)*
Right Clip
Sarot bronchus clamp
Secu clip
Selverstone clamp
side-biting clamp
Verbrugge bone clamp
Wertheim clamp
Zinnanti Z-clamp
Z-clamp

clamshell brace (Ortho).

clamshell incision—same as transverse anterior thoracotomy incision.

Clancy test—also called the circumduction-adduction shoulder maneuver. It is said to be 95% sensitive and specific for diagnosing rotator cuff tendinopathy, including partial tears.

Clarion (ENT)—a hearing implant for pediatric patients.

Clarion cochlear implant—bypasses ear damage, sending electric signals directly to the auditory nerve. These signals are then interpreted by the brain as sounds.

Clarion multi-strategy cochlear implant (ENT)—for use in post-lingually deafened adults.

clarithromycin (Biaxin)—an antibiotic belonging to the macrolide class of drugs, similar in effectiveness to penicillin and erythromycin but with fewer side effects. It is particularly effective against *Mycoplasma pneumoniae*, resistant strains of *Haemophilus influenzae*, and MAC infection.

Claritin (loratadine)—long-acting antihistamine.

Clark classification of malignant melanoma, levels I-IV. Named for the pathologist who devised it, Wallace H. Clark, Jr., M.D.

Clark-Elder classification—a classification of malignant melanoma. See also *Clark* and *Elder*.

Clark perineorrhaphy (Gyn).

Clarus spinescope—a percutaneous spinal endoscope used for treatment of chronic spinal pain by interventional anesthesiologists.

classic abdominal Semm hysterectomy (CASH)—transabdominal hysterectomy done via laparoscopy, pioneered by German surgeon Kurt Semm. It leaves the extrafascial, highly vascularized vascular stem, the corresponding nerves, and the topography of the ureter untouched during extracervical enucleation (removal of part or all of a mass in its entirety) of the fascia of the uterine body, removing the uterus. Because the cardinal ligaments are preserved as well as the nerve supply of the cervical fascia, transvaginal sexual sensations are not impaired. Suspension of the cervical fascia at the supporting ligaments of the uterus can be performed in this procedure.

classification, grade, or **stage**
Altmann congenital aural atresia
Astler-Coller modification of Dukes' classification
Baylor bleeding score
Behavioral Pathology in Alzheimer's Disease Rating Scale
Bethesda rating scale for Pap smears
Blaivas urinary incontinence
Breslow classification for malignant melanoma
Broders' tumor index
Brooker periarticular heterotopic ossification (PHO)
burns classification

classification *(cont.)*
CEAP
chemotherapy code
Child's esophageal varices
Child's hepatic risk criteria
Child-Pugh A, B, C classification
Child-Turcotte classification
CIN (cervical intraepithelial neoplasia)
Clark-Elder malignant melanoma
Clark malignant melanoma
Coleman congenital aural atresia
concussion grades
Couinaud
de la Cruz classification of congenital aural atresia
Delbet fracture classification
diabetes mellitus classification
Dubin and Amelar varicocele
Dukes-Astler-Coller adenocarcinoma
Dukes' carcinoma
Edmondson-Steiner grading of hepatocellular carcinoma
Elder malignant melanoma
Erlanger and Gasser peripheral nerve classification
FAB (French/American/British)
FIGO classification
Floyd peripheral nerve
Framingham criteria for heart failure
Frykman classification of hand fractures
Harvard Criteria for Brain Death
Highet and Sander criteria
Highet and Sander criteria of Mackinnon and Dellon, modified
Highet and Sander criteria of Zachary and Holmes, modified
HIV children classification
Hoehn and Yahr Parkinson's staging
House-Brackmann facial weakness scale

classification *(cont.)*
  Hunt and Hess neurological
  Hyams grading system for
    esthesioneuroblastoma
  hypertension standard
  International Society for Heart and
    Lung Transplantation
  Jewett's classification of bladder
    carcinoma
  Judet epiphyseal fracture
    classification
  Karnofsky performance rating
  Karnofsky status classification
  Kazangia and Converse fracture
  Keith-Wagener classification
    of retinopathy
  Kiel classification of non-Hodgkin's
    lymphoma
  Killip heart failure
  Klatskin tumor classification
  leukemia classification
  Lukes-Collins classification of
    non-Hodgkin's lymphoma
  lymph node location system of neck
  MacKinnon and Dellon criteria
  Marx's classification of microtia
  Masuka staging system, modified
  Mayo Clinic criteria to determine
    patient survival
  Mayo Clinic system for primary
    biliary cirrhosis
  Meurman congenital aural atresia
  Modic's disk abnormality
    classification
  modified Masuka staging system
  MSTS (Musculoskeletal Tumor
    Society) staging system
  murmur grades
  Neer (shoulder fractures I, II, III)
  NYHA (New York Heart
    Association) classification of
    congestive heart failure
  Olerud and Molander fracture
  osteoarthritis grading

classification *(cont.)*
  Pauwel's femoral neck fracture
  Pulec and Freedman congenital
    aural atresia
  Reese-Ellsworth classification
    of retinoblastoma
  Rye histopathologic classification of
    Hodgkin's disease
  Schuknecht congenital aural atresia
  Singh-Vaughn-Williams arrhythmia
  TNM malignant tumor
  tuberculosis
  van Heuven's anatomic classification
    of diabetic retinopathy
  Visick grading system for post-
    gastrectomy carcinoma
    recurrence
  White and Panjabi criteria
  Wiberg classification of patellar
    types
Clauss modified method of plasma fibrinogen measurement.
claustrum—thin layer of gray matter
  lateral to the external capsule of the
  brain. Cf. *colostrum, clostridium.*
**claviculotomy, claviculectomy tech-
  nique**—used for tumors that trans-
  gress the neck, thoracic inlet, and
  axilla, offering maximal exposure
  for excision, vascular control, and
  preservation of vital structures.
clavus (pl., clavi)—a corn on the foot
  or toe.
clean-catch urine specimen—an uncontaminated urine specimen obtained by first thoroughly washing
  the genitalia. The urine stream is
  started and then, midstream, the
  specimen is caught without the urine
  stream or container touching the
  genitalia or perineum.
ClearCut 2—an electrosurgical handpiece by Medtronic used in tissue
  cutting and coagulation.

ClearSite borderless dressing—gauze scrim and a 1 cm printed top film in an open-weave design that allows monitoring of wound healing and complete visualization of the wound site even after extended use. Cf. *Aquasorb, Curasorb, and Ventex.*

ClearSite Hydro Gauze dressing—dressing with a thin layer of Clear-Site gel that maintains a moist environment for healing.

ClearView CO$_2$ laser—includes a device to continually evacuate smoke generated by laser use.

Cleland's ligament—in the hand; keeps the skin sleeve from twisting around the bone of the digit. It may be referred to in operative procedures for Dupuytren's contracture. See also *Grayson's ligament*; they are not synonymous.

clemastine fumarate (Antihist-1).

Cleocin (clindamycin phosphate) **vaginal ovules**—solid, oval-shaped suppositories used as a once-daily, three-day treatment for bacterial vaginosis in nonpregnant women.

Climara (estradiol transdermal system) —a once-a-week estrogen replacement therapy transdermal patch approved both for prevention of osteoporosis and for treatment of menopause symptoms.

clindamycin—antibiotic combined with primaquine, an antimalarial drug, to treat *Pneumocystis carinii* pneumonia in AIDS patients.

Clindoxyl (clindamycin/benzoyl peroxide gel)—new acne treatment.

Clinical Global Impression of Change (CGIC)—measures Alzheimer patient's clinical change relative to baseline.

Clinical Institute Withdrawal Assessment-Alcohol scale (CIWA-A)—a psychological/physiological scale used to assess the degree of alcohol withdrawal that a patient is experiencing. For a score above 10, the patient is given a drug such as chlordiazepoxide (Librium) or diazepam (Valium) to produce sedation and prevent seizures.

CliniCath peripherally inserted catheter.

Clinoril (sulindac)—NSAID; antineoplastic and analgesic. It is found to decrease the number of colon polyps in patients with familial polyposis.

clip—see *clamp.*

Clirans T-series—hollow-fiber-type dialyzer for urea clearance.

clitoridectomy—(also referred to as "excision")—female genital mutilation consisting of removal of entire clitoris, both prepuce and glans, with removal of adjacent labia. See also *infibulation* and *Sunna circumcision.*

CLL (chronic lymphocytic leukemia)—seen primarily in late adulthood, usually after age 50.

CLO (congenital lobar overinflation).

clobazam (Frisium)—antianxiety drug.

Clobetasol E Cream (clobetasol propionate emollient cream 0.05%)—for the topical treatment of inflammatory and pruritic corticosteroid-responsive dermatoses of the scalp.

clofazimine ("klo-fa'-zih-meen") (Lamprene)—for use in treatment of Hansen's disease (leprosy) and now used to treat MAC infection in AIDS patients.

clonidine gel—treatment for peripheral neuropathic pain. It provides concentrated site-specific therapy over a

clonidine gel *(cont.)*
painful area without blocking motor or sensory nerve function.

clonogenic assay—single cell suspensions of tumor cells are cultured in soft agar and then exposed to various chemotherapy agents. The soft agar permits the selective growth of tumor cells. Sensitivity and resistance are estimated by a count of surviving clones of cells.

Clonorchis sinensis—liver fluke.

clonus—see *drawn ankle clonus.*

C-loop of duodenum (Radiol).

closed fracture—one in which there is no break in the skin. Formerly called *simple fracture.*

closed intramedullary pinning (CIMP) —a closed technique for correcting displaced fractures of the epiphysis of the neck of the radius. An incision is made in the shaft of the radius to gain access to the epiphysis. A Kirschner wire is inserted through a drill hole and gently hammered through the medullary canal to the epiphysis. The tip of the K wire secures the fracture fragment. To correct lateral displacement of the fragment, the wire may be rotated 180° on its long axis, creating torque which slides the fragment back in its place. The K wire is then cut at the other end where it exits from the shaft, and the skin incision is closed.

CloseSure procedure kit—used in full-thickness suturing of trocar wounds.

closing base wedge osteotomy (CBWO).

clostridial bacteremia—in cancer patients, most frequently associated with *Clostridium perfringens* and *C. septicum.*

clostridial collagenase—derived from *Clostridium histolyticum* and used for enzymatic wound debridement in preparation for skin grafting.

Clostridium botulinum **toxin, type A** (Dysport, Oculinum)—injected into eye muscles to treat blepharospasm. See *botulinum toxin type A.*

Clostridium difficile—organism isolated from meconium and feces of infants, from wounds, and from the urogenital tract of asymptomatic people.

Clostridium difficile-**associated diarrhea** (CDAC).

Closure System by VNUS—catheters used for endovascular coagulation of blood vessels in patients with superficial vein reflux.

CLOtest (*Campylobacter*-like organism)—a trademark term for the test for *H. pylori. Campylobacter* is the former name of *Helicobacter.*

Clot Stop drain—a drain with an antithrombogenic covering, used in cosmetic surgery.

clotrimazole (Mycelex)—used as treatment to prevent oral fungal infections and vaginal *Candida* infections in AIDS patients. Mycelex troches are dissolved in the mouth three times daily.

clove hitch—a sailor's knot; also used in surgery.

cloverleaf skull (Ger., Kleeblattschädel).

clozapine (Clozaril)—an antipsychotic drug that provides symptomatic relief for many patients who fail to improve sufficiently or cannot tolerate the standard medications prescribed for schizophrenia.

CLSE (calf lung surfactant extract)— see *surfactant, heterologous.*

CLS (Cementless Sportorno) **stem insertion.**

clubbing, cyanosis, and edema.

clubbing of the fingers and toes—thickening and bulbous enlargement of the tissue at the base of the nail; often seen in patients with cystic fibrosis, ulcerative colitis, cirrhosis of the liver, and cardiopulmonary disease.

clubfoot splint—see *Denis Browne.*

clue cells—a term used in reference to a Pap smear. They are so-called because their presence is a clue to possible infection with *Gardnerella vaginalis* (formerly *Haemophilus vaginalis*).

CME (cystoid macular edema) (Oph).

CMF-HBSS (calcium and magnesium-free Hanks' balanced salt solution).

CMFP (cyclophosphamide, methotrexate, fluorouracil, prednisone)—chemotherapy protocol for treating breast cancer.

CMFPT (cyclophosphamide, methotrexate, fluorouracil, prednisone, tamoxifen)—chemotherapy protocol used for inflammatory breast carcinoma.

CMFPTH (cyclophosphamide, methotrexate, fluorouracil, prednisone, tamoxifen, Halotestin)—chemotherapy protocol.

CMFVP (cyclophosphamide, methotrexate, fluorouracil, vincristine, and prednisone)—chemotherapy protocol used for advanced breast cancer.

CMH (cyclophosphamide, m-AMSA, hydroxyurea)—chemotherapy protocol.

CMI (cell-mediated immunity).

CMI/Mityvac cup (Ob-Gyn)—a rigid traction handle attached to a semi-rigid cup, with the vacuum port located at the end of a traction handle. Shaped like a Dixie cup.

CMI/O'Neil cup (Ob-Gyn)—attached to a vacuum source to facilitate vacuum-assisted vaginal deliveries. Available in both anterior and posterior presentations.

CMJ (corticomedullary junction) phase imaging on CT scan.

CML (chronic myelocytic leukemia)—mostly in adults age 20 to 50.

CML (chronic myeloid leukemia).

CMML (chronic myelomonocytic leukemia).

CMOPP (cyclophosphamide, mechlorethamine, Oncovin, procarbazine, prednisone)—chemotherapy protocol for adult non-Hodgkin's lymphoma.

CMRNG (chromosomally mediated-resistant *Neisseria gonorrhoeae*)—a penicillin-resistant gonococcus.

CMT (Certified Medical Transcriptionist).

CMT (circus-movement tachycardia).

CMV (cisplatin, methotrexate, vinblastine)—chemotherapy protocol for transitional cell carcinoma of the bladder.

CMV (cytomegalovirus).

CNM (Certified Nurse Midwife).

CNOP (cyclophosphamide, Novantrone, Oncovin, prednisone)—chemotherapy protocol for non-Hodgkin's lymphoma.

C/N ratio (contrast-to-noise)—a term used in MRI scans.

CNS (central nervous system). Not to be confused with C&S (culture and sensitivity). See *C&S.*

CNV (choroidal neovascularization).

CNVM (choroidal neovascular membrane) (Oph).

coags—slang for coagulation studies.

CoaguChek—self-testing device that measures blood coagulation levels (prothrombin time).

coagulation factors (blood)
I fibrinogen
II prothrombin
III thromboplastin
IV calcium ions
V proaccelerin (accelerator globulin, AcG)
VI factor VI (which is rapidly destroyed by thrombin; hence, it cannot be identified by its activity in the serum) is assumed to be the active form
VII proconvertin (or serum prothrombin conversion accelerator, SPCA)
VIII antihemophilic factor (or von Willebrand's factor)
IX plasma thromboplastin component (Christmas factor)
X Stuart factor (or Stuart-Prower factor)
XI plasma thromboplastin antecedent
XII Hageman factor
XIII fibrin stabilizing factor

Coagulin-B—adeno-associated virus-based gene therapy for the treatment of hemophilia B.

Coaguloop resection electrode (new use)—an instrument used for resection, ablation, and fulguration in the bladder.

coagulum pyelolithotomy—procedure for removal of kidney stones. Coagulum is introduced through two Intracaths, and cryoprecipitate and calcium chloride mixture are instilled simultaneously. After 7 minutes an incision is made in the pelvis of the kidney, and the stones, now surrounded by the gel that has formed, are easily scooped out without rough edges traumatizing the renal tissues.

coal tar, crude—*not* cold tar.

COAP (cyclophosphamide, Oncovin, ara-C, prednisone)—chemotherapy protocol for acute lymphoblastic leukemia.

Coats' disease (Oph)—unilateral, congenital (but not familial) vascular anomalies of the retina. It is sometimes confused with retinoblastoma, but fluorescein angiography and ultrasound help differentiate between the two entities. Coats' disease is frequently seen in young boys.

coaxial sheath cut-biopsy needle—see *PercuCut cut-biopsy needles.*

Cobacter luendi.

CobactinE—a proprietary strain of *Lactobacillus acidophilus* that inhibits *E. coli* 0157:H7.

cobalamin C methylmalonic acidemia—a nutritional deficiency thought to be responsible for certain skin diseases.

Coban dressing, wrapping—an elastic dressing.

Cobb angle—measurement in kyphoscoliosis. "Seven patients had a thoracic curve with a mean preoperative Cobb angle of 69° (range 47 to 112°)." "Instrumentation begins with a convex compression force to shorten not only the posterior column but also the convexity of the scoliotic deformity while reducing the Cobb angle."

Cobb-Ragde needle—a double-prong ligature carrier for bladder neck suspension.

Cobb's syndrome—characterized by the presence of spinal and vertebral angiomas.

cobblestoning—coarsely lumpy appearance of a mucosal surface, such as the tongue, nasal mucosa, or conjunctiva, caused by inflammation.

Cobe gun—a staple gun.

Cobe Optima—a hollow-fiber membrane oxygenator for use in ECMO (extracorporeal membrane oxygenation) systems.

COBE Spectra Apheresis System—an instrument for bone marrow cell processing.

COBE 2991 Cell Processor—an instrument for bone marrow cell processing.

Coblation (trademark coined from "cool ablation")—a patented process that uses radiofrequency (RF) energy applied to a conductive medium, like saline, to remove target tissue in a relatively cool process without damage to surrounding tissue as might occur with heat-driven electrosurgical techniques. Used in orthopedics, plastic surgery, and ears, nose, and throat procedures, and investigationally in cardiovascular procedures.

Coblation Channeling—a minimally invasive procedure for volumetric reduction of tissue, used primarily for treating a variety of upper airway disorders, including snoring, but also in knee and spinal surgery.

cobra head plate (Ortho).

Coburn equiconvex lens—an intraocular lens with an equal curvature from anterior to posterior.

cocaine-induced respiratory failure (CIRF)—the sudden onset of dyspnea, pulmonary edema, and respiratory failure caused by cocaine.

coccygodynia—pain in the coccyx and neighboring region.

cochineal extract—see *carmine dye.*

Cochlea Dynamics sound processing technology—digitally programmable products for persons with hearing loss.

cochlear blood flow (CBF).

cochlear implant—electronic device that provides direct electrical stimulation to the auditory fibers in the inner ear. See *Clarion; Contigen Bard.*

cochleosacculotomy—see *Schuknecht.*

Cockcroft-Gault equation or **formula** —used to quickly calculate renal function by estimating creatinine clearance from serum creatinine. This equation takes into account the patient's age, weight, and sex. It is used to adjust the dosage of certain drugs which are excreted by the kidneys. It is of particular value in elderly patients whose kidney function may be compromised but whose therapy cannot be postponed until a 24-hour urine collection for creatinine clearance is completed.

Co-Cr-Mo pin—named after the chemical symbols of its components (cobalt, chromium, molybdenum).

Codere orbital floor implant (Oph).

Codman exercises—to increase range of motion in a stiff shoulder. The patient bends over at a 90° angle at the waist and, with a weight held in each hand, moves the arms in arcs.

Codman triangle—an abrupt cutoff of periosteal new bone at the edge of a lesion, representing a mass elevating the periosteum, and often associated with malignancy.

Cody tack operation—for treatment of progressive endolymphatic hydrops (Ménière's disease). Similar to the Fick sacculotomy.

Coe-pak—hard- and fast-set periodontal paste.

COF/COM (cyclophosphamide, Oncovin, fluorouracil + cyclophosphamide, Oncovin, methotrexate)—a chemotherapy protocol for nonmetastatic breast carcinoma.

coffee-grounds material, vomitus, emesis—indicative of blood in the gastric contents. "She has vomited twice. This was productive of stomach contents and bile, no hemoptysis, hematemesis, or coffee-grounds material." The appearance of the vomitus is similar to that of the grounds left over after roasting coffee. Note: Coffee grounds, *not* coffee ground.

Coffey ureterointestinal anastomosis.

Coffin-Lowry syndrome—mental retardation and congenital deformities.

Cofield total shoulder system.

Cognex (tacrine)—drug used to treat Alzheimer's disease.

CO₂Guard (typed as one word)—filters gas in laparoscopy and hysteroscopy.

cogwheel breathing—jerkiness or intermittency of breath sounds on inspiration, due to sudden expansion of previously collapsed air sacs.

cogwheel gait—muscle jerkiness due to spasticity in patients with Parkinson's disease.

cogwheel rigidity—seen in Parkinson's disease.

Coherent CO₂ (carbon dioxide) **surgical laser**—Series 2000 Ultima or Novus photocoagulators used in eye surgery.

Coherent UltraPulse 5000C laser—used for aesthetic facial resurfacing and treatment of acne scars, superficial skin cancers, moles, and warts.

Coherent Versapulse device.

Cohn cardiac stabilizer—for retraction and stabilization of the heart during minimally invasive beating-heart surgical procedures.

coin test—for pneumothorax. One coin is pressed against the anterior chest and tapped with another, while the posterior chest is auscultated. A characteristic sound is diagnostic of pneumothorax.

CO₂ject system—allows for routine use of carbon dioxide gas as a replacement for the more expensive iodinated contrast media currently used in angiographic procedures.

Colapinto needle—transjugular liver biopsy needle used in interventional radiology.

CO₂ laser (carbon dioxide laser). See *argon laser, laser, Nd:YAG laser.*

Colazide (balsalazide disodium)—orally administered anti-inflammatory drug for the treatment of acute ulcerative colitis.

colchicine—commonly used to treat gout. Helpful in decreasing the progression of neurological symptoms in patients with multiple sclerosis.

colchicine poisoning—drug intoxication resulting from toxic doses of colchicine used primarily in the treatment of gout.

cold cup biopsy—a method of obtaining tissue for histologic examination. Cold cup biopsies of the lower urinary tract require rigid endoscopic access and the use of biopsy forceps and Bugbee electrodes.

cold knife cone (CKC) **biopsy**.

cold water calorics—a test for vertigo, nystagmus, and vestibular function, with cold water gently injected by syringe into the ear canal. Also, *ice water calorics test.*

Coleman classification of congenital aural atresia.

CollaCote—collagen wound dressing.

collagen hemostatic material for wounds—initially acts as a hemostatic agent when applied to a wound. Continued application seems to aid and hasten the body's own repair mechanisms. The most abundant collagen is type 1, extracted from bovine hide. Other sources include porcine, chicken, and bovine tendon. See also *dressing*.

Avitene
bucrylate
Collastat
Contigen glutaraldehyde
    cross-linked
cryoprecipitate
Endo-Avitene
Hemaflex sheath
Helitene
Hemopad
Hemotene
Instat
Surgical Nu-Knit hemostatic material
Surgicel
Unilab Surgibone
Zyclast
Zyderm I or II

collagen absorbable suture—made of beef tendon.

collagenase (Santyl).

collagen injection, periurethral—given to women for stress urinary incontinence.

collagen injection, transurethral—given for stress incontinence after radical prostatectomy, although not in men with severe bladder neck dysfunction or scarring.

collagen meniscus implant (CMI)—tissue-engineered biological meniscus implant designed to regenerate damaged meniscal tissue.

Collagraft bone graft matrix—non-osteoconductive bone-void filler that provides healing and fusion rates equivalent to an autograft without the risks of viral transmission and donor-site morbidity problems.

CollaPlug (Oral Surg)—wound dressing.

collar—see *cervical collar*.

collar-button abscess of the palm.

collar-button appearance in colon (Radiol).

Collastat—collagen hemostatic sponge with proposed advantages over Avitene. It is said not to shred or pull apart after absorbing tissue fluids, and it costs less.

CollaTape—tape used with wound dressing.

collateralization—formation of collateral vessels.

collateral vessels—vascular channels that are newly formed from existing ones to maintain the circulation of a tissue or organ whose normal blood supply has been impaired by disease or injury. Cf. *collateralization*.

CollectFirst System—used for intraoperative and postoperative autotransfusion.

collecting system (Radiol)—on an intravenous pyelogram (IVP), the nonexcretory portions of the kidney, which collect newly formed urine and conduct it to the ureter; the minor and major calices and the renal pelvis.

colliculus—a small protuberance. Cf. *canaliculus*.

Collier's sign—when the upper lid is elevated, showing more sclera above the iris than is usually seen, producing the so-called thyroid stare; a sign of thyroid disease. Cf. *Dalrymple's sign*.

collimation (Radiol)—in scanning.

Collin-Beard procedure—resection of the levator muscle, with advancement onto the tarsal plate.

Collins' solution—used for preservation of a liver which is to be transplanted; the liver may be kept in this solution for about six hours before implantation. Ringer's solution may be used for this purpose if the liver is to be kept for a shorter period.

Collis-Nissen fundoplication—used in association with transthoracic parietal cell vagotomy for advanced gastroesophageal reflux with peptic stricture and Barrett metaplasia.

Collis-Nissen gastroplasty—a procedure for gastroesophageal reflux.

collodion—a topical protectant used to keep a surgical wound dry.

colloidal bismuth subcitrate—used for reduction of *H. pylori* in the mouth.

colloid oncotic pressure (COP)—measurement of brain edema after cryogenic (vasogenic) brain injury.

colloids—used as blood replacement, including dextrose, hetastarch, plasma protein fraction, and serum albumin. See *crystalloid*.

colloid shift on liver-spleen scan.

ColoCARE—a noninvasive home test to detect early warning signs of colorectal disease.

colocolic intussusception—a term that may be confusing because *colocolic* might be misunderstood as *colonic* or simply stuttering. *Intussusception* is the prolapse of one part of the intestine into an adjoining part. In colocolic intussusception, the colon prolapses into itself rather than the intestine prolapsing into the colon.

colocolponeopoiesis—technique used to create a new vagina in females with congenital vaginal aplasia or in males having a sex change operation. A portion of the sigmoid colon is resected, carefully preserving its blood supply. Using sutures or a stapler, the colonic segment is formed into a conduit for use as a vagina. Also called *modified Kun colocolpopoiesis*.

Colomed—an enema containing short-chain fatty acids, used for treatment of chronic radiation proctitis.

colony-forming unit (CFU).

colony-forming unit–granulocyte, monocyte (CFU-GM).

colony-forming unit–megakaryocyte (CFU-meg or CFU-MK).

Colorado microdissection needle (Neuro).

color Doppler—a computer used with sonography of blood vessels computes the speed of the blood flow and demonstrates it in different colors to the radiologist.

colorectal cancer (CRC).

colorectal cancer screening—includes fecal occult blood testing, flexible sigmoidoscopy, barium enema, and colonoscopy.

Colorgene DNA Hybridization Test—a DNA probe test to detect herpes simplex virus in two hours rather than waiting days for culture results.

Colormate TLc BiliTest system—transcutaneous bilirubinometer for monitoring newborn jaundice.

colostrum (Ob-Gyn)—a thin, milky fluid which is secreted by the mammary glands around the time of parturition. It contains antibodies which provide the baby with passive immunization. Cf. *claustrum*.

colpocystourethropexy (CCUP).

colpoperineopexy—see *abdominal-sacral colpoperineopexy*.

Colyte—a bowel preparation used before colonoscopy or barium enema x-ray examination.

CombiDerm absorbent cover dressing.

Combidex—a multifunctional MRI contrast agent used in the imaging of liver and spleen, the detection and characterization of liver lesions, the diagnosis and staging of metastatic disease in lymph nodes, and the imaging of breast tumors.

combined androgen blockade (CAB).

CombiPatch (estradiol/norethindrone acetate)—delivers a continuous dose of both estrogen and progestogen transdermally via a single patch.

Combitube—a relatively new device used for blind insertion emergency intubation.

Combivent (ipratropium bromide/albuterol sulfate)—used to treat bronchospasm.

Combivir (lamivudine/zidovudine)—used for treatment of HIV infection.

combretastatin A-4—used for treatment of solid malignant tumors.

Comed—a line of post-traumatic and postsurgical footgear.

Comfeel Ulcus—a synthetic (hydrocolloid) occlusive dressing for lower extremity ulcers.

Comfort Cast, Comfort Cast Stirrup—foot and ankle casting system with four adjustable parts, reducing the need for crutches.

Comfort Cath I or II—male external catheter.

ComfortFlex—see *Hanger Comfort-Flex.*

comitant—accompanying, following, related to deviation of the eye. Here is the definition supplied by an ophthalmologist: *Comitant* refers to the eye's deviation in the same amount in all positions of gaze. Let's say it's an in-turning eye and it deviates 10 diopters of inward deviation, and that deviation is the same in upgaze, downgaze, right gaze, and left gaze; we call that *comitant deviation* or *comitant esotropia.* If the deviation varies in different gaze positions, we call it *noncomitant*; it is more likely to be paralytic. Cf. *concomitant.*

Commander PTCA wire line.

Command instrument system—cutting instruments used in the femoral canal for joint replacement.

Command PS pacemaker.

commissure of Gudden—located within the optic chiasm.

Companion 314—a nasal CPAP system designed for in-home use to treat adults with obstructive sleep apnea.

Companion 2 self blood glucose monitoring device. See *SBGM.*

compartment syndrome of the hand or anterior compartment of leg—a condition characterized by raised pressure within a closed space with a potential to cause irreversible damage to the contents of the closed compartment.

Compass hinge—used to prevent joint contractures following elbow or finger trauma or surgery. This external device measures the degree of passive and active range of motion exercises. The numbered calibrations for degrees of motion at the outside of the edge of this circular device resemble those on a compass.

Compassia (dronabinol)—used to reduce agitated behavior in people with dementia.

compensated—corrected or mitigated; said of a defect or disability, as in

compensated *(cont.)*
compensated congestive heart failure; compensated hearing loss, hearing loss improved with a hearing aid; edentulous and compensated, toothless but fitted with dentures.

compensated dysphagia for solid foods—the patient's attempt to deal with the effects of congenital esophageal stenosis. Stenosis may be treated by endoscopic bougienage or balloon dilatation.

Comperm tubular elastic bandage—provides 360° compression and support for sports injuries, postcast support, postburn scarring, sprains, and strains.

complement fixation—a type of serologic test in which the consumption of a serum protein, called complement, is taken as evidence that the expected antigen-antibody reaction has occurred. Cf. *compliment*.

complementary DNA (cDNA).

completely in the [ear] **canal** (CIC)—hearing aids, referring to the ear canal, particularly suited to patients with presbycusis.

complex
AIDS-related (ARC)
anisoylated plasminogen streptokinase activator (APSAC)
Battey-avium
Eisenmenger's
Ghon
Golgi
MAC (*Mycobacterium avium* complex)
MAI (*Mycobacterium avium-intracellulare*) complex
Ranke
sling ring
triangular fibrocartilage (TFCC)

compliance—a patient's following of physician's directions and advice regarding diet or medicinal treatment. *Noncompliance*, when the patient is not cooperative.

Compliant pre-stress system—a prosthetic bone implant device that helps native bone grow into implant and heal.

compliment—an expression of admiration or praise. Cf. *complement*.

Composite Cultured Skin—treatment for severe burns.

composite dressings—products which combine physically distinct components into a single dressing. See *dressing*.

compound Q (trichosanthin)—a highly purified protein from a Chinese cucumber plant. It has been shown in cell cultures to selectively kill cells that are already infected with HIV, and inhibits further production of the virus without adversely affecting normal cells. Studies have shown that HIV-infected macrophages are a reservoir of infected cells in AIDS patients, and that trichosanthin appears to block reproduction of infected T-cells and kills HIV-infected macrophages.

Comprecin (enoxacin)—antibiotic effective against gram-negative bacteria.

compromise—impairment or damage to a normal structure or function, as in neural compromise, circulatory compromise, and compromise of the immune system.

CompuCam—digital intraoral camera.

Compuscan Hittman computerized electrocardioscanner—used in studies of ventricular septal defect, pulmonary stenosis, and Ebstein's

Compuscan *(cont.)*
anomaly of the atrioventricular valve. Example: "Tapes were analyzed with a Compuscan Hittman computerized electrocardioscanner and graded according to the method of Lown and Woolf."

computed dental radiography (CDR) —computerized imaging system that utilizes an electronic sensor where dentists would normally use x-ray film. Images appear almost instantly on a computer monitor.

computed tomography angiographic portography (CTAP).

computed tomography angiography (CTA).

computed tomography laser mammography (CTLM)—breast imaging device that creates contiguous cross-sectional slice images of the breast, without compression of the breast or x-rays.

computed tomography (CT) **scan** (also called *computerized axial tomography,* or *CAT scan*)—an application of computer technology to diagnostic radiology. Instead of exposing a film after passing through the patient, x-rays are detected and recorded by a scintillation counter. The x-ray tube moves around the patient on a frame called a *gantry,* rotating through an arc and "cutting" across one plane of the patient. A series of scintillation counters are so placed that each detects the rays passing through the patient at a different angle. (Alternatively, a single counter may rotate in perfect alignment with the x-ray source.) Data on the amount of x-ray that penetrates the patient at each angle are collected from the counters, digitized,

stored, and analyzed by a minicomputer programmed to generate a cross-sectional image of the patient corresponding to the plane cut by the moving x-ray beam. Contrast medium may be injected into the circulation immediately before CT scanning. Intravenous contrast enhances the sensitivity of CT scanning of certain structures and body regions and improves the visibility of some tumors.

computer-aided diagnosis (CAD).

computer-assisted arthritis detection —see *amorphous silicon filmless digital x-ray detection technology.*

computer-assisted minimally invasive surgery (CAMIS).

computerized dynamic posturography (CDP)—used to evaluate the presence of vestibular and balance disorders.

computerized phonoenterography—a system using computerized analysis of bowel sounds to aid in diagnosis of intestinal obstruction and paralytic ileus.

computerized texture analysis of lung nodules and lung parenchyma—a viable alternative to a histologic examination in patients with focal or diffuse lung diseases.

computerized tomographic hepatic angiography (CTHA).

COMT (catechol-O-methyltransferase) —inhibitors that work to enhance the effectiveness of levodopa by blocking one of the main enzymes responsible for breaking down levodopa in the bloodstream before it reaches the brain.

Comtan (entacapone)—drug to treat Parkinson's disease in patients taking levodopa.

Comvax—combination vaccine that fights both hepatitis B and childhood bacterial meningitis.

concealed straight leg raising test—a method for the physician to determine the extent of the patient's disability. If it appears that the patient is not cooperating in the straight leg raising test or is malingering, the examining physician will pretend to examine the patient's feet but actually will be noting how high up the patient's feet will go with the legs extended. Example: "There is negative concealed straight leg raising at 90° bilaterally."

Conceive Fertility Planner—a software program that uses the natural fertility signs of a woman's body to assist couples who are trying to conceive.

concentric plaques in carotid arteries.

Concept bipolar coagulator—an electronic coagulator for hemostasis of tiny bleeders; effective in a wet field (under irrigation or in a bloody field).

Conceptus Robust guide wire—used for fallopian tube catheterization.

Conceptus Soft Seal cervical catheter—designed for atraumatic transcervical access to the uterus.

Conceptus Soft Torque uterine catheter—designed to allow easy, accurate placement at tubal ostium.

Conceptus VS (variable softness) **catheter**—used for fallopian tube catheterization.

Concerta (methylphenidate HCl)—extended-release tablets used for treatment of children with attention-deficit disorder or attention-deficit/hyperactivity disorder.

Concise cementing sculps—a series of disposable spoon and trowel-shaped instruments that are used to remove excess cement while it is still soft, without scratching the prosthesis.

Concise compression hip screw system.

concomitant—together, along with, accompanying, associated with. Cf. *comitant*.

concussion grades

grade 1—no loss of consciousness, but symptoms may include some transient confusion, inability to maintain a thought process, dizziness, headache, nausea, vomiting, and blurred vision; may resolve within 15 minutes.

grade 2—no loss of consciousness, but symptoms may include transient confusion, amnesia, dizziness, headache, and general disorientation; may persist for 15 minutes or more.

grade 3—a brief or prolonged loss of consciousness, but symptoms of confusion, amnesia, and general disorientation may persist from a few minutes to 24 hours.

condition—see *disease* or *syndrome*.

conduit—see *ileal conduit*.

coned-down view—a study limited to a small area by the use of a cone that narrows and "focuses" the x-ray beam.

C100-3—hepatitis C virus antibody (anti-HIV), diagnostic of hepatitis C.

C1q ("C-one-q") **assay**—one of a series of complement components or inhibitor proteins, numbered C1 to C9 (not a subscript), related to antibody-antigen reactions. The test is used to detect immune complexes in rheumatoid arthritis.

cone of extraocular muscles—an anatomical structure referred to in MRI reports on cavernous hemangioma and other orbital pathology.

Confide HIV test kit—a home collection HIV testing kit. A kit is sent confidentially to a home address, the recipient takes a blood sample, returns the specimen by mail, and phones for results.

confocal microscope (Oph).

Conformant contact-layer wound dressing.

conformer—that part of an eye prosthesis which covers the surface of an artificial eye sphere.

congenital dysplasia (or dislocation) **of hip** (CDH).

congenital esophageal stenosis—considered a diagnosis of exclusion. It is suggested on the basis of barium studies when a long, smooth, concentric area of esophageal narrowing is seen radiographically in patients with a life-long history of dysphagia for solids (often associated with recurrent food impactions) and with no other risk factors for the development of esophageal strictures. Symptoms are usually relieved by endoscopic bougienage or balloon dilatation.

congenital glenoid dysplasia (Ortho).

congenital lobar overinflation (CLO).

Congo red—a dye used in the laboratory to stain amyloids. Has been found to prevent the formation of memory-robbing plaques in Alzheimer's disease and may stop the cell-killing that leads to adult-onset diabetes mellitus. The discovery of Congo red's effect may also provide fundamental information about the aging process.

conical cecum—cone-shaped appearance of the cecum on radiography, indicative of Crohn's disease or colonic tuberculosis.

conjugated estrogens (CE)—given to renal transplant patients to decrease bleeding complications secondary to uremic coagulopathy. Favored over fresh frozen plasma.

conjunctivodacryocystorhinostomy (CDCR).

consensual light reflex—constriction of the pupil of one eye in response to stimulation by light of the retina of the other eye. See *direct light reflex*.

consensus (*not* concensus and *not* consensus of opinion). Consensus means general opinion, or conclusion after discussion with a number of people, so the word *opinion* is redundant.

conserved helix-loop-helix ubiquitous kinase—see *CHUK*.

consolidative process (Radiol)—abnormal process that increases the density of a tissue or region.

Constellation—an advanced mapping catheter for electrical mapping of complex right atrial tachycardias.

construction artifact (Radiol)—also called *superimposition artifact*. See *summation shadow artifact*.

contact-layer wound dressings—thin, nonadherent sheets placed directly on an open wound bed to protect the wound tissue from direct contact with other agents or dressings applied to the wound. They are porous to allow wound fluid to pass through for absorption by an overlying dressing. See *dressing*.

Contigen Bard collagen implant.

Contigen glutaraldehyde cross-linked collagen—used for urethral injection for urinary incontinence.

Contigen implant—an alternative to surgical procedures or wearing external pads for urinary incontinence. Via periurethral or transurethral

Contigen *(cont.)*
cystoscopy, this liquid collagen implant is injected submucosally on either side of the urethra near the bladder neck until the urethral lumen is just occluded and offers normal resistance to the flow of urine from the bladder.

contiguous images (in computed tomography scan)—a series of scans without intervals of unexamined tissue between them.

continent supravesical bowel urinary diversion—for bladder reconstruction to treat invasive bladder cancer. Examples: Camey reservoir, continent urinary diversion, Kock pouch, Mainz pouch, Rowland pouch, and sigmoid colon reservoir.

continuous arteriovenous hemofiltration (CAVH)—a procedure that filters toxins from the blood of patients in renal failure. It has a lower risk of side effects than hemodialysis because the equipment is simpler and blood is removed from the patient's body at a much slower rate.

continuous circular capsulorrhexis technique (Oph).

continuous cyclical peritoneal dialysis (CCPD).

continuous passive motion (CPM).

continuous positive airway pressure (CPAP).

continuous wave Doppler examination.

contoured tilting compression mammography—uses a paddle-shaped rather than flat compression component in the mammography unit. This technique is said to provide more comfort for the patient, since the paddles conform more to the individual's breast shape.

Contour MD implantable single-lead cardioverter-defibrillator.

Contour Profile—anatomically shaped silicone breast implant for breast reconstruction or augmentation.

Contour V-145D and **LTV-135D** implantable cardioverter-defibrillator devices.

contraction fasciculations—rhythmic, brief twitching of a muscle during weak voluntary or postural contractions. Seen in some elderly patients and those with neurogenic muscle atrophy.

contractions—see *Braxton Hicks contractions*.

contracture—see *Volkmann's contracture*.

contralateral acoustic stimulation (CAS)—used in studies of comparative hearing.

contrast echocardiography—ultrasound technique used to diagnose blood flow abnormalities in heart muscle. It uses Optison contrast agent.

contrast material-enhanced scan—MRI term.

contrast medium—see *medication*.

contrast-to-noise (C/N) **ratio**—MRI term.

contrecoup injury—referring to an injury, as to the brain, occurring at a site opposite the point of contact.

Control-Release pop-off needle.

conus medullaris—cone-shaped lower end of spinal cord.

conventional spin-echo MR imaging vs. breath-hold fast spin-echo or multishot spin-echo echo-planar imaging—MRI term.

convergence test (Oph)—locates breaking point of fusion at near vision.

Convergent color Doppler—a more powerful color imaging capability

Convergent *(cont.)*
that is reportedly easier to use, and a more sensitive way to image blood flow dynamics.

conversion disorder—a psychiatric diagnosis in which the loss of function on presentation mimics organic disease. Although rare, it is most common in adolescents and young adults. A patient with conversion disorder may present with progressive bilateral lower-extremity weakness and impaired gait.

convertible slip knot—a knot that converts between a locking and slipping configuration, useful in microsurgical, endoscopic, and laparoscopic applications. See *Aberdeen knot.*

convex linear array—term used in B-scan, Doppler, and color Doppler imaging. See *B-scan.*

convolutions of Gratiolet ("grah-tee-olay")—small convolutions that are buried beneath the lateral surface of the occipital lobe of the brain.

convulsions
benign familial neonatal (BFNC)
benign infantile familial (BIFC)

ConXn (recombinant human relaxin)—for treatment of peripheral vascular disease as well as kidney and cardiovascular disease.

Cook endoscopic curved needle driver—allows endoscopic suturing using standard curved needle sutures so that tissue approximation, anatomical reconstruction, and hemostasis can be performed endoscopically.

Cook TPN (total parenteral nutrition) **catheters** (single and double lumen).

cookie—see *Gelfoam cookie.*

cookie cutter—see *Freeman.*

CoolSpot—skin-cooling device that provides surface cooling to upper layers of skin during dermatological laser treatments.

Cool Tip catheter—used in catheter ablation treatment of atrial arrhythmias.

Coomassie-blue stain.

Cooperman event probability—a clinical scoring system used to predict cardiac morbidity.

Cooper's syndrome—see *fibrocystic breast syndrome.*

Coopervision irrigation/aspiration handpiece. "The residual cortex was aspirated with the Coopervision irrigation/aspiration handpiece."

COP (colloid oncotic pressure).

COPA (cyclophosphamide, oncovin, prednisone, and Adriamycin) **plus cytokine interferon**—used to treat non-Hodgkin's lymphoma.

Copalis—acronym for **co**upled **pa**rticle **li**ght **s**cattering, trademarked by Sienna Biotech, Inc. See *Copalis ToRC.*

Copalis ToRC—completely automated total antibody assay that detects *Toxoplasma gondii*, rubella, and cytomegalovirus in human serum.

Copaxone (glatiramer acetate)—used in treatment of relapsing-remitting multiple sclerosis.

COP-BLEO (cyclophosphamide, Oncovin, prednisone, bleomycin)—chemotherapy protocol.

COPE (cyclophosphamide, Oncovin, Platinol, etoposide)—chemotherapy protocol.

Cope crushing clamp—used in bowel resection.

Cope modification of a Martel intestinal clamp—used in GI surgery.

Copolymer 1 (COP 1)—trademark for random polymer of levorotatory alanine, glutamic acid, lysine, and

Copolymer *(cont.)*
tyrosine. Daily injections early in the course of multiple sclerosis may reduce the number of exacerbations.

copper-binding protein (CBP) **test**.

copper-vapor pulsed laser.

copper wire effect, copper-wiring— narrowing of arterioles in the retina; seen in some patients with arteriosclerosis in the funduscopic examination.

cor (noun)—the heart. Cf. *core, corps.*

coracoacromial—pertaining to coracoid and acromial processes.

coralline hydroxyapatite Goniopora (CHAG).

Cordarone (amiodarone hydrochloride) —given for cardiac arrhythmias.

Cordase (collagenase)—injectable collagenase for treatment of Dupuytren's disease.

cordate—heart-shaped. Cf. *caudate, chordate.*

cord blood—blood drawn from the umbilical cord at birth; used to determine blood type, chemistries, and blood gases.

Cordguard II—a device used by an obstetrician to clamp and cut the umbilical cord and obtain an uncontaminated neonatal blood sample immediately after birth.

Cordis Bioptone sheath.

Cordis-Hakim shunt—used in the Kasai procedure for biliary atresia. See *Kasai procedure.*

Cordis Predator PTCA balloon catheter—used in interventional cardiac treatment.

Cordis Trakstar PTCA balloon catheter—used in interventional cardiac treatment.

cordotomy, chordotomy—words used interchangeably by many dictionaries and journals, although *cordotomy* seems to be the preferred spelling. See *Rosamoff cordotomy.*

Cordox (fructose-1,6-diphosphate)— cardioprotective drug for pretreatment of patients undergoing coronary artery bypass grafting procedures, valve repair and replacement, and a variety of other open heart surgeries.

corduroy artifact (Radiol)—results from grid synchronization problems.

cord, vocal (*not* chord) (ENT).

core (noun)—the central part of something; (verb)—to take out the core of something. Cf. *cor, corps.*

Core aspiration/injection needle—for laparoscopic surgery.

Core CO_2 insufflation needle for laparoscopic surgery.

Coreg (carvedilol)—a beta blocker and vasodilator used in the treatment of congestive heart failure.

Core trocar and cannula systems for laparoscopic surgery.

Cor-Flex wire guides—used with Cook Micropuncture catheter system.

Corin hip system—total hip arthroplasty and hemiarthroplasty cemented system.

Cormed ambulatory infusion pump —permits outpatient therapy in patients receiving chemotherapy, heparin, hyperalimentation, or other ambulatory infusion treatment.

corneae, limbus—see *limbus corneae.*

cornea guttata—degenerative condition of the cornea caused by dystrophy of the endothelial cells.

corneal exhaustion syndrome—a result of long-time wear of contact lens.

corneal impression test (CIT)—allows cells from the cornea to be tested for signs of rabies before blood, skin, or saliva tests can pick up the disease.

corneal reflex—closure of the eyes on stimulating the cornea.

Corneal Ring (Oph)—a product designed to correct myopia by reshaping the curvature of the cornea.

CorneaSparing LTK (laser thermal keratoplasty) **system**—a noncontact simultaneous laser application for correction of hyperopia, presbyopia, and overcorrection resulting from laser treatments for myopia.

corner fracture—metaphyseal lesion commonly found in abused infants.

corner mouth lift—a plastic surgery procedure in which a triangle is excised just above the commissure, with the suture line following the upper lip vermilion border and extending slightly beyond the corner. It may or may not be performed as an adjunct to lip lift. See *lip lift*.

corn picker's pupil—unilateral mydriasis afflicting workers exposed to belladonna or jimsonweed.

Corometrics maternal/fetal monitor.

coronal orientation—MRI term.

coronal SPIR image (MRI). See *SPIR*.

coronal T1-weighted MR image (spin echo).

coronary anastomotic shunt—used in cardiopulmonary bypass surgery to keep the operating field clear of blood while protecting the heart through distal perfusion.

coronary artery scan (CAS) by Ultrafast CT—a simple, low-cost, and noninvasive diagnostic scan that identifies patients at risk for atherosclerosis and coronary disease episodes by detecting and quantifying calcium in the coronary arteries.

coronary atherectomy—an alternative to balloon angioplasty. It works on the Roto-Rooter principle, with suc-

tion apparatus utilized to remove the excised plaque.

coronary devices for treatment of ischemic heart disease include *stents* (Palmaz-Schatz and Gianturco-Roubin), *atherectomy* (directional, rotational, and extraction), and *excimer laser angioplasty*.

coronary radiation therapy (CRT).

coronary remodeling—focal enlargement or shrinkage of the lumina of atherosclerotic arteries during plaque formation. Shrinkage has also been demonstrated as a mechanism of arterial remodeling in vessels that have undergone balloon angioplasty and directional atherectomy.

coronary-subclavian steal syndrome—a rarely occurring retrograde blood flow seen postoperatively in patients who have had a coronary artery bypass graft (CABG).

corps ("core") (noun)—corpus; also, a group or body of individuals organized and under common direction (e.g., the medical corps). Cf. *cor, core, corpse*.

corpse—a dead body. Cf. *corps*.

corpus callosum—mass of white matter in the depths of the longitudinal fissure connecting the two cerebral hemispheres.

corpus cavernosum penile electromyography—predicts cavernous smooth muscle function.

corpuscles—see *malpighian corpuscles*.

corpus Luysii—see *body of Luys*.

corset platysmaplasty—cosmetic surgery for the aging neck. The platysma is used to contour the neck like a corset, producing fewer contour irregularities.

Corti—see *organ of Corti*.

cortical mapping (of the brain).

cortical spoking.

cortical thumb. The thumb lies flat on the palm, with the fingers over it; this is suggestive of a corticospinal lesion.

corticomedullary junction (CMJ) phase imaging on CT scan.

corticotropin-releasing factor (CRF)— a human peptide used for the reduction of edema and inflammation in patients with brain cancer, asthma, and rheumatoid arthritis.

cor triatriatum—a cardiac anomaly in which there are three atria. Also, *triatrial heart*.

cor triatriatum dexter—rare congenital anomaly in which an obstructive membrane is located in the right atrium.

Corvert (ibutilide fumarate)—used for rapid conversion of atrial fibrillation and atrial flutter to normal sinus rhythm.

Corynebacterium—gram-positive organism that causes infection in immunosuppressed patients, particularly pneumonia in AIDS patients.

CoSeal—resorbable synthetic sealant for use in sealing vascular grafts.

Cosgrove-Edwards annuloplasty system.

Cosman ICP Tele-Sensor—implantable telemetric pressure sensor used in hydrocephalus shunts to measure intracranial pressure and to diagnose shunt blockage and function. Also, *Cosman Tele-Monitor System*.

Cosmederm-7—patented anti-irritant said to minimize or eliminate the itching, burning, and stinging commonly associated with high-performance skin care products.

Cosmos II pacemaker—a dual chamber or DDD pacemaker.

Cosopt—used in treatment of glaucoma or ocular hypertension.

Costello's protocol—laser ablation of prostate in benign prostatic hypertrophy.

costosternal angle.

cot—see *finger cot*.

Cotrel-Dubousset instrumentation (CDI)—used for posterior spine stabilization and fusion (with bone graft). See *Kaneda device*. Kaneda and Cotrel-Dubousset procedures may be performed at the same time or separately.

Cotrel traction—treatment for adult scoliosis. Uses a leather head halter, pelvic girdle, and a system of pulleys. Also, *Cotrel-Dubousset*.

Cottle elevator (Neuro).

Cotton-Berg syndrome—proximal end tibia fracture; fender fracture.

Cotton-Loader position cast (Ortho).

cottonoid patty (pattie)—used to stem hemorrhage and to protect the exposed brain in surgery. Cf. *Cellolite*.

Cotton procedure—a cartilage graft to the cricolaryngeal area; for subglottic stenosis.

cotton-wool exudates of retina—microinfarcts of nerve fiber layer that resemble tufts of cotton.

cotyledon—subdivision of the uterine surface of a discoidal placenta.

coudé catheter—bent (or elbowed).

cough CPR—a technique used in cardiac catheterization and emergency medicine in which the patient forcefully and repeatedly coughs. Coughing converts ventricular arrhythmias to a normal sinus rhythm.

Couinaud classification—a grading system for liver disease, using roman numerals that correspond to the segment of liver involved. "The hepa-

Couinaud *(cont.)*
tectomy consisted of a segmentectomy VIII (according to Couinaud's classification)." This means that segment VIII of the liver was involved in the procedure.

Coulter counter—for platelet count.

Coulter HIV-1 p24 antigen assay—an antigen test kit for screening of blood donors for HIV-1 during the initial period when donors may actually be infected but still have negative antibody tests with current testing.

Coumadin (warfarin)—anticoagulant used to prevent thromboembolic events, strokes, and heart failure in patients with mechanical heart valves, atrial fibrillation, post myocardial infarction, and deep vein thrombosis.

coumarin pulsed-dye laser (Pulsolith) —used in lithotripsy.

Councilman bodies—seen in hepatocytes in viral hepatitis.

countercurrent immunoelectrophoresis test (CIE).

counterflow centrifugal elutriation—a technique which removes some lymphocytes from patients who had allogenic bone marrow transplant to decrease the incidence of graft-versus-host disease.

counting fingers (or *count fingers*) (CF)—a term used in eye examinations. "Visual acuity was limited to counting fingers in the right eye, and hand movements in the left eye."

counts, kick—see *kick counts*.

coup de sabre (Fr., stroke of a sword) —linear scleroderma usually found over the scalp or forehead.

coupled suturing—technique for microvascular anastomosis which is an adaptation of a type of continuous stitch used in the garment industry, generally using 9-0 and 10-0 nylon.

COUP-TF—thyroid hormone receptor auxiliary protein.

Cournand cardiac device.

Courvoisier's sign—palpably enlarged gallbladder, sometimes a sign of pancreatic carcinoma.

CoVac 50 and **CoVac 70**—suction ArthroWand.

Covaderm composite wound dressing.

Covera-HS (verapamil)—calcium channel blocker used for the treatment of hypertension and angina. Taken at bedtime, it is designed to lower blood pressure by releasing active drug in concert with the body's natural circadian rhythms. Uses a controlled onset extended release (COER-24) delivery system.

Coverlet—an adhesive dressing.

Cover-Roll—adhesive gauze.

Cover-Strip wound closure strips— uses a hypoallergenic adhesive. In some wounds these may be an alternative to sutures. They have a porous gauze strip that permits air to enter and exudate to pass through.

CoverTip safety syringe—designed to protect against accidental needle sticks.

cover-uncover test (Oph)—assesses eye muscle deviation.

Cowboy Collar—brachial plexus injury control.

COWS (cold to the opposite, warm to the same)—a mnemonic device to help remember the Hallpike caloric stimulation response. "Caloric testing produced COWS." See *caloric testing*.

coxarthrosis—see *end-stage coxarthrosis* (Ortho).

Coxiella burnetii—rickettsia that causes Q fever. See *Q fever.*

COX (cyclo-oxygenase) **pathway**—a prostaglandin.

coxsackievirus, A and B—a virus that causes meningitis and paralytic disease.

COX-2 inhibitors—a class of non-steroidal anti-inflamatory drugs for osteoarthritis, rheumatoid arthritis, acute pain, and primary dysmenorrhea. They work by inhibiting cyclo-oxygenase-2 (COX-2), responsible for producing pain and inflammation, without affecting COX-1, which protects the stomach lining. Inhibition of COX-1 is thought to be the cause of serious GI side effects in NSAIDs.

Cozaar (losartan potassium)—an angiotensin-II inhibitor for treatment of hypertension, volume depletion, and hepatic failure, alone or in combination with other agents.

CP angle (costophrenic).

CPAP (continuous positive airway pressure) ("see-pap")—provides positive pressure in lungs even when the patient exhales fully, to prevent lungs from collapsing.

CPB (cyclophosphamide, Platinol, BCNU)—chemotherapy protocol.

CPC (cyclophosphamide, Platinol, carboplatin)—chemotherapy protocol.

CP-Cardiosol—used in cardiopulmonary bypass.

CPD (cephalopelvic disproportion).

CPD (chorioretinopathy and pituitary dysfunction) **syndrome**—characterized by severe, early-onset chorioretinopathy, trichosis, and evidence of pituitary dysfunction.

CPE (chronic pulmonary emphysema).

CPHV OptiForm mitral valve—used in patients requiring mitral valve replacement. The OptiForm mitral valve has a flexible sewing cuff that can be sculpted to fit mitral annular anatomy, thus ensuring tissue compliance with the valve. *CPHV* is an acronym for *Carbomedics prosthetic heart valve.*

CPI (conventional planar imaging).

CPK (creatine phosphokinase)—serum enzyme that can be chemically distinguished into three isoenzymes or fractions: the MB isoenzyme, elevated in myocardial infarction; the MM isoenzyme, elevated in cerebral infarction; and the BB isoenzyme, sometimes elevated in uremia and other conditions. When separated in the laboratory by electrophoresis, these isoenzymes appear as distinct bands in a visual display. Hence the expression "*MB band* is roughly synonymous with *MB isoenzyme.*" Do not confuse *creatine* with *creatinine.*

CPM (continuous passive motion) **devices**—see *Autoflex II.*

CPP (cerebral perfusion pressure).

CPPD (calcium pyrophosphate deposition; disease).

CPS (cardiopulmonary support) **system**—heart-lung machine.

CPT hip system.

CPVG (cryopreserved vein graft).

crack—street name for rock cocaine, a concentrated, smokable form of the drug which is highly addicting. Cf. *crank.*

cracked pot sound—(1) a percussion sound like that heard when striking a cracked pot and indicates a pulmonary cavity; (2) a sound on percussion caused by the separation of cranial sutures in children with increased cranial pressure, e.g., as seen in hydrocephalus. Also called *Macewen's sign.*

cracker test (for the presence of Sjö-gren's disease). "She has a negative cracker test in the sense that if we were to give her a soda cracker, she would easily be able to swallow without drinking water."

cradle cap—seborrheic dermatitis manifested as thick yellowish scales, often seen on the scalp of infants.

Crafoord-Senning heart-lung machine.

Cragg endoluminal graft—see *Cragg Endopro System 1*.

Cragg Endopro System I—a covered stent design, used in Cragg endoluminal graft procedure as adjunct to balloon angioplasty of long complex iliac stenosis. The stent is covered with woven fabric graft and is a flexible, self-expanding endoprosthesis of nitinol wire.

Cragg thrombolytic brush—a mechanical thrombolysis system to dissolve clots in hemodialysis access grafts.

cranial electrical stimulation (CES)—introduced by Saul Liss for relief of pain and anxiety, there being a noted correlation between depression and chronic pain. The Liss CES device is used for chronic headache pain and is similar to TENS application.

cranial nerves, twelve—written with roman numerals, I to XII.
  I   olfactory
  II   optic
  III   oculomotor
  IV   trochlear
  V   trigeminal
  VI   abducens
  VII   facial
  VIII   vestibulocochlear (acoustic)
  IX   glossopharyngeal
  X   vagal

cranial nerves *(cont.)*
  XI   accessory
  XII   hypoglossal

cranioplastic powder—used for repair of cranial defects.

craniosacral therapy (CST)—a hands-on light-touch method of assisting in the natural flow of cerebrospinal fluid within the system. The CST method of evaluating and enhancing the function of the physiological body system called the craniosacral system was developed by John E. Upledger, an osteopathic physician, and is referred to as *Upledger CST*.

craniosynostosis (craniostosis)—premature closure of the sagittal suture in newborns, resulting in scaphocephaly and other associated compensatory deformational changes. When treated early (less than 2-3 months of age), a simple suturectomy or resection of the synostotic suture provides correction. By 6 months of age, patients require major craniofacial reconstructive procedures. See also *endoscopic strip craniectomy, helmet-molding therapy,* and *scaphocephaly.*

crank—slang term for the street drug methamphetamine ("speed"), which is snorted or injected. Cf. *crack.*

Crawford's graft inclusion technique (Cardio)—with direct branch vessel reattachment.

CRC (colorectal cancer).

CR/CO (centric relation-centric occlusion)—used in maxillofacial surgery when discussing bite patterns.

CRE (cAMP response element)—a DNA sequence that acts as a binding site for proteins.

C-reactive protein (CRP)—a protein which is high when there is an

C-reactive *(cont.)* inflammatory response and returns to undetectable as the response clears.

creatine—a nitrogenous substance that is found in muscles, brain, and blood of vertebrates. Cf. *carotene, creatinine, keratin.*

creatine phosphokinase—see *CPK.*

creatinine clearance, 24-hour—a measure of kidney function, calculated from the serum creatinine level and the amount of creatinine excreted in the urine in 24 hours. Cf. *creatine, creatinine.*

creatinine, serum—a waste product of protein metabolism, elevated in kidney disease. Cf. *creatine.*

CREB (cAMP response element binding) **protein**—regulates genes for neurotransmitter synthetic enzymes.

Credé ("kre-day") **maneuver**—massaging the lower abdomen over the bladder to promote complete emptying in patients with neurological damage. "Bladder Credé was ordered." Cf. *Credé method.*

Credé method—expressing the placenta from the uterus by pushing the uterus down into the pelvis and squeezing it. Cf. *Credé maneuver.*

creola bodies (lowercase *c*)—balls of desquamated epithelium. Often found in the sputa of asthmatics.

crepitant rales—fine crackling or bubbling sounds heard on auscultation of the breath sounds.

crescendo-decrescendo murmur—increases from quiet to louder and then decreases again. May be diagnostic of aortic stenosis when heard as a systolic murmur. In aortic insufficiency it is heard as a diastolic murmur. Also, *diamond-shaped murmur.*

crescent artifact—see *kink artifact.*

crescentic base wedge osteotomy—a rotational osteotomy whose axis is near the first metatarsal base. Used for correction of hallux valgus and similar to an opening base wedge osteotomy.

CREST syndrome—see also *CRST.*

C calcinosis cutis
R Raynaud's phenomenon
E esophageal dysmotility
S sclerodactyly
T telangiectasia

cribogram—a special mattress wired with sensing devices. An infant who is suspected of hearing loss is placed on it and a computer compares the baby's movements with the stimulation.

crick—painful spasm, usually in the neck.

Cricket—small, light pulse oximeter.

cri du chat (cat's cry)—an indication of a chromosomal irregularity causing mental retardation; the name derives from the catlike cry emitted by these children.

Crigler-Najjar syndrome—one of the reasons for liver transplant in children.

Crikelair otoplasty (ENT).

crinkle artifact—see *kink artifact.*

Crinone bioadhesive progesterone gel —vaginally delivered to administer progesterone directly to uterus for treatment of infertility, maximizing therapeutic benefits and eliminating pain of IM injection and messiness of vaginal suppositories.

crisis—see *Dietl's crisis.*

crisscross heart—a heart with crossing of the atrioventricular valves.

"crit"—slang for hematocrit.

criteria (pl.)—standards or means by which conclusions are arrived at. "On EKG there were voltage criteria for left ventricular hypertrophy." See *Jones criteria, revised.*

Crixivan (indinavir sulfate)—a protease inhibitor used as an AIDS drug.

Crohn's disease—regional enteritis; a chronic granulomatous inflammatory disease.

Cröhnlein procedure (Oph).

cross-chest adduction test—also referred to as horizontal adduction test. It is used for diagnosing rotator cuff tendinitis.

cross-cover test—measures degree of eye deviation.

crossed coil—MRI term.

crossed reflex—in which stimulus applied to one side produces a response on the contralateral side.

crossed-swords technique (Oph)— "The inferior oblique muscle was reattached using the crossed-swords technique."

crossfire radiation therapy—a procedure for treating brain tumors. Doctors attach a metal frame to the skull with screws to hold the head still and help aim the beams. The beams are fired from hundreds of points, following paths that intersect only at the tumor. Working together, they kill the tumor while sparing other tissue.

CrossFlex LC coronary stent—for improving luminal diameter and maintaining patency in ischemic coronary arteries secondary to discrete de novo stenosis or restenosis of native coronary arteries. It is an over-the-wire product that is placed via a balloon catheter during PTCA procedures.

crosshatch pattern (Oph)—see *fishbone pattern.*

CrossSail—coronary dilatation catheter.

cross-talk effect—MRI term.

cross-tunneling incision—used in performance of lipectomy. "A cross-tunneling incision was made and a 1.8 and a 2.4 mm triple-hole cannula used."

crowncork tympanoplasty (ENT)—a total reconstruction of the tympanic membrane. A composite graft of tragal cartilage and perichondrium is fashioned. It looks like a crown on top of a bottle cork. It is used in correcting subtotal or total defects of the tympanic membrane, found in surgery for middle ear malformation.

CRP (canalith repositioning procedure)—measures vertigo. A vibrational device is held against the mastoid process of the ear that is affected with benign paroxysmal positional vertigo.

CRS (Cell Recovery System).

CRS (Counter Rotation System)—type of brace used to correct internal and external tibial torsion in children. Consists of a hinged device with rods that attach to footplates glued onto both shoes. It allows kicking and crawling, and children can sleep in it comfortably.

CRST syndrome—see also *CREST.*
C calcinosis cutis
R Raynaud's phenomenon
S sclerodactyly
T telangiectasia

CRT (coronary radiation therapy).

cruciate incision—cross-shaped.

crude coal tar (*not* cold tar)—used in treatment of psoriasis.

Cruiser hip abduction brace—polypropylene hip abduction brace for treating hip dysplasia in toddlers up to 2¹/₂ years of age.

crutched-stick-type endoprosthesis—a descriptive term used for a biliary duct stent.

Crutchfield skeletal traction tongs.

cry, uterine (Ob-Gyn)—as in "Curettage was done, with good uterine cry." "Uterine cry" refers to the sound of the uterus as it is being scraped clean of debris, during the curettage. The uterus is a smooth and firm muscle, and once all the lining and debris are removed by sharp curettage, the smooth muscle emits a "cry" when it is clean and smooth once again. Note: Some physicians pronounce "cree" (probably from French *cri*, as in *cri du chat*), others "cry" (long *i*).

cryoablation for prostate cancer—a minimally invasive procedure performed under general or local anesthesia. It involves freezing and destroying cancerous tumors inside the body, using advanced ultrasound technology to locate the tumor and a cryoprobe to freeze tissue. The body absorbs the dead tissue over time.

CRYOcare system—used in endometrial cryoablation as treatment for dysfunctional uterine bleeding.

cryocrit—the percentage of red and white blood cells re-added to arrive at this value. Cf. *cytocrit*.

Cryo/Cuff ankle dressing—reduces swelling and pain by applying cryotherapy and compression.

Cryo/Cuff boot—boot filled with ice and water, covering foot and ankle. Exerts pressure up to 40 mmHg.

cryogens—supercooled gases such as helium or nitrogen, used to cool the magnet at the heart of a magnetic resonance scanner.

CryoHit—allows surgeons to ablate localized tumors by freezing diseased cells during a minimally invasive procedure using ultra-thin probes. The system is compatible with interventional MRI (I-MRI), which provides real-time video images of the tissue during surgery.

CryoLife-O'Brien valve—a stentless porcine heart valve.

cryomagnet—MRI term.

cryophake (Oph)—an instrument using extremely cold temperatures to remove a cataract. Example: *Keeler cryophake*.

cryoprecipitate—used to control bleeding in patients with uremia and prolonged bleeding time. Contains fibrinogen, factor VIII, fibronectin, and factor XIII. It is used as a last resort in life-threatening bleeding because of the risk of viral transmission. See *DDAVP.*

cryopreserved vein graft (CVG).

cryoprobe—instrument used to apply extreme cold to tissues, as in cryosurgery.

cryostat—a device containing a microtome for sectioning frozen tissue.

cryosurgery—a treatment that kills some types of cancer cells by freezing them with liquid nitrogen. It is used in prostate cancer if there has been no spread to other tissue. Cryosurgery is performed under spinal or general anesthesia, with the aid of an ultrasound probe that is inserted into the rectum. The ultrasound converts sound waves into images on a TV monitor; this functions as a guide for inserting the probes, through

cryosurgery *(cont.)*
which the liquid nitrogen is administered. The iceball that is formed within the prostatic tissue and tumor can be seen on the screen. And the neat thing (in the housekeeping sense) is that the dead cells are absorbed by the body. This is a form of therapy that can be repeated, if the cancer should recur.

CryoValve-SG—human allograft heart valve processing method. It depopulates the native cells of a donor heart valve, leaving a collagen matrix with the same functionality as other cryopreserved heart valves.

Cryptaz (nitazoxanide)—anti-infective for AIDS-related cryptosporidial diarrhea.

"crypto"—slang term for cryptococcosis, infection with *Cryptococcus neoformans*, or cryptosporidiosis, which is seen in AIDS patients. As with all slang, when in doubt, ask the dictator for clarification.

cryptochrome—a newly discovered light-sensitive pigment in the eye that has been found to mediate the circadian rhythm, the biological timer regulating many body functions.

Cryptococcus neoformans—rare cause of lytic bone lesions; an AIDS infection.

cryptosporidiosis antibody—immunostimulant for AIDS patients, obtained from cow's milk.

Cryptosporidium—a protozoan parasite. Sometimes referred to as the slang term "crypto."

crystalloid—a substance in solution that can pass through a semipermeable membrane. "Fluids: 1600 cc of crystalloid." Normal saline solution and lactated Ringer's solution are crystalloids used as blood replacement.

CSD (cat-scratch disease).

CSDH (chronic subdural hematoma).

CSF (cerebrospinal fluid).

CSF (colony-stimulating factor).

CS-5 cryosurgical system—used for cryoablation of prostatic tissue and liver metastases and other gynecological, urological, and general surgical applications.

C-shaped curves.

CSQI (continuous subcutaneous infusion)—pain-control method utilizing a butterfly needle inserted subcutaneously and connected to an intravenous line. It is used for patients who will receive narcotic medication for more than 48 hours and who cannot receive intravenous medication due to poor veins or other problems. The system can be coupled with a patient-controlled analgesia pump which allows the patient to select the time when the medication is most needed for pain control and administer it. *Sub-Q-Set* is the trade name for one continuous subcutaneous infusion device.

CSVT (central splanchnic venous thrombosis).

CSWT (cardiac shock wave therapy).

CT (computed tomography).

CTA (computed tomographic angiography).

CTAP (CT angiographic portography).

CTCb (cyclophosphamide, thiotepa, carboplatin)—chemotherapy protocol used to treat metastatic breast carcinoma.

CTCL (cutaneous T-cell lymphoma)—also called *mycosis fungoides*.

CTD (connective tissue disease).

CTDx electrostimulation system—helps decrease symptoms associated with repetitive stress injury of the wrist while providing wrist support.

C-terminal assay for PTH (parathormone; parathyroid hormone).

CTE:YAG (CrTmEr:YAG) **laser**.

CTFC (corrected TIMI frame count)—a quantitative method of assessing coronary artery flow during angiography.

CT gantry—the bridgelike frame on a CT scanner on which the traveling crane of the scanner moves.

CTHA (computerized tomographic hepatic angiography).

C.Ti. Brace—a six-point knee support especially for ACL (anterior cruciate ligament) deficient knees.

CT laser mammography (CTLM)—a "painless mammogram" that requires no breast compression, uses no x-rays, and produces detailed cross-sectional images of the tissue.

CTLC (contact transscleral laser cytophotocoagulation).

CTLM (computed tomography laser mammography).

CTMP (contrast threshold for motion perception).

CTNS—a gene associated with cystinosis. Neuropathic cystinosis is characterized by an accumulation of the amino acid cystine in cells, leading to severe organ damage, primarily in the kidneys. Most patients develop the disease within their first year of life, and many die of kidney disease before the age of 10.

CT PEG (CT-guided percutaneous endoscopic gastrostomy)—for placement of a gastric feeding tube without open surgery.

CTR (cardiothoracic ratio).

C-TRAK handheld gamma detector—measures the accumulated radioactivity in a nodule after radionuclide injection.

CTS (carpal tunnel syndrome).

CT scanner—see *scanner.*

CT/SPECT fusion—digitally fused CT and radiolabeled monoclonal antibody SPECT images. Used to detect tumors.

CT with slip-ring technology.

C225—monoclonal antibody antineoplastic.

C-type acupuncture needle—used with a guiding tube to assure straight entry into the skin. B-type needles are used without guiding tubes.

cubital tunnel syndrome—caused by compression of the ulnar nerve at the elbow. Cf. *carpal tunnel syndrome.*

Cueva cranial nerve electrode monitoring device.

cuirass ("kwe-ras´")—a covering for the chest. Also, *cuirass respirator.*

CUI (Cox-Uphoff International) **tissue expander**.

culdoplasty, modified McCall posterior—performed at the time of abdominal hysterectomy to decrease the incidence of posthysterectomy vaginal vault prolapse and enterocele formation.

cul-de-sac—a blind pouch; a saclike cavity or tube open at only one end, e.g., the rectouterine pouch, or pouch of Douglas.

Cullen's sign—a bluish discoloration around the umbilicus, indicative of a ruptured ectopic pregnancy or acute hemorrhagic pancreatitis.

culture and sensitivity (C&S)—a lab test in which an organism is grown

culture *(cont.)*
on a nutrient medium containing several antibiotic-laden disks. A lack of growth around a disk shows that the organism is sensitive to that antibiotic. Do not confuse *C&S* with *CNS* (central nervous system).

cultured autologous melanocytes—applied to superficially dermabraded skin for treatment of vitiligo.

cultured epithelial autografting—a technique to cover a burn wound in patients with massive burns, who do not have enough skin of their own for grafting. Small pieces of their remaining skin are cultured into new skin.

Cun-Meter—a mathematical search square which is a point-search aid used to assess position of acupuncture points. Measurements are registered in Cun, which is the width of the thumb joint. With these measuring instruments, width is first measured, after which readings can be taken at any time from a scale of 0.5 to 2.5 Cun.

Cunningham clamp—for male urinary incontinence.

cupping—method of stimulating acupuncture points by applying suction through a metal, wood, or glass jar in which a partial vacuum has been created. This technique produces blood congestion at the site and therefore stimulates it. Used for low backache, sprains, soft-tissue injuries, and helping remove fluid from lungs in chronic bronchitis.

cup-to-disk ratio (Oph).

Curaderm hydrocolloid dressing material.

Curafil hydrogel dressing.

Curafoam foam wound dressing.

Curagel Hydrogel dressing—absorbs excess exudate while it cools and cushions a wound. It has a top layer of polyurethane designed to help control evaporation and leave no residue to irritate the wound when removed.

Curasorb calcium alginate dressing—reacts with sodium ions in wound exudate to form a nonadherent gel that provides a moist healing environment, reducing possible maceration of healthy skin surrounding a wound. It can be trimmed and customized for a variety of wound shapes and sizes and can be used for packing deep wounds. Cf. *Aquasorb, Ventex*.

Curdy blade (Oph).

C-urea breath excretion test—highly sensitive test, diagnostic for *Helicobacter pylori*. Patients are given a dose of C-urea and "cold" urea, with breath samples taken at 30- and 60-minute intervals, and C-urea measured in exhaled CO_2. See also *breath pentane test, C-cholyl-glycine breath test, C-urinary excretion, Helicobacter pyloric breath test*.

C-urinary excretion—measurement of C-urea in urine after oral dose, correlates with C-urea breath test for diagnosis of *H. pylori*. See also *C-urea breath test*.

Curling's ulcer—gastric or duodenal ulcers seen in patients who have suffered severe burns over large areas of the body.

Curosurf (poractant alpha) **intratracheal suspension**—porcine-derived lung surfactant for the treatment of respiratory distress syndrome (hyaline membrane disease) in premature infants.

Curretab (medroxyprogesterone).

Curschmann's spirals—formed elements that have been found in the sputa of asthmatic patients.

curve of Spee—a curved line extending along the summits of the buccal cusps from the first premolar to the third molar. Named for a German embryologist, Ferdinand von Spee.

curvilinear incision (*not* curvalinear)—a curved incision.

CUSA (Cavitron ultrasonic aspirator).

Cu-Safe 300—IUD specifically designed to decrease unwanted side effects, such as bleeding, pain, and expulsion, while providing simplicity of insertion, ease of removal, and fair contraceptive protection.

CUSALap—ultrasonic accessory that provides simultaneous fragmentation, irrigation, and aspiration.

Cushieri maneuver, two-hand—a maneuver used in laparoscopic cholecystectomies.

cushingoid (*not* cushinoid)—having the appearance or symptoms of Cushing's disease, as in "cushingoid facies."

Cushing's response—a neurologic indication of intracranial pressure. As intracranial pressure increases, the systolic blood pressure increases noticeably, while the diastolic pressure changes little, if at all. The increased difference between the two blood pressures is significant as an indication of the onset of late-stage intracranial pressure. Cf. *Cushing's triad.*

Cushing's syndrome—a symptom complex including moon facies, buffalo hump, abdominal distention, hypertension, amenorrhea (in women), impotence (in men), muscle wasting and weakness, fat pad formation, skin darkening, and skin thinning. More common in women than men. Caused by taking large amounts of steroids for long periods of time or by the excess production of cortisol. Cf. *Cushing's response.*

Cushing's triad—rising blood pressure, bradycardia, and widening pulse pressure are indicative of cerebral hemorrhage and cerebral edema. See *Cushing's response.*

CustomCornea Wavefront system—see *wavefront measurement.*

cut—a CT (computed tomography) section or image; a scan. See *tangential cut.*

cutaneous T-cell lymphoma (CTCL).

cut-biopsy needle—see *PercuCut.*

cut, clamp, and tie—the basic operating program: first, make or extend an incision or dissection; second, clamp with hemostats any vessels severed in the process ("bleeders"); third, tie ligatures around the ends of the severed vessels and remove the hemostats. Alternatively, bleeding vessels may be coagulated with electric current or sealed with metal clips.

cutdown catheter—inserted in the cutdown to a vein when no veins are accessible to a needle in an emergency situation.

Cutinova Cavity wound filling material.

Cutinova Hydro—hydrocolloid transparent and flexible dressing that does not leave a residue on the wound.

Cutivate cream (fluticasone propionate)—a topical corticosteroid used for treatment of atopic dermatitis in infants 3 months of age or older.

Cutler-Beard bridge flap procedure —for reconstructing large defects of

Cutler-Beard *(cont.)*
the upper eyelid, with flaps from the lower lid and the median forehead. Similar to the modified Hughes procedure of the lower eyelid.

Cutting Balloon microsurgical dilatation catheter system for treatment of coronary artery disease. It uses microsurgical blades mounted longitudinally on an angioplasty balloon to open narrowed arteries.

cutting loops—used with resectoscopes.

CVA (cerebrovascular accident, called *stroke* or *brain attack*)—the result of a severe cerebrovascular occlusion in which symptoms do not resolve within 24 hours, and in which there is a long-term residual deficit. See *TIA*.

CVAD (cyclophosphamide, vincristine, Adriamycin, dexamethasone)—chemotherapy protocol used to treat non-Hodgkin's lymphoma.

CVB (chorionic villi biopsy)—used in prenatal diagnosis of many birth defects. It can be performed at 8 to 11 weeks, rather than the 17 to 20 weeks needed for amniocentesis.

CVC—see *central venous catheter*.

CVD (cisplatin, vinblastine, dacarbazine)—chemotherapy protocol for metastatic malignant melanoma.

CVP (cyclophosphamide, vincristine, and prednisone)—chemotherapy protocol for adult non-Hodgkin's lymphoma and breast carcinoma.

CVPP (cyclophosphamide, vinblastine, procarbazine, prednisone)—chemotherapy protocol.

CVT-124—a highly selective adenosine A_1 receptor antagonist used in the treatment of edema associated with congestive heart failure.

C-wire Serter—a handheld, battery-driven device for inserting C-wires into place in bones in hand and foot surgery.

cyanoacrylate (Superglue)—a tissue adhesive.

CyberKnife stereotactic radiosurgery/ radiotherapy system—uses a linear accelerator, robotic arm, and image-guided technology to provide non-invasive treatment of tumors and other conditions affecting the brain, head, neck, and cervicothoracic spine.

Cybex test—apparatus used in testing and measuring the strength of a muscle as it is involved by a joint going through range-of-motion testing, as in shoulder girdle muscles or hip and thigh muscles.

cyclic adenosine monophosphate (cAMP).

cyclic vomiting syndrome—digestive disorder that for the most part affects children, characterized by chronic nausea, vomiting, extreme fatigue, motion sickness, abdominal pain and, in some cases, vertigo that may last for hours to days. The exact cause of cyclic vomiting syndrome is not known.

cycloplegia—pathologic or induced paralysis of the ciliary muscle of the eye; paralysis of accommodation.

cyclops lesion—localized anterior fibrosis of the knee, often occurring after anterior cruciate ligament reconstruction and leading to loss of knee extension.

Cyclops procedure—technique used to cover a large soft tissue defect after excision of a breast, chest wall muscles, and clavicle or ribs. The opposite breast, which must be large, is

Cyclops *(cont.)*
rotated intact across the chest wall to completely cover the surgical defect.

cyclosporine (Sandimmune)—approved for treating psoriasis unresponsive to any other therapies or drugs. In use for years as an antirejection drug in transplantation.

Cycrin (medroxyprogesterone).

cyesis ("si-e'-sis")—pregnancy. "Her symptoms of acute nausea and vomiting are probably secondary to cyesis."

CYFRA 21-1—a tumor marker detected in the serum of patients with non-small cell lung cancer. May also be useful as a tumor marker for breast carcinoma and gynecology neoplasm.

CyHOP (cyclophosphamide, Halotestin, Oncovin, prednisone)—chemotherapy protocol for lymphoma.

Cylexin—a selectin blocker used to prevent reperfusion injury in infants undergoing heart surgery.

Cyma line—a term used in foot x-ray reports.

cymba conchal cartilage graft—a graft harvested from the upper part of the concha of the auricle, used in rhinoplasty. See also *cavum conchal cartilage graft*.

Cymetra—brand name for LifeCell's micronized AlloDerm, a nonsurgical soft tissue replacement material used in facial plastic surgery.

CyPat—treatment for hot flashes experienced by prostate cancer patients following surgical or chemical castration.

CYP3A4—naturally occurring enzyme present in the small intestine that can interfere with drug metabolism. Grapefruit juice has been found to decrease levels of CYP3A4 and improve drug efficacy.

Cyriax physiotherapy—for treatment of tennis elbow, consisting of deep transverse friction over the extensor origin and manipulations.

Cystadane (betaine anhydrous)—oral solution for homocystinuria, a genetic disease.

Cystagon (cysteamine bitartrate)—for treatment of nephropathic cystinosis.

cystic adenomatoid malformation.

cysticercosis—infestation with a larval form of tapeworm.

cystitome (Oph)—an instrument used to open the capsule of the lens of the eye. Cf. *cystotome*.

cystocolpoproctography—fluoroscopic imaging for the detection and measurement of prolapse of pelvic organs.

cystoid macular edema (CME).

cystometrogram (CMG).

cystotome (Urol)—an instrument used for incising the bladder. Cf. *cystitome*.

Cytadren (aminoglutethimide)—used to treat advanced breast and prostatic carcinomas.

cytarabine (ara-C, Cytosar-U)—chemotherapy drug.

cytoblast—the cell nucleus. Cf. *cytoplast*.

cytocidal—cell-killing or destroying. "The cytocidal properties of this drug could be useful if those we are trying should prove less than effective." See *cidal*.

cytocrit—the sum of the percentage of white blood cells and the percentage of red blood cells. Cf. *cryocrit*.

CytoGam (cytomegalovirus immune globulin)—used to treat CMV infections and CMV enteritis.

cytokeratins—proteins that form the intermediate filaments of the cytoskeleton.

cytokines—proteins produced by the body in response to HIV infection and other stressors. Their action is not yet well understood. Tumor necrosis factor (TNF) and interleukins 1 and 6 are cytokines. Examples of cytokines under development for AIDS treatment:
Alferon LDO (interferon alfa-n3)
Alferon N injection
   (interferon alfa-n3)
Hivid (zalcitabine)
Intron A (interferon alfa-2b, recombinant) with Retrovir (AZT)
Leucomax (molgramostim,
   GM-CSF) with Retrovir (AZT)
Leukine (sargramostim)
Neupogen (filgrastim)
Proleukin (aldesleukin)
Veldona
Wellferon (alpha interferon)
   with Retrovir (AZT)

Cytolex—1% topical antibiotic cream (MSI-78) for treatment of infection in diabetic foot ulcers.

cytomegalic inclusion body.

cytomegalovirus (CMV)—herpesvirus that causes several diseases in AIDS patients, including intestinal disease, retinitis that can lead to blindness, and other problems.

cytomegalovirus encephalitis—an opportunistic infection of the brain by cytomegalovirus, seen in patients with immunodeficiency. Variable symptoms include seizures, clouding of consciousness, and other symptoms similar to those of the HIV dementia complex.

cytomegalovirus hepatitis.

cytomegalovirus immune globulin (CytoGam).

cytomegalovirus retinitis—an infection of the retina caused by one of a group of herpesviruses. This is one of a number of opportunistic infections seen in AIDS.

cytoplasmic inclusion body.

cytoplast—a cell whose nucleus has been removed, but which remains viable for a period of time. Cf. *cytoblast*.

CytoPorter—drug delivery system that transports drugs across lipid barriers (e.g., skin, cellular membranes) into the interior of cells for optimal therapeutic effect.

cytoreductive surgery—surgical removal of malignant tissue, also called *debulking*.

CytoRich preservative—fixative and preservative used in cell pathology.

cytoskeleton—the cells that comprise the bony skeleton.

cytostatic—bringing to a halt; stopping or suppressing the growth of cells and their reproduction; also, an agent that accomplishes this.

CytoTAb (TAb stands for Therapeutic Antibodies, Inc., the drug manufacturer)—a purified polyclonal antibody used to prevent and treat kidney transplant rejection.

cytotoxic cells—"killer" T-cell lymphocytes, also called *T-8 cells*. T-4 cells are the lymphocytes affected by the virus, but they are needed to activate the cytotoxic cells. As AIDS research has shown, loss of one piece of the immune system makes it ineffective, as the interactions are multiple and complex.

Cytovene (ganciclovir).

Czaja-McCaffrey rigid stent introducer/endoscope—used for insertion of tracheal stents.

D, d

dacliximab—a monoclonal antibody used to help prevent acute kidney transplant rejection. See *Zenapax*.

Dacomed snap gauge—used in testing impotence; will break if an erection occurs during sleep, thus indicating that the impotence is not organic in nature. See *snap gauge band*.

Dacron synthetic ligament material.

Dafilon suture—nonabsorbable polyamide surgical suture for skin closure. Used in plastic, ophthalmic, and microsurgery procedures.

Dagrofil suture—nonabsorbable polyester braided suture for use on muscles and in orthopedic procedures.

Dakin's solution—used as an antibacterial agent and in irrigating wounds.

Dale Foley catheter holder.

Dalgan (dezocine)—a narcotic-like drug which relieves pain as well as morphine but is not derived from natural opium, and is not a controlled substance like morphine. Given to orthopedic patients for trauma and postoperative pain control.

Dalkon shield—intrauterine device.

Dall-Miles cable grip system—cerclage application for bone grafting and fracture fixation.

Dalrymple's sign ("dal-rimplz")—the widened eyelid opening typical of the "stare" in hyperthyroidism. Cf. *Collier's sign*.

dalton—unit of measurement of the molecular weight of proteins (measured in kilodaltons), which constitute aeroallergens.

Damus-Kaye-Stansel operation—for repair of congenital heart defect.

DANA (designed after natural anatomy) shoulder prosthesis.

dance medicine—holistic multidisciplinary approach to on-site treatment of injured dancers beyond traditional orthopedic care, often using a staff of orthopedic surgeons, physical therapists, massage therapists, a psychologist, a nutritionist, a podiatrist, a naturopathic physician who performs acupuncture, a family medicine practitioner, and a chiropractor.

Dance's sign—a slight retraction of the tissue in the right iliac region in some cases of intussusception.

Dandy-Walker syndrome—congenital hydrocephalus caused by blockage of the foramina of Magendie and Luschka. Can be diagnosed on fetal ultrasound.

DAP/TMP (dapsone plus trimethoprim) —used in therapy for *Pneumocystis carinii* pneumonia.

dapiprazole (Rev-Eyes)—an ophthalmic solution used to reverse mydriasis.

dapsone—previously used to treat leprosy; now used against *Pneumocystis carinii* pneumonia in AIDS patients.

dapsone plus trimethoprim (DAP/TMP).

Darco shoe—brand name for postop podiatric shoe.

Dardik Biograft—modified human umbilical vein graft; used as a substitute for saphenous vein graft in revascularization procedures on the lower extremities.

Dardik clamp—used in liver transplantation surgery.

dark-field microscopy—a microscopic technique using special lighting that makes it easier to identify *Treponema pallidum*, the organism that causes syphilis.

Darkschewitsch, nucleus of—also, depending on which dictionary you consult, spelled *Darkshevich, Darkschevich*.

Darrach procedure—extensor carpi ulnaris tenodesis, or surgery on distal radioulnar joint.

"dashboard" knee—a knee injury in a motor vehicle accident.

Dash pacemaker—a single-chamber rate-adaptive pacemaker.

DAT (daunomycin, ara-C, thioguanine) —chemotherapy protocol for acute myeloid leukemia.

data clipping detection error—MRI term.

Datascope catheter—used to position an intra-aortic balloon pump.

data spike detection error—MRI term.

DaTSCAN—radiopharmaceutical imaging agent for diagnosis of Parkinson's disease.

DATVP (daunomycin, ara-C, thioguanine, vincristine, prednisone)—chemotherapy protocol.

daunorubicin HCl (Cerubidine, Dauno-Xome)—chemotherapy drug.

DaunoXome (liposomal daunorubicin HCl)—for Kaposi's sarcoma, colorectal and endometrial cancer, and other solid tumors. Cf. *liposomes, daunorubicin, DATVP.*

Dautery osteotome.

DAVA (desacetyl vinblastine amide)— see *vindesine sulfate*.

David Letterman sign—in which the scapholunate dissociation distance is wider than 2 mm on x-ray. Also known as Terry-Thomas sign (for actor Terry-Thomas).

daVinci surgical system—allows totally endoscopic mitral valve repair.

Davol drain—see *Relia-Vac.*

Davydov vagina construction (Ob-Gyn) —a technique used to create a new vagina in patients with congenital vaginal aplasia, or males having a sex-change operation. See also *colocolpo-neopoiesis, Frank and McIndoe, Abbe-McIndoe procedures.*

dawn phenomenon—hyperglycemia occurring before dawn in both type 1 (insulin dependent) and type 2 (non-insulin dependent) diabetics; an early morning hyperglycemia.

Daypro (oxaprozin).

DayTimer carpal tunnel support— prevents wrist flexion while allowing useful range of motion.

DBM (demineralized bone matrix).

DC (direct current) **offset**—MRI term.

DCA (directional coronary atherectomy) —treatment for coronary artery disease.

DCA (directional coronary angioplasty) (also, atherectomy).

DCC (deleted in colorectal carcinoma) **gene**—implicated in the development of colorectal carcinoma.

DCH (diffuse choroidal hemangioma).

D-chiro-inositol—a drug that is found naturally in fruits and vegetables. It helps the body use insulin and may be effective in promoting ovulation in patients with polycystic ovary syndrome, thus reducing the risk for diabetes and heart attacks due to high levels of insulin, blood pressure, and triglycerides.

DCIA (deep circumflex iliac artery).

DCIS (ductal carcinoma in situ).

D$_{CO}$—pulmonary diffusion capacity.

DCP (dynamic compression plate).

DCR (dacryocystorhinostomy)—a laser endonasal procedure.

DCS (decompression sickness).

DCS (dorsal column stimulator, or stimulation)—implanted for relief of pain.

DDAVP (desmopressin acetate)—synthetic analog of vasopressin used in controlling bleeding in uremic patients; the treatment of choice, rather than cryoprecipitate. Also used to treat diabetes insipidus, which can be a complication of hypophysectomy (pituitary removal).

DDAVP nasal spray (desmopressin acetate)—treatment for bedwetting.

ddC or **DDC** (dideoxycytidine, Hivid, zalcitabine)—an antiviral drug used in treating AIDS. Also used in patients who cannot tolerate Retrovir.

DDD pacemaker (Cardio).

ddI or **DDI** (dideoxyinosine, Videx)— see *didanosine.*

DDT ([fluorescein] **dye disappearance test)**.

DeBakey woven Dacron.

debris ("duh-bree")—amorphous and necrotic material.

debulking—a process in which the inner "core" (or bulk) of a tumor is removed. This permits the outer portion to, in effect, "cave in" a bit, thereby permitting easier removal of the whole tumor. If the "outer wall" portion of the tumor does not readily separate from the attached tissue, at least the total volume of the tumor is somewhat reduced and hence does not exert as much pressure on the adjacent structures as it did before.

DECAL (dexamethasone, etoposide, cisplatin, ara-C, L-asparaginase)— chemotherapy protocol.

deceleration—slowing, as in "deceleration of contractions."

decerebrate rigidity—seen in metabolic disorders that affect upper brain stem function, evidenced by clenched teeth, and arms and legs stiffly extended. Cf. *decorticate rigidity.*

decidua—that part of the endometrium of the pregnant uterus that is shed at parturition.

decision—the settling of a controversy; a conclusion arrived at or a choice made. Cf. *discission.*

de Clérambault's syndrome—erotomanic delusions; a psychosis in which a person is under the delusion that another person, often famous or celebrated, is engaged in erotic communication with the subject and that the object of the delusion was the first

de Clérambault's syndrome *(cont.)*
to fall in love and the first to make advances. The amorous delusion is always directed toward the same individual throughout the episode, and the subject rationalizes the object's paradoxical behavior (such as failing to respond to phone calls or letters). Celebrities are frequently victims of persons with de Clérambault's syndrome.

decompression sickness (DCS)—see *caisson disease.*

decorticate rigidity—seen in lesions which damage the internal capsule of the brain and nearby structures, evidenced by flexion of the fingers, wrist, and arm, plantar flexion, and internal rotation of the leg. Cf. *decerebrate rigidity.*

decubitus ulcer—bed sore, pressure sore, trophic ulcer. Decubitus means "lying down" and these synonymous terms refer to the ulcerated areas of ischemic necrosis on the tissues that overlie bony prominences (sacrum, hips, greater trochanters, lateral malleoli, heels, and other areas where there may be pressure and friction). They are usually seen in patients who have been bedridden for long periods of time, who are emaciated or paralyzed, or in whom pain sensation is absent.

deep tendon reflexes:
4+   brisk, hyperactive, clonus
3+   is more brisk than normal, but does not necessarily indicate a pathologic process
2+   normal
1+   is low normal, with slight diminution in response
0   no response

deep venous insufficiency (DVI).

deep venous thrombosis (DVT).

defensins—naturally occurring peptides with antimicrobial activity. Investigators have for the first time found defensins in tissues of the eye and in tears, suggesting that purified defensins may be useful in treating eye infections.

defibrillation threshold (DFT).

Definition PM (Pre-Mantle) **femoral component**—used in orthopedic surgery.

deglutition mechanism (Radiol)—the coordinated sequence of muscular contractions in the mouth, pharynx, and esophagus involved in normal swallowing, as demonstrated in a barium swallow or upper GI series.

degradable starch microspheres (DSM)—injected into an artery at the same time as a chemotherapy drug to temporarily block the blood flow at the capillary level (chemoembolization). The chemotherapy drug is then concentrated in the region of the cancer, and high tissue uptake is achieved. DSM has a short half-life and does not occlude the local circulation long enough to produce ischemia, and in conjunction with a chemotherapy drug can be administered repeatedly.

DEHOP (diethylhomospermine)—for treatment of refractory AIDS-related diarrhea.

dehydroemetine (Mebadin)—used to treat amebiasis in immunocompromised patients.

DEI (diffraction-enhanced imaging).

Deiters' cells (ENT)—in the organ of Corti.

déjà vu (Fr., already seen)—the incorrect feeling that one has seen or experienced something before, a

déjà vu *(cont.)*
feeling which frequently precedes seizures. Cf. *jamais vu.*

Dejerine's onion peel sensory loss—sensory loss starting from mouth and nose and extending concentrically outward in an "onion peel" distribution.

De Juan forceps.

Deklene—blue monofilament polypropylene suture used in cardiovascular surgery and in neurosurgery.

Deknatel (Shur-Strip)—a sterile wound closure tape.

de la Cruz classification—congenital aural atresia.

Delaprem (hexoprenaline sulfate).

delayed pulmonary toxicity syndrome (DPTS)—a lung disorder seen in breast cancer patients in the weeks following treatment with a combination of chemotherapy and bone marrow transplantation. If the inflammation is detected early and the body's inflammatory response modified through steroids, lung toxicity can be prevented or significantly minimized.

delayed xenograft rejection (DXR)—delayed rejection reaction in response to transplantation of cells, tissue, or solid organ of animal origin.

Delbet fracture classification, types I-IV—the most widely accepted system of classification of femoral head and neck fractures in children.

Delbet splint—used for heel fractures.

De Lee retractor (Ob-Gyn).

"dellovibrio"—a phonetic spelling of *Bdellovibrio*, a genus of parasitic gram-negative organisms that live on certain other gram-negative bacteria. Although this is not a word you will often hear, who would think to look under the *B*'s?

Delrin joint replacement biomaterial.

delta—When a dictator gives a lab value such as "delta of 35," the reference is to the anion gap.

delta OD$_{450}$—in amniocentesis, testing for bilirubinemia in erythroblastosis fetalis.

Demadex (torsemide).

De Mayo two-point discrimination device.

Dementia Rating Scale (DRS)—used in detecting patients with dementia of the Alzheimer type.

demineralization—reduction in the amount of calcium present in bone, due to disease or immobilization, as seen on x-ray.

demineralized bone matrix (DBM).

de Morsier's syndrome—agenesis of the olfactory lobes, hypoplasia of the thalamus, dystrophy of the cerebral hemispheres, and absence of development of the gonads at puberty. Also, *de Morsier-Gauthier syndrome.*

Demser (metyrosine)—for patients with pheochromocytoma. Also used for preoperative preparation, for management of patients for whom surgery is contraindicated, and long-term treatment in patients with malignant pheochromocytoma.

de Musset's sign—rhythmic shaking of the head caused by carotid artery pulsations; a sign of aortic insufficiency. Cf. *bishop's nod.*

denatured homograft (Surg).

Denavir (penciclovir)—a topical prescription treatment for cold sores.

dendritic lesion—having a branched appearance.

dengue hemorrhagic fever (DHF)—a disease on the increase in the U.S. and Latin America. The recent introduction of the *Aedes albopictus* mosquito to the U.S. will increase

dengue *(cont.)*
the probability of more severe disease, according to the CDC.

Denis Browne clubfoot splint—talipes hobble splint. Named for Dr. Denis (pronounced "Denny") Browne, Hospital for Sick Children, London, England.

Dennis-Brown pouch (Urol).

Dennis-Varco pancreaticoduodenostomy.

Dennyson-Fulford extra-articular subtalar arthrodesis—for correction of supple hindfoot valgus deformities in children.

de novo inflammatory growth—beginning, recurring, or new inflammatory growth. "De novo tissue was generated from mesenchymal precursors."

densitometry—determination of variations in density (for example, bone density) by comparison with that of another material or with a certain standard. See *dual photon densitometry*.

dens view of cervical spine (Radiol)—a view of the odontoid process of the second cervical vertebra on x-ray. The word *dens* is not an eponym.

dental bonding materials
Aquasil Smart Wetting impression
In-Ceram Alumina
In-Ceram Cerestore
In-Ceram Dicor
In-Ceram Empress
In-Ceram Fortress
In-Ceram Optec
In-Ceram Spinell

dental implant
Amelogen
Bioceram two-stage series II
Bioceram type S
Geristore

dental implant *(cont.)*
Omniloc
OsteoGen HA (hydroxyapatite)
Steri-Oss
Sustain

DentaScan—a program for multiplanar reformation that processes axial CT scan information to obtain true cross-sectional images and panoramic views of the mandible and maxilla; this optimizes the ability to detect tumor involvement in the mandible and maxilla.

DentiPatch lidocaine transoral delivery system—dental anesthetic patch for the prevention of pain from oral injections and soft tissue dental procedures.

Dento-Infuser—an instrument used by dentists to infuse Astringedent, a topical hemostatic solution.

DENT-X—intraoral dental x-ray unit.

Denver Developmental Screening Test—rating scale for development of fine motor skills, gross motor skills, language, and personal/social skills in infants and preschool children.

Denver nasal splint—a quickly applied adhesive nasal splint.

Denver PAK (percutaneous access kit) includes a Denver ascites shunt designed for subclavian vein placement.

Denver pleuroperitoneal shunt—for control of chronic pleural effusions.

Denys-Drash syndrome—an inherited renal disease.

Deon hip prosthesis—made of a titanium alloy which can be implanted with or without cement.

deoxy-D-glucose—an antiviral glucose analogue which may be useful in treating herpes.

deoxynojirimycin (butyl-DNJ)—for patients with AIDS and ARC.

deoxyspergualin—a lymphocyte transformation inhibitor to decrease the incidence of organ transplant rejection.

Depacon (valproate sodium injection) —drug used for the temporary treatment of certain types of epilepsy.

DepoAmikacin—injectable sustained-release formulation of amikacin, a potent broad-spectrum aminoglycoside antibiotic. It is intended to be administered into tissues for the local treatment of bacterial infections.

DepoCyt—anticancer therapeutic for treatment of neoplastic meningitis arising from solid tumors or non-Hodgkin's lymphoma.

DepoMorphine—sustained-release encapsulated morphine sulfate used to treat acute post-surgical pain.

depth-resolved NIRS—permits the noninvasive assessment and quantification of certain characteristics of specific blood and tissue that is deep in the body and surrounded, or behind, other more superficial blood and tissue (e.g., in the brain and behind the scalp and skull). See *NIRS.*

DePuy total hip system with porous coating. Also, Profile.

de Quervain's disease—inflammation of the long abductor and short extensor tendons of the thumb, with accompanying tenderness and swelling. Also called *Quervain's disease.*

Dercum's disease—see *adiposis dolorosa.*

Dermablend—a cover cream used to cover vitiligo, birthmarks, etc.

Dermabond—a topical skin adhesive (2-octyl cyanoacrylate) which is an alternative to sutures or staples. Used to close incisions made to repair facial deformities such as cleft lip and palate.

dermabrasion—an abrasion procedure for acne scars, performed after anesthetizing and freezing the skin with Freon; scars are abraded with fine sandpaper, diamond fraises, or abrasive brushes. See *diamond fraise.*

Dermacea—wound and skin care product line.

Derma-Gel hydrogel sheet.

Dermagraft-TC—a human fibroblast-derived temporary skin substitute, used as a short-term wound covering for severe burns. Also used for diabetic foot ulcers.

Dermagran ointments and dressings —used to treat decubitus ulcers.

Derma K laser (Surg)—uses both pulsed Er:YAG and CO_2 laser energy to perform skin rejuvenation.

DermaLase laser system (Surg)—used in surgical procedures that involve incision, excision, ablation, vaporization, and/or coagulation of soft tissue.

Dermalene—linear polyethylene monofilament suture material.

Dermalon—monofilament nylon suture material.

Dermal Regeneration Template—used in conjunction with Integra artificial skin.

DermaMend foam wound dressing.

DermaMend hydrogel dressing.

DermaNet contact-layer wound dressing.

Dermapor glove—allows the escape of water and heat from hand perspiration but keeps out water and external irritants, resulting in drier and less irritated hands.

DermaPulse—pressure control zone therapy for pressure sores.

DermaScan—used with skin rejuvenation devices.

DermaSeptic—small electronic device that delivers broad-spectrum antimicrobial ions directly into the skin in a process known as iontophoresis, providing highly effective treatment for conditions such as cold sores, pimples, and warts, where infection lies on or beneath the skin surface.

Derma-Smoothe/FS—low- to medium-potency corticosteroid for treatment of atopic dermatitis in pediatric patients six years of age and older.

Dermasof—semiocclusive reinforced gel sheeting for treatment of hypertrophic and keloid scar tissue.

DermAssist hydrocolloid dressing material.

DermAssist wound filling material.

Dermatell hydrocolloid dressing material.

Dermatology Index of Disease Severity (DIDS)—a severity-of-illness index for inflammatory skin diseases.

Dermatop (prednicarbonate).

Dermatophagoides farinae—a mite; it may be one of the principal sources of antigen in house dust in some areas. Cf. *Dermatophagoides pteronyssinus.*

Dermatophagoides pteronyssinus—a mite that may be one of the principal sources of antigen in house dust in some areas. Cf. *Dermatophagoides farinae.*

dermatophyton control—used as a control with PPD testing.

dermatoscope—handheld microscope that allows magnification of the skin x 10 and replaces previously used inflexible and expensive stereomicroscopes which were cumbersome and time-consuming. Important in the diagnosis of malignant melanoma for which an oil or disinfectant solution is applied to the skin and a halogen light at an angle of 20° is used to make the horny layer of the skin more translucent.

Derma 20 laser system (Surg)—pulsed Er:Yag laser intended for general dermatological applications, including skin surfacing.

DermMaster—first macroabrasion system for skin resurfacing and other aesthetic/dermatology applications that does not use aluminum oxide.

Descemet's membrane—between the endothelial layer of the cornea and the substantia propria.

descemetocele—herniation of Descemet's membrane.

Deschamps ligature carrier.

describe—to explain or characterize in words. Cf. *ascribe.*

DES (diethylstilbestrol) **daughter**—a female exposed in utero to diethylstilbestrol, formerly prescribed for bleeding and other complications of pregnancy and now known to affect fetal development of the genital tract.

desflurane (Suprane)—a general anesthetic, rapid-acting, inhaled as a vaporized solution. Awakening time after surgery is said to be significantly faster than with other inhaled general anesthetics.

desiccated (*not* dessicated)—dried.

Desilets-Hoffman introducer—used to introduce balloon, electrode, and other catheters.

desloratadine—nonsedating, long-acting antihistamine for treatment of seasonal allergic rhinitis.

desmoplastic small round-cell tumor (DSRCT)—a histologic entity that is

desmoplastic *(cont.)*
uniform in appearance and is characterized by the presence of poorly differentiated small round cells, but also abundant fibrous stroma and a specific multidirectional immunohistochemical profile.

desmopressin acetate (DDAVP; Stimate) nasal spray.

Desogen (ethinyl estradiol, desogestrel) —an oral contraceptive. Of note, progestin desogestrel is derived from the root of a wild yam found in the Mexican jungle.

DeSouza exercises—to encourage position change of fetus.

detergent worker's lung—extrinsic allergic alveolitis caused by exposure to detergent powder.

Detoxahol—used to lower blood alcohol levels.

Detrol (tolterodine tartrate)—used in treatment of overactive bladder.

Detsky modified risk index score—a clinical scoring system used to predict cardiac morbidity.

De Vega tricuspid annuloplasty—performed on children.

developer artifact (Radiol)—flawed images with areas resembling lesions resulting from darkroom problems.

developmental causes of limb-length discrepancy—avascular necrosis of hip, hip dislocation, idiopathic, Klippel-Trenaunay-Weber syndrome, linear scleroderma, local tumor, melorheostosis, neuromusculature, osteomyelitis, slipped capital femoral epiphysis, talectomy, trauma.

developmental milestones—the mastery of activities or skills expected at a certain age for normal child development.

Devic's disease—neuromyelitis optica, a form of acute multiple sclerosis.

device—a quick-reference list of medical devices and systems found in medical and surgical dictation. Common devices such as *catheter, endoscope, pacemaker, stent, tube,* and many others appear as main entries throughout the book.

ABI Vest Airway Clearance System (the "Vest")

ablatherm HIFU (high-intensity focused ultrasound)

Absolok endoscopic clip applicator

Ac'cents permanent lash liner

Accellon Combi biopsampler

Accel stopcock

Access MV system

Accu-Chek InstantPlus system

Accu-Chek II Freedom blood glucose system

accuDEXA bone densitometer

AccuGuide injection monitor

AccuLength arthroplasty measuring system

Accu-Line knee instrumentation

AccuSharp instrument

AccuSpan tissue expander

AccuSway balance measurement system

Accutom low-speed diamond saw

ACD (active compression-decompression) resuscitator

ACG knee instrumentation

ACL (anterior cruciate ligament) drill guide

Acland-Banis arteriotomy set

ACM (automated cardiac flow measurement) technology

Acro-Flex artificial disk

Acryl-X ultrasonic orthopedic cement removal

ACS Anchor Exchange device

ACTID (analgesic cell therapy implantable device)

Actis venous flow controller (VFC)

device *(cont.)*

Active Compression-Decompression (ACD) resuscitator
actocardiotocograph
Acufex arthroscopic instruments
Acufex biosabsorbable suture anchor
AcuFix anterior cervical plate
AcuPressor myotherapy tool
Acuson V5M monitor
Acusyst-Xcell monoclonal antibody culturing system
Acutrak fusion system
Acutrainer electronic bladder retraining
Adaptive Focusing Technology (AFT)
Add-On Bucky digital system
Adjustable Leg and Ankle Repositioning Mechanism (ALARM)
Adkin's strut
Adolescent and Pediatric Pain Tool
ADTRA composite external fixator ring
advanced cardiac life support (ACLS)
AdvanTeq II TENS unit
Advantim revision knee system
Advantx LC+ cardiovascular imaging system
Aerochamber
AeroTech II nebulizer
AERx electronic inhaler
Aescula left ventricular (LV) lead
Aesop 2000 surgical robot
Affymetrix GeneChip system
Agee carpal tunnel release system
Agee-WristJack fracture reduction system
Agris-Dingman submammary dissector
Air-Limb
AirMax external nasal dilator
Air Supply

device *(cont.)*

air trousers
Akros extended care mattress
Alexa 1000 breast lesion diagnostic
AlloDerm
Allon
Aloka color Doppler system
Aloka SSD ultrasound system and probes
AlphaStar operating room table
Alphatec mini lag-screw system (MLS)
Alphatec small fragment system (SFS)
Alta reconstruction rod
Alta tibial/humeral rod
ALVAD (abdominal left ventricular assist device)
Amadeus microkeratome
Ambu bag
Ambulator shoe
AME bone growth stimulators
AME PinSite Shields
Amicus separator
Amis 2000 respiratory mass spectrometer
AMK (Anatomic Modular Knee) total knee system
AML (Anatomic Medullary Locking) total hip system
amorphous silicon filmless digital x-ray detection technology
Amset ALPS (anterior locking plate system)
Amsler grid
anal EMG PerryMeter sensor
anatomic graduated components (AGC)
Anchorlok soft-tissue anchor
Ancure endovascular repair
Andrews spinal frame/table
AneuRx stent graft
AngeCool RF (radiofrequency) catheter ablation system

device *(cont.)*
AngeFlex leads
AngioJet Rheolytic thrombectomy
  system
Angio-Seal hemostatic puncture
  closure
Angstrom MD defibrillator
ankle air stirrup
AnkleCiser exerciser
AnnuloFlo annuloplasty ring system
Anspach surgery instruments
anterior chamber maintainer (ACM)
Aortic Connector System
APACHE CV Risk Predictor
  Internet-based product
Apex irrigation system
Apex universal drive
Apollo triple lumen papillotome
applanometer
Appraise diabetes monitoring
APR total hip system
Aqua-Flow collagen glaucoma
  drainage
AquaShield
arch bar
Arcometer instrument
AREx inhaler
argon beam coagulator (ABC)
Argosy Cameo CIC (completely-in-
  the-canal) hearing aid
Argyle CPAP nasal cannula
Argyle Turkel safety thoracentesis
  system
Arnett-TMP (trimandibular plate)
  system
Aromapatch nasal inhaler
AromaScan
Arrequi laparoscopic knot pusher
  ligator
arrhythmia mapping system
Arrow PICC system
Arrow pneumothorax kit
Arrowsmith corneal marker

device *(cont.)*
Arthro-BST arthroscopic probe
ArthroCare Coblation-based
  cosmetic surgery
Arthro-Flo system
Arthro-Lok system
Arthopor acetabular cup
ArthroSew arthroscopic suturing
ArthroWand
ARTMA virtual patient technology
ARUM pin
AS-800 artificial sphincter
Asnis 2 guided screw system
Aspen electrocautery
Aspen laparoscopy electrode
Aspen ultrasound system
aspiration-tulip device
Assistant Free calibrated femoral
  tibial spreader
ASSI wire pass drill
Aston cartilage reduction system
Atrial View Ventak AV implantable
  cardioverter-defibrillator
Atrigel drug delivery
Atrioverter
augmentative communication device
Augustine guide and scope
Aurora dedicated breast MRI
  system
AutoCat automatic intra-aortic
  balloon pump
Autoclix fingerstick device
Autoflex II CPM unit
Autolet fingerstick device
Automated Cellular Imaging System
  (ACIS)
automated external defibrillator
  (AED)
Automator
AutoPap 300 QC automatic Pap
  screener
AVA (advanced venous access) 3Xi
Avitene Ultrafoam collagen hemostat

device *(cont.)*

AvocetPT (prothrombin time) meter
Aware breast self-examination pad
Axostim nerve stimulator
AxyaWeld bone anchor
BabyFace 3-D surface rendering
    accessory
Babytherm IC gel mattress
BackBiter orthopedic instrument
BackTracker
BACTEC blood culture system
Baculovirus Expression Vector
    System (BEVS)
Baim-Turi cardiac device
Bair Hugger warming body cover
BAK/C (cervical) and BAK/T
    (thoracic) interbody fusion
    system
Bakelite material
Bakes dilator
Baladi Inverter
balloon dissector
Balloon-on-a-Wire cardiac device
band-ligator
Bard biopty gun
Bard Clamshell Septal Umbrella
Bard Composix mesh
Bard endoscopic suturing
Bard PDA (patent ductus arteriosus)
    Umbrella
Bard TransAct intra-aortic balloon
    pump
Barouk button space
Barouk microscrew
Barouk microstaple
Barron disposable trephine
Barron donor corneal punch
Barron pump
Barron radial vacuum trephine
Baton laser pointer
BDProbeTec ET
Beacon incontinence surgical line
beam splitter
beating-heart bypass system

device *(cont.)*

Bedge antireflux mattress
Bellucci scissors
Belos compression pin
Bentley Duraflo II perfusion circuit
Berkeley optic zone marker
Berman locator
Beta-Cath radiation therapy
Betaseron needle-free delivery
    system
Biad SPECT imaging system
Bilibed phototherapy system
BiliBottoms phototherapy diaper
BiliCheck handheld battery-
    powered system
Bili mask
bilirubinometer
bioabsorbable closure device
Biobrane glove
BioBypass
Biocor 200 oxygenator
Biofilter hemoconcentrator
biofragmentable anastomotic ring
bio-interference screw
Biologically Quiet Screw
Biologically Quiet suture anchor
Biolox ball head
Bionicare 1000 stimulator
Bioplus dispersive electrode
BioRCI orthopedic screw
BioScrew bio-absorbable interference
    screw
Bio-Tense relaxation tool
Biotrack coagulation monitor
BioZ system
biplane sector probe
bipolar urological loop
Bird cup
Bird's Nest filter (BNF)
birthing ball
BIS (bispectral index) Sensor
Blood Shield
Blumenthal irrigating cystitome
Bluntport disposable trocar

device *(cont.)*
BMP cable
boat hook
Bone Bullet suture anchor
Bookler swivel-ball laparoscopic
   instrument holder
Bores radial marker
Bovie ultrasound aspirator
bovine pericardium strips
Bowen wire tightener
Boyle uterine elevator
Boynton needle holder
Brackmann facial nerve monitor
Brackmann II EMG system
Brandt cytology balloon
BreastAlert differential temperature
   sensor (DTS) screening device
breast bolster
BreastCheck handheld electronic
   device for breast self-exam
BreastExam breast exam device
Breast Imaging and Reporting Data
   System of the American College
   of Radiology (BI-RADS)
Breathe Right nasal strips
Bremer AirFlo Vest
Bremer Halo Crown system
Brent pressure earring
Brockenbrough cardiac device
Browlift BoneBridge
Brown dermatome
Brown-McHardy pneumatic dilator
Brown-Roberts-Wells (BRW)
   stereotactic system
Bruel-Kjaer transvaginal ultrasound
   probe
Bruening syringe
Bruns bone curette
BRW (Brown-Roberts-Wells) CT
   stereotaxic guide
BSD-2000
Button and Button-One Step gastros-
   tomy devices
BVM (bag-valve-mask)

device *(cont.)*
bypass circuit
CA (cardiac-apnea) monitor for
   newborns
CADD-Prizm pain control system
   (PCS)
Cadence AICD (automatic implant-
   able cardioverter-defibrillator)
Cadet cardioverter-defibrillator
Calandruccio triangular compres-
   sion fixation device
calcar reamer
Calcitek drill system
Calcitek spline dental implant
calipers
calorimeter
Cam (controlled ankle motion)
   walker
CAM tent
Canal Finder System
Cannulated Plus screw system
Capio CL transvaginal suture-
   capturing
CAPS ArthroWand
CAPSure ArthroWand
Capsure steroid-eluting electrode
CAPS X
cardiac sling
CardioBeeper CB-12L
Cardiocap 5 patient monitor
CardioCard
Cardiofreezer cryosurgical system
cardiopulmonary support system
   (CPS)
CardioSEAL septal occluder
C-arm fluoroscopy portable x-ray
   unit
Carolina rocker wheelchair
Carpentier-Edwards Physio annulo-
   plasty ring
Carter pillow
Carter-Thomason suture passer
Castanares face-lift scissors
Castaneda bottle

device *(cont.)*
  Catarex surgical
  catheter vitrector
  Cath-Finder
  CathLink
  CathTrack catheter locator system
  CaverMap surgical device
  Cavitron ultrasonic surgical aspirator (CUSA)
  C-bar web-spacer
  C Cap (compliance cap)
  CD8 AIS CELLector
  Cellpatch drug delivery
  cell recovery system (CRS)
  Cellugel ophthalmic viscosurgical (OVD)
  Centauri Er:YAG laser dental
  Ceresine pyruvate dehydrogenase stimulator
  ChemTrak AccuMeter
  chest shell
  Christoudias fascial closure
  ChromaVision digital analyzer
  Chronicle implantable hemodynamic monitor
  CicaCare topical gel sheeting
  CIC (completely-in-the-canal) hearing aid
  ClearCut 2
  CoaguChek
  Coaguloop resection electrode
  Coblation technology
  Cochlea Dynamics sound processing technology
  Cohn cardiac stabilizer
  Colormate TLc BiliTest bilirubinometer
  Combitube
  ComfortFlex
  Command cutting instrument
  Commander PTCA wire line
  completely-in-the-ear hearing aid
  Compliant
  CompuCam digital intraoral camera
  Conceive Fertility Planner

device *(cont.)*
  Conceptus Robust guide wire
  Concise compression hip screw system
  confocal microscope
  Contigen Bard collagen implant
  Contour MD implantable single-lead cardioverter-defibrillator
  Contour V-145D and LTV-135D implantable cardioverter-defibrillator
  Convergent color Doppler imaging technology
  CoolSpot skin-cooling
  Core trocar and cannula
  CorneaSparing LTK (laser thermal keratoplasty)
  Cotrel-Dubousset instrumentation (CDI)
  Cottle elevator
  Cournand cardiac device
  CoVac 50
  CoVac 70
  CoverTip safety syringe
  Cowboy Collar
  CPM (continuous passive motion) devices
  CPS (cardiopulmonary support) heart-lung machine
  CPT hip system
  Crafoord-Senning heart-lung machine
  Cragg thrombolytic brush
  cribogram
  Cricket oximeter
  Crutchfield skeletal traction tongs
  CRYOcare endometrial cryoablation
  Cryo/Cuff boot
  CryoHit
  cryophake
  cryoprobe
  cryostat
  CS-5 cryosurgical system
  CT with slip-ring technology

device *(cont.)*
  C-TRAK handheld gamma detector
  Cueva cranial nerve electrode
    monitoring device
  CUI (Cox-Uphoff International)
    tissue expander
  Cun-Meter
  Cu-Safe 300
  CUSALap
  CustomCornea Wavefront System
  Cutting Balloon microsurgical
    dilatation catheter
  C-wire Serter
  CyberKnife stereotactic radiosurgery/
    radiotherapy
  cystitome
  cystotome
  CytoPorter drug delivery
  Dacomed snap gauge
  Dalkon shield
  Dall-Miles cable grip system
  Darco shoe
  Dautery osteotome
  daVinci surgical
  DayTimer carpal tunnel support
  Definition PM (pre-mantle) femoral
    component
  De Lorme quadriceps boot
  De Mayo two-point discrimination
    device
  DentiPatch lidocaine transoral
    delivery system
  Dento-Infuser
  DENT-X intraoral dental x-ray unit
  DePuy total hip system with porous
    coating
  Dermapor glove
  DermaSeptic
  DermMaster macroabrasion
  Deschamps ligature carrier
  Desilets-Hoffman introducer
  DEXAscan bone densitometer
  diamond bur
  diamond fraise

device *(cont.)*
  Diamond-Lite
  DiaPhine corneal trephination
    device
  Diasensor 1000 for blood glucose
  DICOM (Digital Imaging and Com-
    munications in Medicine)
  Digikit pneumatic tourniquet
  DigiMatch
  Digirad 2020 TC Imager
  DigiSound
  digital Add-On Bucky image
    acquisition
  Digital Fundus Imager
  digital holography system
  digital ICG (iodocyanine green)
    fluorescein dye videoangi-
    ography
  Digital OsteoView 2000
  digital signal processing (DSP)
  DIGIT-grip
  Digitrapper MKIII esophageal
    sphincter pressure assessment
  Digitron digital subtraction imaging
  Dilamezinsert (DMI)
  DIMAQ integrated ultrasound
    workstation
  DirectFlow arterial cannula
  DirectRay direct-to-digital
    technology
  Disetronic Insulin Pen
  Disk-Criminator
  disposable aortic rotating punch
  Diva laparoscopic morcellator
  domino connectors
  Dormia noose
  dorsal column stimulator (DCS)
  double umbrella device
  Douvas roto-extractor
  DPAP Stealth
  Draeger high vacuum erysiphake
  Draeger tonometer
  Drake-Willock automatic delivery
    system

device *(cont.)*
  DSP Micro Diamond-Point
  Dualine digital hearing instrument
  Dubecq-Princeteau angulating needle
    holder
  Ducor tip
  Duette instruments
  Duet vascular sealing device
  Dura-Kold ice wrap
  Durasul large diameter head
  Durathane cardiac device
  Duval disposable dermatome
  Dyna-Lok plating system
  dynamic compression plate
  Dynamic Cooling Device (DCD)
  Dynamic Optical Breast Imaging
    System (DOBI)
  DynaPulse 5000A blood pressure
    monitor
  Dynasplint knee extension unit
  Dynasplint shoulder system
  DynaVox 2 communication device
  DynaWell spinal compression
  DyoVac suction punch
  Eagle II survey spirometer
  Eagle Vision-Freeman punctum
    plug
  EarCheck Pro reflectometer
  ear oximeter
  Easi-Lav gastric lavage system
  EBI bone healing system
  EBI SPF-2 implantable bone
    stimulator
  E.CAM photon emission camera
  Eccovision acoustic rhinometry
    system
  EchoEye 3-D ultrasound imaging
    system
  EchoFlow blood velocity meter
    (BVM-1)
  Eclipse TENS unit
  ECTA (enzyme-catalyzed therapeutic
    activation) technology
  Ectra system

device *(cont.)*
  EDA (extravasation detection
    accessory)
  Elasto-Gel shoulder therapy wrap
  electron-beam CT technology
  electro-oculogram apparatus
  Electroscope disposable scissors
  El Gamal cardiac device
  Eliminator dilatation balloon
  Ellik kidney stone basket,
    evacuator, elevator
  Elmor tissue morcellator
  Embol-X arterial cannula and filter
  Embosphere microspheres
  Emergency Infusion Device (EID)
  EMI scanner
  EnAbl thermal ablation system
  Ender nail
  End-Flo laparoscopic irrigating
    system
  Endius endoscopic access
  Endius Trifix thoracolumbar pedicle
    screw
  endoanal coil
  Endo Clip applier
  Endodissect instrument
  endoesophageal MRI coil
  EndoFix absorbable interference
    screw
  Endo-Gauge tissue thickness
    measurement device
  Endoloop suture instrument
  Endo Lumenal Gastroplication
  EndoLumina bougie
  EndoMate Grab Bag
  EndoMed LSS laparoscopic system
  Endopath ES endoscopic stapler
  Endopath laparoscopic trocar
  Endopath Linear Cutter
  Endopath Optiview optical surgical
    obturator
  Endopath TriStar trocar
  Endopearl
  Endo-P-Probe

device *(cont.)*
  endorectal coil
  EndoSaph vein harvest system
  EndoShears
  Endo Stitch endoscopic suturing
  Endotak lead defibrillation system
  Endotrac endoscopic instruments
  endotracheal cardiac output
    monitoring (ECOM)
  endovaginal coil
  endovaginal ultrasound (EVUS)
  EndoWrist
  Enduron acetabular liner
  Ensemble contrast imaging (ECI)
  ENTec Coblator Plasma Surgery
  ENTec Plasma Wand
  Entera-Flo
  Entree Plus and Entree II trocar and
    cannula system
  Entree thoracoscopy trocar and
    cannula
  EPIC-C or EPICS Profile flow
    cytometer
  EpiE-ZPen auto injector
  Epi-Grip device
  Epistat double balloon
  Epitrain elbow support
  Equinox occlusion balloon
  ErecAid system
  Eros-CTD (clitoral therapy device)
  Esclim estradiol transdermal
  E-Scope electronic stethoscope
  Escort balloon stone extractor
  esophageal pill electrode
  estrogen/progesterone transdermal
    delivery
  ESU (electrosurgical unit) dispersive
    (grounding) pad
  Euro-Collins multiorgan perfusion
    kit
  EVac wand
  Evershears
  Evolve Cardiac Continuum
  ExacTech blood glucose meter

device *(cont.)*
  Exact-Fit ATH hip replacement
  Excelart MRI
  eXcel-DR (disposable/reusable)
    instruments
  Excel GE glucose monitoring strip
  EX-FI-RE external fixation system
  Extractor three-lumen retrieval
    balloon
  eXtract (trademark) specimen bag
  extravasation detection accessory
    (EDA)
  Extra View balloon
  ExtreSafe needles, lancets, phlebot-
    omy devices, catheters, syringes
  E-Z Flap system
  E-Z Flex jaw therapy device
  E-Z Tac soft-tissue reattachment
  eZY WRAP orthopedic products
  FACScan (fluorescence-activated
    cell sorter) flow cytometer
  FACSVantage cell sorter
  FastTake electrochemical blood
    glucose monitoring system
  FASTak suture anchor system
  F.A.S.T. (First Access for Shock
    and Trauma) 1 intraosseous
    infusion system
  Faulkner folder
  FeatherTouch automated rasp
  Felig insulin pump
  femoral canal restrictor
  FemoStop femoral artery
    compression arch
  FemSoft insert continent
  Femtosecond laser keratome
  fenestrated Drake clip
  Filcard temporary removable vena
    cava filter
  filiforms and followers
  Finesse cardiac device
  Finger Blocking Tree
  finger cot
  fingerstick blood glucose testing

device *(cont.)*

Firm D-Ring wrist support (Rolyan)
FirstSave automated external
  defibrillator (AED)
Fisch drill
fixation
FlashPoint optical localizer
Fletcher-Suit applicator
Fletcher-Suit-Delclos (FSD) mini
  colpostat tandem and ovoids
Flexicath silicone subclavian
  cannula
Flexiflo Lap G laparoscopic
  gastrostomy kit
Flexiflo Lap J
F. L. Fischer microsurgical neurec-
  tomy bayonet scissors
Flimm Fighter percussor machine
Flocor (poloxamer 188)
Flo-Restor
Flo-Stat fluid management system
FlowGun
FloWire ultrasound device
Flowtron DVT pump system
Flu-Glow fluorescein-impregnated
  paper strip
Fluorescence activated cell sorter
  (FACS)
Fluor-i-Strip
FluoroCatcher
FluoroPlus Angiography
FluoroPlus Cardiac digital imaging
FluoroPlus Roadmapper
FluoroScan
Fluoro Tip cannula
Flutter chest percussion therapy
"flying spot" excimer laser
ForeRunner automatic external
  defibrillator
Forma water-jacketed incubator
Freedom arthritis support
FreeDop
Freehand neuroprosthetic system
Freeman cookie cutter areola
  marker

device *(cont.)*

Freeman femoral component with
  a Rotalok cup
Freeman Punctum Plug
Freer elevator
Free-standing Tissue Retraction
  Bridge system
Freezor cryocatheter
fria pelvic continent aid
Friedländer marker
Frigitronics probe
Fujinon Sonoprobe system
Fukushima cranial retraction
Fukushima-Giannotta instruments
Gaffney joint
GAIT (great toe arthroplasty
  implant technique) spacer
Galileo intravasular radiotherapy
Gamma Knife radiosurgical
  instrument
Gammex RMI DAP meter
Gardner chair
Garrett dilator
Gatch bed
Geenan cytology brush
gelatin compression boot
Gelfoam cookie
Gellhorn pessary
gel pads
Gem DR implantable defibrillator
Gemini paired helical wire basket
GEM-Premier analyzer
GeneChip system
Generation 6 integrated radiotherapy
GenESA system
Gen-Probe hybridization kit
Gensini cardiac device
GenStent biologic gene-based
  therapeutic
GentlePeel skin exfoliation
Gentle Touch appliance
Genutrain P3
Georgiade visor
GE Senographe 2000D digital
  mammography

device *(cont.)*
Ghajar guide
Gherini-Kauffman endo-otoprobe
Gianturco-Roehm bird's nest vena
cava filter
Gianturco wool-tufted wire coil
Gingrass and Messer pins
Girard Fragmatome
Glassman stone extractor
GliaSite radiation therapy
glide
Glidewire
Glucometer DEX blood glucose
monitor
GlucoWatch
Goldmann applanation tonometer
Goodale-Lubin cardiac device
GoodKnight 418A, 418G, 418P
CPAP
Gore cast liner
Gore Smoother Crucial Tool
gossypiboma (cotton) laparotomy
pad
gouge
Gould electromagnetic flowmeter
Gould polygraph
GraNee needle (Riza-Ribe grasper
needle)
Greenfield IVC filter
Greenwald cutting loop
Greenwald flexible endoscopic
electrodes
Grieshaber manipulator
Grinfeld cannula
Grosse and Kempf locking nail
system
G-suit
GTS great toe system
Guardsman femoral screw
Guardwire angioplasty
Guglielmi Detachable Coil
Guidant's TRIAD three-electrode
energy defibrillation system
Gullstrand's slit lamp
gurney

device *(cont.)*
Gynecare Verascope hysteroscopy
system
Gyroscan ACS NT MRI scanner
Gyrus endourology
HAART (highly active antiretroviral
therapy)
Haemonetics Cell Saver
Haid Universal bone plate system
Hakim-Cordis pump
Halifax interlaminar clamp system
Hall dermatome
Hall valvulotome
Hammer mini-tubular external
fixation valve
Hancock II tissue valve
Hanger ComfortFlex knee
prosthesis
Hardy-Sella punch
Harmonic Scalpel
Harpoon suture anchor
Harrington rod
Harris-Galante porous-coated
femoral component
Harrison-Nicolle polypropylene
pegs
Harvard 2 dual syringe pump
Harvard pump
Hasson blunt-end cannula
Hasson graspers
Hasson open laparoscopy cannula
Hasson SAC (stable access cannula)
Hasson trocar
Hastings frame
HDI 1000 ultrasound system
HDI 5000 ultrasound system
Healey revision acetabular
component
HeartMate vented electric LVAS
(left ventricular assist system)
Heartport Port-Access system
HeartSaver VAD artificial heart
Heartstream ForeRunner automatic
external defibrillator
HearTwave EP (electrophysiology)

device *(cont.)*

HeatProbe
Hedrocel
Heffington lumbar seat spinal
   surgery frame
Helios diagnostic imaging systems
heliX knot pusher
Helmholtz coil
Hemaflex PTCA sheath with
   obturator
Hemaquet PTCA sheath with
   obturator
HemAssist
Hemasure r/LS red blood cell
   filtration
Hemi Sling
Hemoccult Sensa
HemoCue photometer
hemodialyzer
Hemopad
Hemopump
hemostatic eraser
Hemotherapies liver dialysis unit
Henning instruments
Herbert bone screw
Herbert-Whipple bone screw
HercepTest HER2 protein
   expression
Hewlett-Packard ear oximeter
Hexcelite
Hexcel total condylar knee system
Hex-Fix
Heyer-Schulte tissue expander
high-resolution multileaf collimator
Hilger facial nerve stimulator
Hi-Per cardiac device
HipNav process
HiSonic ultrasonic bone conduction
   hearing device
Hi Speed Pulse Lavage
Histofreezer cryosurgical wart
   treatment
HMWPe (ultra-high molecular
   weight polyethylene) ball liner

device *(cont.)*

Hoffmann external fixation device
Hoffmann mini-lengthening fixation
   device
HomeChoice Pro with PD Link
HomeTrak Plus compact cardiac
   event recorder
HomMed Monitoring System
Honan balloon
Honan manometer
Hopkins 70° rigid telescope for
   laryngoscopy
Horizon AutoAdjust CPAP system
Horn endo-otoprobe
Hot and Cold Sensory System
Hot/Ice Cold Therapy Cooler
Hotsy Cautery
Housecall transtelephonic
   monitoring
Houston Halo
Howmedica Universal compression
   screw
HPCD (hemostatic puncture closure
   device)
Hp Chek
HP SONOS 5500 ultrasound
   imaging system
HRL (Hardy-Rand-Littler)
   screening plates
H-TRON insulin pump
Hubbard hydrotherapy tank
Hulka tenaculum
Humalog Mix 75/25 Pen (insulin
   lispro protamine suspension,
   insulin lispro injection)
HumatroPen
HumidAire heated humidifier
HUMI uterine manipulator/injector
Hummer microdebrider
Hummingbird wand
Humulin 70/30, Humulin R,
   and Humalog Pens
Hunter-Sessions balloon
HydroBlade keratome

device *(cont.)*
HydroBrush keratome
Hydrocollator
HydroFlex arthroscopy irrigating
    system
hydrogel sheets
Hydromer coagulation probe
HydroSurg laparoscopic irrigator
HydroThermAblator
Hyfrecator coagulator
Hylashield, Hylashield Nite
Hypafix nonwoven tape
hyperbaric chambers
Hyperion LTK (laser thermal
    keratoplasty)
IceSeeds
ICLH (Imperial College, London
    Hospital) orthopedic apparatus
Ideal cardiac device
I-Flow nerve block infusion kit
Ilizarov system
Illi intracranial pressure monitoring
    and fixation device
Illumina PROSeries laparoscopy
    system
ImageChecker detection system
    for mammography
IMED infusion device
Imount instruments
IMP-Capello arm support
Import vascular access port with
    BioGlide
Import vascular access port with
    dual lumen
Impress Softpatch
incentive spirometer
Incert
In Charge diabetes control
Indigo LaserOptic treatment
In-Exsufflator cough machine
Infant Flow nasal CPAP system
In-Fast bone screw system
InFix interbody fusion
Infuse-a-port

device *(cont.)*
Injex
InnerVasc sheath
Innova home therapy system
InnovaTome microkeratome
Innovator Holter system
INRO surgical nails
Insall/Burstein II system
Inspiron
InstaTrak
Insuflon
InSurg laparoscopic stone baskets
InSync cardiac stimulator
Intacs
Integrated Wound Manager
Integris 3-D RA (rotational
    angiography)
Integrity AFx AutoCapture
    pacemaker
intense pulsed light source (IPLS)
interferential stimulator
Inter Fix RP (reduced profile)
    threaded spinal fusion cage
Inter Fix spinal fusion cage
InterStim neurostimulation
Inter-Vial drug delivery system
Intrabeam intraoperative
    radiotherapy (IORT)
Intracell
intracoronary Doppler flow wire
IntraDop
Intra–Op autotransfusion
Intrel II spinal cord stimulation
    system
INVOS 3100 (and 3100A) cerebral
    oximeter
Ioban antimicrobial incise drape
iodophor-impregnated adhesive
    drape
Iowa trumpet
I-Plant brachytherapy seeds
iris hook
IRIS (Intensified Radiographic
    Imaging System)

device *(cont.)*
Irrijet DS
Ishihara plates
ISI laparoscopic instruments
Isocam SPECT imaging system
Isola spinal instrumentation system
Isolex system
Isovis wound protector
i-STAT system
Itrel 3 spinal cord stimulation
IVAC electronic thermometer
IVAC volumetric infusion pump
JACE W550
Jackson spinal surgery and imaging
   table
Jaeger eye chart
Jaeger lid plate
Jako facial nerve monitor
Jamar dynamometer
Jameson calipers
Jarit Rotator
Jay seating system
Jeter lag screws or position screws
Jewel AF implantable defibrillator
Joe's hoe
Joystick
J-wire
Kambin and Gellman instrumenta-
   tion
KAM Super Sucker
Kanavel brain-exploring cannula
Kaneda spine stabilizing system
Karl Storz Calcutript
Kaycel towels
Kaye tamponade balloon
K-Caps
KCD (kinestatic charge detector)
K-Centrum anterior spinal fixation
Kellan hydrodissection cannula
Kempf internal screw fixation
Ken nail
KeraVision Intacs intracorneal ring
Key-Med dilator
Kid-Kart

device *(cont.)*
Killip wire
Kim-Ray Greenfield caval filter
kinestatic charge detector (KCD)
KineTec hip CPM machine
KinetiX ventilation monitor
King cardiac device
Kirklin fence
Kirschenbaum foot positioner
Kirschner Medical Dimension
Kish urethral illuminated catheter
   set
Kitano knot
Klein pump
Kleinsasser anterior commissure
   laryngoscope
KLS Centre-Drive screws
Knee Signature System (KSS)
K9 Scooter
Knodt rod
Koch phaco manipulator/splitter
KOH colpotomizer system
Kold Kap
Köper Knit
Kostuik internal spine fixation
   system
Kraff nucleus splitter
K-Sponge
Kuhn-Bolger seeker
Kusch'kin Ace wheelchair
Küttner blunt dissector
Lactosorb plating system
LADARVision
Laerdal resuscitator
Laitinen CT guidance system and
   stereotactic head frame
laminaria applicator
Landolt pituitary speculum
Landolt ring
Lange skin-fold calipers
LaparoLith
LaparoSAC single-use obturator and
   cannula
laparoscopic Doppler probe

device *(cont.)*
Laparosonic coagulating shears
Lap-Band adjustable gastric banding
(LAGB)
Lapro-Clip ligating clip system
Lap Sac
lap tape
LapTie
Lapwall
laser Doppler flowmetry (LDF)
Laserflo blood perfusion monitor
(BPM)
Laser Lancet
LaserPen
LaserTweezers
Lasette laser finger perforator
Lawrence Add-A-Cath trocar
and sheath
LazerSmile tooth-whitening
leading bar
Legasus Sport CPM device
Lehman cardiac device
Leibinger miniplate system
Leibinger Profyle system
Leksell stereotaxic frame
LeMaitre Glow 'N Tell tape
Leonard Arm
LeukoNet Filter
Levulan Kerastick
Lexer gouge
Lido Lift
LifeGuide blood glucose monitor
LIFE-Lung fluorescence endoscopy
system
Life-Pack 5 cardiac monitor
LifeSite hemodialysis access
LiftMate patient transfer device
Ligaclip
LightSheer diode laser
Light Talker
Lilliput neonatal oxygenator
LIMA-Lift
LIMA-Loop
Lindorf lag screws or position
screws

device *(cont.)*
Lindstrom arcuate incision marker
Link Lubinus SP II hip replacement
Linvatec cannulated interference
screw
Linvotec microdebrider
LINX-EZ cardiac device
lion jaw tenaculum
liposhaver
Liss CES (cranial electrical stimula-
tion) device
LiteNest portable seating system
lithotrite
Littleford/Spector introducer
Lloyd-Davies scissors
LMA-Unique
long taper/stiff shaft Glidewire
LoPro ArthroWand
LORAD StereoGuide stereotactic
breast biopsy system
low-resistance rolling seal
spirometer
LPI (Laser Photonics, Inc.) laser
Luhr fixation system
Lunderquist-Ring torque guide
Luque rods and sublaminar wires
Lusk instruments
Lutrin photosensitizer
Luxtec fiberoptic system
LVAS (left ventricular assist
system) implantable pump
Lymphedema Alert Bracelet
lyodura loop
Lyo-Ject syringe
Lyra laser
MAC (Miami Acute Care) collar
Mackay-Marg tonometer
MacKinnon-Dellon Diskriminator
Macroplastique continent implant
Maddacrawler
MagnaPod pain relief magnets
Magnes 2500 WH (whole head)
imager
Magnetic Surgery System
Magnetom MRI system

device *(cont.)*
Mainstay urologic soft tissue anchor
Makler insemination device
Malis CMC-II bipolar coagulator
malleus nipper
Mallinckrodt sensor systems
Malmstrom cup
Maloney endo-otoprobe
MammoSite RTS (radiation therapy
   system)
Mammotest breast biopsy system
Mammotome handheld breast biopsy
Mandibular Excursiometer
Mark II Kodros radiolucent awl
Mark II Sorrells
Mark VII cooling vest
Marlow Primus instrument
   collection device
Marsupial pouch-like belt
Marx bridging plate system
Maryland dissector
Mascot indirect ophthalmoscope
Masimo SET (signal extraction
   technology)
Master Flow Pumpette
Matritech NMP22 test kit
Matroc femoral head
Maxilift Combi patient lifting
   system
Maxima Forté blood oxygenator
Maxima II TENS unit
Maxim modular knee system
May anatomical bone plates
Mayfield-Kees headholder
Mayo-Gibbon heart-lung machine
McCain TMJ arthroscopic system
McGaw volumetric pump
McGee platinum/stainless steel
   piston
McGlamry elevator
McIvor mouth gag
McKinley EpM pump
McNeill-Goldmann blepharostat
MDILO medication intake monitor

device *(cont.)*
Mectra Tissue Sample Retainer
Medela breast pump
Medelec DMG 50 Teflon-coated
   monopolar electrode
Medfusion 2001 syringe infusion
   pump
medical holography
Medicon surgical instruments
Medigraphics 2000 analyzer
Medi-Ject needle-free insulin
   injection system
Medi-Jector Choice
MediPort
Medisense Pen 2 blood glucose
   monitor
Medisorb drug delivery system
MedJet microkeratome
Mednext bone dissecting system
Medoff sliding fracture plate
Medrad automated power injector
Medrad MRinnervu endorectal
   colon probe
Medstone STS shock-wave
   generator
Medtronic Activa tremor control
   therapy
Medtronic Gem automatic
   implantable defibrillator
Medtronic Hemopump
Medtronic Inspire
Medtronic Jewel AF implantable
Medtronic Micro Jewel II
Medtronic Octopus
Medtronic Sprint lead for
   cardioverter-defibrillator
Medtronic SynchroMed pump
Medtronic tremor control therapy
   device
MedX physical therapy device
Megadyne/Fann E-Z clean
   laparoscopic electrodes
MegaDyne all-in-one hand control
membrane delamination wedge

device *(cont.)*

MemoryTrace AT cardiac device
Mentor BVAT computer screen
    chart
Mercedes tip cannula
Merocel sponge
Merry Walker ambulation device
Messerklinger sinus endoscopy set
Metrix implantable atrial
    defibrillation system
Miami J collar
MIC disposable cytology brush
Micro-Aire pulse lavage system
Microblator
Micro Diamond-Point microsurgery
    instruments
microendoscopic diskectomy
    (MED) instrumentation
MicroGlide reciprocating osteotome
Micro-Imager
MicroLap and MicroLap Gold
    microlaparoscopy system
Micron Res-Q implantable
    cardioverter-defibrillator
Microny SR+ pulse generator
MicroPlaner soft tissue shaver
Micropuncture Peel-Away
    introducer
microSelectron-HDR (high dose
    rate) afterloader
MicroSmooth probe
MicroSpan microhysteroscopy
    system
MicroTeq portable belt
microtome
Microvasic Rigiflex TTS balloon
Microvit cutter
microwave cardiac ablation system
Micro-Z stimulator
Midas Rex pneumatic instruments
Mijnhard electrical cycloergometer
Miltex surgical instruments
MIMCOM (multimode imaging
    confocal optical microscope)

device *(cont.)*

Minerva neurosurgical robot
Mini-Acutrak
mini Hoffmann external fixation
    system
Mini-Med Continuous Glucose
    Sensor
Mirage nasal ventilation mask
    system
Mitek anchor system
Miya hook ligament carrier
MKM AutoPilot stereotactic system
MMS-10 Tympanic Displacement
    Analyzer
Mobetron intraoperative radiation
    therapy (IORT) treatment system
    (linear accelerator)
Mobin-Uddin umbrella filter
Modulap probe
Modulock posterior spinal fixation
Moe instrumentation
Molnar disk
Molt periosteal elevator
Monolyth oxygenator
Monoscopy locking trocar with
    Woodford spike
monster rongeur
Monticelli-Spinelli system
Morscher titanium cervical plate
Morse taper stem
Moss Miami load-sharing spinal
    implant system
Moss T-anchor needle introducer
    gun
Mullins cardiac device
Multibite biopsy forceps
Multifire Endohernia clip applier
Multileaf Collimator (MLC)
Multilok hand operating table
Multi-Operatory Dentalaser (MOD)
Multi Podus (boot)
MultiVac ArthroWand
MUSE (medicated urethral system
    for erection) urethral suppository

device *(cont.)*
MUSTPAC
Myers Solution instrument and
   technique
MYOterm XP
MyoTrac and MyoTrac 2 EMG
   monitoring
Nagahara phaco chopper and phaco
   chop technique
Nakao snare I and II
nanowalker
Nashold TC electrode
National Notifiable Disease
   Surveillance System (NNDSS)
Natural-Knee system
Navarre interventional radiology
NBIH cardiac device
Nellcor Symphony
Neocontrol magnet technology
NeoNaze
Neoprobe 1000 detector
Neoprobe 1500 portable
   radioisotope detector
Neoprobe detector
Neotrend system
nerve block infusion kit
NervePace
NeuroCybernetic Prosthesis
NeuroLink II
NeuroMate robotic technology
Neuromed Octrode implantable
   device
Neuromeet nerve approximator
Neuroperfusion pump
neuroprobe
Neuro-Trace
Neurotrend system
New England Baptist acetabular cup
NexGen complete knee replacement
Nezhat-Dorsey Trumpet Valve
   hydrodissector
Nibbler
Nibblit laparoscopic device
Nicolet Nerve Integrity Monitor-2
   (NIM-2)

device *(cont.)*
Nidek MK-2000 keratome
NightOwl pocket polygraph
ninety-ninety (90/90) intraosseous
   wiring
NIRS (near infrared spectroscopy)
nitinol mesh-covered frame
Nomos pin-free attachment
   stereotactic system
NonSpil drug delivery
NordiPen human growth hormone
   injection
Nottingham introducer
Novacor left ventricular assist
   system (LVAS) implantable
   pump
NovolinPen device
Novus Verdi diode-pumped green
   photocoagulator
Nucleotome Endoflex
Nucleotome Flex II
Nu-Tip disposable scissor tip
Nycore cardiac device
Nylok self-locking nail
Oasis thrombectomy
obturator
Obwegeser-Dalpont internal screw
   fixation
Ocutech Vision Enhancing System
ocutome
Ogden anchor
olive ring
olive wire
Olympia VACPAC support device
Olympus forward-viewing
   CF-1T100L video colonoscope
Olympus UM-1W endoscopic probe
Olympus URF-P2 translaparoscopic
   choledochofiberscope
Omega splinting material
OmniFilter
Omnifit Plus hip system
Omni-Flexor
One-Shot anastomotic instrument
One Touch blood glucose meter

device *(cont.)*
OnLineABG monitoring system
Onyx finger pulse oximeter
Opal Photoactivator
OPERA STAR (specialized tissue
  aspirating resectoscope) SL
Operating Arm System
Opsis DistalCam video system
optical pachometer
Optical Tracking System
Opti-Gard patient eye protector
Optipore wound-cleaning sponge
Optistat power injector
Orbasone noninvasive therapeutic
Orfizip wrist cast
Origin balloon, tacker, trocar
Orion anterior cervical plate
OR1 electronic
Ortho Dx
Orthofix Cervical-Stim
Orthofix intramedullary nail
Ortho-Ice Multipaks
Ortholav equipment
Ortholoc Advantim knee revision
  system
OrthoNail
OrthoPak II bone growth stimulator
orthoplast jacket
Orthosorb absorbable pin
OSCAR bone cement removal
Osciflator balloon inflation syringe
oscillating saw
OSI arthroscopic leg holder
OSI extremity elevator
OSI well leg holder
Osteo-Clage cable system
Osteonics Omnifit-HA hip stem
OsteoStim implantable bone growth
  stimulator
OsteoView 2000
OutBound
Oves cervical cap
Oves fertility cap
OV-1 surgical keratometer
Oxifirst fetal oxygen monitoring

device *(cont.)*
oximeter
Oxylator EM-100 resuscitation
Oxymizer
Oxytrak pulse oximeter and
  Dinamap blood pressure monitor
Pacesetter APS pacemaker
  programmer
Pacesetter Trilogy DR+
pachometer
Pach-Pen
PACS (Picture Archiving and
  Communications Systems)
Padgett baseline pinch gauge
Padgett hydraulic hand
  dynamometer
pallidal brain stimulation
Panje voice button
Panoramic 200 nonmydriatic
  ophthalmoscope
Papercuff
Paramax cruciate guide
Parasmillie double-bladed knife
Paratrend 7 and 7+
Parietex composite mesh
P.A.S. Port Fluoro-Free
Passager introducing sheath
Patil stereotaxic system
Pavlik harness
PCD Transvene implantable
  cardioverter-defibrillator system
PC Polygraf HR device
P.D. Access with Peel-Away
  needle introducer
peakometer
Pearce nucleus hydrodissector
Pelorus stereotactic system
Pennig dynamic wrist fixator
Pennig minifixator
People-Finder
Perclose closure device
PercuGuide
PercuPump disposable syringe and
  injector
percutaneous gastroenterostomy

device *(cont.)*

Percutaneous Stoller Afferent Nerve
   Stimulation System (PerQ SANS)
PerDUCER pericardial access
   device
PerFixation screws
PerFix Marlex mesh plug
peripheral access system (PAS) port
Peri-Strips Dry
Perkins Brailler
Perkins tonometer
PERM (Electropneumatic Platform
   for Motor Rehabilitation)
Persona monitoring kit
Peyman vitrector
PFC Sigma total knee system
Phaco-Emulsifier
Phantom nasal mask
Philips ultrasound machines
photocatalytic air filtration system
PhotoDerm PL
PhotoDerm VL
Photon cataract removal
Photon Radiosurgery System (PRS)
Photopic Imaging ultrasound
Phylax AV cardioverter-defibrillator
Physios CTM 01
Picasso phone
Picker Magnascanner
piezo electrical stimulator
Pigg-O-Stat
Pilot audiometer
PINC polymer
Pinn.ACL guide
Pinpoint stereotactic arm
Pittman IMA retractor
Pixsys Flashpoint
Plasma Scalpel
Plastizote collar
platinum coil
Pleatman sac
PlegiaGuard
PMT AccuSpan tissue expander
Pneumo Sleeve

device *(cont.)*

PocketDop
point-search acupuncture
   instruments
Polaris cage
Polarus proximal humeral fixation
   system
Polar Vantage XL heart rate
   monitor
Poly-Dial insert
polylactide absorbable screw
Polyrox
Polystan cannula
pondylophyte impaction set
Poppen Ridge Sensitometer
portable blood irradiator
Port-A-Cath
Porta Pulse 3 defibrillator
Positrol cardiac device
Posture S'port
potential acuity meter (PAM)
Potts scissors
Powerheart
PowerSculpt cosmetic surgery
Precision Osteolock
Precision QID
Premium Plus CEEA disposable
   stapler
preperitoneal distention balloon
   (PDB)
PREP Pap smear
PressureSense Monitor
Presto cardiac device
Prima laser guide wire
Primbs-Circon indirect video
   ophthalmoscope
Prime ECG (electrocardiographic)
   mapping
Prisma digital hearing aid
Probe cardiac device
Prodigy bone densitometer
Prodigy lens inserter
Profile total hip system with porous
   coating

device *(cont.)*

Profore four-layer bandaging
ProForma double-lumen
  papillotome
ProLease
PROloop electrosurgical
Propaq Encore vital signs monitor
Propel cannulated interference
  screws
ProPoint
Prosorba column pheresis device
Prostar, Prostar Plus, and Prostar
  XL percutaneous closure devices
Prostatron
Prosthetic Disc Nucleus (PDN)
ProtectaCap
Protectaid contraceptive sponge
Protect-a-Pass suture passer
Protector suturing system
Protocult
Protouch
Pro-Trac
Protractor
public access defibrillation (PAD)
PulmoSphere
Pulsavac III wound debridement
  system
PulseDose technology
pulse oximetry devices
Pulse Pro heart rate monitor
PulseSpray
punctum plug
Pursuer CBD Helical or
  Mini-Helical stone basket
Pylon intramedullary nail
PZT (plumbeous zirconate titanate)
  tip
QuantX color quantification tools
Quartet system
Questus Leading Edge arthroscopic
  grasper-cutter
Questus Leading Edge sheathed
  arthroscopy knife
QuickDraw venous cannula

device *(cont.)*

Quikheel lancet
RAD55 self-irrigating suction bur
radioimmunoluminography (RILG)
radiolucent spine frame
RadiStop radial compression
Radstat
rake
Ranawat/Burstein total hip system
Rancho cube
Rancho fixation system
Rand microballoon
RAP (remote access perfusion)
  cannula
RapidFlap cranial fixation
Rashkind cardiac device
Rashkind double umbrella device
Rasor blood pumping system
  (RBPS)
Raulerson syringe
Ray-Tec sponge
Ray threaded fusion cage (TFC)
Razi cannula introducer
RDX coronary radiation catheter
  delivery
ReAct NMES device
real-time color flow Doppler
real-time position management
  (REAL) tracking
reciprocating saw
Reddick-Saye screw
Reese dermatome
Reese stimulator
Refinity Coblation
ReFlex Wand
Regency SR+
Reichert/Mundinger stereotactic
  device
Reliance CM femoral component
Reliance urinary control insert
ReliefBand NST (nerve stimulation
  therapy)
Relton-Hall spine frame
Repela surgical glove

device *(cont.)*

Repose surgical
Res-Q ACD (arrhythmia control device)
Res-Q Micron
resipump
Resolve Quickanchor
ReSound Digital 2000 hearing aid
Respiradyne
Respironics CPAP (continuous positive airway pressure) machine
Respitrace machine
Response GM
Restore ACL guide system
Retcam 120 digital camera
retrospectoscope
Retrox Fractal active fixation lead
Reuter suprapubic trocar and cannula system
Reveal Plus insertable loop recorder
Revo retrievable cancellous screw
Revo rotator cuff repair
Rhinoline endoscopic system
Rhino Rocket
Richards Solcotrans Plus
Riester otoscope
RigiScan
RIGS system
RinoFlow
Risser localizer cast
Risser table
RLS (rhinolaryngostroboscopy) system
R-Med Plug
RM (Reichert/Mundinger) stereotaxic system
Robicsek Vascular Probe (RVP)
Robodoc
Robotrac passive retraction system
ROC and ROC XS suture fasteners
Rochester bone trephine
Roeder loop
roentgen knife

device *(cont.)*

Rogozinski spinal fixation system
Roho air-filled mattress
Rolyan Firm D-Ring wrist support
Romano surgical curved drilling system
Rossiter stretching program
Rotablator RotaLink rotational atherectomy
Rotalok cup
Roth Grip-Tip suture guide
Rothman Gilbard corneal punch
Roth retrieval net
roticulating endograsper
Roto-Rest bed
Roy-Camille plates
Ruiz-Cohen round expander
Ruiz microkeratome
Rumi uterine manipulator and injector
Russel (one *L*) gastrostomy kit
Russell-Taylor (R-T) nail
Rutzen ileostomy bag
Rx5000 cardiac pacing system
RX stent delivery system
SACH (solid-ankle, cushioned heel) heels
sacral nerve stimulation (SNS) implantable device
Sadowsky hook wire
SAF-T shield
Sahara Clinical Bone Sonometer
Sahara densitometer
Salz nuclear splitter
Sand process
SANS (Stoller afferent nerve stimulation)
SaphFinder surgical balloon dissector
SAPHtrak balloon dissector
Sarns aortic arch cannula
SatinCrescent tunneler
SatinShortcut
SatinSlit keratome

device *(cont.)*
SB Charité III intervertebral
dynamic disc system
scalp electrode
Scanmaster DX x-ray film digitizer
Scanning-Beam Digital X-ray
(SBDX)
Scaphoid-Microstaple system
Schantz screw
Schiek back support
Scholten endomyocardial bioptome
and biopsy forceps
SciTojet needle-free injector
scleral expansion band (SEB)
Scopette
Scorpio total knee
Scully Hip S'port
SEA (side entry access) port
Secur-Fit HA (hydroxyapatite) hip
SeedNet cryotherapy
Segura CBD (common bile duct)
basket
Seidel humeral locking nail
Seidel intramedullary fixation
Semmes-Weinstein nylon
monofilaments
Senning intra-atrial baffle
Senographe 2000D digital
mammography imaging
Sensability lubricated plastic sheet
Sens-A-Ray dental imaging system
SensiCath optical sensor
Sensi-Touch anesthesia delivery
system
Sentinel implantable cardioverter-
defibrillator
Seprafilm
SergiScope robotic microscope
Servo pump
SharpShooter
Shaw I and Shaw II scalpel
Shepherd internal screw fixation
Sherwood intrascopic suction/
irrigation system
Shuffors internal screw fixation

device *(cont.)*
SI (sacroiliac) belt
Side Branch Occlusion system
side-cutting Swanson bur
Side-Fire reflecting dish
SieScape imaging technology
Silhouette therapeutic massage
system
silicone flexor rod
Silipos Distal Dip
SI-LOC
Silon tent
Silverstein facial nerve monitor
Silverstein stimulator probe
Simal cervical stabilization
Simplicity spirometer
Single-Day Baxter infuser
Sinskey hook
Sinuscope or SinuScope
SiteSelect percutaneous breast
biopsy system
SJM-Seguin annuloplasty ring
Skil saw
Skimmer RRP laryngeal shaver
Skin Skribe
SKY epidural pain control system
Skylight gamma camera
slip-ring CT technology
SLS (Spectranetics laser sheath)
"smart" defibrillator
SmartKard digital Holter system
SmartMist
Smart Scalpel
SmokEvac electrosurgical probe
SODAS (spheroidal oral drug
absorption system)
Soehendra dilator
Sofamor spinal instrumentation
device
SoftLight
Soft N Dry Merocel sponge
Soft Shield collagen corneal shield
soft tissue shaving cannula
(liposhaver)
Soft Touch cup

device *(cont.)*
Soluset
SomaSensor
SOMATOM Volume Zoom CT
Somer uterine elevator
Somnoplasty system
Sonablate 200
sonic-accelerated fracture healing
   system (SAFHS)
sonicator
SonoCT real-time compound
   imaging
SonoHeart handheld digital
   echocardiography
SONOLINE Sierra ultrasound
   imaging
SonoSite 180 hand-carried
   ultrasound
Sonotron
Sophy programmable pressure valve
Soprano cryoablation system
Sorbie Questor elbow
Spacemaker balloon dissector
Space*Saver volumetric pump
SpaTouch PhotoEpilation System
Spectranetics Laser Sheath (SLS)
Spectraprobe-Max probe
Spectrum tissue repair
Speculite
SP-501 Sonoprobe endoscopy
   system
SpF Spinal Fusion Stimulator
Sphygmocorder
Spiessel lag screws, position screws,
   internal screw fixation
SpinaLogic 1000 bone growth
   stimulator
Splintrex
sponge dissector
SprayGel adhesion barrier
spud dissector
Squirt wound irrigation
S-ROM femoral stem prosthesis
SRT (smoke removal tube) vaginal
   speculum

device *(cont.)*
S.S.T. small bone locking nail
Stability total hip system
Stableloc external wrist fixation
   system
STARRT (selective tubal assess-
   ment to refine reproductive
   therapy) falloposcopy system
Statak
Statham electromagnetic flow meter
StatLock Universal Plus
Stat 2 Pumpette
Steeper powered Gripper
Steffee plates and screws
Steinhauser lag screws, position
   screws, or internal screw fixation
Steinmann pin
StereoGuide
Steri-Drape
steroid-eluting electrode
Stim Plus
St. Jude Medical Port-Access
Stomeasure
STOO Series Ten Thousand
   Ocutome
STOP (selective tubal occlusion
   procedure) contraceptive
Storz Calcutript
Storz cholangiograsper
Storz infant bronchoscope
Storz radial incision marker
Straight-In surgical system
StraightShot arterial cannula
Strata hip system
STRETCH cardiac device
Stryker leg exerciser
Stryker microdebrider
Stulberg hip positioner
Stylet esophageal MRI coil
Summit LoDose collimator
Super-9 guiding cardiac device
Super Pinky
SuperQuad assistive device
Supramesh
SureCell Chlamydia test kit

device *(cont.)*
SureCell herpes (SC-HSV) test kit
Sure-Closure
Suretac
SureTrans autotransfusion system
surgical isolation bubble (SIBS)
Surgical No Bounce Mallet
SurgiLav Plus machine
Surg-I-Loop
Surgiport
SurgiScope
Surgitron
Suture/VesiBand organizer
Sweet Tip pacing lead
Swenson papillotome
SwingAlong walker caddie
Symbion J-7-70-mL-ventricle total
    artificial heart
Symmetra I-125 brachytherapy seeds
Symmetry EndoBipolar Generator
Symphonix Vibrant soundbridge
SynchroMed infusion system
Synergy neurostimulation
Synthes CerviFix
Synthes compression hip screw
Synthes dorsal distal radius plate
Synthes drill
Synthes mini L-plate
Synthes transbuccal trocar
Syringe Avitene
Szabo-Berci needle drivers
TAG (tissue anchor guide) system
Tagarno 3SD cine projector
Take-apart scissors and forceps
Talent LPS endoluminal stent-graft
Tanne corneal punch
Tanner mesher
Tanner-Vandeput mesh dermatome
tantalum mesh, plate, ring, wire
TAPET (tumor amplified protein
    expression therapy)
targeted cryoablation
Targis microwave catheter-based
Targis system

device *(cont.)*
Taylor pinwheel
TCPM pneumatic tourniquet system
TCu380A IUD (intrauterine device)
Tebbetts rhinoplasty set
Techstar and Techstar XL
Techstar percutaneous closure
TeleCaption decoder
Telescopic Plate Spacer (TPS)
telesensor
Teller acuity card (TAC)
Tender Touch Ultra cup
Tendril DX
Tendril SDX
Tennant nuclear ball rotator
Tenzel calipers
Terry keratometer
Tetrax interactive balance system
ThAIRapy Vest
Therabite jaw motion rehabilitation
    system
TheraGym exercise balls
thermistor
ThermoChem system
Thermoflex
Thermophore
Thermoscan Pro-1-Instant
    thermometer
Thermoskin arthritic knee wrap
Thermo-STAT
TherOx 0.014 infusion guide wire
The Viewing Wand surgical
    digitizer
ThinLine EZ
Thora-Port
Thoratec VAD (ventricular assist
    device)
Thornton double corneal ruler
Thornton 360° arcuate marker
THORP (titanium hollow-screw
    osseointegrating reconstruction
    plate) system
threaded interbody fusion cage
threadwire saw

device *(cont.)*

thrombolytic assessment system (TAS)

TiMesh

tissue morcellator

TMS 3-dimensional radiation therapy treatment planning system

Todd-Wells guide

Tono-Pen tonometer

Toomey syringe kit

TOTAL O2 system

Tracer Blood Glucose Micro-monitor

TracerCAD

Tracer hybrid wire guide

Trachlight

Trak Back

transesophageal pacing system

transvaginal suturing (TVS) system

TraumaJet

Travenol infuser

Triangle gelatin-sealed sling material

TriFix spinal instrumentation

Trilogy acetabular cup

Trippi-Wells tongs

Trocan disposable CO_2 trocar and cannula

Tru-Area Determination wound-measuring device

Tru-Close wound drainage system

TruJect

Trumpet Valve hydrodissector

TruWave pressure transducer

T-Span tissue expander

T3 system

Tubex injector

tulip probe

tulip tip

Tum-E-Vac

turnbuckle functional position splint

Turvy internal screw fixation

Tutofix cervical pin

2010 Plus Holter

device *(cont.)*

Twisk needle holder, forceps, scissors combination instrument

Two-Photon Excitation (TPE)

Tylok cerclage cabling system

UC strip catheter tubing fastener

Ulson fixator system

Ultima C femoral component

Ultra-Drive bone cement removal system

Ultraject

Ultraseed ultrasound brachytherapy

Ultratome

Uniflex femoral nail

Uniflex intramedullary nail

UNILINK system

UniPuls electro-stimulation instrument

UniShaper keratome

Unitron Esteem CIC (completely-in-the-canal) hearing aid

Universal fixation screws

University of Akron artificial heart

unreamed femoral nail (UFN)

Urologic Targis

Uroloop

UroVive balloon

USCI cannula

USCI Goetz bipolar electrodes

USCI NBIH bipolar electrodes

U-Titer

Vabra aspirator

V.A.C. (vacuum-assisted closure)

Vac-Lok cushion

Vac-Pak Pad

Vacurette

Vacutainer

Vairox high compression vascular stocking

Validyne manometer

Valle hysteroscope

Vancenase Pockethaler

Vannas capsulotomy scissors

VaporTrode electrode

device *(cont.)*
VariLift spinal cage
VasoSeal VHD (vascular hemostatic device)
VasoView balloon dissection system
Vasoview Uniport
Vbeam pulsed dye laser
VCS vascular clip applier
vectis lever
Vector intertrochanteric nail
VED (vacuum erection device)
Veley headrest
VenaFlow compression
Vena Tech LGM filter
Ventak AV III DR implantable cardioverter defibrillator
Ventak Mini III implantable defibrillator
Ventak Prizm defibrillator
VentCheck ventilator monitor
ventilation-exchange bougie
Ventritex Angstrom MD
ventroposterolateral thalamic electrode
venturi mask
VeriFlex cardiac device
Vernier calipers
VerreScope
Versadopp 10 probe
Versa-Fx femoral fixation
Versalok fixation system
VersaPoint system
Versaport trocar system
vertebral body impactor
Vertetrac ambulatory traction system
Vesica bladder neck stabilization kit
V5M Multiplane transducer
V510B Biplane TEE transducers
VHS variable-angle hip fixation
Vibracare percussor machine
Vibram-soled rockerbottom shoe
videoendoscopic surgical equipment
Viewing Wand

device *(cont.)*
ViewPoint CK (conductive keratoplasty) system
Viratrol
Viringe vascular access flush device
virtual labor monitor (VLM)
Virtuoso imaging system
Visijet hydrokeratome
Visilex mesh
Visuflo blood flow device
VISX Star S2 excimer laser
VISX WaveScan Wavefront System
VitaCuff antimicrobial cuff
VitaCuff attachable cuff
Vitalograph spirometer
Vitatron catheter electrode
Vitrax viscoelastic
vitrector probe
vitreous cutter
V-MAX
VNUS Closure catheter/ radiofrequency generator
VNUS Restore catheter/system
Vocare bladder
Volutrol
Von Lackum surcingle
Voptix corneal
Vortex router
Vortex stabilization
Voxgram
Voyager Aortic IntraClusion
Vozzle Vacu-Irrigator
VPL (ventroposterolateral) thalamic electrode
WACH (wedge adjustable cushioned heel) shoe
Wagner's distraction
Wallaby phototherapy system
Wallace Flexihub central venous pressure cannula
Wallace pipette
Wallach pencil
Warm 'n Form lumbosacral corset
WarmTouch patient warming system

device *(cont.)*
Wartenberg pinwheel
Water-Pik irrigator
Watzke Silicone sleeve
wavefront measurement
Wedeen wire passers
Wedge electrosurgical resection device
Wehbe arm holder
WEST-foot
Wholey wire
Williams cardiac device
Wilson-Cook (modified) wire-guided sphincterotome
Wiltse pedical screw
Wiltse rods
WinABP ambulatory blood pressure monitor
Wissinger rod
Wixson hip positioner
Wizard cardiac
Wizard microdebrider
wobble board
Wolvek sternal approximation fixation instrument
Wound Stick measuring
Wrightlock posterior fixation
Wristaleve
Wurzburg plating system
WuScope
Xillix LIFE endoscopic system
Xillix LIFE-Lung system
XKnife software
XPS Sculpture system
XPS Straightshot
XT cardiac
Yankauer curette (curet)
Yasargil bayonet scissors
Yellow IRIS workstation
Yperwatch gamma control watch
Zebra exchange guide wire
Zeiss ophthalmology instruments
Zenith AAA (abdominal aortic aneurysm) endovascular graft

device *(cont.)*
Zest Anchor Advanced Generation (ZAAG) bone anchoring system
Zeus robotic system
Zielke instrumentation
Zimmer CPT (collarless polished taper) hip system
Zipper Medical neck band
Ziramic femoral head
Zirconia orthopedic prosthetic heads
ZMS intramedullary fixation system
Zoll defibrillator
Zone Specific II meniscal repair
ZTT I and ZTT II acetabular cups
Zucker and Myler cardiac
ZUMI uterine manipulator

"devil's grip"—see *Bornholm disease.*

devil's pinches—factitious purpura; purpura psychogenica. Recurrent painful bruising, consciously or unconsciously self-inflicted.

dewlap—redundant skin hanging below the chin.

DEXA (dual energy x-ray absorptiometry) **scan**—for bone density determination.

dexfenfluramine (Redux).

Dexon mesh—a synthetic (polyglycolic acid filaments) and stretchable fabric used in surgery on soft-tissue organs, e.g., liver, spleen, that do not hold sutures well. The idea is to salvage the organ by enclosing it within the mesh, suturing the mesh to the organ at 1/2 to 1/4 inch intervals. The mesh is absorbed by the body tissues in four to six weeks, by which time healing should have taken place.

Dexon Plus suture—a coated synthetic absorbable suture with a timed coating that lasts for 7 hours.

Dexon II suture—an improved Dexon suture which, according to the

Dexon II *(cont.)*
manufacturer, ties more securely and has better overall strength.

dexrazoxane (Zinecard)—used to prevent cardiomyopathy caused by the chemotherapy drug doxorubicin.

dextran sulfate (Uendex)—for treatment of AIDS patients.

Dextrostix—trade name of plastic strip with reagent areas that change color in the presence of glucose in a drop of capillary blood (usually obtained from the ear lobe or finger stick). Used in monitoring and control of diabetes. Cf. *Chemstrip bG.*

Dey-Wash skin wound cleanser—a saline solution in an aerosol can which sprays under pressure to gently debride and cleanse wounds.

dexrazoxane (Zinecard)—a drug used to prevent cardiotoxicity in pediatric patients with sarcoma receiving Adriamycin chemotherapy.

dezocine (Dalgan).

DFA test (direct fluorescent antibody)—for *Legionella pneumophila*. See also *IFA.*

d4T (didehydrodideoxythymidine, stavudine, Zerit)—antiretroviral agent for HIV patients.

DFT (defibrillation threshold).

DFV (DDP [cisplatin], fluorouracil, VePesid)—chemotherapy protocol.

DG (Davis & Geck) **Softgut suture**—surgical chromic suture.

DHAC (dihydro-5-azacitidine)—chemotherapy drug.

DHAP (dexamethasone, high-dose ara-C, Platinol)—chemotherapy protocol for Hodgkin's lymphoma.

DHE-45 (dihydroergotamine)—for headaches, including migraine; a positive response is diagnostic of migraine.

"The patient uses daily ergotamine and lithium for his cluster headaches, and took two doses of DHE prior to coming to the hospital."

DHPG (dihydroxypropoxymethylguanine; ganciclovir)—for treatment of cytomegalovirus infections in immunosuppressed patients and those with AIDS.

DiaBeta (glyburide)—oral drug for type 2 (non-insulin-dependent diabetes mellitus) diabetics who do not respond to diet alone. In advertisements the *B* is written as the Greek letter *beta* (Diaßeta). The beta cells of the pancreas produce insulin.

diabetes, bronze—see *bronze diabetes.*

diabetes mellitus classifications—from the American Diabetes Association to replace the terms *juvenile onset* and *adult onset,* as follows:

type 1, IDDM (insulin dependent diabetes mellitus) refers to the type of diabetes that requires insulin to sustain life.

type 2, NIDDM (non-insulin-dependent diabetes mellitus) refers to the type of diabetes that does not require insulin to sustain life. This category includes two subgroups: obese and non-obese.

Other redefined categories: *impaired glucose tolerance* which replaces borderline, chemical, or latent as a description of glucose levels which fall between normal and diabetic; *gestational diabetes* that refers to women who develop diabetes during pregnancy; and *diabetes associated with certain conditions or syndromes,* such as diabetes secondary to pancreatic disease or endocrine disease.

diabetes mellitus, pregnancy classifications:

class A (gestational diabetes)—transient diabetes that reverts to normal after the delivery. Usually is well controlled by diet.

class B—onset after age 20, duration less than 10 years; has been controlled by diet, but patient may become insulin dependent during the pregnancy; may not need insulin after the delivery.

class C—onset between 10 and 19 years of age (formerly called juvenile-onset diabetes). The patient has been insulin dependent and will need increased doses during pregnancy, but will usually return to the pre-pregnancy dosage after delivery.

class D—onset at less than 10 years of age, with duration more than 20 years. Hypertension, diabetic retinopathy, and peripheral vascular disease are noted.

class E—calcification of pelvic vessels is present.

class F—diabetic nephropathy is present.

Infants of class A, B, and C diabetic mothers are likely to be large for gestational age (LGA).

Infants of class D, E, and F diabetic mothers are likely to be small for gestational age (SGA).

DiabetiSweet sugar substitute—an artificial sweetener.

DiabGel hydrogel dressing.

DiabKlenz wound cleanser.

Diab II—a prescription treatment for diabetes type 2 and impaired glucose tolerance.

Diacol—a tablet formulation of sodium phosphate for use as a gastrointestinal cleansing agent taken prior to colonoscopic evaluation.

Diacyte DNA ploidy analysis—a way to identify aneuploid tumor of the prostate which may require aggressive treatment, such as tumors with intermediate Gleason scores.

Diagnex Blue test—lab test for gastric acid. (Diagnex Blue is a trademark.)

dial a haptic (Oph).

diamagnetic—MRI term.

diamond bur—instrument used to abrade or smooth; for example, to resect an osteophyte.

diamond fraise—an instrument used in dermabrasion.

Diamond-Lite—titanium cardiovascular surgical instruments.

diamond-shaped murmur—a systolic heart murmur that first grows louder and then softer, the same as a crescendo-decrescendo murmur. Named for diamond-shaped tracing on phonocardiogram.

Dianon prostate profile and diagraph —an oncology trend report showing results over time of PSA, PAP, and LASA-P in patients with prostate cancer.

diaphanography—transillumination of the breast, with photography of the transilluminated light on infrared-sensitive film.

diaphanoscope—instrument for transilluminating a body cavity.

diaphanous—see-through, transparent. See *diaphanoscope*.

DiaPhine corneal trephination device —uses a diamond dissection blade.

diaphragmatic hump—a finding on radiography, due to distortion of the diaphragm by enlarged liver or liver tumor.

diaphysis—the shaft of a long bone between the ends (the epiphyses). *Cf. diastasis, diathesis.*

DIAPPERS—an acronym for causes of transient urinary incontinence:
D delirium
I infection
A atrophic urethritis, vaginitis
P pharmaceuticals
P psychological (especially severe depression)
E excess urine output
R restricted mobility
S stool impaction

Diasensor 1000—a sensor that measures the blood glucose level using near-infrared technology, without the need of a finger prick for a blood sample.

diastasis—separation (or dislocation) of two bones that are normally attached without the presence of a true joint; sometimes refers to the separation of muscles, as in diastasis recti abdominis. Cf. *diaphysis, diathesis.*

Diastat (diazepam, Valium)—can be given rectally to patients experiencing continuous seizures called status epilepticus or acute repetitive seizure disorder.

diastatic fracture—involves separation of the bones at the suture line of the skull, or marked separation of the bone fragments.

Diastat vascular access graft—used for dialysis access.

diathermy—see *ultrasound diathermy.*

diathesis—constitution of the body that predisposes one to certain diseases or conditions, as "The patient appeared to have a hemorrhagic diathesis, although there was no family history of hemophilia." Cf. *diaphysis, diastasis.*

diaziquone (AZQ)—a chemotherapy drug for lymphoma, leukemia, brain tumors (astrocytomas).

Dibbell unilateral cleft lip nasal reconstruction.

dibenzodiazepines—a class of antipsychotic drugs. See *clozapine.*

dibromodulcitol (DBD, mitolactol)—a chemotherapy agent.

DIC (disseminated intravascular coagulation).

DIC (drip infusion cholangiography)

diclofenac potassium (Cataflam)—nonsteroidal anti-inflammatory drug for arthritis, pain, and dysmenorrhea.

diclofenac sodium (Voltaren)—a nonsteroidal anti-inflammatory drug for pain in trauma, dysmenorrhea, rheumatoid arthritis, osteoarthritis, ankylosing spondylitis, degenerative joint disease, rheumatoid arthritis, renal and biliary colic. Cf. *diclofenac potassium* (Cataflam).

DIC (differential interference contrast) **microscopy**.

DICOM (Digital Imaging and Communications in Medicine) (teleradiology)—the industry standard for transfer of radiologic images and other medical information between computers.

DID (delayed ischemic deficit).

didanosine (ddI, Videx)—a drug for HIV-positive patients who cannot tolerate zidovudine (Retrovir) or who have strains of HIV that are resistant to zidovudine.

didehydrodideoxythymidine (d4T)—see *d4T* and *stavudine.*

didelphys—see *uterus didelphys.*

dideoxycytidine (ddC, Hivid, zalcitabine)—a drug approved by the FDA to treat patients with AIDS.

dideoxyinosine (ddI)—see *didanosine.*

Didronel (etidronate).

Dieckmann intraosseous needle—used to deliver drugs and fluids through the bone marrow. Because children's

Dieckmann *(cont.)*

veins are so small, administering drugs intravenously is very difficult and slow, but, in an emergency, using this needle, the physician can get to the bone marrow within 30 seconds. The easiest point to access the marrow (which is said to be much like a noncollapsible vein) is just below the knee.

diener ("dee-ner")—an assistant in a laboratory or morgue.

diethyldithiocarbamate (Imuthiol)—a drug used to treat AIDS.

Dietl's crisis—when a kidney twists on its pedicle, cutting off blood flow.

Dieulafoy's gastric lesion—a congenital defect in a submucosal artery lining the stomach. It can burst and cause massive hemorrhage. Also referred to as a *cirsoid aneurysm, caliber-persistent artery, submucosal arterial malformation,* or *vascular malformation.*

"diff"—medical slang for WBC differential. See *differential.*

differential interference contrast microscopy (DIC).

differential in white blood cell count:
eosinophils—range 5-6%
basophils—range 0-1%
lymphocytes—range 20-40%
monocytes—range 0-7%
polymorphonuclear neutrophils
　(PMNs or polys)—range 50-70%
　of total white blood cells

Differin (adapalene) **gel**—0.1% topical prescription anti-acne medication.

DiffGAM—bovine anti-*Clostridium difficile* immunoglobulin. It is used for treatment of *C. difficile*-associated diarrhea.

Diffistat-G—uses a polyclonal antibody in a test for *C. difficile* diarrhea.

Diff-Quik stain—see *"diff."*

diffraction-enhanced imaging (DEI)—imaging method using a single-energy x-ray source to detect breast tumors. The method produces sharply defined pictures by reducing scattering and helping visualize low-contrast areas not visible with traditional mammography.

diffusion-weighted imaging—ultrafast MRI technique that shows exactly which brain tissue is dead following a stroke and helps to determine whether the patient has had a transient ischemic attack (TIA). Victims of TIA usually recover fully but run a high risk of major strokes at a later time. It is also useful in diagnosing Alzheimer's disease. See *perfusion-weighted imaging.*

Diflucan (fluconazole)—for oral treatment of vaginal candidiasis.

diflunisal (Dolobid)—a nonsteroidal anti-inflammatory drug.

difluorodeoxycytidine (gemcitabine).

difluoromethylornithine (DFMO)—a drug used to treat AIDS.

"dig" ("dij")—slang for *digoxin, digitoxin,* and *digitalis.* If you cannot ask the dictator and the chart does not show which drug is intended, you may transcribe *digitalis* or type the brief form dictated.

DiGeorge's anomaly (DGA). Also, *DiGeorge's syndrome.*

DiGeorge's syndrome—thymic hypoplasia. Congenital aplasia of the thymus and parathyroid glands; pure T-cell deficiency, but with B-cell function intact. Cf. *Nezelof syndrome.*

digestive-respiratory fistula (DRF)—a coated Wallstent used for palliative treatment.

Digibar 190 (barium sulfate for suspension)—contrast agent specifically for use in digital fluoroscopic studies of the gastrointestinal tract.

Digibind (digoxin immune Fab [ovine] fragments)—for treatment of life-threatening digoxin intoxication.

Digidote (digoxin immune Fab)—see *Digibind*.

Digikit—finger and toe pneumatic tourniquet that prevents nerve trauma that could occur with the use of a Penrose drain as a tourniquet.

DigiMatch—"pinless" technology for performing Robodoc robotic surgeries without using any fiducial reference system.

Digirad 2020 TC Imager—solid-state gamma camera for use in nuclear medicine.

DigiScope—automated camera used to identify diabetics with diabetic retinopathy before they sustain permanent damage and lose vision.

DigiSound—two-channel digital signal processing hearing instrument.

digital Add-On Bucky—x-ray image acquisition system that produces filmless, digitized images.

Digital Fundus Imager—digital camera and recording system for color and/or fluorescein angiography by ophthalmologists and optometrists.

digital holography system—uses data collected by computed tomography and magnetic resonance scanners to produce a three-dimensional image called a Voxgram. These images help clinicians diagnose craniofacial problems, create the surgical treatment plan and templates, and intraoperatively measure and reconstruct deformities.

digital ICG (iodocyanine green) fluorescein dye) **videoangiography**—provides enhanced imaging of subretinal diseases.

digital movement analysis (DMA)—a new instrumental approach to assessing oral tardive dyskinesia by means of digital image processing of a video signal, which tracks five paper dots placed around the patient's mouth and detects perioral tremor as a sign of parkinsonism.

Digital OsteoView 2000—amorphous silicon flat panel x-ray detection system, capable of detecting both osteoporosis and arthritis.

digital parabola (Radiol)—term related to toe lengths in x-ray reports.

digital radiography—low-dose, reduced-dose digital technique for follow-up radiographs in pediatric orthopedic patients.

digital signal processing (DSP)—technology for hearing aids.

digital storage—a term used in cineangiography. "High resolution images from magnetic tape were transmitted to digital storage to serve as guiding or map views for subsequent angioplasty."

digital subtraction angiography (DSA) —an interventional radiological procedure which allows visualization of the small vessels. Iodinated contrast material is injected via venous catheter, and a computer subtracts out all the tissues until only the vessels visualized by contrast material are left; any vessels blocked by occlusion or stenosis are then readily apparent.

digital subtraction macrodacryocystography (Oph).

digital-to-analog converter—MRI term.

DIGIT-grip—a computer-based device used by physical therapists to rehabilitate patients with hand injuries. It displays a digital readout of either total grip strength or the strength of the middle/index fingers or ring/little fingers.

Digitrapper MKIII—device for ambulatory assessment of lower esophageal sphincter (LES) pressures and esophageal motility disorders.

Digitron—a digital subtraction imaging system.

digoxin immune Fab (Digibind, Digidote).

digoxin-specific Fab antibody fragments.

dihematoporphyrin ether (DHE).

dihydroergotamine (DHE-45).

Dilacor XR (diltiazem hydrochloride extended-release capsules)—used to treat hypertension and angina.

Dilamezinsert (DMI)—urologic instrument consisting of a dilator and inserter to aid in penile prosthesis implantation.

Dilapan—synthetic laminaria for cervical dilatation. See *Laminaria.*

DILE (drug-induced lupus erythematosus).

dilevalol—a beta blocker drug used to treat mild to moderate hypertension.

Diltia XT (diltiazem hydrochloride extended-release capsules)—used to treat hypertension and angina.

dilutional hematocrit—when too much water or crystalloid dilutes the blood, lowering the hematocrit. *Not* delusional.

DIMAQ integrated ultrasound workstation.

DIMOAD syndrome—diabetes insipidus, diabetes mellitus, optic atrophy, and deafness.

Dinamap blood pressure monitor and Oxytrak pulse oximeter—to measure oxygen saturation.

dinoprostone (Prepidil)—prostaglandin E_2 in a gel form that is applied topically to "ripen" the cervix in women who are at or near term and have medical indications for induction but also have an unfavorable cervix (Bishop's score of less than or equal to 4). Use of Prepidil results in increased Bishop's scores, with many patients progressing to labor within 24 hours of treatment. Prepidil is given prior to oxytocin to increase the chance of successful induction of labor.

diode laser.

DioPexy probe—for treatment of retinal detachment, an alternative treatment to cryopexy. The procedure employs transscleral retinal photocoagulation.

Diovan (valsartan)—angiotensin II AT receptor blocker for hypertension control, with once-daily dosing.

Dipentum (olsalazine)—anti-inflammatory for ulcerative colitis.

dipslide—see *Uricult dipslide.*

dipstick technique—topical application of liquid nitrogen to skin warts. Although it can cause intense pain, the cure rate is said to be 93 to 97%.

dipyridamole (Persantine)—coronary vasodilator.

dipyridamole echocardiography test—may demonstrate exercise-induced myocardial ischemia, which might be "EKG-silent," by providing evidence of the ischemic event. Also an agent to reduce blood viscosity.

dipyridamole thallium stress test—a chemical equivalent of the treadmill stress test, used when patients cannot take the standard treadmill test.

dipyridamole *(cont.)*

Dipyridamole (Persantine), given orally or intravenously, dilates the coronary arteries and increases the blood flow to the heart, reproducing the effects of exercise. A radioisotope, thallium, is then injected into a vein. A scanning device will record the passage of the thallium and demonstrate the areas that receive adequate amounts of blood and which are occluded. See *thallium stress test.*

Dirame (propiram)—an orally administered opioid analgesic for the treatment of moderate to severe pain.

DirectFlow arterial cannula—introduced through a thoracic trocar or incision and used to deliver oxygenated blood during cardiopulmonary bypass surgery. Also used to introduce and remove the Heartport EndoClamp aortic catheter.

direct fluorescent antibody test (DFA).

Directigen latex agglutination test—identifies pathogens by detecting specific antigens in cerebrospinal fluid and urine.

directional coronary angioplasty (DCA)—method of treating stenosis of a saphenous vein free-graft coronary artery bypass graft. Alternative treatment to percutaneous transluminal coronary balloon angioplasty.

directional coronary atherectomy (DCA)—cardiac catheterization procedure in which a catheter with a small mechanically driven cutter is inserted into the plaque-containing artery. A rotating blade shaves off the plaque, which is pushed into a storage chamber in the catheter and removed with the catheter. Also, *rotational coronary atherectomy.*

direct light reflex—light reflex in which the response occurs in the eye that was stimulated. See *consensual light reflex.*

direct myocardial revascularization (DMR).

DirectRay—uses direct-to-digital technology to capture and convert x-ray energy into digital images using a full-field (14" x 17") digital image-detector array.

direct vision internal urethrotomy (DVIU).

dis-, see *dys-.*

disc—alternate spelling of *disk.* See *disk.*

discission—the incision, or cutting into, as of a capsule of a cataract, or of the cervix uteri. Cf. *decision.*

disconjugate gaze—when the eyes do not work in unison. Alternate spelling, *dysconjugate.* Apparently either spelling is acceptable.

discordant cellular xenograft—transplantation of tissue from a distantly related species, such as the pig.

discordant organ xenograft—transplantation of a solid organ from a distantly related species, such as the pig.

discreet—circumspect, prudent, using or showing good judgment in conduct and in speech, as "I hope you will be most discreet in using this information." Cf. *discrete.*

discrete—separate, composed of distinct parts or discontinuous elements, as "There were large, discrete nodules noted in the neck." (A mnemonic device to help remember this spelling: *discrete* means separate; note that the *t* separates the two *e*'s.) Cf. *discreet.*

disease, disorder, or **condition**
(see also *lesion*)
ACAD (atherosclerotic carotid
artery disease)
acanthosis
ACD (allergic contact dermatitis)
achondroplastic dwarfism
acrodysostosis
acromesomelic dysplasia
acute inflammatory demyelinating
polyradicular (AIDP) neuropathy
acute promyelocytic leukemia
(APML)
acute repetitive seizure (ARS)
disorder
acute zonal occult outer retinopathy
(AZOOR)
adenocarcinoma in situ (AIS)
of the cervix
adenomatous hyperplasia (AH)
adiposis dolorosa
adolescent idiopathic scoliosis (AIS)
adRP (autosomal-dominant retinitis
pigmentosa)
adult chronic immune thrombocytopenic purpura (ITP)
age-associated memory impairment
(AAMI)
age-related macular degeneration
(AMD)
aggressive angiomyxoma
AILD (angioimmunoblastic
lymphadenopathy with
dysproteinemia).
AIOD (aortoiliac obstructive
disease)
AIP (acute intermittent porphyria)
air-space disease
aldosterone-producing adenoma
(APA)
allergic bronchopulmonary
aspergillosis (ABPA)
Alström's disease
alveolar soft-part sarcoma (ASPS)
AML (acute myeloblastic leukemia)

disease *(cont.)*
AML (angiomyolipoma)
AMMOL (acute myelomonoblastic
leukemia)
AMOL (acute monoblastic
leukemia)
AMPPE (acute multifocal placoid
pigment epitheliopathy)
anterolisthesis
Antopol-Goldman lesion
AOIVM (angiographically occult
intracranial vascular
malformation)
aortoiliac obstructive (or occlusive)
disease (AIOD)
aphtha
apical impulse
apocrine metaplasia
appendicular ataxia
APSGN (acute poststreptococcal
glomerulonephritis)
argentaffin carcinoma
ARS (acute repetitive seizure)
disorder
Arthus reaction
ash leaf spots in the eye
astasia–abasia
asthenopia
asymmetric septal hypertrophy
(ASH)
auricular perichondritis
babesiosis
bacillary angiomatosis (BA)
bacterial endophthalmitis
basidiobolomycosis
Bassen-Kornzweig abetalipoproteinemia
Batten disease
beaver fever
Bellini's duct carcinoma
benign intracranial hypertension
(BIH)
benign necrotizing otitis externa
(BNOE)

disease *(cont.)*
  benign paroxysmal positional
    vertigo
  benign prostatic hypertrophy or
    hyperplasia (BPH)
  Berger's disease
  bipolar affective illness
  birdshot chorioretinopathy
  black patch delirium
  body dysmorphic disorder (BDD)
  bone surface lesion
  Bornholm disease ("devil's grip")
  bovine spongiform encephalopathy
    (BSE)
  brittle bone disease (osteogenesis
    imperfecta)
  broad beta
  bronchiolitis obliterans with
    organizing pneumonia (BOOP)
  bronze (Addison's) disease
  bubble boy disease
  Buerger's disease
  bull's eye lesion
  buried penis
  Burkitt's lymphoma
  C. difficile-associated diarrhea
    (CDAD)
  caisson disease
  calcium pyrophosphate deposition
    (CPPD)
  cameral fistula
  Campbell de Morgan spots
  carcinoma ex pleomorphic adenoma
  carcinoma in situ (CIS)
  cardiac allograft vascular disease
    (CAVD)
  Caroli disease
  Carrión's disease
  Castleman's disease
  CATCH 22 (microdeletion of
    chromosome 22q11)
  cat-scratch (CSD)
  central splanchnic venous
    thrombosis (CSVT)

disease *(cont.)*
  Chester-Erdheim disease
  chronic bacterial prostatitis (CBP)
  chronic subdural hematoma (CSDH)
  circinate-pattern interstitial
    keratopathy
  cobalamin C methylmalonic
    acidemia
  combined hernia
  common acute lymphoblastic
    leukemia antigen (CALLA)
  compound volvulus
  congenital esophageal stenosis
  cradle cap
  craniosynostosis (craniostosis)
  Curling's ulcer
  cutaneous T-cell lymphoma
  cyclops lesion
  cystic adenomatoid malformation
    (CAM)
  cytomegalovirus retinitis
  de Quervain's disease
  Dercum's disease
  desmoplastic small round-cell tumor
    (DSRCT)
  detergent worker's lung
  Devic's disease
  "devil's grip"
  devil's pinches
  Dieulafoy's gastric lesion
  "dry" age-related macular
    degeneration (ARMD)
  dumbbell tumor
  duodenal ulcer perforation (DUP)
  dysfibrinogenemia
  dyskaryosis
  dyskeratosis
  dysphagia lusoria
  dysthymia
  Eales disease
  ENL (erythema nodosum leprosum)
  eosinophilic pustular folliculitis
  ependymitis granularis
  epidermodysplasia verruciformis

disease *(cont.)*

epidermolysis bullosa acquisita
equilibratory ataxia
Erb's palsy
Erdheim-Chester disease
erythema migrans (EM)
erythematous vulvitis en plaque
erythroplasia of Queyrat
esophageal achalasia
Ewing's sarcoma
extrahepatic cholangiocarcinoma
Fabry's lipid storage disease
facioscapulohumeral dystrophy
(FSHD)
farmer's lung disease
female sexual arousal disorder
(FSAD)
fibrodysplasia ossificans progressiva
(FOP)
fingerprint dystrophy
fish meal lung disease
fish tank granuloma
foamy esophagus
Fournier's gangrene
Freiberg's disease
furrier's lung disease
gas-forming liver abscess
GAVE (gastric antral vascular
ectasia)
germ cell tumor (GCT)
gestational trophoblastic
disease (GTD)
giant anorectal condyloma
acuminatum
giant cell arteritis (GCA)
glioblastoma multiforme
glomus tumor
graft versus host disease
granulomatous mastitis
Grover's skin
GTD (gestational trophoblastic
disease)
Gudden's atrophy
Haglund's deformity

disease *(cont.)*

hairy-cell leukemia
hemangiopericytoma
hepatic venous web disease
hepatitis A (infectious hepatitis)
hepatitis B (serum hepatitis)
hepatitis C (chronic hepatitis)
hepatitis D
hepatitis E
hepatitis F
herpes whitlow infection
herpesencephalitis
herpesvirus
HGD (high grade dysplasia)
HIB (*Haemophilus influenzae*
type B) disease
Hill-Sachs lesion or deformity
HIV-associated thrombocytopenia
Hollenhorst plaques
Holt-Oram atriodigital dysplasia
hordeolum
human granulocytic ehrlichiosis
(HGE)
Hunner's interstitial cystitis
Hunner's ulcer
ICE (immunoglobulin-complexed
enzyme) disorders
idiopathic CD4+ lymphocytopenia
(ICL)
idiosyncratic asthma
ileosigmoid knot
inflammatory bowel disease (IBD)
interstitial cystitis (IC)
intracranial aneurysm (ICA)
intraepidermal blistering disease
(pemphigus)
intramural duodenal hematoma after
blunt abdominal trauma
intraosseous pneumatocyst, cervical
spine
iron storage disease
ischemic penile gangrene
Janeway lesions
kaposiform hemangioendothelioma

disease *(cont.)*

Kawasaki disease
Kienböck's lunatomalacia disease
Kimmelstiel-Wilson disease
König disease
kraurosis vulvae
Krukenberg's tumor
Kugelberg-Welander disease
Kussmaul's respiration
Lafora body disease
Lassa fever
late luteal phase dysphoric disorder
(LLPDD)
lateral hypopharyngeal pouches
(LHPs)
leather-bottle stomach gastric
carcinoma
Leber's disease
legionnaires' disease
Letterer-Siwe disease
Lewis upper limb cardiovascular
disease
Lhermitte-Duclos disease
lichen planus
lipid storage disease
Listeria meningitis
Little League elbow
littoral cell angioma
longitudinal melanonychia
low-grade dysplasia (LGD)
low-grade squamous intraepithelial
lesion (LSIL)
lupus pernio
Lyme disease
Lyme lymphocytic meningo-
radiculitis
lymphocytic interstitial pneumonitis
(LIP)
lymphogranuloma venereum (LGV)
lymphomatoid papulosis (LyP)
Lynch and Crues Type 2 lesion
lytic (or osteolytic) lesion
MAC (*Mycobacterium avium*
complex) infection
macro-orchidism lesion

disease *(cont.)*

macular degeneration
mad cow disease (bovine spongiform
encephalopathy) (BSE)
Madura foot
MAI (*Mycobacterium avium-*
intracellulare) infection
malacoplakia of kidney
Malassezia furfur pustulosis
MALToma
maple bark stripper's disease
maple-syrup urine disease (MSUD)
Marburg hemorrhagic fever
Marchiafava-Bignami disease
Martorell hypertensive ulcer
Masson's tumor
MC (multifocal choroiditis)
meat wrapper's asthma
Mediterranean lymphoma
Meige's disease or syndrome
melorheostosis
membranous croup
MEN (multiple endocrine neoplasia)
meningococcal supraglottitis
meralgia paresthetica
Merkel cell carcinoma (MCC)
metaphyseal lesion of the distal
femur
methylmalonic acidemia
microchimerism
"micro-dots"
Miescher's cheilitis granulomatosa
milk leg disease
Milroy's disease
moccasin-type tinea pedis
Mondini's dysplasia
Mondor's disease
mucormycosis
multifocal chorioretinitis
multigenic carcinogenesis
multiple endocrine neoplasia
(MEN), type 2b
mushroom worker's disease
(or lung)
Mycobacterium abscessus

disease *(cont.)*

mycosis fungoides palmaris et plantaris
myocardial remodeling
myositis ossificans (MO)
NANB (non-A/non-B) hepatitis
nasal T-cell/natural killer cell lymphoma
necrotizing enterocolitis (NEC)
necrotizing fasciitis
neonatal acne
neural tube defects (NTD)
neuro-Behçet's disease
neuroimmune dysfunction
new variant Creutzfeldt-Jakob disease (nvCJD)
NHL (non-Hodgkin's lymphoma) tumors
Niemann-Pick disease
nil disease (lipoid nephrosis)
non-nasal CD56+T/NK (natural killer) cell lymphoma
non-small cell lung carcinoma (or cancer) (NSCLC)
nonseminomatous germ cell tumor
nonspecific esophageal motility disorder (NEMD)
nonspecific urethritis (NSU)
nosocomial disease
NTG (normal-tension glaucoma)
obliterative bronchiolitis
obsessive-compulsive disorder (OCD)
ocular rosacea
onychopachydermoperiostitis
ophthalmic pneumocystosis, AIDS-associated
optic neuritis
Ormond's disease
osteomesopyknosis
painter's encephalopathy
pantaloon hernia
paroxysmal nocturnal hemoglobinuria (PNH)

disease *(cont.)*

Patella's disease
peliosis hepatis
Pelizaeus-Merzbacher disease
penile gangrene and penile necrosis
peptic ulcer (PUD)
periarticular heterotopic ossification (PHO)
periorbital infantile myofibromatosis
pes anserine bursitis
PID (primary immune deficiency)
pilomatrix carcinoma
"pizza" lung
plus disease
Pneumocystis carinii pneumonia (PCP)
pneumocystis choroidopathy
pneumoparotitis
pollybeak nasal deformity
polymorphous light eruption
Pompe's glycogen storage disease, type II
portal hypertensive gastropathy (PHG)
post-transplantation lymphoproliferative disorders (PTLD)
post-transplant diabetes mellitus (PTDM)
Pott's puffy tumor
preinvasive urothelial neoplasia
primary biliary cirrhosis (PBC)
primary immune deficiency (PID)
primary pure teratoma
primary sclerosing cholangitis (PSC)
primary trimethylaminuria (fish-odor syndrome)
progressive multifocal leukoencephalopathy (PML)
progressive osseous heteroplasia
progressive parenchymal restriction
pseudodermachalasis
pseudo-Hurler deformity
pseudomembranous colitis (PMC)

disease *(cont.)*

psoriatic onychopachydermo-
    periostitis
pulmonary sequestration
pyogenic granuloma
Q fever
Quervain's disease
raccoon eyes
rachitic rosary
radiation-related optic neuropathy
    (RON)
reactive airways disease (RAD)
reactive perforating collagenosis
    (RPC)
rectal linitis plastica (RLP)
Rector-Gordon-Healey-Mendoza-
    Spitzer type IV renal tubular
    acidosis
recurrent respiratory papillomatosis
    (RRP)
Reese's retinal telangiectasia
reflex sympathetic dystrophy (RSD)
Regnauld-type degeneration
Reis-Bückler's corneal dystrophy
renal cell carcinoma (RCC)
repetitive strain injury (RSI)
retrobulbar neuritis
reversible obstructive airway disease
    (ROAD)
rhabdomyolysis
rhagades
rhinocerebral aspergillosis (RA)
Richter's hernia
Riedel's struma
rippling muscle disease
Roger's disease
Rosai Dorfman disease
Roth-Bernhardt disease
sabre shin deformity
"sagging brain"
salmon-patch hemorrhages
"salon sink" radiculopathy
satellite lesion
scaphocephaly (sagittal synostosis)

disease *(cont.)*

Scheuermann's disease
schizencephaly
schneiderian papilloma, inverted
Schönlein-Henoch purpura
scleroderma
sclerosing encapsulating peritonitis
sebaceous miliaria
severe childhood autosomal
    recessive muscular dystrophy
    (SCARMD)
sexually transmitted disease (STD)
short-limb dwarfism
short-segment Barrett's esophagus
    (SSBE)
silent prostatism
Sinding Larsen–Johannson disease
single-stripe colitis (SSC)
sink-trap malformation
"skier's" tear
skip metastasis
Sly disease
small cell lung carcinoma
    (or cancer) (SCLC)
solar keratosis
spondylodiskitis
squamous cell carcinoma (SCC)
Staphylococcus aureus septicemia
Stargardt's dystrophy
Still's disease
streptococcus A infection
string phlebitis
subcortical atherosclerotic
    encephalopathy (SAE)
subcortical dementia
subepithelial hematoma of the renal
    pelvis
suberosis
systemic lupus erythematosus
talcosis
Takayasu's arteritis
"terrible triad" of the shoulder
Terrien's degeneration
thoracic splenosis

disease *(cont.)*
thromboembolic disease (TED)
Tis disease
Tornwaldt's bursitis
transient aplastic crisis (TAC)
transitional cell carcinoma of the
bladder (TCCB)
trichinosis
trichosis
tularemia
tumoral calcinosis
typhlitis
Van Bogaert's disease
veno-occlusive disease (VOD)
vestibular adenitis
vestibulodynia
VHL (von Hippel-Lindau) disease
Vincent's infection
vipoma endocrine tumor
Voerner's disease
Vogt-Koyanagi-Harada disease
von Hippel-Lindau (VHL) disease
von Recklinghausen's disease
wandering spleen
Warthin's tumor
watermelon stomach
Wegener's granulomatosis
Werdnig-Hoffmann disease
Wernicke's disease
"wet" age-related macular
degeneration (ARMD)
Wharton's tumor
wheat weevil disease
Whipple's disease
wood pulp worker's lung disease
Woringer-Kolopp disease
xanthelasma
xanthogranulomatous cholecystitis
X-linked familial spastic paraparesis
X-linked SCID
Disetronic Insulin Pen—does not use a
prefilled cartridge but allows a diabetic patient to fill the insulin reservoir with economical vial insulin.

DISH (diffuse idiopathic skeletal hyperostosis).
disk, disc (Gr., diskos, L., discus)—a
circular or rounded flat plate. Note:
Disk appears to be the preferred
spelling, although *disc* is also used,
especially in names of anatomic
structures.
Disk-Criminator—used to check localization of stimuli.
disk diameter (dd or DD)—1.5 mm
(the diameter of the optic nerve
head); used in measuring the size of
a fundal lesion or in describing its
location. Also, *disc diameter.*
diskectomy
APLD (automated percutaneous
lumbar)
SMALL (same-day microsurgical
arthroscopic lateral-approach
laser-assisted) fluoroscopic
diskectomy with Cloward fusion.
disorder—see *disease.*
disposable aortic rotating punch—
used in cardiovascular bypass surgery. It has a patented rotating blade
and is said to have unique cutting
action.
disproportion—see *cephalopelvic.*
dissecans—see *osteochondritis.*
dissection
blunt
Cavitron
Creed
Desmarres corneal
Dingman breast
dissector
Falcao suction
finger
Kitner
Küttner blunt
Neivert
Nezhat-Dorsey Trumpet Valve
hydrodissector

dissection *(cont.)*
Pearce nucleus hydrodissector
Rhoton
sharp and blunt
spontaneous coronary artery (SCAD)
spud
Trumpet Valve

disseminated intravascular coagulation
(DIC)—results from imbalance between the mechanisms of coagulation and of fibrinolysis. Can be induced by infection (meningococcal meningitis, Rocky Mountain spotted fever, septicemia), trauma, shock, complications of pregnancy and parturition, and myelocytic leukemia. Clinical manifestations range from widespread bleeding to widespread intravascular thrombosis, and both of these may occur together.

disseminated lupus erythematosus *(not* erythematosis)—see *systemic lupus erythematosus.*

dissociated vertical divergence (DVD).

Distaflo bypass graft—used an alternative to vein cuffs and patches when adequate autologous saphenous vein is not available.

distal articular set angle (DASA).

distention—the state of being expanded, stretched. Also, *distension.*

distortion product otoacoustic emission (DPOAE)—used in studies of comparative hearing.

Ditropan XL (oxybutynin chloride)—extended-release tablets for once-a-day treatment of overactive bladder characterized by urge urinary incontinence, urgency, and frequency.

Diva laparoscopic morcellator—used in SMART (surgical myomectomy as reproductive therapy) procedures to remove uterine fibroids.

Dix-Hallpike position (ENT)—for Epley's canalith repositioning.

Dix-Hallpike test—for paroxysmal positional nystagmus.

DJD (degenerative joint disease).

DJJ (duodenojejunal junction).

DLCO (diffusing capacity of the lung for CO) (carbon monoxide).

DLT (double lung transplant) **recipient**.

DMA (digital movement analysis).

DMARDs (disease-modifying antirheumatic drugs)—thought to slow down the basic destructive rheumatoid arthritis process, e.g., oral or injectable gold, methotrexate, azathioprine (Imuran), cyclophosphamide (Cytoxan), hydroxychloroquine (Plaquenil).

DMAST (Dyna Med Anti-Shock Trousers)—an antishock garment that is noninflatable, has no tubes or valves, and has no risk of puncture. Used by NASA, the military, and paramedics. See also *MAST.*

DMI (Dilamezinsert).

DMR (direct myocardial revascularization)—a minimally invasive cardiac catheterization procedure using laser technology to revascularize ischemic heart muscle.

DMVA (direct mechanical ventricular actuation)—ventricular assist device that can begin biventricular support in as little as three minutes, because insertion is technically easy. There is no need for systemic anticoagulation as it has no cannulas in any blood vessels. It is said to decrease the need for drug support for a failing heart, provide prolonged circulatory support without cardiac trauma, and increase cardiac output. Currently DMVA is used as a temporary measure to sustain patients whose hearts fail while they wait for a suitable donor heart for heart transplantation.

DNA ploidy analysis—a test on biopsy tissue of the prostate that correlates

DNA ploidy *(cont.)*
well with the Gleason score for severity of cancer. The test may help physicians and patients make more informed decisions about whether radical prostatectomy should be performed.

DNA polymerase-alpha—tumor marker. When found in frozen tissue sections of patients who have had an exploratory thoracotomy for early non-small cell lung carcinoma, the presence of this marker can be used to indicate those patients who will most likely suffer an early relapse of the disease and a poorer prognosis.

DNA sequencing—method of genetic testing that identifies mutations not found by other methods.

DNJ (N-butyl-deoxynojirimycin)—drug for treating AIDS and ARC patients.

DNS (dysplastic nevus syndrome)—can lead to malignant melanoma.

Dobbhoff gastrectomy feeding tube.

DOBI (Dynamic Optical Breast Imaging System)—uses dynamic functional imaging to detect angiogenesis associated with growth of malignant lesions and is designed to offer a noninvasive and pain-free method to distinguish between malignant and benign breast lesions.

dobutamine stress echocardiography (DSE).

docetaxel (Taxotere)—for cancer treatment.

Docke's murmur—diastolic murmur associated with stenosis of left anterior descending artery of the coronary distribution.

Döderlein's bacillus—a strain of lactobacillus normally seen in the vagina. It is considered a benign bacterium and maintains the normal acid pH of the vagina. Also, Doederlein.

Döderlein laparoscopic hysterectomy—vaginal hysterectomy combined with laparoscopic technique to dissect uterus and adnexa and develop bladder flap. Can be used for patients with adhesions or previous cesarean sections, who might not otherwise be candidates for vaginal hysterectomy. Also, Doederlein.

dog boning—a surgical complication caused when an angioplasty balloon becomes excessively expanded at either end of a stent (similar in appearance to a dog bone).

Dohlman plug—used to treat perforated corneal ulcers.

dolichocephalic—long head.

DoLi S—extracorporeal shock wave lithotriptor by Dornier.

doll's eye sign—dissociation between movements of the eyes and those of the head. A positive sign indicates damage to cranial nerves III, IV, and VI.

domino connectors—descriptive term for connectors on a spinal instrumentation device used to correct scoliosis.

domperidone (Motilium)—enhances gastric emptying and improves gastric-duodenal coordination. Blocks the side effects of nausea, vomiting, weight loss, and anorexia of dopamine therapy in Parkinson's patients without reducing dopamine's central antiparkinsonian effect.

DonJoy Goldpoint knee brace—for resisting tibial translation in a patient with deficient anterior or posterior ligaments.

DonJoy knee splint—"A dry sterile dressing was then applied, followed by a DonJoy splint holding the knee out in extension."

donor island harvesting—a method of obtaining micro- and minigrafts from a hairbearing strip.

donor-specific transfusion (DST).

DOOR syndrome—inherited disorder characterized by hearing impairment, malformations of the nails and certain bones, mental retardation, and other abnormalities. DOOR is an acronym for the characteristic abnormalities associated with the disorder: deafness, onychodystrophy, osteodystrophy, and mild to severe mental retardation.

Dopascan—a radiopharmaceutical used in imaging to diagnose Parkinson's disease.

dopexamine—an inotropic agent found to improve splanchnic oxygen delivery to the gut, liver, and skeletal muscle in septic shock.

Doppler echocardiography—useful for assessment of left ventricular diastolic function in ischemic heart disease.

Doppler instruments
blood flow detector
fetal heart monitor
IntraDop intraoperative
intraoperative
ultrasonic blood flow detector
ultrasonic fetal heart monitor

Doppler Perfusion Index (DPI)—the ratio of hepatic arterial-to-total liver blood flow. May be a prognostic indicator of early death in colorectal cancer patients who have undergone supposedly curative surgery.

Doppler sonography of the SMA (superior mesenteric artery)—noninvasive method to detect inflammatory disease of the small bowel.

Doppler tissue imaging (DTI) (Cardio)—used for transesophageal echo-cardiography (TEE) imaging on the V5M Multiplane and V510B Biplane TEE transducers. TEE imaging with DTI shows tissue motion with high resolution, which may enable cardiologists to differentiate normal versus ischemic or infarcted tissue; visualization and timing of contractile impulse; qualitative measurement of myocardial wall velocity; quantification in M-mode for high temporal resolution and reduced subjectivity of wall motion analysis.

Doppler waveform analysis (Radiol)—noninvasive study of blood vessels. See *duplex ultrasound* and *ultrasound*.

Dopplette—a small Doppler monitor.

Doptone monitoring—of fetal heart tones.

Doral (quazepam)—sedative.

Dorc surgical instruments.

Dorello's canal—an opening in the temporal bone which is the point of entry of the sixth cranial nerve into the cavernous sinus.

Dorendorf's sign—of aortic arch aneurysm, evidenced by fullness of supraclavicular groove.

Dormia noose—a surgical device used for grasping, e.g., "The ligamentum teres hepatis was grasped with a Dormia noose and pulled up through the gastric tube to close the perforated ulcer." The Dormia noose can be left in place, secured with Kocher forceps for several days until closure is certain.

dornase alfa (Pulmozyme)—a mucolytic for cystic fibrosis patients. It breaks up the thick secretions that clog the lungs and favor respiratory tract infections. Improved breathing and lung function lead to lower mortality and better quality of life.

Dornier compact lithotriptor—a much smaller, less expensive, mobile, and user-friendly lithotriptor. Effective for treatment of kidney stones, with a low incidence of complications and adverse effects.

Dorros—infusion and probing catheter.

dorsal (adj.)—referring to the back or to any posterior part or surface, e.g., the dorsal surface of the hand is the back of the hand. See *dorsum.*

dorsal column stimulator (DCS) (also *spinal cord stimulation*)—a controversial and risk-prone procedure for pain relief. It is said by some to be a procedure of last resort. One of the pioneers in percutaneous and transcutaneous electrical nerve stimulation no longer uses it, but other surgeons and anesthesiologists do.

dorsal lithotomy position *(not* dorso-lithotomy).

dorsal penile nerve block (DPNB)—a technique to reduce behavioral stress and modify the adrenocortical stress response in neonates undergoing circumcision.

dorsum (noun)—back; posterior aspect. See *dorsal.*

Dos Santos needle—for aortography.

Dostinex (cabergoline) **tablets**—for treatment of hyperprolactinemic disorders, either idiopathic or due to pituitary adenomas (tumors). Utilizes only twice-weekly dosing.

dothiepin HCl (Prothiaden)—an antidepressant drug that appears to have significant analgesic activity. It is similar in composition and effectiveness to amitriptyline (Elavil) and doxepin (Sinequan).

Dotter-Judkins PTA (percutaneous transluminal angioplasty)—involves dilatation of the lumen of a stenotic femoral artery in patients who are not good risks for femoral-popliteal bypass surgery. A special catheter is directed to the site of the atheromatous lesion under fluoroscopy, and then progressively larger catheters are introduced over a guide wire. See *PTA.*

double anterior horn sign—knee meniscal displacement. Can be seen with either medial or lateral bucket-handle tears or in association with double posterior cruciate ligament or fragment-in-notch signs.

double-armed suture—a suture with a needle at each end. See *suture.*

double-blind study—a study in which neither the patient nor the physician knows if the drug administered is a test medication or a placebo.

double bubble flushing reservoir—in patients with hydrocephalus.

double bubble sign—seen in infants with choledochal cysts and obstructive jaundice. "Plain films show the double bubble sign, with a large air bubble that represents the stomach; the second bubble represents air dilating the duodenum that is proximal to the point of blockage." Also, ultrasound appearance of a fetus with fluid-filled stomach and duodenum which, along with polyhydramnios, indicates duodenal atresia.

double contrast arthrography—used for evaluation of ligamentous injuries of the knee, but thought to be not as accurate as single-contrast arthrography or the newer arthroscopic techniques. With the double contrast technique, more time is available for air to enter the joint, causing misleading findings.

double contrast barium enema (Radiol)—a modification of the barium enema procedure. After the standard barium enema examination has been completed, the patient expels most of the barium, and the colon is then inflated with air. The coating of barium remaining on the surface may outline masses or defects not seen during the standard examination.

double dose delay (DDD)—contrast studies.

doubled semitendinosus and gracilis autograft (DST&G).

double exposure artifact (Radiol)—a darkroom error.

double exposure drift—MRI term.

double helix acquisition—used in CT scanning.

Double J indwelling catheter stent—trademark, from Surgitek (Urol).

Double J ureteral stent (Urol).

double lung transplant (DLT) **recipient**.

double-orifice repair—a reliable and safe surgical correction of mitral regurgitation in Barlow disease.

double PCL (posterior cruciate ligament) **sign** (Ortho).

double plate Molteno implant (Oph).

DoubleStent biliary endoprosthesis.

double umbrella device—used in closure of a patent ductus arteriosus.

double whammy syndrome (Oph)—voluntary eye propulsion; the ability to voluntarily propel and retract one or both eyes.

Douek-MED Bioglass middle ear device (ENT)—enables surgeons to reconstruct the ossicular chain, using a biocompatible, nonporous material that forms a physiochemical bond with soft tissue and bone.

doula—an individual contracted to provide either labor or postpartum support for a pregnant woman. Doulas often work under the supervision of midwives but do not perform nursing jobs or deliveries.

Douvas roto-extractor (Oph).

Dovonex (calcipotriene).

dowager's hump—kyphosis due to osteoporosis of the spine.

Downey texture discrimination test.

downgoing toes—in a normal response to the Babinski test, the great toe curls downward when the sole of the foot is stroked; thus, a negative Babinski is a flexor plantar response: "The toes are downgoing." Cf. *upgoing*.

doxacurium chloride (Nuromax)—a long-acting neuromuscular blocker used in conjunction with a general anesthetic to provide skeletal muscle relaxation. Most useful in patients with heart disease undergoing surgery because, unlike Pavulon, it does not cause tachycardia.

doxazosin mesylate (Cardura)—an antihypertensive drug.

doxepin hydrochloride cream (Zonalon)—for dermatitis.

Doxil (doxorubicin HCl liposome injection)—an old drug now delivered in a new way. Enclosed in tiny fatty bubbles, the drug travels to a malignant ovarian tumor, where the bubble ruptures, and the drug then attacks the tumor cells. It selects out the tumor cells and blocks the normal toxic effect on normal tissue, with less nausea and side effects. See *liposome encapsulated doxorubicin (LED); liposomes, encapsulated.*

DOX-SL (sublingual) (liposomal doxorubicin)—used to treat AIDS-related Kaposi's sarcoma. See *Doxil*.

Doyle Shark nasal splint—maintains a patent nasal airway and prevents synechiae and postsurgical adhesions.

DPA (Designated Power of Attorney) for Health Care.

DPAP Stealth—a real-time interactive positive airway pressure device used for treatment of sleep apnea. It uses a flow-sensing and measurement device to monitor all air moving through the breathing circuit. It responds with a rapid increase in air pressure when a critical reduction is detected, as in sleep apnea. The device intermittently assists the breathing process and restores patency before oxyhemoglobin desaturation and/or arousal from sleep occurs.

DPI (Doppler Perfusion Index)

DPOAE (distortion product otoacoustic emission).

DPPC (dipalmitoyl phosphatidylcholine) **test**—an accurate predictor of respiratory distress syndrome and fetal lung maturity. DPPC is the major surface-active component of the mature fetal lung surfactant.

DPTS (delayed pulmonary toxicity syndrome).

Draeger high vacuum erysiphake (Oph).

Draeger tonometer—a handheld applanation tonometer; used to measure intraocular pressure.

drain
Blair silicone
Blake wound
butterfly
Chaffin-Pratt
Clot Stop
Davol
endoscopic retrograde biliary (ERBD)
J-Vac closed wound drainage

drain *(cont.)*
Molteno implant drainage
Nélaton rubber tube
Penrose
Quad-Lumen
Relia-Vac
Shirley wound
Solcotrans closed vacuum-drainage
Stryker
Thora-Drain III three-bottle chest drainage unit
Thora-Klex chest drainage system

Drake clip—used in clipping intracranial aneurysms.

Drake-Willock automatic delivery system—used in peritoneal dialysis with Tenckhoff catheter.

DRAM (de-epithelialized rectus abdominis muscle) **graft**—a free flap that can be used in reconstruction in patients with cranial-dural defects.

Draw-a-Bicycle test—a mental status examination. Also, *DAB test*.

Draw-a-Flower test—a mental status examination. Also, *DAF test*.

Draw-a-House test—a mental status examination. Also, *DAH test*.

Draw-a-Person test—a mental status examination. Also, *DAP test*.

drawer sign—in testing for ligamentous instability or for rupture of the cruciate ligaments of the knee.

drawn ankle clonus.

DRC (dynamic range control) **algorithm**—see *dynamic range control algorithm*.

DRD (dopa-responsive dystonia).

DRD2 (D2 dopamine receptor)—see *bromocriptine*.

DRE (digital rectal examination).

dressing—see also *adhesive, bandage*.
AcryDerm border island
AcryDerm Strands absorbent wound
Acticoat silver-based burn

dressing *(cont.)*
>   Acu-Derm I.V./TPN
>   AlgiDERM alginate wound
>   AlgiSite alginate wound
>   Algosteril alginate wound
>   Allevyn
>   Aquacel hydrofiber wound packing
>   Aquaphor gauze
>   Aquasorb transparent hydrogel
>   ArtAssist
>   Bioclusive transparent
>   Biopatch foam wound
>   BreakAway absorptive wound
>   BlisterFilm transparent
>   Carra Film adhesive film
>   CarraSmart foam
>   Carra Sorb H
>   Carra Sorb M
>   Carrasyn Hydrogel wound
>   CircPlus compression
>   ClearSite Hydro Gauze
>   ClearSite transparent wound
>   Coban
>   CollaCote
>   CollaPlug
>   CollaTape
>   CombiDerm absorbent cover
>   CombiDerm hydrocolloid
>   Comfeel Ulcus
>   composite
>   contact-layer wound
>   Covaderm
>   Coverlet adhesive surgical
>   Cryo/Cuff ankle
>   Curaderm
>   Curafil
>   Curafoam
>   Curagel Hydrogel
>   Curasol
>   Curasorb calcium alginate
>   Cutinova Cavity
>   Cutinova Hydro
>   Dermacea alginate wound
>   Derma-Gel hydrogel sheet

dressing *(cont.)*
>   Dermagran hydrogel
>   DermaMend hydrogel
>   DermaNet contact-layer wound
>   DermAssist glycerin hydrogel
>   DermAssist hydrocolloid
>   Dermatell hydrocolloid
>   DiabGel hydrogel
>   DuoDerm compression
>   Dyna-Flex compression
>   Elastikon elastic tape
>   Elasto-Gel hydrogel
>   Elastomull
>   Elta Dermal hydrogel
>   EpiFilm otologic lamina
>   Epi-lock polyurethane foam wound
>   ExuDerm hydrocolloid
>   Exu-Dry absorptive
>   Fibracol collagen-alginate
>   Fibracol collagen hemostatic wound
>   FlexDerm hydrogel sheet
>   Flexzan foam wound
>   foam
>   Fuller shield
>   FyBron alginate wound
>   Gelocast Unna boot compression
>   Gentell alginate wound
>   GraftCyte gauze wound
>   Handages
>   Humatrix Microclysmic Gel
>   hyCure collagen hemostatic wound
>   hyCare G hydrogel
>   Hydrasorb wound
>   Hydrocol hydrocolloid
>   hydrocolloid
>   hydrofiber
>   hydrogel
>   hydrophilic semipermeable
>   absorbent polyurethane foam
>   Hydrosorb foam wound
>   Hypergel
>   Iamin Gel wound
>   Iamin hydrogel
>   Inerpan

dressing *(cont.)*
  Intelligent Dressing
  IntraSite gel
  Iodoflex absorptive
  Iodosorb absorptive
  Kalginate alginate wound
  Kaltostat wound packing
  Kling adhesive
  Kling fluff rolls and sponges
  Liquiderm liquid healing bandage
  Lyofoam C
  Lyofoam tracheostomy
  Maxorb alginate wound
  Medifil collagen hemostatic wound
  Medipore Dress-it
  Mepitel contact-layer wound
  Mepore absorptive
  Mesalt
  Mitraflex foam wound
  Mitraflex multilayer wound
  MPM hydrogel
  Multidex wound filling material
  MultiPad absorptive
  Normigel hydrogel
  N-Terface contact-layer wound
  Nu-Derm hydrocolloid
  Nu Gauze
  Nu-Gel hydrogel
  Oasis wound dressing
  O'Donoghue
  Omiderm transparent adhesive film
  OpSite Flexigrid transparent
    adhesive film
  OsmoCyte pillow
  PanoGauze hydrogel-impregnated
    gauze
  PanoPlex hydrogel
  Polyderm foam wound
  PolyMem foam wound
  Polyskin II
  PolyWic wound filling
  Primapore absorptive wound
  Primer compression
  Pro-Clude transparent adhesive film

dressing *(cont.)*
  ProCyte transparent adhesive film
  Profore four-layer bandage system
  RepliCare hydrocolloid
  Repliderm
  Reston foam wound
  Restore alginate wound
  Saf-Gel hydrogel
  SignaDress hydrocolloid
  Silverlon wound packing strips
  SiteGuard MVP transparent
    adhesive film
  SkinTegrity hydrogel
  SofSorb absorptive
  SoftCloth absorptive
  SofWick
  SoloSite hydrogel
  SorbaView composite wound
  Sorbsan topical wound
  StrataSorb composite wound
  SurePress compression
  SureSite transparent adhesive film
  Synthaderm
  TAB (tumescent absorbent bandage)
  Tegaderm transparent
  Tegagel hydrogel
  Tegagen HG alginate wound
  Tegagen HI alginate wound
  Tegapore contact-layer wound
  Tegasorb
  Thera-Boot compression
  THINSite with BioFilm
  3M Clean Seals
  Tielle absorptive
  Transeal transparent adhesive film
  TransiGel hydrogel-impregnated
    gauze
  Transorbent
  transparent adhesive film
  TubeLok tracheotomy
  tumescent absorbent bandage (TAB)
  Ultec hydrocolloid
  Uniflex polyurethane adhesive
    surgical

dressing *(cont.)*
Unna-Flex compression
Unna-Pak compression
Vari/moist
Veingard
Velpeau
Ventex
Viasorb
Vigilon
wet-to-dry
Woun'Dres hydrogel
WoundSpan Bridge II
Xeroform
Zipzoc stocking compression
DREZ (dorsal root entry zone) **lesion** (Neuro).
DREZ-otomy—a surgical procedure to treat spasticity and pain in the lower limbs.
DRF (digestive-respiratory fistula).
drip infusion cholangiography (DIC) —not to be confused with diffuse intravascular coagulopathy.
Dripps-American Surgical Association score—a clinical scoring system to predict cardiac morbidity.
droloxifene—an antiestrogen used to test for breast cancer.
dronarinol (Marinol)—an antiemetic drug given with chemotherapy; also used to treat loss of appetite in AIDS patients. The active ingredient is derived from the marijuana plant.
drop attacks—episodes of dropping objects but remaining conscious; a form of petit mal epilepsy. Also may be experienced by narcoleptics who have sudden brief periods of unconsciousness.
Droxia (hydroxyurea)—a decades-old cancer drug that has recently been approved by the FDA as a treatment for adults suffering from sickle cell anemia. It is believed to reduce the frequency of sickle cell crises and the need for blood transfusions.
DRS (Dementia Rating Scale).
DR-70 tumor marker test—for detecting lung cancer tumors and quantifying levels of tumor marker in patients. The DR-70 is a noninvasive procedure compared to other cancer detection methods such as biopsies. It is a biochemical probe that has shown early indications of being one of the most sensitive tumor marker tests in current use. The test is based on the detection of submicroscopic ring-shaped particles (RSP) that appear to be shed in detectable quantities by malignant cells, both in the lab and in the human body.
drug-induced lupus erythematosus (DILE).
DRUJ (distal radioulnar joint) **prosthesis**—for painful radioulnar joint instability after failure of Kapandji-Sauve or Moore-Darrach procedure.
drusen—small hyaline globular pathological growths formed on Bruch's membrane.
"dry" age-related macular degeneration (Oph)—breakdown or thinning of retinal pigment epithelial cells, leading to atrophy of these light-sensitive, photoreceptor cells.
dry eye—keratoconjunctivitis sicca. See *Schirmer's test.*
dry heaves—gagging or retching without emesis.
DS (duplex sonography).
DSA (digital subtraction angiography).
DSE (dobutamine stress echocardiography).
DSM (degradable starch microspheres).
DSP (digital signal processing).
DSP Micro Diamond-Point microsurgery instruments.

DSRCT (desmoplastic small round-cell tumor).

DST (donor-specific transfusion)—used before kidney transplantation, to identify any possible incompatibility between donor and recipient and thus possibly prevent rejection of a transplant.

DST&G (doubled semitendinosus and gracilis) **autograft**—a technique for anterior cruciate ligament (ACL) reconstruction in which the ACL autograft consists of the semitendinosus and gracilis tendons. Both tendons are dissected, placed side by side, sutured together, and then folded, using a weaving Krackow-type stitch of Tycron. One end of the doubled tendons is attached to a screw in the femur, the other end to a screw in the tibia.

D-Tach removable needle—separates from the suture with a slight pull, but does resist inadvertent removal of the needle, which makes for faster interrupted suturing. See *pop-off needle*.

DTAFA (descending thoracic aorta-to-femoral artery) **bypass graft**—used for treatment of aortoiliac disease when opening the abdomen is contraindicated or ill advised.

DTaP vaccine—diphtheria, tetanus (toxoids), and accelerated pertussis (vaccine), given to children beginning at 2 months of age. Studies have shown that adults are often misdiagnosed as having bronchitis when they in fact have pertussis; there is no pertussis vaccine for adults, who often transmit the disease to the young and vulnerable before the infants are old enough for the vaccine.

DTC-101—an extended-release formulation of cytarabine.

DTI (Doppler tissue imaging).

DTIC-Dome (dacarbazine)—single drug used in the treatment of malignant melanoma.

DTICH (delayed traumatic intracerebral hematoma)—a frequent complication following closed head trauma. The patient is relatively asymptomatic after the head injury for several hours to several days, but then suddenly presents with a neurological deficit. A CT scan is diagnostic, revealing either the presence of a new intracranial hematoma or enlargement of an existing one. Proposed causes of DTICH include poor clotting as shown by the prolonged PT and PTT noted in head-injury patients or local cerebral ischemia which leads to necrosis and blood vessel rupture.

D-stix—slang for Dextrostix.

DTPA (diethylenetriamine-penta-acetic acid or acetate)—used in combination with gadolinium as a contrast medium in MRI scans.

DU (duplex ultrasound).

dual chamber Medtronic.Kappa 400 pacemaker (yes, a period between Medtronic and Kappa).

dual chamber pacemaker (Cardio).

dual energy x-ray absorptiometry (DEXA).

Dualer Plus—system for documenting range of motion and completing AMA impairment ratings for spine and extremities.

Dualine digital hearing instrument—uses digital signal processing (DSP) and a digital loudness control.

DualMesh—a biomaterial by Gore-Tex, used for repair of hernias and soft tissue deficiencies to permit a secure closure.

dual photon densitometry—test recommended for diagnosis of osteoporosis through comparative height measurements. Loss of height means the patient is losing trabecular bone and should undergo further testing for osteoporosis.

dual switch valve (DSV)—a valve for shunting hydrocephalus that avoids overdrainage-related problems such as subdural hygromas/hematomas or slit-like ventricles with the high risk of proximal catheter obstruction.

Duane's retraction syndrome—a congenital, usually unilateral, disorder of eye movement, affecting females more often than males. The affected eye usually has complete absence of abduction, and partial absence of adduction (sometimes the reverse). The involved eye retracts into the orbit on adduction, and demonstrates pseudoptosis. There is also paresis or failure of convergence. Also known as *Stilling-Türk-Duane syndrome.*

Dubecq-Princeteau angulating needle holder—a 5 mm needle holder indicated for use in laparoscopic procedures.

Dubin and Amelar—classification of varicocele.

Dubowitz scale for infant maturity—a 24-hour test to correlate the neurological function with fetal gestational age. "The infant was 38 weeks' gestational age by Dubowitz."

duck waddle—a test of the integrity of the knee joints and menisci, in which the patient is required to "walk" in a squatting position.

Ducor tip—a blend of two polyurethane materials, used as a catheter tip in coronary arteriography. It is said to be softer than the "standard" multipurpose catheter tip.

Ducrey's bacillus—see *Haemophilus ducreyi.*

ductal carcinoma in situ (DCIS).

duct ectasia—an inflammatory lesion that possibly accounts for 1% of all operative breast lesions. Also called *plasma cell mastitis.* See also *granulomatous mastitis.*

ductions—monocular rotations (with the other eye covered):
abduction—outward rotation
adduction—inward rotation
infraduction—downward movement
supraduction—upward movement

ductions and versions (Oph).

Duecollement maneuver—in hemicolectomy.

Duette—collective trade name for catheters, probes, and baskets used in endoscopic retrograde cholangiopancreatography. Each instrument has a double lumen (hence the name) to facilitate multiple procedures: insertion of guide wires and other instruments as well as injections of drugs.

Duet vascular sealing device—used to seal the arterial access site following catheterization procedures such as angiography, angioplasty, and stenting.

Duffy blood antibody type—factor in agglutination. See also *Kell, Kidd, Lewis, Lutheran.*

Duhamel pull-through procedure—for correction of Hirschsprung's disease. It involves excision of the aganglionic segment of the proximal colon and anastomosis between the normal remaining bowel and the posterior wall of the healthy segment of the rectum. Also, Duhamel laparoscopic

Duhamel *(cont.)*
pull-through anastomosis. Cf. *Lester Martin modification of Duhamel procedure.*

Duke bleeding time—the number of minutes it takes for a small incision in the skin (by puncture of the earlobe), made with a lancet, to stop bleeding.

Duke pouch—for continent urinary diversion. A resected segment of colon is used to form the pouch.

Dukes-Astler-Coller adenocarcinoma classification—uses letters and arabic numbers (A1, B1, etc.). See *Dukes' classification.*

Dukes' classification of carcinoma, named for Cuthbert E. Dukes, a British pathologist. Classes:
A invading mucosa and submucosa
B invading muscularis
C spread to regional lymph nodes; distant metastasis

Duke treadmill exercise score—of prognostic value in patients with suspected coronary artery disease.

Dulaney intraocular implant lens.

dullness—see *shifting dullness.*

Dumas-Duport glioma pathology grading scale.

dumbbell-shaped shadow (Radiol).

dumbbell tumor—a tumor that penetrates two nearby anatomic structures with a narrow bridge in between.

Dumon tracheobronchial stent.

dumping syndrome—symptoms of palpitations, sweating, and weakness, sometimes seen after gastrectomy, and caused by rapid emptying of gastric contents into the small intestine (hence "dumping").

Dunlop synoptophore test—for eye vergence.

duodenal bulb (Radiol)—onion-shaped dilatation of the duodenum immediately below its origin at the pylorus.

duodenal C-loop (Radiol)—C-shaped loop of the duodenum as it courses around the head of the pancreas.

duodenal seromyectomy—a partial denudation procedure to clear the duodenum of metastatic tumor. "Right hemicolectomy and seromyectomy of the duodenum at the site of adhesion was performed in this patient with Dukes' class C primary adenocarcinoma of the ascending colon adherent to the duodenum."

duodenal sweep (Radiol)—the normal course of the duodenum, from the pylorus and around the head of the pancreas to the ligament of Treitz, as visualized with contrast medium in an upper GI series.

duodenal switch—a procedure for pancreaticobiliary diversion that eliminates the need for the antrectomy and vagotomy that is done with a Roux-en-Y gastrojejunostomy.

duodenal ulcer perforation (DUP).

duodenojejunal junction (DJJ).

duodenum deformed by scarring.

DuoDerm dressing—a wound dressing used in treatment of leg ulcers, pressure sores, and superficial wounds. Also, *DuoDerm CGF* (control gel formula) *dressing.*

DuoDerm hydroactive gel for wound hydration.

Duodopa (levodopa/carbidopa)—liquid preparation for intraduodenal infusion. It is used for the treatment of patients with late-stage Parkinson's disease when treatment with conventional oral levodopa is difficult.

DUP (duodenal ulcer perforation).

DUPEL—iontophoretic drug delivery system allowing for simultaneous treatment at two sites, thus cutting treatment time in half.

Du Pen long-term epidural catheter—used for long-term access to the epidural space for the delivery of preservative-free morphine sulfate to relieve intractable pain in cancer patients.

duplex pulsed-Doppler sonography.

duplex ultrasound—simultaneous high resolution real-time sonography and Doppler color spectral analysis. Used to diagnose a variety of conditions, including deep venous thrombosis. Shows areas of blood flow in color contrast on a video screen to demonstrate movement of blood. Since sonography does not require use of contrast media, it is less painful, less expensive, and quicker than contrast studies such as venograms. Individuals allergic to certain contrast media are thus spared allergic reactions. See also *Doppler* and *ultrasound*.

Dupont distal humeral plate.

Duraclon (clonidine HCl injection)—a nonopioid analgesic solution for continuous epidural administration as adjunctive therapy with intraspinal opiates for the treatment of severe pain in cancer patients not adequately relieved by opioid analgesics alone.

Duracon total knee system.

Duract (bromfenac sodium capsules) —non-narcotic analgesic belonging to the nonsteroidal anti-inflammatory drug class.

DuraGen—an absorbable dural graft matrix used as a dura substitute for repair of the dura mater in spinal and cranial surgical procedures. It is used for the closure of the dural membrane that covers the brain and spinal cord.

Duragesic (fentanyl).

Duraglide stone balloon catheter.

DURAglide3 stone balloon—single-use triple-lumen balloon catheter for removal of biliary stones from the common bile duct.

Dura-Kold wrap—reusable ice wrap for postoperative and rehabilitation cold therapy.

Durapatite (hydroxyapatite).

Duraphase prosthesis—inflatable penile prosthesis.

DuraPrep surgical solution—an iodophor scrub.

DuraScreen—a waterproof, long-lasting sunscreen.

Durasphere—an injectable bulking agent for the treatment of stress urinary incontinence due to intrinsic sphincter deficiency. It is injected under the mucosal lining of the bladder neck and urethra, expands, and then closes the bladder neck.

Durasul large diameter head system —for orthopedic hip implant applications.

Durathane cardiac device.

Dura-II positional penile prosthesis.

Duret hemorrhage—blood effusion in the brain stem due to herniation.

Durie and Salmon—classification of multiple myeloma in three stages.

Durkan CTS (carpal tunnel syndrome) **gauge**—a positive screening test for carpal tunnel syndrome.

dusky, duskiness—a bluish skin color from cyanosis.

Duval disposable dermatome.

DuVal distal (caudal) **pancreaticojejunostomy**—a drainage technique that

DuVal *(cont.)*
was used more in the past than at present. The term may be encountered in a patient's past history.

Duvall lung-grasping clamp.

DuVries hammer toe repair.

DVA (dynamic visual acuity).

DVD (dissociated vertical divergence) —when the eyes do not move together and the deviating eye tends to move up and out.

DVI (deep venous insufficiency)—see *Hunter tendon rod.*

DVI (digital vascular imaging).

DVIU (direct vision internal urethrotomy).

DVP (daunorubicin, vincristine, prednisone)—chemotherapy protocol.

DVP (draining vein pressure).

DVT (deep venous thrombosis).

Dwyer correction of scoliosis—a procedure using an internal device of clips, screws, and a cable to straighten the spinal column. A clip is applied to each vertebra involved; a screw with a screwhead that has a hole in it is screwed through a hole in the clip and into the bone. A braided titanium cable is run through the holes protruding from the screw heads and tightened (after grafts of cancellous iliac bone or pieces of rib bone have been placed between the vertebrae). Tension is then applied to the cable.

Dwyer osteotomy—calcaneal osteotomy as seen in ankle surgery.

DXR (delayed xenograft rejection).

dye exclusion test—measures bone marrow viability.

dye laser—a type of laser used to remove birthmarks such as port wine stains by pinpointing and vaporizing the abnormal blood vessels which cause these marks. No anesthesia is necessary, as the procedure is essentially painless. The yellow-orange dye inside the laser is sensitive to the color red, therefore zeroing-in on the blood vessels with light energy that turns into heat, thus vaporizing the vessels or skin tumors consisting of blood vessels. It cannot be used for correction of varicose veins.

Dynabac (dirithromycin)—a macrolide antibiotic used once daily to treat lower respiratory tract infections, pharyngitis, tonsillitis, skin and skin structure infections.

Dynacin (minocycline)—prescription drug for treatment of severe acne.

DynaCirc (isradipine)—antihypertensive.

Dyna-Flex compression dressing or wrap.

Dynaflex penile prosthesis—for male impotence.

Dyna-Lok system—a plating system incorporating the advantages of both the rigid and semirigid system for spinal instrumentation.

Dyna Med Anti-Shock Trousers (DMAST)—see *DMAST.*

dynamic compression plate (DCP) (Ortho)—"When the reduction was considered satisfactory, DCPs were bent to conform with the patient's anatomy and secured in place with an assortment of cortical and cancellous screws."

dynamic computerized tomography— rapid sequential CT scanning after an intravenous bolus injection of contrast medium for detection of microadenomas that are isodense with surrounding tissues on conventional (delayed) CT scans.

dynamic conformal therapy—an irradiation technique focusing radiation precisely on malignancies, no matter how irregular the shape. This technique allows physicians to deliver more effective treatments with fewer side effects and minimizes radiation effects on healthy tissue surrounding the tumors under treatment.

Dynamic Cooling Device (DCD)—reduces pain and trauma to patients during laser therapy by delivering a short burst of the cooling agent to the target area immediately prior to the laser treatment.

Dynamic Flotation pressure control zone therapy for pressure sores.

dynamic graciloplasty—a technique for correcting fecal incontinence in which the gracilis muscle is wrapped around the anus to create a new sphincter. Several weeks later, a standard cardiac pacemaker is implanted in the lower abdomen and electrodes placed on the gracilis muscle. Continued stimulation of the muscle by the pacemaker actually changes the type of muscle fibers to ones which resist fatigue and can maintain a sustained contraction around the anus. When the patient needs to defecate, the pacemaker is temporarily turned off with an external magnet.

Dynamic Optical Breast Imaging System (DOBI).

dynamic range control (DRC) **algorithm**—used in digital radiography. It has been shown to improve image quality and contrast in poorly penetrated regions of digital chest images.

dynamic spiral CT lung densitometry—used to differentiate air trapping from compensatory hyperinflation in children.

DynaPulse 5000A—ambulatory blood pressure monitor.

Dynasplint knee extension unit—a device that provides ongoing dynamic stress while patients are asleep or at rest.

Dynasplint shoulder system—applied for treatment of adhesive capsulitis (frozen shoulder).

DynaVox 2—an augmentative communication device that uses a wireless computer connection and software designed to aid nonverbal communication.

DynaWell—medical compression device used with MRI or CT to provide a more accurate diagnosis of spinal conditions by providing the weight and load of upright posture.

Dyonics disposable arthroscope blade.

DyoVac suction punch for arthroscopy.

dysconjugate gaze—see *disconjugate.*

dysfibrinogenemia—a condition in which there is abnormality of fibrinogen, an essential clotting factor.

dysfunctional *(not* dis-*)*—abnormality of function of an organ.

dysgeusia—persistent alteration in taste perception.

dyskaryosis—aberrant nuclear arrangement or structure; may be seen in malignancy or cell death. Cf. *dyskeratosis.*

dyskeratosis—aberrant keratin production and/or deposition. Cf. *dyskaryosis.*

dysphagia—difficulty in swallowing due to mechanical problems with the GI tract, esophageal infection or ulcers, or strokes. Cf. *dysphasia.*

dysphagia lusoria (from *lusus naturae,* freak of nature)—esophageal compression by anomalous right subclavian artery. An aberrant right subclavian artery is the most common aortic arch anomaly in adults.

dysphasia—impairment or loss of the power to use or understand speech; caused by disease of, or injury to, the brain. Cf. *dysphagia.*

Dysport (*Clostridium botulinum* toxin*).*

dysprosody—change in the rhythm of speech due to neurologic or psychiatric disease. Cf. *hyperprosody.*

dysthymia—mood disorder. "Secondary to her disabling organic illness, she has developed a chronic dysthymia."

dystrophy
Reis-Buckler's corneal
SCARMID (severe childhood autosomal recessive muscular dystrophy)
Stargardt's

E, e

EAAT2 protein—a gene deficiency present in amyotrophic lateral sclerosis (ALS) (Lou Gehrig's disease), due to aberrant ribonucleic acid which halts the production of this protein. A new test is being developed to detect this aberrant ribonucleic acid in the hopes of early detection of ALS.

EAC (expandable access catheter)—facilitates embolectomy and angioplasty procedures. In its collapsed state, the EAC is inserted into either the iliac, femoral, or popliteal artery. In its expanded state, the EAC's lumen is wide enough so that an angioscope with either a Fogarty embolectomy catheter or an angioplasty balloon can be placed inside it.

Eagle-Barrett syndrome ("prune-belly syndrome")—congenital absence of one or more layers of the abdominal wall musculature, often accompanied by other congenital anomalies.

Eagle equation—a scoring system used to predict cardiac morbidity.

Eagle straight-ahead arthroscope.

Eagle II survey spirometer.

Eagle Vision-Freeman punctum plug (Oph)—see *Freeman punctum plug*.

Eales disease—characterized by neovascularization and recurrent hemorrhage of retinal vessels. Seen principally in young men.

EAP (etoposide, Adriamycin, Platinol) —chemotherapy protocol for gastric adenocarcinoma.

ear—may easily be confused with "air" when the dictator says "air-bone-gap" in audiology (*never* "ear bone gap" or "airborne gap"). Cf. *ear oximeter*.

EarCheck Pro—an instrument that can detect the presence of middle ear effusion through acoustic reflectometry (sonar-like technology). It is reported to be comparable in accuracy to a tympanometer but does not require an airtight seal or pressurization of the ear canal.

ear lobe crease (ELC)—diagonal ear lobe creases are associated, in a graded fashion, with higher rates of cardiac events in patients admitted to the hospital with suspected coronary disease.

ear oximeter (*not* air)—a photoelectric device that is attached to the ear and measures oxygen saturation of the blood that passes through the ear. See *Hewlett-Packard ear oximeter*.

earring, Brent pressure—used to treat earlobe keloids.

Easi-Lav—a system for gastric lavage. Used in patients with upper GI bleeding, it delivers a greater volume of lavage in less time than standard methods.

Eastern Cooperative Oncology Group (ECOG) performance status in cancer patients.

EAST test (Vasc Surg)—an acronym for external rotation, abduction, stress test. With the hands/arms held straight up (as in a holdup), the hands are opened and closed. In a positive EAST test, the patient reproduces the symptoms for which medical care was sought.

eating cell (phagocyte).

EATL (enteropathy-associated T-cell lymphoma).

Eaton agent (*Mycoplasma pneumoniae*) —used thus in dictation: "primary atypical pneumonia, possibly due to the Eaton agent."

Ebastel (ebastine)—used to treat allergies.

ebastine—an antiallergic agent.

EBI bone healing system—noninvasive system for treating nonunion and failed arthrodesis with electromagnetic fields. (EBI, Electro Biology, Inc.).

EBIORT (electron beam intraoperative radiotherapy) **procedure**—bypasses the radiosensitive skin and the superficial structures, thus allowing radiation to be administered to the surgically exposed tumor.

EBI SPF-2 implantable bone stimulator.

EBL (endoscopic band ligation)—a procedure for treating bleeding esophageal varices, said to have fewer side effects than sclerotherapy. Also, *endoscopic variceal ligation* (EVL).

EBL (estimated blood loss)—estimated by measuring blood in the suction bottle and weighing the sponges that have soaked up blood.

EBNA (Epstein-Barr nuclear antigen) **test**.

Ebola virus—acute hemorrhagic febrile disease, highly fatal, endemic to areas of Africa at this time. See also *Marburg fever*.

EBRT (external beam radiation therapy).

Ebstein's cardiac anomaly (*not* Epstein, as in Epstein-Barr virus).

EBT (electron beam tomography).

eburnated bone; eburnation.

EBV (Epstein-Barr virus).

E-CABG (endarterectomy and coronary artery bypass grafting).

E-CABG (endoscopic coronary artery bypass graft).

E.CAM—photon emission camera used for whole-body emission tomography and general imaging procedures with variable angle techniques. Also referred to as *E.CAM positron emission tomography* (PET) *imaging system*.

ECC (emergency cardiac care).

ECCE (extracapsular cataract extraction).

Eccentric "Y" retractor—adjustable finger retractor for use in laparoscopic procedures.

Eccocee—a mid-range compact ultrasound diagnostic system.

Eccovision acoustic rhinometry system—used to obtain quantitative measurements of the nasal cavity.

E-CFC (erythroid colony-forming cells).

echocardiographic automated border detection—a technique that allows continuous measuring of left ventricular cavity area (and thus volume) by differentiating the acoustic backscatter characteristics of blood from myocardial tissue within a defined area of the heart, replacing more invasive techniques such as catheter insertion.

echocardiography—a noninvasive cardiac diagnostic procedure. From the sonographic pattern are determined the dimensions, position, and movements of the chamber walls and valve leaflets, and any possible deformities. See *dobutamine stress echocardiography*, *M-mode, sector scan, transesophageal echocardiogram*, and *two-dimensional echocardiography*.

echo characteristics (ultrasonography) —the frequency, intensity, and distribution of echoes produced by a structure or region.

Echo-Coat ultrasound biopsy needles.

echocolonoscope—endoscopic sonographic transducer in combination with a colonoscope.

EchoEye—3-D ultrasound imaging system that is placed in front of a catheter or probe to provide tissue imaging during surgery.

EchoFlow blood velocity meter system (BVM-1)—enables physicians to evaluate and quantify blood flow in vessels using ultrasound technology.

EchoGen emulsion (perflenapent injectable emulsion)—contrast agent for use in echocardiographic evaluation of left ventricular endocardial border delineation and left ventricular chamber opacification.

echogastroscope—used for endoscopic ultrasonography.

Echols retractor (Neuro).

EchoMark catheter—an angiographic catheter that contains a wire and transducer sensitive to ultrasound signals. As the catheter is advanced, ultrasound (rather than x-rays) is used to correctly position the catheter in the vessel.

echo planar imaging (EPI)—MRI term.

echo sign (Neuro)—repetition of the last word of a sentence or phrase, indicating brain pathology.

echo time (TE)—given in milliseconds (msec)—MRI term.

Echovist (galactose)—ultrasound contrast medium for gynecological imaging.

ECI (Ensemble contrast imaging).

EC-IC (extracranial-intracranial) **bypass**—for complete carotid occlusions or intracranial carotid stenosis not treatable by endarterectomy.

Eckhout vertical gastroplasty (named for Clifford V. Eckhout, M.D.).

Eclipse TENS unit—see *TENS*.

Eclipse TMR laser—a holmium laser device used in transmyocardial revascularization (TMR) to create pathways within the heart muscle.

ECM (extracellular matrix).

ECMO (extracorporeal membrane oxygenation) ("ek-mo")—a technique used in infants with serious lung problems at birth with poor prognosis for survival. The baby's blood is circulated through a machine that removes carbon dioxide and adds oxygen, thereby functioning for the lungs while they mature or heal.

ECMV (etoposide, cyclophosphamide, methotrexate, vincristine)—chemotherapy protocol for small cell lung carcinoma.

ECochG (electrocochleography)—test to estimate hearing loss.

ECOG (Eastern Cooperative Oncology Group) performance status in cancer patients.

ECoG (electrocorticographic) **data**.

E. coli 0157:H7—a strain of *Escherichia coli,* causing recent outbreaks of severe diarrheal disease in the U.S. Transmission occurs through contaminated food and water and directly from person to person. It is particularly dangerous for children and the elderly.

E. coli L-asparaginase—a chemotherapy drug for acute lymphoblastic leukemia. *E. coli* is a gram-negative bacterium which provides the enzyme L-asparaginase aminohydrolase contained in this version of L-asparaginase. Some people who are allergic to the *E. coli*-derived version of the drug can be given *Erwinia* L-asparaginase, from the gram-negative bacterium *Erwinia*.

ECOM (endotracheal cardiac output monitoring).

EcoNail—a nail lacquer that contains the antifungal drug econazole and a drug-absorption-enhancement compound. It is used to treat fungal infections of the fingernails and toenails.

Ecovia (remacemide)—a low-affinity NMDA channel blocker for the treatment of Parkinson's and Huntington's diseases.

ECRB (extensor carpi radialis brevis).

ECRL (extensor carpi radialis longus).

ECS (extracellular-like, calcium-free solution)—see *cardioplegic solution.*

ecstatic—exhibiting great elation or enthusiasm. Cf. *ectatic.*

ECT (electroconvulsive therapy).

ECTA (enzyme-catalyzed therapeutic activation) **technology**—focuses on treatment of drug resistance in cancer.

ectatic—stretched or distended. Cf. *ecstatic.*

ectodermal groove—embryonic feature that lies between the maxillary and mandibular facial prominences. Incomplete fusion is thought to cause facial aplasia cutis (failure of development of skin).

Ectra system—for endoscopic release of the transverse carpal ligament in carpal tunnel syndrome.

ECU (environmental control unit)—enables severely disabled individuals to perform everyday functions with use of computer commands activated by blow tubes or mouth sticks. Each system is designed to meet the needs of the individual.

ECV (external cephalic version).

EDA (extravasation detection accessory).

EDAM (10-ethyl-deaza-aminopterin, 10-EDAM)—a single agent chemotherapy drug.

EDAP (etoposide, dexamethasone, ara-C, Platinol)—chemotherapy protocol used to treat multiple myeloma.

EDAS (encephaloduroarteriosynangiosis).

EDC (extensor digitorum communis).

eddy currents; eddies—MRI terms.

edema—see cystoid macular edema (CME).

Edex (alprostadil)—injectable used for treatment of erectile dysfunction.

EdgeAhead phaco slit knife—used in cataract surgery. Note: *EdgeAhead* is one word.

edge detection (ED)—a term used in MRI scans.

edge ringing artifact (Gibbs phenomenon, truncation band)—an MRI artifact caused by limitation of the image reconstruction algorithm.

edible vaccines—created from a genetically engineered food product (e.g., potato) containing a toxin produced by *E. coli.* Volunteers who ate portions of the potato in separate doses over a 21-day period showed an increase in antibodies in the blood, and some had increase in antibodies in the lining of the digestive tract. The director of the government agency funding the study stated, "Edible vaccines offer exciting possibilities for significantly reducing the burden of diseases like hepatitis and diarrhea . . . in the developing world where storing and administering vaccines are often major problems."

Edinger-Westphal nucleus—the parasympathetic nucleus from which arises the oculomotor nerve (cranial nerve III), for constriction of the pupil and accommodation of the lens for near vision.

Edmondson Grading System—in small hepatocellular carcinoma; it is written EdGr II, etc.

Edmondson-Steiner histologic grading of hepatocellular carcinoma (grades I, II, II, IVa).

Edronax tablets (reboxetine)—an antidepressant used to treat acute depressive illness or major depression.

EDRT (endothelium-derived relaxant factor).

Edwards woven Teflon aortic bifurcation graft.

EEA stapler (end-to-end anastomosis).

EECP (enhanced external counterpulsation).

EEC (ectrodactyly–ectodermal dysplasia–clefting) **syndrome**—including hypertelorism, cleft lip or palate, or both, and possibly seizures.

EEPLND (extraperitoneal endoscopic pelvic lymph node dissection).

EES (expandable esophageal stent).

efface—used in plastic and reconstructive surgery to describe obliteration of a deformity by covering it with a graft. "A flat onlay graft was inserted through an intercartilaginous incision into a precise pocket to efface the deformity."

effacement—abnormal flattening of the contour of a structure.

effect (noun)—an immediate result produced by an agent or cause, as "The surgical procedure produced a good cosmetic effect." Examples: proarrhythmic effect, Somogyi effect, Tyndall effect.

effect (verb)—to execute, accomplish, bring to pass, as "This therapy should effect a cure" or, in surgery, "closure was effected." *Effect* is most often used as a noun. Cf. *affect.*

efferent—moving away from the center. Cf. *afferent.*

Effexor XR (venlafaxine HCl)—once-a-day dosing alternative for Effexor in treatment of generalized anxiety disorder.

effusion—escape of a fluid into a part. Examples: pericardial and pleural. Cf. *infusion.*

Efidac/24—a 24-hour over-the-counter cold remedy containing pseudoephedrine decongestant.

E5 monoclonal antibody—a drug obtained from mice and found to be effective against gram-negative sepsis (a virulent and deadly multisystem disease caused by the endotoxins released in the bloodstream by gram-negative bacteria). E5 binds to the endotoxins, inactivating them.

eflornithine (Ornidyl)—used to treat *Pneumocystis carinii* pneumonia in AIDS patients. It has an antiprotozoal action and is also used to treat sleeping sickness.

EFM (electronic fetal monitoring)—uses telephone transmission of data and remote sensory devices for patient monitoring.

Egan's mammography—a set of procedures for mammographic examination developed by Robert L. Egan, M.D., the author of a standard textbook and many articles on mammography.

EG/BUS (external genitalia/Bartholin's glands, urethra, and Skene's glands).

EGCg (epigallocatechin gallate)—a compound in green tea that inhibits activity of an enzyme required for cancer cell growth.

EGD (esophagogastroduodenoscopy).

EGF (epidermal growth factor).

EGF-R (endothelial growth factor receptor) **small molecule inhibitors**—used in the treatment of psoriasis.

egoisme à deux—a phenomenon sometimes seen when both members of a couple deny they have a problem, such as one individual's dementia.

EGTA (esophageal gastric tube airways).

EHL (electrohydraulic lithotripsy).

Ehlers-Danlos syndrome—increased laxity and elasticity in the supporting structures of the joints; can also follow neurosyphilis or severe rheumatoid arthritis.

EIA (enzyme-linked immunoassay)—used in the detection of AIDS-associated retroviruses.

EIA-2 (enzyme-linked immunoassay)—detects the presence of the hepatitis C virus in blood.

EIB (exercise-induced bronchospasm).

EIC (extensive intraductal carcinoma).

eicosapentaenoic acid (EPA)—a marine fatty acid, analogue of arachidonic acid that is found in fish, some other marine oils, and also possibly in seaweeds. Some researchers think that a diet rich in EPA may be protection against thrombosis in patients with high serum cholesterol and triglyceride levels.

EID (Emergency Infusion Device)—percutaneous central venous large-bore catheter.

EIFT (embryo intrafallopian transfer).

800 Series Blood Gas and Critical Analyte System—provides diagnostic measurements of blood gas, electrolytes, metabolites, and CO-oximetry from a single blood sample in a compact and user-friendly format.

EIP (extensor indicis proprius).

Eisenmenger complex—congenital heart anomaly.

EIT (endoscopic injection therapy).

EIWA (Escala Inteligencia Wechsler Para Adultos)—the Wechsler Adult Intelligence Scale for administration to adults who speak only Spanish.

EKG (electrocardiograph) **leads**
augmented leads: aVF, aVL, aVR
cardiac leads: I, II, III, V1 to V6

ELA (euglobulin lysis activity).

Elase (fibrinolysin; desoxyribonuclease)—topical enzymatic debriding agent for treatment of inflammatory and infected wounds, ulcers, and burns.

Elastalloy Ultraflex Strecker nitinol stent.

elastic fibers stain (Weigert)—a special tissue stain to reveal the presence of elastin (a fibrous microscopic cell protein) found in skin and vessels.

Elastikon elastic tape—for pressure dressings.

Elasto-Gel hydrogel sheet.

Elasto-Gel shoulder therapy wrap—used for giving heat treatments for shoulder injuries.

Elastomull—an elastic gauze bandage, a double-woven stretch dressing.

ELC (ear lobe crease).

ELCA (excimer laser coronary angioplasty).

Eldepryl (selegiline)—used as an adjunct in management of Parkinson's disease patients. It shows promise as a treatment for Alzheimer's disease.

Elder classification—a classification of tumor-infiltrating lymphocytes in malignant melanoma. Named for pathologist D. E. Elder, M.D.

Eldisine (vindesine sulfate)—chemotherapy drug.

elective lymph node dissection(ELND).

electrically generated pain management techniques—see *pain management techniques*.

electric zone—see *triangle of pain*.

electroacuscope—a feedback-oriented microcurrent stimulator that generates complex waveforms that automatically adjust to meet the needs of injured tissue. Used in treating carpal tunnel syndrome.

electrocardiogram—see *signal-averaged electrocardiogram* (SAECG).

electrocardiographic gating with electron-beam CT technology.

electrocautery—see *cautery*.

electrochemotherapy—a therapy in which a split-second electrical impulse is applied to the skin in combination with topical chemotherapy. It opens up skin pores, allowing the chemotherapeutic agent to seep in and more effectively target cancerous cells. It is relatively painless and involves no cutting or stitching, so there is none of the disfigurement that might be associated with surgery.

electroconvulsive therapy (ECT).

electrocorticography—procedure performed to clarify the origin of tumor-related seizures.

electrode data—When a neurosurgeon dictates: "The electrode was connected with zero two zero negative polarity," it should be written *0-2/0 negative*.

electroejaculation—an infertility procedure on anejaculatory males under anesthesia. A probe inserted into the rectum administers an electric shock, causing ejaculation.

electrogalvanic stimulation—used in treatment of fractures. See *pulsing current*.

electromechanical dissociation (EMD) **of the heart**.

electromyography of penile corpus cavernosum muscles—a diagnostic tool to evaluate cavernous smooth muscle and its autonomic innervation.

electron-beam angiography of coronary arteries—minimally invasive procedure performed on the electron-beam tomography scanner.

electron-beam computed tomography (CT)—method of examining the cardiovascular system.

electronic fetal monitoring (EFM).

electro-oculogram apparatus (Oph)— used in determining saccadic velocity.

electrophoresis—a process in which charged particles (such as ions), suspended in liquid, are moved under the influence of an applied electrical field. Note the different root words in electrophoresis (*phoresis*, carrying, transmission) and plasmapheresis (*apheresis*, separation).

electrophysiologic study (EPS).

electroporation therapy—application of high electric field pulses of short duration to create temporary pores (holes) in membranes of cells for easier and more efficient entrance of potential tumor-killing drugs.

electroretinogram, -graphy (ERG).

Electroscope disposable scissors used in laparoscopic procedures.

electrostimulation—see *pulsing current.*

electrotransfer test—see *Western blot electrotransfer test.*

elemental diet—for burn patients, a high-nitrogen liquid diet that requires almost no digestion and produces little residue.

ELF (etoposide, leucovorin, fluorouracil)—chemotherapy protocol for gastric carcinoma.

El Gamal cardiac device.

elicit—to draw out, as "We could elicit little information as to the patient's past medical history." Cf. *illicit.*

Eligoy metal alloy—used in joint replacement.

Eliminator dilatation balloon.

Eliminator—right angle ArthroWand.

eliprodil—investigational drug that appears to help nerve demyelination associated with multiple sclerosis.

ELISA (enzyme-linked immunosorbent assay)—the first "AIDS test" used by blood banks to diminish the chance of HIV infection through a blood transfusion. ELISA can also be used as a screening test for hepatitis C.

Elite dual chamber rate-responsive pacemaker—marketed by Medtronic, weighing only $1^1/2$ oz., and using CapSure SP leads.

Elite Farley retractor—adjustable retractor for all types of spinal surgery.

Ellence (epirubicin)—treatment for node-positive early-stage breast cancer.

Ellestad protocol—treadmill stress test.

Ellik kidney stone basket, evacuator, elevator.

Elmiron (pentosan polysulfate sodium) —used for the relief of pain and discomfort associated with interstitial cystitis, which causes severe bladder and pelvic pain, and urinary frequency.

Elmor tissue morcellator—a tissue morcellator powered by radiofrequency energy that is used to isolate, contain, and remove large tissue masses during laparoscopic surgery.

Elmslie triple arthrodesis—used for podiatric surgical correction of post polio pes calcaneovalgus deformity.

ELND (elective lymph node dissection).

"eloquent" areas of the brain—seizures starting from a focus in these areas will produce an aura.

Eloxatin (oxaliplatin)—first-line treatment of patients with advanced colorectal cancer in combination with 5-FU-based chemotherapy.

Elta Dermal hydrogel dressing.

EL2-LS2 flexible video laparoscope.

elusion—an adroit or clever escape; escape notice of, as "Elusion of a fourth parathyroid gland indicated its

elusion *(cont.)*
possible congenital absence." Cf. *allusion, illusion.*

EMA (epithelial membrane antigen).

EMACO (etoposide, methotrexate, actinomycin D, cyclophosphamide, and Oncovin)—chemotherapy regimen for metastatic choriocarcinoma.

embolotherapy—embolization of hypervascularized tumors and arteriovenous malformations, cutting off blood supply.

Embosphere microspheres—device for occluding the blood supply to uterine fibroids during uterine artery embolization. The device is also used to treat hypervascularized tumors and arteriovenous malformations with embolization, or embolotherapy.

Embol-X arterial cannula and filter system—protects against the risk of stroke and other neurologic deficits during cardiovascular procedures by capturing emboli (including aortic plaque) that may be released into systemic circulation.

EMBP (estramustine binding protein) (Neuro).

embryo biopsy—involves the testing of fertilized human eggs to check whether hereditary ailments are carried in the genes following fertilization procedures.

embryo intrafallopian transfer (EIFT).

embryoscopy—the use of a fiberoptic endoscope to visualize a fetus in the first trimester. This technique allows greater access to very tiny fetuses than ultrasonographically guided prenatal diagnostic testing.

Emcyt ("m-site") (estramustine phosphate sodium)—used in treatment of prostatic carcinoma that is unresponsive to estrogen therapy.

EMD (electromechanical dissociation) —"He was defibrillated into asystole and treated with atropine, but he went into an EMD and we were unable, despite continued and adequate CPR, to resuscitate him."

Emdogain—periodontal gel product for rejuvenation of tooth-supporting tissues.

Emergency Infusion Device (EID).

emergency medical services (EMS).

EMF (endomyocardial fibrosis)

eminence—a bony projection. Cf. *imminent.*

EMI ("emmy") **scanner**—the original CT scanner. (EMI, Electrical Musical Instruments.)

EMIT (enzyme-multiplication immunoassay technique)—used in toxicology screens on urine samples.

EMLA anesthetic disc—prescription-only adhesive patch designed for children. It contains a combination of lidocaine and prilocaine and releases the anesthetic into the skin to ease the pain of injections, stitches, and related procedures.

EMLA cream (lidocaine and prilocaine) —applied to the skin topically and covered with a dressing for 60 minutes. It provides a level of anesthesia complete enough for dermal procedures that an additional injection of lidocaine is often not needed.

empty nest syndrome—restlessness and depression in parents whose children have grown up and left home.

empty sella syndrome—diagnosed in a patient with an enlarged sella turcica, where there is no tumor present and the sella fills with air on CT or MRI scan.

EMR (endoscopic mucosal resection).

EMS (emergency medical services).

EMS (encephalomyosynangiosis).

EMS (eosinophilia-myalgia syndrome).

E-MVAC (escalated methotrexate, vinblastine, Adriamycin, cisplatin or cyclophosphamide)—chemotherapy protocol for tumors of the urothelial tract.

EMV grading, Glasgow Coma Scale: E = eyes; M = motor; V = voice. Written as $E_2M_4V_2$. The Glasgow Coma Scale goes to 8. See *Glasgow Coma Scale*.

ENA (extractable nuclear antigen).

EnAbl system—a thermal ablation system used to treat excessive uterine bleeding.

Enable (tenidap).

ENANB hepatitis—enterically transmitted non-A, non-B hepatitis.

ENBA (Epstein-Barr virus nuclear antigen).

en bloc laminectomy (Neuro, Ortho).

en bloc transplantation of small pediatric kidneys into adult recipients, using an interposition technique—averts the complication of vascular thrombosis and provides adequate mass to achieve a normal level of renal function. The successful technique places the allografts using vascular anastomoses in continuity.

en bloc vein resection—performed in the treatment of pancreatic adenocarcinoma adherent to the superior mesenteric-portal vein.

Enbrel (etanercept)—used to treat children and teenagers with moderately severe polyarticular juvenile rheumatoid arthritis.

encapsulated liposomes—see *liposomes*.

encephaloduroarteriosynangiosis (abbreviated EDAS)—surgical treatment for moyamoya disease, in which a scalp artery is dissected over the course of several inches, then a small temporary opening in the skull directly beneath the artery is made. The artery is then sutured to the surface of the brain and the bone replaced. Cf. *encephalomyosynangiosis*.

encephalomyosynangiosis (abbreviated EMS)—surgical treatment for moyamoya disease. The temporalis muscle of the forehead region is dissected, and through an opening in the skull it is placed onto the surface of the brain. Cf. *encephaloduroarteriosynangiosis)*.

encephalopathy—see *painter's encephalopathy*.

endarterectomy and coronary artery bypass grafting (E-CABG).

end-biting forceps.

Ender nail, or rod, fixation—used for fixation of long bone fractures.

End-Flo laparoscopic irrigating system.

Endius endoscopic access system—for noninstrumental posterolateral spinal fusion.

Endius Trifix—thoracolumbar pedicle screw system. Uses the Dome screw design and Diamond connectors.

endoanal coil—used in MRI studies to image the lower colon.

Endo-Avitene—a microfibrillar collagen hemostatic material, used in an endoscopic delivery system.

Endo-Babcock—surgical grasping device.

Endobag—laparoscopic specimen retrieval system.

endobronchial needle aspiration—to diagnose endobronchial small cell carcinoma.

Endocare Horizon prostatic stent—for relief of bladder outlet obstruction.

Endocare renal cryoablation—freezes and destroys diseased tissue in place, eliminating the necessity for nephrectomy in patients with renal carcinoma.

Endo Clip applier—laparoscopic clip applier.

EndoCoil biliary stent—for malignant obstruction of the bile duct due to pancreatic cancer.

EndoCoil esophageal stent to treat a stenosis.

EndoCPB (endovascular cardiopulmonary bypass) **catheter**.

Endodissect—reticulating (or roticulating) dissecting instrument.

endoesophageal MRI coil—tiny probe that is inserted through the mouth and nestles in the esophagus, giving an image of the aorta that is nine times sharper than the standard MRI provides.

end-of-dose deterioration—a loss of symptom control in patients, such as those on L-Dopa for Parkinson's disease.

EndoFix absorbable interference screw (Ortho)—bioabsorbable device made of a polyglyconate polymer. Used in bone-tendon-bone fixation in anterior cruciate ligament surgery.

Endoflex—minimally invasive endoscopic lumbar diskectomy scope and instrument system.

Endo-Gauge—device used to measure the thickness of tissue in laparoscopic wedge biopsy of the liver.

endogenous morphine (endorphins).

Endo-GIA suture stapler.

Endo Grasp device—used in minimally invasive lung surgery.

Endo-Hernia stapler—used in laparoscopic hernia repairs.

Endoknot suture—used in minimally invasive surgeries such as laparoscopy.

Endoloop—disposable chromic ligature suture instrument.

Endo Lumenal Gastroplication—device used for treatment of patients with severe gastroesophageal reflux disease. (Note the spelling "lumenal," not luminal.)

EndoLumina bougie—illuminated bougie for transillumination of esophagus, using a silicone-sheathed fiberoptic bundle bonded to a soft, clear, flexible tip. Also for general, colorectal, and gynecological laparoscopic surgery.

endolymphatic hypertension.

EndoMate Grab Bag—an endoscopic specimen retrieval bag.

EndoMed LSS—total laparoscopic system.

endometrial ablation—used as a treatment for dysfunctional uterine bleeding. Ablation of the uterine lining with hysteroscopy is less invasive than hysterectomy.

Endo-Model rotating knee joint prosthesis—permits flexion of the joint up to 165°.

endomyocardial fibrosis (EMF)—a severe and progressively restrictive form of cardiomyopathy.

Endopath EMS hernia stapler.

Endopath ES—reusable endoscopic stapler.

Endopath laparoscopic trocar—used for laparoscopic surgery, as in inguinal hernia repair.

Endopath Linear Cutter—a surgical stapler, used in minimally invasive surgery.

Endopath Optiview optical surgical obturator—allows visually guided trocar entry for laparoscopic surgery.

Endopath TriStar trocar—used in minimally invasive surgery. Allows use of the fingertip technique of placing the trocar precisely and with much less force than conventional trocars.

Endopath Ultra Veress needle—used for insufflation during obstetric and gynecologic laparoscopic procedures.

Endopearl—bioabsorbable device that provides enhanced fixation of soft tissue grafts within the femoral socket during ACL reconstruction of the knee.

endophthalmitis—inflammation of the internal structures of the eye or the adjacent tissues.

Endo-P-Probe—used in combination with standard ultrasound machines for endorectal ultrasonography.

endoprosthesis—crutched-stick type biliary duct stent. See *prosthesis*.

endopyelotomy procedure—minimally invasive procedure for primary ureteropelvic junction obstruction. It has no major negative impact on eventual open pyeloplasty if that should become necessary.

endorectal coil—MRI term.

EndoRetract—a retractor used in minimally invasive surgery.

endorphin (endogenous morphine)—natural morphine-like compound produced by the brain.

EndoSaph vein harvest system—used in minimally invasive harvesting of the saphenous vein for CABG procedures.

endoscope
Agee endoscope
AO (American Optical) indirect ophthalmoscope
AudioScope
Baggish hysteroscope

endoscope *(cont.)*
Benjamin binocular slimline laryngoscope (ENT)
Benjamin pediatric laryngoscope
biomicroscope
CF-200Z Olympus colonoscope
Clarus spinescope
Czaja-McCaffrey rigid stent introducer
dermatoscope
diaphanoscope
DigiScope
Eagle straight-ahead arthroscope
echocolonoscope
echogastroscope
EL2-LS2 flexible video laparoscope
electroacuscope
endometrial resection and ablation (ERA) resectoscope sheath
EVIS 140 endoscope reprocessing system
falloposcope
FG-36UX linear scanning echoendoscope
Flexiblade laryngoscope
flexible steerable nasolaryngopharyngoscope
Futura resectoscope sheath
Gautier ureteroscope
gonioscope
Iglesias fiberoptic resectoscope
indirect laser ophthalmoscope
InjecTx cystoscope
Kantor-Berci video laryngoscope
Karl Storz flexible ureteropyeloscope
Killian-Lynch laryngoscope
Landry vein light venoscope
Lewy suspension laryngoscope
Lindholm operating laryngoscope
lingoscope
Microprobe laser microendoscope
MiniSite laparoscope
Morganstern continuous-flow operating cystoscope

endoscope *(cont.)*
mother and baby endoscope
Navigator flexible endoscope
Olympus CF-200Z colonoscope
Olympus CYF-3 OES cysto-
fiberscope
Olympus ENF-P2 flexible
laryngoscope
Olympus EVIS 140 endoscope
reprocessing system
Olympus EVIS Q-200V video-
endoscope
Olympus GIF-EUM2 echoendo-
scope
Olympus GIF-1T10 and GIF20
echoendoscope
Olympus JF1T10 fiberoptic
duodenoscope
Olympus JF-UM20 echoendoscope
Olympus OSF flexible
sigmoidoscope
Olympus SIF10 enteroscope
Olympus TJF-100 endoscope
Olympus VU-M2 and XIF-UM3
echoendoscope
Olympus XQ230 gastroscope
orascope microfiberoptic
Ossoff-Karlen laryngoscope
Panoramic 200 nonmydriatic
ophthalmoscope
Pentax EUP-EC124 ultrasound
gastroscope
Pentax FG-36UX echoendoscope
Pentax-Hitachi FG32UA
endosonographic system
percutaneous diskoscope
Pixie minilaparoscope
Shapshay/Healy laryngoscope
SIF10 Olympus enteroscope
Sine-U-View nasal endoscope
Sonde enteroscope
STAR (specialized tissue aspirating
resectoscope)
Surgiview multiuse disposable
laparoscope

endoscope *(cont.)*
3-Dscope laparoscope
URF-P2 choledochoscope
van Loonen operating keratoscope
VideoHydro laparoscope
videolaseroscopy
Visicath
visuscope
Weerda distending operating
laryngoscope
Welch Allyn AudioScope
Zeiss Endolive endoscope
endoscopic aspiration mucosectomy.
endoscopic band ligation—see *EBL.*
endoscopic biliary endoprosthesis—a relatively safe and effective palliative procedure for patients with unresectable carcinoma of the gallbladder. The prosthetic stent is placed endoscopically beyond the stricture with the goal of producing free flow of bile, a 30% fall in the patient's bilirubin, and relief of pruritus.
endoscopic brow lift—minimally invasive procedure in which the eyebrows are "lifted" to smooth wrinkles and remove excess fat and skin.
endoscopic coronary artery bypass graft (E-CABG).
endoscopic division of incompetent perforating veins—a minimally invasive procedure for the treatment of venous ulceration of the lower leg. It is said to be as effective as open surgical exploration but leads to fewer wound healing complications with its endoscopic exploration of the subfascial area through a small incision.
endoscopic injection therapy (EIT).
endoscopic laser cholecystectomy—see *laparoscopic laser cholecystectomy.*

endoscopic laser dacryocystorhinostomy.

endoscopic ligation—a surgical treatment for bleeding esophageal varices.

endoscopic mucosal resection (EMR)—surgical therapeutic method based on principles of strip biopsy for resection of flat lesions of the gastrointestinal tract. Researchers believe applying EMR to esophageal dysplasia, a precancerous condition, would decrease incidence of esophageal cancer.

endoscopic mucosectomy for treatment of early gastric carcinoma.

endoscopic papillectomy (EP).

endoscopic retrograde cholangiography (ERC).

endoscopic retrograde cholangiopancreatogram (ERCP).

endoscopic sphincterotomy (ES).

endoscopic strip craniectomy—precedes helmet-molding therapy in infants (less than 3 months of age) to correct sagittal craniosynostosis. Endoscopic technique for early correction of sagittal synostosis is said to be safer, decreases blood loss, operative time, hospital costs, and provides early surgical results. See *craniostosis*, *helmet-molding therapy*, and *scaphocephaly*.

endoscopic transpapillary catheterization of the gallbladder (ETCG)—a procedure to dissolve gallstones. The gallbladder is catheterized using an ERCP catheter. The catheter with a hydrophilic guide wire is passed through the nose and advanced via a retrograde approach through the common bile duct. The ERCP catheter is then exchanged for a radiopaque Teflon biliary dilating catheter that allows the guide wire to be inserted into the cystic duct and gallbladder. The next day the patient undergoes both extracorporeal shockwave lithotripsy and infusion of solvent through the catheter to dissolve gallstones.

endoscopic ultrasound-guided fine needle aspiration (EUS-FNA)—provides visualization of peripancreatic tumors and their relationship to the surrounding structures as well as enabling cytologic diagnosis of the tumor and adjacent lymphadenopathy. It is a tool for the imaging and staging of peripancreatic tumors.

endoscopic ultrasonography (EUS)—examination of the esophagus and stomach with ultrasound using an echogastroscope. It can measure the thickness of the gastric folds and determine the depth to which carcinoma has invaded the stomach wall in order to stage esophageal and gastric carcinomas.

endoscopic ultrasound-assisted band ligation—technique for resection of submucosal tumors.

endoscopic variceal ligation (EVL)—see *EBL*.

endoscopic variceal sclerotherapy (EVS).

EndoShears—used in minimally invasive surgery.

Endosol—balanced salt solution for eye or ENT irrigation in surgery.

endosonography—insertion of sonographic transducers in upper or lower GI endoscopy.

Endosound endoscopic ultrasound catheter.

Endostatin—used in cancer treatment and potentially other diseases that depend upon new blood vessel

Endostatin *(cont.)*
growth, such as in some forms of blindness and arthritis. Endostatin is a natural antiangiogenic protein that has been found to inhibit the growth of blood vessels, thereby "starving" cancerous tumors.

Endo Stitch suturing device for endoscopic suturing.

Endotak lead defibrillator (Cardio)— provides increased electrode surface area and reduced system resistance in an implantable defibrillator. Also, *Endotak C lead* and *Endotak DSP.*

Endotak Picotip cardiac defibrillation lead.

endothelium-derived relaxant factor (EDRT).

Endotrac cannula, elevator, obturator, probe, rasp, retractor—endoscopic instruments used in carpal tunnel procedures.

endotracheal cardiac output monitoring (ECOM)—monitoring devices incorporated into a standard endotracheal tube to allow for continuous cardiac output monitoring of patients undergoing surgery or on respiratory support.

endovaginal coil—MRI term.

endovaginal ultrasound (EVUS)— ultrasound probe is placed directly into the vagina to obtain a measurement of the uterine lining and detailed images of the uterus. This procedure has been found to identify 96% of uterine cancer and 92% of uterine disease in postmenopausal women who experience abnormal vaginal bleeding.

endovascular stent grafting—used for treatment of abdominal aortic aneurysm. A wire and fabric-covered stent are inserted into the body via the catheter system. The delivery catheter is advanced through the leg to the site of the aneurysm, and the sclf-expanding stent graft is released. The graft lines the existing vessel and provides a new path for blood to flow past the aneurysm.

EndoWrist—instruments used with the daVinci surgical system for endoscopic mitral valve repair.

end-stage—referring to a progressively deteriorating condition that has reached the point of lethal (terminal) functional impairment of an organ or organ system, e.g., end-stage renal failure, end-stage lung disease.

end-stage coxarthrosis—treated by total hip arthroplasty.

end-stage liver disease (ESLD).

end-stage renal disease (ESRD).

end-tidal carbon dioxide ($ETCO_2$)— used in addition to arterial blood gas values to assess the patient's ventilatory status.

Enduron acctabular liner—a ball liner made with UHMWPe (ultra-high molecular weight polyethylene) for extra strength to prevent cracking.

en face ("ahn fahs") (Fr., in front, head on). "X-rays revealed left chest wall and diaphragmatic pleural plaques, the former seen both in profile and en face."

engaged, engagement—said of the fetal head as it enters and becomes lodged in the superior pelvic strait.

Engerix-B—a hepatitis B and D vaccine (recombinant).

Englert forceps (Plas Surg).

enhanced external counterpulsation (EECP)—a noninvasive outpatient procedure to relieve angina pectoris by improving perfusion to ischemic areas of the heart.

enisoprost—a drug given in conjunction with cyclosporine (Sandimmune) to decrease its toxicity in organ transplant patients.

Enkaid (encainide).

ENL (erythema nodosum leprosum).

Enlon-Plus (atropine and edrophonium)—blocks the effects of muscle relaxants used in general anesthesia.

enoxacin (Penetrex)—a fluoroquinolone type of broad-spectrum antibiotic used to treat gonorrhea and urinary tract infections.

enoxaparin (Lovenox)—a low molecular weight heparin that is given postoperatively to patients after hip replacement surgery to prevent deep venous thrombosis.

ENP (extractable nucleoprotein).

Ensemble contrast imaging (ECI)—used with Sonoline Elegra ultrasound platform to improve detection and characterization of organ tumors.

EnSite—cardiac catheter and cardiac mapping procedure.

Ensure Plus—a liquid diet formula.

entacapone—drug to treat Parkinson's disease in patients taking levodopa.

Entamoeba histolytica—parasite which can be very virulent in AIDS.

ENTec Coblator Plasma Surgery System—provides precise, rapid incisions and channeling of submucosal tissue with minimal thermal injury to surrounding tissue, using Coblation technology. Used for physician-office tonsillotomy, to debulk the tonsil rather than remove it.

ENTec Plasma Wands—used to apply radiofrequency in Coblation-Channeling techniques.

Entera-Flo—enteral feeding pump for use with Entera closed tube feeding products that look like boxed drink containers.

enteral—pertaining to the small intestine or to administration of a drug or solution via the small intestine. Example: enteral feedings via tube. Cf. *parenteral.*

enterically transmitted non-A, non-B hepatitis (ENANB).

Enterobacter liquefaciens—now *Serratia liquefaciens.*

Enterobacter sakazakii—formerly *E. cloacae.*

enterocleisis—closure of a wound in the intestine. Also, occlusion of the lumen of the intestine. Cf. *enteroclysis.*

enteroclysis—the injection of a nutritional or medicinal liquid into the bowel. Cf. *enterocleisis.*

enterokinase—an enzyme of the small intestine.

enteropathy-associated T-cell lymphoma (EATL)—a highly aggressive neoplasm.

enteroscope vs. endoscope—sound-alikes that can be confused in dictation; the former is used for the small intestine, the latter for upper or lower GI tract.

Entero-Test—a method for retrieving duodenal contents without intubation; the patient swallows a nylon line coiled inside a gelatin capsule.

enterotoxigenic *Escherichia coli* (ETEC).

Entero Vu (barium sulfate for suspension)—low-density contrast medium used in "see-through" radiographic studies of the small bowel.

Enterra—gastrointestinal "pacemaker" that shocks nerves lining the stomach that control how it digests food. Useful in patients with severe gastroparesis that causes continual nausea, vomiting, and pain.

Entity pacemaker.

Entocort CR (budesonide)—a controlled release formulation for the acute treatment of mild-to-moderate Crohn's disease.

Entree Plus and **Entree II** trocar and cannula systems for laparoscopic surgery. Also referred to as *Core trocars and cannulas*.

Entree—thoracoscopy trocar and cannula.

EntriStar PEG (percutaneous endoscopic gastrostomy) **tube**—polyethylene feeding gastrostomy (or jejunostomy) tube inserted using percutaneous endoscopy. It has a larger internal diameter than other tubes to avoid clogging. The catheter end closes for insertion and removal but opens into a flow-through, three-dimensional star shape in the stomach to maintain tube position and prevent tip obstruction.

enucleation—removal of the eyeball, without taking the eye muscles or the remaining orbital contents. Also, shelling out a tumor from its bed without rupturing it. See also *evisceration, exenteration, extirpation*.

enuresis—bed-wetting. Enuresis differs from incontinence in that enuresis more commonly refers to involuntary discharge of urine during sleep. Cf. *anuresis*.

Envacor—a lab test of two HIV proteins.

Enzogenol—antioxidant derived from the bark of the *Pinus radiata* tree in New Zealand.

enzymatic debriding agents—agents that are selective in removing necrotic tissue. They loosen necrotic debris so that surgical debridement may be avoided. Enzymatic agents act on materials such as collagen, protein, fibrin, elastin, and nucleoproteins. See *dressing*.

enzyme immunoassay technique—screens drugs in the urine that have been present for up to 7 days.

enzyme-linked immunoassay (EIA).

enzyme-linked immunosorbent assay (ELISA).

EOA (esophageal obturator airway).

EOG (electro-oculogram)—used in sleep studies, as in "EOG does show some rapid eye movement."

eosinophilia-myalgia syndrome (EMS) —multisystem disease with neuromuscular manifestations, the correct name for the group of symptoms resulting from the use of the amino acid L-tryptophan. The clinical picture of severe myalgia, fever, cramps, weakness, and arthralgias can be confused with myositis or trichinosis unless a history of L-tryptophan use is established.

eosinophilic pustular folliculitis—a pruritic skin condition with sterile follicular pustules on an expanding erythematous plaque. Biopsy of pustules at the advancing edge of the plaque shows an eosinophilic abscess within the follicle or sebaceous gland. Before its association with AIDS, this condition had been reported mostly in Japan and affected mostly males.

Eovist (gadolinium EOB-DTPA)—MRI contrast agent for imaging of liver.

EP (endoscopic papillectomy).

EP (evoked potential).

EPA (eicosapentaenoic acid).

EPAP (expiratory positive airway pressure).

ependyma—cells lining the fluid-filled central cavity of the brain and spinal cord.

ependymitis granularis—granular inflammation of the lining membrane of the ventricles of the brain.

ependymoma—tumor originating from ependymal cells lining the ventricular system of the central nervous system.

"epi"—slang term for epinephrine (Adrenalin). Can also refer to epithelial cell seen in urinalysis. See *Eppy*.

EPI (echo planar imaging) (MRI term).

EPI (epirubicin).

epi-ADR, epi-Adriamycin (epirubicin).

EPIC-C or EPICS Profile flow cytometer.

Epicel autologous skin cells—a tissue repair product.

Epic ophthalmic 3-in-1 laser system.

epicritic two-point sensation (Neuro).

epidermal growth factor (EGF)—given to increase the rate of corneal healing after corneal transplant surgery. Used to accelerate wound healing in partial-thickness wounds and second-degree burns.

epidermodysplasia verruciformis—a rare lifelong disease that is a model of cutaneous genetic cancer induced by specific human papillomaviruses.

epidermolysis bullosa acquisita (Derm)—an acquired blistering skin disease caused by autoantibodies to the dermoepidermal junction of the skin.

epididymal sperm aspiration (ESA).

epididymovasostomy—see *microsurgical epididymovasostomy*.

epidural blood patch—injection of the patient's own blood into space around the spine. This is done to repair holes or tears in the spinal fluid sac; it leads to a temporary blood clot that allows time for the sac wall to repair itself.

EpiE-ZPen (epinephrine 0.3 mg and 0.15 mg)—an autoinjector for use by patients in the emergency treatment of allergic reactions. The device resembles a fountain pen, with a pocket clip for easy carrying. It is disposable and contains a cartridge filled with epinephrine with push-button activation.

EpiFilm otologic lamina—a biological dressing used to enhance healing of exposed bone during otologic surgery.

Epi-Grip—a medical device used in cardiopulmonary bypass surgery to improve the presentation and isolation of the bypass site.

epihidrosis—excessive perspiration.

EpiLaser—laser-based hair removal system.

epileptic equivalent—as in migraine equivalent, some or all of the symptom complex without the convulsion. See *migraine equivalent*.

epileptogenic focus—the area in which tumor-related seizures originate.

Epi-lock—polyurethane foam wound dressing.

epinephrine—used as an adjunct with local anesthetic to prolong the effectiveness of the anesthetic agent used and to constrict superficial blood vessels. Also, *racemic epinephrine*. Cf. *"epi," Eppy*.

epiphysis—the end of a long bone, usually wider than the long portion of the bone. Cf. *apophysis, hypophysis, hypothesis*.

epirubicin (epi-Adriamycin, epi-ADR, EPI)—a chemotherapy drug.

episcleral plaque brachytherapy—treatment of subretinal fluid caused by circumscribed choroidal hemangiomas. Cf. *lens-sparing external beam radiation therapy*.

Epistat double balloon—used in treatment of uncontrolled epistaxis.

epistaxis—nasal bleeding.

epithelial membrane antigen (EMA) —pathologic finding in benign cystic mesothelioma.

epithelial turn-in flap (ENT)—used for reconstruction of the internal lining in full-thickness nasal defects.

EpiTouch—a laser used for hair removal and in the treatment of tattoos and pigmented lesions.

Epitrain (Ortho)—an elastic elbow support with contoured silicone inserts.

Epivir (lamivudine)—oral antiviral drug used to treat HIV.

Epivir-HBV (lamivudine)—oral antiviral drug used for treatment of adults with chronic hepatitis B.

Epivir/Retrovir (lamivudine/zidovudine)—combination AIDS drug.

EPL (extracorporeal piezoelectric lithotriptor)—see *Piezolith-EPL*.

EPO—a synthetic form of erythropoietin. It is given to stimulate red blood cell production in AIDS patients taking zidovudine (Retrovir). See also *epoetin alfa*.

EPOCH (etoposide, prednisone, Oncovin, cyclophosphamide, Halotestin) —chemotherapy protocol for refractory lymphoma.

epoetin alfa (*not* alpha) (erythropoietin; Epogen; Procrit)—a genetically engineered erythropoietin used in treatment of severe anemias (such as those that are a side effect of dialysis or AZT therapy), and anemia found in patients who are in chronic kidney failure.

epoetin beta (Marogen)—used to treat the anemia associated with end-stage renal disease.

Epogen (epoetin alfa).

epoxyeicosatrienoic acids—compounds produced naturally in the body that trigger arteries to dilate and help prevent adhesion of monocytes to artery walls, thus lessening atherosclerotic plaque build-up.

eprosartan mesylate (Teveten).

EPS (electrophysiologic study)—used to assess ventricular arrhythmias.

Epstein-Barr virus (EBV)—the herpeslike virus known to cause mononucleosis, with evidence that it plays a part in susceptibility to Burkitt's lymphoma, and possibly to AIDS.

ePTFE (expanded polytetrafluoroethylene)—used for facial implants in plastic and reconstructive surgery.

eptifibatide—an antiangina drug that works by inhibiting the receptor that causes platelets to bind together and form a clot.

Equate *Legionella* water test—an on-site detection of *Legionella* bacteria in water supplies.

equilibratory ataxia—the disturbance of equilibratory coordination, with abnormal gait and station. On testing gait and station, the physician is ruling in/out lesions of the vermis, labyrinthine-vestibular apparatus, and frontopontocerebellar pathways.

Equinox occlusion balloon system— for occluding and controlling distal blood flow during vascular procedures. The balloon is introduced via the SilverSpeed guide wire.

equipment artifact (Radiol)—produced by some equipment, such as surgical sponges or pillows used for patient positioning, that is not radiopaque as advertised.

equivalent—as in anginal equivalent, migraine equivalent, epilepsy equivalent. An atypical pain syndrome in

equivalent *(cont.)*
which the location or character of the pain differs from that usually experienced. "It is not clear whether this left shoulder discomfort radiating down his arm is arthritic or may be an anginal equivalent." Cf. *milli-equivalent.*

ER (estrogen receptor).

ER (evoked response) (Neuro).

ERA (endometrial resection and ablation) **resectoscope sheath**—used for minimally invasive procedures such as endometrial resection and ablation, myomectomy, and polypectomy.

ERBD (endoscopic retrograde biliary drainage).

Erb-Duchenne paralysis—see *Erb's palsy.*

erbium:YAG infrared laser (Er: YAG) —now approved for use directly on teeth. The laser has been shown to be as safe and effective as high-speed drills for removing dental decay.

Erb's palsy—injury to the fifth and sixth cervical roots, causing flaccid paralysis of the entire arm, without involving the small muscles of the hand. Also called *Erb-Duchenne paralysis* and *Duchenne's paralysis.*

ERC (endoscopic retrograde cholangiography).

ERCP (endoscopic retrograde cholangiopancreatogram)—study of the gallbladder, pancreas, and biliary system through an endoscope and a special cannula.

ErCr:YAG (erbium chromium: yttrium-aluminum-garnet) **laser**.

Erdheim-Chester disease—a rare lipid storage disorder characterized by hardening of the growth areas of the long bones of the body. Lipid cell deposits (histiocytes) are found in various vital organs of the body such as heart, lungs, peritoneum, kidneys, and other tissues. Severity of the disease differs with each patient, but the cause is unknown and the outcome is generally fatal.

ErecAid system—nonsurgical treatment for erectile impotence.

ERG (electroretinogram)—see *flicker electroretinogram.*

Ergamisol (levamisole)—for detection of coronary artery disease.

Ergoset tablets—used to reduce blood sugar levels while lowering certain blood lipids in obese type 2 diabetics.

Ergos O$_2$ pacemaker—a dual chamber rate-responsive pacemaker.

Erich arch bar (Oral Surg).

Erlanger and Gasser—classification of peripheral nerves.

Ernest-McDonald soft IOL folding forceps—used for placement of thin, soft intraocular lenses.

erogenous zones—areas of the body that produce feelings of sexual desire when stimulated. Cf. *aerogenous.*

Eros-CTD (clitoral therapy device)— treatment for female sexual dysfunction (FSD).

ERT (estrogen replacement therapy).

ERT patch—for treatment of vasomotor symptoms related to menopause.

Erwinase—trade name for *Erwinia* L-asparaginase, for acute lymphocytic leukemia.

Erwinia **L-asparaginase**—a chemotherapy drug used to treat acute lymphoblastic leukemia. *Erwinia* is a gram-negative bacterium which provides the enzyme L-asparaginase

Erwinia (cont.)
aminohydrolase contained in this version of L-asparaginase. *Erwinia* is used as a source of this enzyme rather than the original source, the gram-negative bacterium *E. coli*, because some patients exhibit sensitivity to the *E. coli*-derived version of L-asparaginase.

ERYC (pronounced "Eric" or "airy-C")—an erythromycin capsule containing enteric-coated little pellets, or beads; an antibiotic.

Ery-Tab—trade name for an enteric-coated erythromycin tablet.

erythema migrans (EM)—a rash that appears after a bite of the tick (*Ixodes dammini*) that transmits the organism (*Borrelia burgdorferi*) that causes Lyme disease. The rash is circular in form, target-like, may disappear and reappear, often in another site (hence migrans). It may be the first symptom of Lyme disease. See *target lesion*.

erythema nodosum leprosum (ENL) —a skin complication of leprosy.

erythematous vulvitis en plaque—see *vulvar vestibulitis syndrome*.

Erythroflex—a hydromer-coated central venous catheter that resists thrombus formation.

erythroplasia of Queyrat—an intraepidermal squamous cell carcinoma that presents as a well-demarcated moist red patch on the penis. Also referred to as *carcinoma in situ of the glans penis*.

erythropoietin, recombinant human (Eprex, Marogen)—for anemia in patients with AIDS or end-stage renal failure.

ES (endoscopic sphincterotomy).

ESA (epididymal sperm aspiration).

ESAT-6 protein—may be effective in diagnosing *Mycobacterium tuberculosis*.

Escala Inteligencia Wechsler Para Adultos (EIWA).

escape pacemaker (Cardiol). Unless an escape pacemaker takes over pacing the ventricles, ventricular standstill occurs and there will be only P waves on the EKG tracing.

Esclim—estradiol transdermal system for treatment of vasomotor symptoms of menopause, vulvar and vaginal atrophy, and abnormal vaginal bleeding.

E-Scope—electronic stethoscope that allows amplification of heart, breath, and Korotkoff sounds without accentuation of background noise. Can be used with hearing aid or second listener.

Escort balloon stone extractor—designed for easy cannulation and fluoroscopic visibility.

ESLD (end-stage liver disease).

Esmarch ("Ez-mark") **bandage**—used as a tourniquet.

esmolol HCl (Brevibloc)—a cardiac medication for control, or conversion, of atrial fibrillation or flutter.

esodeviation ("ee-so")—inward deviation of the eye; also, *esotropia, esophoria*.

EsophaCoil self-expanding esophageal stent—used to minimize dysphagia and help restore swallowing and nutritional intake for patients with malignant strictures.

esophageal achalasia—failure of the esophagogastric sphincter to relax in swallowing, resulting in dilation. It is treated with laparoscopic Heller myotomy and Toupet fundoplication.

esophageal dysmotility (Radiol)—seen on upper GI series; abnormality in the strength or coordination of peristaltic movements in the esophagus.

esophageal gastric tube airways (EGTA).

esophageal obturator airways (EOA).

esophageal pill electrode—a disposable EKG lead encased in a gelatin capsule which is swallowed by the patient. Two attached wires exit through the patient's mouth and are attached to an EKG machine. When the gelatin capsule dissolves, electrical activity from the heart can be detected. The esophageal electrode is thus better able to record the electrical activity of the atrial contraction which is obscured with standard EKG leads.

esophageal sling procedure—see *ligamentum teres cardiopexy*.

esophageal stenosis, congenital—see *congenital esophageal stenosis*.

esophagogastroduodenoscopy (EGD) —examination of the esophagus, stomach, and duodenum using an endoscope.

esotropia—turning inward of the eye; crossed-eye or cross-eyed.

ESP—automated blood culture system.

esprolol—potent, rapid-acting sublingual beta-blocker; possible indications are for treatment of migraine, anxiety attacks, and tachycardia.

esprolol plus Viagra (sildenafil citrate) —medication regimen thought to protect men with heart disease who are also taking Viagra.

ESRD (end-stage renal disease).

Essiac—one of the most popular herbal cancer alternatives in North America, comprised of four herbs—burdock, Turkey rhubarb, sorrel, and slippery elm. Although illegal in the U.S., it is nevertheless widely available. Researchers at the Memorial Slone-Kettering Cancer Center claim it has no anticancer effect.

Estalis—combination estrogen/progesterone transdermal delivery system.

estazolam (ProSom)—a sedative drug of the benzodiazepine group (similar to Dalmane and Restoril). Used for short-term treatment of insomnia.

Esterman visual function score—used as the standard, adopted by the American Medical Association, for rating visual field disability (glaucoma). Obtained from the patient's responses to a disability questionnaire. Scores range from I-4-e to V-4-e. (Benjamin Esterman, M.D.)

esthetic(s)—relating to pleasing appearance, beautiful. While *aesthetic* is preferred in artistic contexts, *esthetic* is often seen in plastic, dental, and maxillofacial surgery journals.

estramustine—a conjugate of estradiol with nitrogen mustard.

estramustine binding protein (EMBP).

estramustine phosphate sodium (Emcyt)—hormonal chemotherapy drug. See *Emcyt*.

Estring—an estradiol-loaded silicone vaginal ring for treatment of postmenopausal women with symptoms of urogenital aging.

estrogen—may prevent stress-induced constriction in the arteries, as estrogen opens arteries and allows blood to flow freely in conditions of cold-related stress. Angina and heart attacks occur more often in cold weather.

estrogen receptor (ER)—a cytoplasmic protein. Estrogen receptor tests of breast cancer tissue reflect the degree

estrogen *(cont.)*
of hormone dependency of that particular breast cancer. If there is a high degree of hormone dependency, an oophorectomy may be performed to alter the course of the disease.

estrogen replacement therapy (ERT) —now used to treat symptoms of stress urinary incontinence. Estrogen (given orally, as a transdermal patch, or applied vaginally as a topical cream) has long been used to counteract the symptoms of vaginal dryness, hot flashes, and fatigue experienced by postmenopausal women. It is now known that decreased levels of estrogen have an adverse effect on the function of the urethra as well as the genitalia. The urethra has a concentration of estrogen receptors similar to that of the vagina. Decreased estrogen levels alter nerve conduction and elasticity of the urethral mucosa. Restoring estrogen levels to normal appears to decrease stress urinary incontinence in some women.

estropipate (Ortho-est)—a drug given to postmenopausal women to treat symptoms of vaginal atrophy and hot flashes.

Estrostep (norethindrone acetate and ethinyl estradiol)—oral contraceptive pill that works by releasing low but graduated doses of estrogen, in conjunction with a constant dose of progestin, over the course of a woman's menstrual cycle.

ESU (electrosurgical unit) **dispersive** (grounding) **pad**.

ESWL (extracorporeal shock-wave lithotripsy). See *lithotriptor*.

ET (embryo transfer).

etafilcon A (Acuvue)—disposable contact lens.

ETCG (endoscopic transpapillary catheterization of the gallbladder).

ETCO$_2$ (end-tidal carbon dioxide).

ETEC (enterotoxigenic *Escherichia coli*).

Ethalloy TruTaper cardiovascular needle.

ethambutol (Myambutol)—a drug used to treat tuberculosis, and now used to treat MAC infection in AIDS patients.

ethanol—alcohol, EtOH.

ethers—see *dihematoporphyrin ethers*.

Ethibond—polyester suture with prethreaded Teflon pledgets.

Ethicon—manufacturer of Teflon paste and numerous surgical products.

Ethiflex—a synthetic suture material. Ethibond, Ethiflex, and Ethilon sutures are all manufactured by Ethicon, but they have different coating materials.

Ethilon—a monofilament nylon suture with extremely low tissue reactions. It comes in black, green, and clear and is a nonabsorbable suture.

Ethmozine (moricizine)—antiarrhythmic.

Ethodian (iophendylate)—a radiopaque contrast medium and diagnostic aid.

ethylene vinyl alcohol (EVAL).

Ethyol (amifostine)—injection for reduction of moderate to severe xerostomia in patients undergoing postoperative radiation treatment for head and neck cancer.

etidronate (Didronel)—a drug that, when taken with calcium supplements, has been found to increase bone mass in women with osteoporosis; it can also reduce the inci-

etidronate *(cont.)*
dence of spontaneous fractures experienced by these patients.

E to A changes—on chest examination the patient's "e" sounds like "a" through a stethoscope. The sound of "e" indicates normal lung, "a" indicates consolidated lung.

etodolac (Apo-Etodolac, Lodine, Lodine XL)—an analgesic and nonsteroidal anti-inflammatory drug for use in pain relief and for patients with osteoarthritis.

etoglucid (also ethoglucid)—a chemotherapy drug for transitional cell bladder carcinoma, administered intravesically.

EtOH (lowercase "t")—ethanol, ethyl alcohol.

etoposide injection (VePesid, VP-16)—chemotherapy agent for use in the treatment of refractory testicular tumors and small cell lung carcinoma (or cancer), as well as Kaposi's sarcoma.

e-TRAIN 110 AngioJet catheter.

ETT (exercise tolerance test)—see *MPHR and Bruce protocol.*

EUA (examination under anesthesia).

Eucerin—proprietary name of wool fat-based cream.

euglobulin lysis activity (ELA).

eukaryotic cells—cells with a true nucleus.

Eulexin (flutamide)—drug therapy for patients with prostate cancer and minimal metastatic bone disease.

Eulexin plus LHRH-A—a protocol for treating advanced prostate carcinoma patients. It combines drug therapy with radiation therapy to provide improved clinical outcomes.

Euro-Collins multiorgan perfusion kit—used for organ procurement and preservation.

EUS (endoscopic ultrasonography).

EUS-FNA (endoscopic ultrasound-guided fine needle aspiration).

euthymic—normal thymus gland function.

euthyroid—normal thyroid gland function.

EVA (etoposide, vinblastine, Adriamycin)—chemotherapy protocol for Hodgkin's disease.

EVac—wet field wand for tissue ablation, coagulation, and suction in tonsillotomy.

EVac CAT—minimally invasive procedure for the treatment of snoring, with the creation of channels in the soft palate.

Evacet—liposome-encapsulated doxorubicin for treatment of metastatic breast cancer.

Evac-Q-Kwik (bisacodyl)—administered orally as a bowel prep to clean the colon prior to x-ray.

EVAL (ethylene vinyl alcohol)—used for liquid embolization of spinal angiomas (as in Cobb's syndrome). EVAL (not a glue) is used in the same way as cyanoacrylate.

Evalose—lactulose solution used as a laxative.

Evans-Burkhalter protocol—rehabilitation following tendon repair.

Evans tenodesis—reconstruction of the peroneus brevis tendon to treat chronic lateral ankle instability by reattaching the tendon to the muscle in a slightly overlapped fashion.

Eve procedure—the transfer of vascularized seventh rib, fascia, cartilage, and serratus muscle to other anatomic areas to reconstruct severe defects. The procedure is named for Eve, who in the Bible was said to be created from one of Adam's ribs.

Evershears—a surgical instrument that combines a curved scissors tip at the end of a bipolar electrocautery. Used in laparoscopic surgery.

Evershears II bipolar curved scissors—bipolar curved scissors with cutting and coagulating capability indicated for use in laparoscopic surgical procedures.

Evert-O-Cath—drug delivery catheter.

evisceration—(1) removal of the contents of the eyeball, but leaving the shell of sclera—see *enucleation*; (2) disemboweling; exenteration; extirpation; splitting open of a surgical wound and subsequent spillage of its contents.

EVIS 140 endoscope reprocessing system.

Evista (raloxifene hydrochloride)—a selective estrogen receptor modulator (SERM) used to prevent osteoporosis in postmenopausal women.

EVL (endoscopic variceal ligation).

evoked potential (EP)—a noninvasive way to examine the functional integrity of the central nervous system. It demonstrates the response of the brain to electrical stimulation. EPs are used as indicators, both diagnostic and prognostic, in patients with head injuries. See *brain tests, noninvasive*.

evoked response (ER) (Neuro)—see *brain tests, noninvasive*; also *EP*.

Evolution XP scanner—an ultrafast CT scanner.

Evolve Cardiac Continuum—designed to support physicians in a systematic approach from open-chest surgery to endoscopic beating-heart surgery, integrating computer and robotic technology.

Evoxac (cevimeline hydrochloride)—for treatment of dry mouth in patients with Sjögren's syndrome.

EVS (endoscopic variceal sclerotherapy)—to control variceal hemorrhage, particularly due to portal hypertension.

EVUS (endovaginal ultrasound).

Ewald tube—used in gastric lavage.

Ewart's sign—pericardial effusion.

Ewing's sarcoma—osteosarcoma.

Exact-Fit ATH—hip replacement system.

ExacTech blood glucose meter—for self-testing by diabetics.

examination—see *test*.

eXamine cholangiography catheter.

excavatum, pectus—*not* excurvatum.

Excelart—short-bore MRI with wide opening, said to be very quiet.

eXcel-DR (disposable/reusable) **instruments**
a-fiX cannula seals
eXcel-DR pneumo needle
cXpose retractor
eXtract specimen bag
hcliX knot pusher

Excel GE—electrochemical glucose monitoring test strip for use with Glucometer Elite R meters.

excess—the degree or state of surplus, or beyond the usual, as "There was excess peritoneal fluid present." See *base excess*. Cf. *access, axis*.

excimer laser—*excimer,* a word coined from *excited dimer*. The laser uses ultraviolet light.

excimer laser coronary angioplasty (ELCA)—used in percutaneous revascularization for coronary artery disease.

excision—removal, as of an organ, by cutting. Cf. *incision*.

Exelderm (sulconazole nitrate).

Exelon (rivastigmine tartrate)—cholinesterase inhibitor for treatment of mild to moderate Alzheimer's disease.

exenterative surgery for pelvic cancer —removal of organs and adjacent structures of the pelvis. Usually performed to surgically ablate cancer involving urinary bladder, uterine cervix, and/or rectum.

exercise tolerance test (ETT).

EX-FI-RE external fixation system— for reduction and fixation of long bones and for limb lengthening.

Exidine (chlorhexidine gluconate 4%) —a preoperative prep solution; a broad spectrum antimicrobial. Also Exidine Skin Cleanser; Exidine-2 Scrub; Exidine-4 Scrub.

exodeviation—outward deviation of the eye; also, exotropia, exophoria.

Exogen SAFHS (sonic accelerated fracture healing system)—a low-intensity ultrasound therapy in an in-home, non-invasive, portable unit.

Exorcist—a respiratory compensation technique—MRI term.

Exosurf Neonatal (colfosceril palmitate) —a synthetic surfactant used to supplement low levels of natural surfactant in the lungs of premature infants suffering from respiratory distress syndrome, also known as *hyaline membrane disease.* Surfactant maintains surface tension to prevent the lungs from collapsing with each breath. It is administered via an endotracheal tube. It is also being tested in patients with cystic fibrosis, apnea of prematurity, adult respiratory distress syndrome, and asthma. See *RDS, Survanta.*

expandable access catheter (EAC).

expandable esophageal stent (EES).

expandable metallic stent—used as an alternative to the plastic stent. It offers ease of insertion and lack of migration. Its risks include erosion of adjacent vital structures, difficulty in adjustment or removal, and overgrowth of malignant tissue.

expiratory positive airway pressure (EPAP).

expire—to exhale, or to take one's last breath, i.e., to die.

eXpose (trademark) **retractor**—comes in three shapes: inflatable triangle, U, and wand shapes. (Note the initial lowercase *e* and capital *X*.)

Express PTCA catheter (percutaneous transluminal coronary angioplasty).

exquisite—said of extremely severe pain or tenderness, as exquisite tenderness of the breast.

exstrophy—congenital eversion of an organ, as of the bladder.

extended right hepatectomy—a surgical option in patients with hilar bile duct cancer.

extension (*not* extention).

extensive intraductal component (EIC) —risk factor leading to recurrence in young women with breast cancer.

external beam radiation therapy (EBRT)—using linear accelerator or cobalt machine, to irradiate internal structures from an external source.

external cephalic version (ECV) (Ob-Gyn)—repositioning of a fetus using I.V. terbutaline and vibroacoustic stimulation. It is performed to avoid vaginal breech delivery or cesarean section.

extinction phenomenon—when the patient is touched in the same area on both sides of the body and perceives it on only one side. May be indicative of a lesion of the sensory cortex.

extirpation—see *evisceration*.

extracapsular cataract extraction (ECCE).

extracellular-like, calcium-free solution (ECS).

extracellular matrix (ECM).

extracorporeal circulation—using the heart-lung machine to provide circulation outside the body during heart surgery.

extracorporeal membrane oxygenation therapy (ECMO).

extracorporeal photoimmune therapy —involves use of ultraviolet or visible light and compounds that are activated by such light to alter function of blood cells or blood components. See also *photophoresis*.

extracorporeal piezoelectric lithotriptor (Piezolith-EPL)—device with a single-focus dish which directs all of the shock waves to the renal stone or gallstone, eliminating any unfocused shock waves that could cause the patient pain or discomfort (thus eliminating the need for anesthesia). The stone is reduced to fragments 2 mm or less in size which are then readily passed by the patient.

extracorporeal shock-wave lithotripsy (ESWL)—see *lithotriptor*.

extractor—an instrument to remove a metal implant from bone. See *Glassman stone extractor*.

Extractor three-lumen retrieval balloon.

eXtract specimen bag—an expandable bag for isolating organs or specimens retrieved during laparoscopic surgery, e.g., a gallbladder with stones, to prevent stone spillage in abdomen.

extraperitoneal excision of lower one-third of ureter—a urologic procedure making a bladder cuff without an initial vesicotomy, without injury to the opposite ureteric orifice. It is used to treat urothelial tumors of the kidney and ureter. Advantages of this procedure are said to be minimal blood loss, a small vesicotomy, and easy suturing of the bladder.

extrapyramidal signs (or symptoms)— involuntary movements such as tics or tremors, or impairment of involuntary movement such as rigidity, secondary to antipsychotic drugs or chemical imbalances in the brain. See *tardive dyskinesia*. Cf. *pyramidal signs, akathisia*.

Extra Sport coronary guide wire— coronary guide wire marketed under the ACS Hi-Torque group of guide wires.

extravasation detection accessory (EDA)—for use during contrast-enhanced CT studies performed with a power injector. The EDA keeps contrast material from leaking into surrounding soft tissues by halting the infusion when extravasation is detected.

extravasation of contrast—leakage of contrast medium from the structure into which it is injected through a perforation or other abnormal orifice.

Extra View balloon—used in laparoscopic procedures to create extraperitoneal space.

extremis, in—at the point of death.

ExtreSafe—needles, lancets, phlebotomy devices, catheters, syringes, and butterflies that minimize the risk of accidental needle sticks.

exudate, cotton-wool.

ExuDerm hydrocolloid dressing material.

Exu-Dry absorptive dressing.

ex vivo (L., outside of the living body). "He mentioned that in the near future there will be a commercial concern which is able to grow blood ex vivo and to have the cells then harvested for therapeutic transfusions."

ex vivo liver-directed gene therapy—used for the treatment of familial hypercholesterolemia. A liver segmentectomy is performed and the specimen delivered to the laboratory, where hepatocytes are isolated and exposed to a recombinant retrovirus. The hepatocytes are then harvested and infused back into the patient via the mesenteric vein.

eye movement tracking techniques—electro-oculography, infrared scleral reflection technique, Purkinje image tracking, scleral search coil, and video pupil scanning. They are valuable for early detection and localization of central nervous system lesions.

E-Z Flap—a mini-plate system constructed from titanium, used in neurosurgical procedures.

E-Z Flex jaw therapy—patented mandibular rehabilitation exercise system designed to treat pain in jaws and the sides of the face.

EZ-Screen Profile—urine drug screening test for marijuana, cocaine, opiates, arnphetamines, and PCP. The device was developed primarily for employers. The screening device is about the size of a credit card, no laboratory evaluation is required, and results are available in less than 10 minutes on site.

E-Z Tac soft-tissue reattachment system—cuts operative procedure time by securing soft tissues without sutures, without knot tying, and without the need for a guide wire.

eZY WRAP—orthopedic products including splints, abdominal binders, elbow supports, rib belts, and foam positioners.

F, f

F—Plasma F is plasma cortisol, or a dictator may speak of "free F in the urine."

FA (femoral anteversion)—hip dysplasia measurement in children with cerebral palsy.

Fab (fragment, antigen-binding)—acronym, as used in Fab fragment, Fab region, Fab segment. See *digoxin immune Fab (ovine) fragments*.

FAB (French/American/British)—morphologic classification of acute non-lymphoid leukemia, as used in the format, FAB T2N1M0 (no subscripts). See *TNM classification*.
M1 myeloblastic, with no differentiation
M2 myeloblastic, with differentiation
M3 promyelocytic
M4 myelomonocytic
M5 monocytic
M6 erythroleukemia

fabere sign—acronym for the maneuvers of Patrick's test for hip-joint disease: flexion, abduction, external rotation, extension.

Fabry's lipid storage disease (Oph)—verticillate (whorl-shaped) keratopathy.

facial—pertaining to the face. Cf. *falcial, fascial*.

facilitated angioplasty—so-called when adjunctive angioplasty is performed immediately after atherectomy or excimer laser angioplasty.

facioscapulohumeral dystrophy (FSHD).

facioscapulohumeral (FSH) muscular dystrophy.

faciotomy, medial (*not* fasciotomy)—a term coined for a somewhat rare procedure, also referred to as four-walled osteotomy or facial bipartition, for the skeletal treatment of orbital hypertelorism.

FAC-M (fluorouracil, Adriamycin, cyclophosphamide, methotrexate)—chemotherapy protocol.

FACS (fluorescence-activated cell sorter)—FACS-sorted cells.

FACScan (fluorescence-activated cell sorter) flow cytometer.

FACSVantage cell sorter.

Factive (gemifloxacin)—a potent quinolone antibiotic for the treatment of
respiratory and urinary tract infections.
factor—see also *cogulation factors*.
autocrine motility (AMF)
basic fibroblast growth (bFGF)
BeneFix hemophilia B blood clotting
blood coagulation
brain-derived neutrotrophic (BDNF)
cardiac risk
coagulation
corticotropin-releasing (CRF)
epidermal growth
fibroblast growth
human fibroblast growth factor-I
(FGF-I)
IGF-1 (insulin-like growth factor 1)
IL4-PE (interleukin-4-*Pseudomonas*
exotoxin fusion protein)
leukemia inhibitory (LIF)
megakaryocyte growth and
development (MGDF)
nerve growth (NGF)
recombinant human insulin-like
growth (rhIGF)
recombinant platelet-derived growth
(rPDGF)
ReFacto antihemophilic (recombinant)
Repifermin (keratinocyte growth
factor 2 [KGF-2])
Rh (Rhesus)
rheumatoid (RF)
Stuart
thymic humoral
tumor necrosis (TNF)
vascular endothelial growth (VEGF)
von Willebrand's (vWF)
FACT (Focal Angioplasty Catheter
Technology) coronary balloon angioplasty catheters.
FACT (Functional Assessment of Cancer Therapy)—a scale for assessing
the functional capabilities of cancer
patients while undergoing therapy.
factor V Leiden mutation test—uses
the power of the polymerase chain
reaction to amplify DNA from a
patient's blood to detect the presence
or absence of factor V Leiden mutation, which is the most common
inherited cause of a thrombotic tendency.
Factor III multimer assay.
Faden retropexy—posterior fixation
suture procedure used in strabismus
surgery.
Fader Tip ureteral stent—a Percuflex
stent with a tip that dissolves in one
to two hours in the body, leaving a
wide hole for maximum drainage.
fadir sign—acronym for maneuvers
used to test the hip joint: **f**lexion,
adduction, **i**nternal **r**otation.
Fagan test—used to detect retardation
in infants. A six-month-old is shown
a picture for a certain period of time.
Later, the infant is shown the same
picture and a new picture. The amount
of time the infant looks at the new picture correlates with overall intelligence.
failed back surgery syndrome (FBSS)
—seen in patients who have persistent
back pain following back surgery.
Further testing often reveals a migrat-
ed disk fragment, another disk herniation at a different level, previously
undetected lateral recess syndrome
(stenosis), a tethered nerve root, an
anomalous root, or tumor above the
level of the previous surgery.
failure to thrive (FTT)—in infants or
the severely debilitated, or a patient
making no progress despite treatment.
Fajersztajn's crossed sciatic sign.

falcial—see *falcine region*. Cf. *facial, fascial*.

falcine region—either the region of the falx cerebelli or the falx cerebri. Also *falcial*.

Falcon coronary catheter.

falloposcope (flexible fallopian tube endoscope).

falloposcopy—an imaging method used in diagnosis and treatment of infertility by providing views of the interior of the fallopian tube. In this procedure, a flexible catheter is inserted into the fallopian tube, after which a flexible fallopian tube endoscope (falloposcope) with imaging fibers is inserted and slowly withdrawn while taking images of the lumen of the tube.

Fallot's pentalogy—tetralogy of Fallot plus atrial septal defect. See *Fallot's trilogy, tetralogy of Fallot*.

Fallot's trilogy—congenital cyanotic heart disease that includes pulmonary stenosis and atrial septal defect, but does not have any ventricular septal defect. See *Fallot's pentalogy, tetralogy of Fallot*.

Falope ring (Ob-Gyn).

false labor—see *Braxton Hicks contractions*.

false memory syndrome (Psych)—a controversial condition in which an adult patient "recalls" episodes of childhood sexual abuse and sometimes memories of satanic ritual and child sacrifice for which there is no documentation available. The psychiatric community is split over the issue, some believing the patient's memories are of actual events; others believe the memories to have been prompted by overzealous counselors and the patient's desire to please the counselor. The American Psychiatric Association has issued a position statement on the syndrome and guidelines for evaluating patients with restored memories of traumatic events from infancy and childhood.

false negative—a test result that is normal or negative despite the presence in the patient of a disease or condition that would be expected to produce an abnormal or positive test result.

false positive—an abnormal or positive test result in a patient who is healthy or free from the condition tested for.

falx cerebri—a sickle-shaped fold of tough connective tissue partially separating the two cerebral hemispheres.

FAM (5-fluorouracil, Adriamycin, and mitomycin C)—chemotherapy protocol for recurrent gastric carcinoma, biliary tract carcinoma, and large-cell undifferentiated carcinomas.

FAM-CF (fluorouracil, Adriamycin, mitomycin, citrovorum factor)—chemotherapy protocol.

famciclovir (Famvir)—antiviral agent used for treatment of varicella-zoster virus (VZV) and herpes simplex virus types 1 and 2 (HSV-1, HSV-2) infections. Also for use in immunocompromised patients.

FAME (fluorouracil, Adriamycin, MeCCNU)—chemotherapy protocol.

familial visceral neuropathy—an inherited disorder characterized by polyneuropathy, ophthalmoplegia, leukoencephalopathy, and intestinal pseudo-obstruction. The latter is caused by destruction of the gastrointestinal myenteric plexus resulting in dysmotility, early satiety, bloating, nausea and vomiting, abdominal distention, diarrhea, weight

familial *(cont.)*
loss, and malnutrition. Neuronal destruction of other parts of the peripheral and central nervous system may be present as well. This syndrome can be fatal.

FAMMM (familial atypical multiple mole melanoma) **syndrome.**

FAMP (fludarabine monophosphate).

FAMTX (fluorouracil, Adriamycin, methotrexate [MTX] [with leucovorin rescue])—chemotherapy protocol for gastric carcinoma.

Famvir (famciclovir)—an antiviral drug used in the treatment of recurrent genital herpes and herpes zoster.

FANA (fluorescent antinuclear antibody).

Fansidar (sulfadoxine-pyrimethamine). Used for prophylaxis and treatment of chloroquine-resistant falciparum malaria. Also used as an AIDS drug.

FAP (5-fluorouracil, Adriamycin, and Platinol)—a standard chemotherapy protocol for gastric carcinoma.

FAPGAR—Family APGAR questionnaire. See *APGAR.*

FAPs (fibrillating action potentials).

Faraday shield—MRI term.

faradic (electrical) **stimulation**—named for Michael Faraday, English physicist, 1791-1867.

Fareston (toremifine citrate)—oral antiestrogen designed for treatment of metastatic breast cancer in postmenopausal women who are estrogen-receptor-positive or with unknown tumors.

farmer's lung disease—extrinsic allergic alveolitis caused by exposure to moldy hay.

Farr test—a specific test for anti-DNA antibodies in screening for systemic lupus erythematosus (SLE). High titers of anti-DNA antibodies would be diagnostic of SLE.

farsightedness—see *presbyopia.*

Fas—one of a family of cell-surface death receptors. One of the better known of this family is the smaller type 1 receptor for the cytokine tumor necrosis factor (TNF).

fascial—pertaining to the subcutaneous layer of fascia found throughout the body and encountered during surgery. Cf. *facial, falcial.*

fascia lata suburethral sling—used in treating recurrent urinary stress incontinence.

Fast-Cath introducer catheter.

Fastex—proprioceptive and agility test.

fast-Fourier transform (FFT)—MRI term.

fast low-angle shot (FLASH)—MRI term.

F.A.S.T. (First Access for Shock and Trauma) **1 System**—provides rapid, reliable access to a patient's blood stream to administer drugs and fluids for intraosseous infusion through a sternal insertion site.

fast spin-echo acquisition (MRI)—2-D or 3-D technique used in MR cholangiography.

FastTake electrochemical blood glucose monitoring system.

FASTak suture anchor system—used in arthroscopic surgery.

fast track product—a designation by FDA that means the agency will facilitate the development and expedite the review of a drug if it is intended for the treatment of a serious or life-threatening condition and it demonstrates the potential to address unmet medical needs for such a condition.

fast-twitch fibers (Sports Med)—fast runners have relatively more of these in their skeletal muscles than the rest of the population.

FasTrac guide wire—hydrophilic-coated guide wire for smooth tracking.

fat- and water-suppressed T2-weighted images (MRI)—used in the diagnosis of optic neuritis.

fat depot ("de-po")—area in the body of deposit of stored fat. "The face was very bony, showing loss of fat depots."

fat embolism syndrome (FES)—a type of adult respiratory distress syndrome. A complication of long-bone fracture or trauma to fatty tissues, FES occurs when an embolus of fat lodges in the lungs.

fat pad sign—distention and displacement of fat adjacent to a joint capsule, in elbow or knee, visible on x-ray with joint flexion. A sign of fracture within the joint. Example: "X-rays of the right elbow show no acute bony injury or any posterior fat pad sign per the radiologist's interpretation."

FAT SAT (fat saturation) technique.

fat towels (or wound towels)—used in surgery to protect tissues, to keep them from losing moisture.

Faulkner folder—an instrument that holds an intraocular lens in a folded position for insertion in cataract surgery.

faulty RF (radiofrequency) **shielding** in MRI scanner room.

FAZ (foveal avascular zone) (Oph).

FBI (food-borne illness).

FBSS (failed back surgery syndrome).

FCAP (fluorouracil, cyclophosphamide, Adriamycin, Platinol)—chemotherapy protocol for breast carcinoma.

FCE—see *Functional Capacity Evaluation.*

FCIS (Flint Colon Injury Scale).

F_ECO_2 (fraction of expired carbon dioxide)—recorded numerically on a capnograph.

FCR 9501HQ—a high-resolution storage phosphor imaging agent.

FCU (flexor carpi ulnaris).

FDI (frequency domain imaging)—in ultrasound.

FDP (fibrin degradation products).

FDT (fluorescein disappearance test).

FeatherTouch—CO_2 laser used in skin resurfacing to treat deep lines, wrinkles, scars, and hair transplantation.

FEB (fluorinated ethylene propylene).

FEC (fluorouracil, epirubicin, cyclophosphamide)—chemotherapy protocol for breast carcinoma.

fecal occult blood test (FEOT)—blood present in stool in too small an amount to be detected by naked-eye observation, but detectable by chemical testing or microscopic examination. See *guaiac*; *Hemoccult Sensa*; *Hemoccult II*; *occult blood.*

Fechtner syndrome—a form of hereditary thrombocytopenia associated with giant platelets, characterized by interstitial nephritis, congenital cataracts, and neurosensory deafness associated with Alport syndrome.

FDG (18-fluorodeoxyglucose) **positron emission tomography**.

FeatherTouch automated rasp—used in rhinoplasty procedures.

FED (fluorouracil, etoposide, DDP [cisplatin])—chemotherapy protocol.

Federici's sign—a sign of gas in the abdomen, or peritonitis, when cardiac sounds are heard on abdominal auscultation.

feeding mean arterial pressure (FMAP).

feeding solution—see *medication*.

feeding tube—see *tube*.

FEF$_{25-75}$ (forced midexpiratory flow).

Felbatol (felbamate)—an oral anticonvulsant. It is said to be more effective than other agents with fewer side effects, and is used for treatment of partial and generalized seizures, plus Lennox-Gastaut syndrome.

Felig insulin pump—worn externally.

fellow—the holder of a fellowship for teaching or research, an academic appointment carrying a stipend and providing facilities for postdoctoral study or research. Teaching fellow, research fellow.

felodipine (Plendil).

felon—an abscess of the fingertip. See *herpes whitlow*.

female genital mutilation—see *Sunna circumcision*, *clitoridectomy*, and *infibulation*.

female sexual dysfunction (FSD)—including symptoms such as lack of lubrication and lack of blood flow to the genital area.

Femara (letrozole) **tablets**—once-a-day therapy for postmenopausal women with advanced breast cancer. It prevents the body's manufacture of estrogen, a hormone that may stimulate growth of breast cancer in some patients.

femhrt or **FemHRT** (combination tablet containing norethindrone acetate and ethinyl estradiol)—for treatment of moderate to severe vasomotor symptoms associated with menopause, and prevention of postmenopausal osteoporosis.

femoral canal restrictor (Ortho).

FemoStop femoral artery compression arch.

FemPatch—a low-dose, transdermal estrogen replacement system, highly effective in relieving vasomotor menopausal symptoms.

Femprox—an alprostadil-based drug delivered topically to treat female sexual dysfunction, such as lack of lubrication and lack of blood flow to the genital area.

FemSoft insert—small, single-use liquid and silicone device for the treatment of stress urinary incontinence in women. The self-inserted device slides into and conforms to the urethra and creates a seal at the bladder neck to prevent unintended leakage. Available by prescription only.

Femstat 3 (butoconazole nitrate 2%) **vaginal cream**—an over-the-counter treatment for vaginal yeast infections.

femtoliter (fL)—unit of measurement in mean corpuscular volume (MCV). One-quadrillionth of a liter.

Femtosecond laser keratome system—essentially replaces microkeratomes, which use blades to create a corneal flap prior to laser vision correction procedures.

fencing-in—placing of laparoscopic or thoracoscopic ports too close together, which interferes with maneuverability of the instruments. See also *sword-fighting*.

fenestra ovalis; **fenestra vestibuli**—see *vestibular window*.

fenestrated Drake clip—for clipping of intracranial aneurysm.

fenestrated drape—sterile surgical drape with round opening to expose just the operative site.

fenestrated tracheostomy tube—tracheostomy tube with an opening on its upper surface that permits the patient to talk while still keeping the airway open.

fenestrating—the making of openings. Cf. *festinating*.

fenestration—a window-like inclusion in a cell caused by large cellular spaces called *vacuoles*.

fenoprofen (Nalfon)—a nonsteroidal anti-inflammatory drug.

fenoterol (Berotec)—an investigational bronchodilator for exercise-induced bronchospasm, acute asthma attacks, and maintenance therapy for chronic asthma and COPD.

fen-phen or **phen-fen diet**—weight loss program consisting of the anorectic medications fenfluramine (Pondimin) and phentermine (Fastin, Ionamine), and a reduced-calorie ADA diet. Fenfluramine has since been taken off the market due to association with cardiac valvular dysfunction.

fentanyl (Duragesic)—a narcotic available in a transdermal patch designed to provide 72 hours of continuous pain control in patients with cancer. Prior to development of the transdermal patch, fentanyl (Sublimaze) was commonly used in combination with inhaled anesthetics to maintain general anesthesia.

fentanyl citrate (Oralet lollypop)—a narcotic drug previously given by injection with regional or general anesthesia. Available in a candy-like oral tablet (to be sucked) for pediatric patients to relieve severe pain. Also available in lozenge form as a preanesthesia narcotic; patients are told to suck vigorously on the lollypop and usually become sedated in about ten minutes.

Feridex I.V. (ferumoxides injectable solution)—a contrast medium used in MRI scans to aid in detection of primary and metastatic liver cancer, imaging lesions as small as 3 mm.

fern test—used in obstetrics to determine the level of estrogen secretion; so-called because of the fernlike appearance of the cervical and uterine mucus when it dries on the glass slide.

Ferris chart—measures visual acuity.

Ferrlecit (sodium ferric gluconate)—used for iron supplementation in patients with iron-deficiency anemia.

ferromagnetic materials and MRI—a combination resulting in danger to patients having MRI scans. Ferromagnetic materials on or in a patient's body can result in burns and tissue tears during an MRI scan. Usually these are easy to detect, but shrapnel, prostheses, aneurysm clips, or pacemakers may be forgotten. At least one fatality has been reported because a stainless steel neurosurgical clip was actually ferromagnetic (there are several types of stainless steel). This shows once again the importance of accurate medical records, as operative reports should contain exact information about metallic implants.

Fertinex (urofollitropin)—injectable fertility treatment.

ferumoxsil (GastroMark) oral contrast agent.

FES (fat embolism syndrome).

FeSO₄—chemical symbol for iron sulfate.

FESS (functional endoscopic sinus surgery).

FES (functional endoscopic sinus) **surgery**.

festinating gait—the short, accelerating steps seen in patients with Parkinson's disease. Cf. *fenestrating*.

fetal fibronectin (fFN) **test**—a diagnostic test using cervical mucus to detect the presence of the protein, fetal fibronectin, to aid in detecting symptoms in women that may cause premature delivery.

fetal hydantoin syndrome—disorder that is caused by exposure of a fetus to phenytoin (Dilantin), an anticonvulsant drug prescribed for epilepsy. Major symptoms may include abnormalities of the skull and facial features, growth deficiencies, underdeveloped nails of the fingers and toes, and/or developmental delays.

fetal neuron allotransplantation—the implantation of fetal cells of human origin into adult brains; used successfully to treat patients with Parkinson's disease.

fetal-pelvic index—a method of determining the presence of fetal-pelvic disproportion which is said to be more accurate than estimated fetal weights by ultrasonography, the use of the Mengert index, or x-ray pelvimetry. A positive fetal-pelvic index indicates fetal-pelvic disproportion and the need for a cesarean section. A false negative result can occur in the presence of a malpositioned fetus.

fetal pig cell transplantation—a procedure in which fetal pig cells are transplanted into the brains of Parkinson's disease patients to restore dopamine to natural levels. (Parkinson's disease patients cannot produce enough dopamine, causing the brain to lose communication with the rest of the body.)

fetal small parts—the extremities of a fetus as felt through the mother's abdominal wall.

fetal ventral mesencephalic tissue transplantation—performed on parkinsonian patients in hopes of improving cognitive function.

FETENDO or **fetendo** (Ob-Gyn)—a coined word used to describe a fetoscopic approach, allowing the surgeon to work not only inside the uterus but also inside the fetus to view, endoscopically, the fetal trachea, esophagus, and bladder.

FEV (forced expiratory volume). The subscript, as in FEV_1, indicates the number of seconds in which the forced expiratory volume is measured.

FFL (floral variant of follicular lymphoma).

FFP (fresh frozen plasma).

FFT (fast-Fourier transform)—MRI term. See *Fourier analysis*.

FGF (fibroblast growth factor).

FGF-I (human fibroblast growth factor-I).

FGFR2 (fibroblast growth factor receptor 2).

FG-36UX linear scanning echoendoscope.

FIAC (fiacitabine).

fiacitabine (FIAC)—drug used to treat patients with HIV/AIDS and CMV infections.

fialuridine (FIAU)—drug used to treat patients with HIV/AIDS and herpesvirus infections; also chronic active hepatitis B.

FIAU (fialuridine).

Fiberlase—flexible and disposable beam delivery system for CO_2 surgical lasers developed for Surgilase unit.

fiberoptic bronchoscopy (FOB).

fiberoptic, fiber optic, fibreoptic—these three different spellings appear in different books and journals, with

fiberoptic *(cont.)*
fiberoptic the most common. *Fibreoptic* is a British spelling. See *Luxtec fiberoptic system*.

fiberoptic intracranial pressure monitor—instrument under development to measure brain temperature.

Fiblast (trafermin)—basic fibroblast growth factor (bFGF) used for the treatment of strokes and coronary artery disease.

Fibracol collagen-alginate dressing—nonadherent dressing that maintains its integrity when wet. It is used for treatment of ulcers, burns, and donor sites.

fibrillating action potentials (FAPs).

Fibrillex (NC-503)—for the treatment of secondary amyloidosis.

Fibrimage—technetium imaging agent used in detection of deep vein thrombosis.

fibrin degradation products (FDP)—important in coagulation process. Also, they show up on MRI scans, indicating that an earlier hemorrhage has occurred.

fibrin glue—a surgical adhesive. An example of usage from dictation: "I reconstituted the anterior wall of the sella with a piece of nasal septal cartilage, and then over this I applied fibrin glue in which I placed a piece of subcutaneous fat."

fibrin sealant—liquid biological tissue glue composed of thrombin and fibrinogen (blood products). It is used to stop air leaks and control bleeding in surgical and orthopedic procedures.

fibroblast growth factor (FGF).

fibrocystic breast syndrome—may be "a rose by any other name." A number of eponyms are used to identify this syndrome, including *Bloodgood's syndrome*, *Cheatle's syndrome*, *Cooper's syndrome*, *Reclus I syndrome* or *disease*, *Schimmelbusch's disease* or *syndrome*, and *Tillaux-Phocas* or *Phocas syndrome*. Cystic breast syndrome may also be called *blue dome syndrome*, *chronic cystic mastitis*, and *mastopathia chronica cystica*. Although there may be minute differences of meaning among these terms, they may also be used less discriminately. See also *breast fibrocystic disease stages*.

fibrodysplasia ossificans progressiva (FOP)—a rare hereditary disorder that manifests as ossification of skeletal muscle and connective tissue and congenital deformity of the bones. Occurs in childhood. No effective therapy is known.

fibrofatty infiltration of the pancreas.

fibroglandular tissue—a term used on mammogram reports, referring to the dense stroma of tissue made up of fibrous glandular tissue.

fibroid embolization—performed by an interventional radiologist, who makes a small incision in the groin (less than one-quarter inch), places a catheter into the femoral artery, and guides it to the uterine artery via x-ray imaging. Small particles are then injected into the uterine artery, cutting off the blood supply to the fibroid and dramatically shrinking it. A general anesthetic is not required.

fibroinflammatory pseudotumor of the middle and inner ear—characterized by total deafness in the affected ear and lack of response to caloric stimulation, destruction of inner ear structures, and atypical widening of parts of the labyrinth. A

fibroinflammatory *(cont.)* pseudotumor is a tumefactive fibroinflammatory lesion.

fibromuscular dysplasia (FMD).

fibrose—a verb meaning to form fibrous tissue. Cf. *fibrous.*

fibrous—an adjective describing something composed of fibers. Cf. *fibrose.*

fibroxanthogranulomatous—see *xanthogranulomatous cholecystitis.*

Fick method—calculates cardiac output. The oxygen content of exhaled air is measured to determine oxygen consumption in a patient undergoing cardiac catheterization. This is then compared to the oxygen levels from an arterial blood sample and a venous blood sample. The differences in oxygenation are used to calculate the cardiac output.

Fick sacculotomy—procedure for treatment of progressive endolymphatic hydrops (Ménière's disease). Picks are introduced through the footplate of the stapes to puncture the saccule, thus producing a permanent fistula in the saccular wall to drain endolymph into the perilymphatic space. See *Cody tack operation.*

FID (free induction decay)—MRI term.

field gradient; field lock—MRI terms.

field of view (FOV)—MRI term.

FiF (Functional Intact Fibrinogen) **test**.

FIGO (Fédération Internationale de Gynécologie et Obstétrique)—used in staging adenocarcinoma of the endometrium, e.g., FIGO II.

figure-4 position—so-called because in this position the patient lies with the right side of the body up and brings the right ankle up to rest on the left knee, forming the figure *4.*

Filcard temporary removable vena cava filter—used in local thrombolytic therapy.

fil d'Arion silicone tube (Oph).

filgrastim (Neupogen)—a white blood cell stimulator that counteracts the myelosuppression caused by chemotherapy. See *G-CSF.*

filiforms and followers—used to dilate a urethral stricture.

filling defect—a zone within a tubular structure that is not filled by injected contrast medium (usually a tumor or abnormal mass).

filling factor—MRI term.

filmy adhesion.

Filshie female sterilization clip—comparable to the Hulka clip and to tubal rings.

filtered-back projection (Radiol).

filtering bleb—a tiny, surgically coated vesicle, or blister, placed over a passageway into the eye to provide drainage in treatment of open-angle glaucoma.

filter replacement fluid (FRF)—given intravenously during CAVH (continuous arteriovenous hemofiltration) to maintain fluid balance.

filum terminale—threadlike extension of the spinal cord from conus medullaris to the tip of the dural sac.

finasteride (Propecia; Proscar)—the first of a class of drugs known as 5-alpha-reductase inhibitors. The drug inhibits the action of 5-alpha reductase, responsible for converting testosterone to dihydrotestosterone, the hormone causing the prostate to enlarge. Thus, the drug is able to reverse the benign prostatic hypertrophy seen in most men over age 50. However, only 50% of patients

finasteride *(cont.)*
taking the drug experience an actual decrease in their urinary symptoms. Patients who do respond positively to finasteride therapy must continue on the drug indefinitely.

fine-angled curet *(not* Fine) (Neuro).

fine-needle aspiration biopsy (FNAB). Also, *Skinny needle, Chiba needle.*

Finesse cardiac device.

Fine-Thornton scleral fixation ring— ophthalmic instrument that provides fixation of globe without injury.

Finger Blocking Tree—a hand therapy product for use during finger or thumb blocking exercises.

finger cot—surgical glove material to fit just one finger.

finger fracture—blunt dissection performed with the surgeon's fingers.

finger friction—"She cannot hear finger friction in either ear." Rubbing thumb and index finger together makes an audible rubbing sound. It may not be heard by someone with hearing loss.

fingerprint dystrophy—a corneal dystrophy characterized by fine, wavy, concentric lines that may be associated with a map- or dot-like pattern.

fingerstick devices for blood glucose testing: Autoclix, Autolet, Monojector.

finger-to-nose test (F to N). The patient is asked to touch his nose with the index finger of one hand and then the other, with the eyes closed, alternating hands and increasing speed. In a variation of this test, the patient is asked to touch his nose and then the examiner's finger at a distance of 12 to 18 inches, with increasing speed. This test is used to evaluate the patient's coordination, and may be

one of the neurologic tests administered in the physical examination.

finger-trap phenomenon (Ortho)—a rise in compartment pressure soon after fracture reduction and fixation.

Finkelstein's sign; test—for synovitis of the abductor pollicis longus tendon.

Finney Flexi-Rod penile prosthesis.

Finn hinged knee replacement prosthesis.

FIRDA (frontal irregular rhythmic delta activity)—in EEG. "Since the amplitude of the FIRDA was greatest over the left hemisphere, it may in this instance also suggest a possible left frontal structural lesion."

Firm D-Ring wrist support—a splint (manufactured by Rolyan) used to restrict wrist flexion and extension to help decrease pain and inflammation associated with severe tendinitis or ligament damage of the wrist.

first pass effect—metabolic action of the liver on drugs. A drug that is taken orally first passes through the liver before reaching the general circulation to exert any systemic effect. For some drugs the first-pass effect is so extensive that almost all of the drug dose is immediately metabolized. Some drugs are not metabolized and are excreted unchanged through the kidneys. A decreased rate of drug metabolism occurs in patients with liver diseases and hepatitis, impaired liver function due to aging, or immature liver function in premature infants.

first pass view (in multiple gated acquisition scan, or MUGA)—an image or set of images obtained immediately after injection of radionuclide into the circulation, when its

first pass view *(cont.)* concentration in the blood pool is at its highest.

FirstSave—automated external defibrillator (AED).

first-toe Jones repair.

Fisch drill (ENT)—named for Professor Ugo Fisch of University of Zurich.

fishbone pattern—seen in sclerotic white retinal arterioles and venules in lattice degeneration of the retina. Also called *crosshatch pattern*.

Fisher's exact test.

fish meal lung disease—extrinsic allergic alveolitis caused by exposure to fish meal.

fish-odor syndrome—primary trimethylaminuria, a rare condition that causes an individual to emit the odor of rotting fish. Caused by excessive bodily emission of trimethylamine (TMA), the problem may be a byproduct of digestion of choline-rich foods such as saltwater fish, eggs, and liver.

FISH (fluorescence in situ hybridization) **protocol in bone marrow transplantation**—a method to monitor engraftment in bone marrow transplantation patients.

fishtank granuloma—a skin infection caused by bacteria that live in aquatic environments. It is contracted by cleaning tanks without using gloves.

fissula—a little groove. Cf. *fissura, fistula.*

fissura—fissure, a general reference to a groove or cleft, e.g., fissura cerebri lateralis (fissure of Sylvius). Cf. *fissula, fistula.*

fistula (cf. *fissula, fissura*)—aberrant passage from one organ to another,

or from an organ through to the outside surface of the body. Types:
AV (arteriovenous)
brachioaxillary bridge graft
brachiosubclavian bridge graft
Brescia-Cimino AV
cameral
colovesical
digestive-respiratory fistula (DRF)
 Wallstent
perilymphatic (PLF)
rectovaginal
vesicovaginal

Fitz-Hugh and Curtis syndrome—gonococcal perihepatitis in women with a history of gonorrheal salpingitis.

5-ASA (5-aminosalicylic acid)—see *mesalamine.*

5-AZA (azacitidine)—a chemotherapy drug for acute myelogenous leukemia.

5-FU (5-fluorouracil)—antineoplastic chemotherapeutic agent.

5-HIAA (hydroxyindoleacetic acid)—substance found in the urine of patients with carcinoid tumors of intestine.

5-HT1, 5-HT2 receptors—two types of serotonin receptors present in the central nervous system which are stimulated by certain drugs such as buspirone (BuSpar) to relieve anxiety. Serotonin is also known as *5-hydroxytryptamine (5-HT).*

5-HT3 receptors—a serotonin receptor found in the chemoreceptor trigger zone of the brain and in the GI tract. The stimulation of these receptors is thought to trigger the vomiting reflex. The antiemetic drug ondansetron (Zofran) is the first drug in the class of 5-HT3 receptor blockers

5-HT3 *(cont.)*
and is used to prevent vomiting in chemotherapy patients.

5′nucleotidase (5′NT) ("five prime nucleotidase").

5-prong (or five-prong) **rake blade**—a self-retaining retractor blade.

566C80—drug used to treat *Pneumocystis carinii* pneumonia and toxoplasmosis in AIDS patients.

five-view chest x-ray (*not* 5-U)—AP, PA, lateral, and both oblique views. "A five-view chest x-ray series was obtained."

fixation device—any appliance placed surgically in or on a bone to stabilize a fracture during healing. See *device, implant, prosthesis.*

fixation switch diplopia—may be experienced by adults with a history of strabismus since childhood, if a change in their refractive error or use of glasses encourages fixation with their nondominant eye. If correctly diagnosed, this seldom-recognized cause of acquired diplopia in adults may be successfully treated with the proper optical management.

fixative (Path)—see *glycol methacrylate, Hollande's solution, Zenker's.*

FK-565—a drug used to treat HIV-positive patients.

fL (femtoliter).

FLAC (5-fluorouracil, leucovorin rescue, Adriamycin, cyclophosphamide)—chemotherapy protocol.

Flack's node—see *sinoatrial node.*

Flagyl ER—extended-release formulation containing 750 mg of the anti-infective agent metronidazole, for treatment of bacterial vaginosis.

flail chest (*not* frail)—movement of the chest wall inconsistent with respirations; caused by rib fractures.

FLAIR (fluid-attenuated inversion recovery) (MRI term).

flap—see also *graft.*
abdominal
axial
Bakanjian
bipedicle
butterfly
Chinese
cross-finger
Cutler-Beard bridge
deltopectoral
distant pedicle
epithelial turn-in
E-Z titanium
free
free flap transfer
gluteus myocutaneous
gracilis myocutaneous
groin
Gunderson conjunctival
Iselin flag
island
Karapandzic lip
Kazanjian midline forehead
lateral island
lateral transverse thigh (LTTF)
latissimus dorsi myocutaneous
liver
"maple leaf"
Martius labial fat pad
Martius urethral repair
McCraw gracilis myocutaneous
Moberg advancement
modified Martius
neurovascular
neurovascular pudendal–thigh
    fasciocutaneous
perineal artery fasciocutaneous
Pontén-type tubed pedicle
random transposition (rhomboid
    or Limberg)
Rubens
sliding plus pivoting

flap *(cont.)*
  thenar
  Thom
  TRAM (transverse rectus abdominis myocutaneous)
  transposition
  transverse rectus abdominis myocutaneous
  triangular island
  tummy tuck
  V-Y island
  Wolfe
  YV advancement

FLAP (fluorouracil, leucovorin rescue, Adriamycin, Platinol)—chemo-therapy protocol used to treat gastric adenocarcinoma.

flap tracheostomy—may be useful in the management of pediatric patients who require long-term bypass of the upper airway.

Flarex (fluorometholone acetate)—a steroid in ophthalmic solution.

flare—sudden exacerbation; a sudden outburst; a spreading out. Also a term used in ophthalmology, as in *aqueous flare, cell and flare, Tyndall effect.* (*Not* flair, which means an aptitude or bent, as in "She has a flair for writing.")

FLASH (fast low-angle shot)—an MRI term. "FLASH images were obtained with gradient echo technique."

flashlamp-pulsed Nd:YAG laser—used in lithotripsy by converting light into thermal energy.

flashlamp-pumped pulsed dye laser—used to treat uncomplicated and recalcitrant warts.

FlashPoint—image-guided surgical instruments that utilize CT and MRI data to provide surgeons with real-time visual localization of surgical instruments relative to a patient's anatomy during image-guided surgical procedures.

flash pulmonary edema with anuria—an atypical presentation of renovascular hypertension.

FlashTab—quick-dissolving oral tablet that requires no intake of liquid. This dosage form may be used in the future with a variety of medications and should be particularly useful for children or the elderly.

flat (or flattened) **affect**—diminished emotional response; apathy.

flat electroencephalogram—flat or isoelectric EEG recorded for at least 10 minutes in the absence of hypothermia or central nervous system depressants.

Flatt finger/thumb prosthesis.

Fleischer ring—a deposit of iron, ring-shaped, in the cornea; seen with keratoconus. See *Kayser-Fleischer ring.*

Fleischner's syndrome (Radiol)—actually not a syndrome. It's a linear or discoid shadow seen on radiographs, located in the lower third of one or both lungs.

"flesh-eating" bacteria—see *streptococcus A infection; necrotizing fasciitis; and toxic shock syndrome.*

Fletcher-Suit applicator—an appliance used for the insertion of radiation sources for treatment of carcinoma of the endometrium. Also, *Fletcher applicator.*

Fletcher-Suit-Delclos (FSD)—a mini-colpostat tandem and ovoids system. It is used for insertion of radioactive seeds for therapy of cervical cancer.

fleur de lis pattern—a breast reconstruction pattern used for latissimus dorsi reconstruction. This technique provides enough skin and fat overlying the muscle to create sufficient

fleur de lis *(cont.)*
volume without necessitating an implant.

FlexDerm hydrogel sheet.

Flexeril—a skeletal muscle relaxant. Often misspelled *Flexoril* because of its association with flexor muscles.

Flexguard tip catheter (Cardio).

Flexiblade laryngoscope—rigid laryngoscope with flexible blade for placement of tracheal tube and for examination and visualization of the upper airway.

flexible fallopian tube endoscope (falloposcope) (Gyn).

flexible steerable nasolaryngopharyngoscope.

Flexicath silicone subclavian cannula.

Flexiflo Lap G laparoscopic gastrostomy kit—believed to be an alternative to surgical gastrostomy and PEG. It uses a T-fastener that helps affix the stomach to the abdominal wall without tedious suturing and which can raise or lower the stomach for better visibility and retract it for stability during tube insertion. See *PEG*.

Flexiflo Lap J—a laparoscopic jejunostomy kit for direct jejunal feeding tube placement. This is fitted with a Brown/Mueller T-Fastener set.

Flexiflo Stomate low-profile gastrostomy tube—does not require endoscopy for removal.

Flexisplint—flexed arm board used as a restraint after brachial embolectomy or placement of an AV fistula in the forearm.

Flexlase 600—laser system for treatment of benign cutaneous vascular and pigmented lesions.

flexor—a muscle that flexes a joint. Cf. *flexure*.

FlexPosure endoscopic retractor—used to facilitate exposure and allow simultaneous use of other instruments during endoscopic spinal surgery.

FlexSure HP test—noninvasive test for serum IgG antibodies to *Helicobacter pylori*.

flexure—the bent part of an organ or structure. Cf. *flexor*.

Flexxicon and **Flexxicon Blue catheters**—dialysis catheters with flexible tips.

Flexzan foam wound dressing.

F. L. Fischer microsurgical neurectomy bayonet scissors—used in electrosurgery, craniofacial surgery, and skull base surgery.

flicker electroretinogram (ERG)—used in predicting outcome in central retinal vein occlusion (such as development of neovascularization of the iris). It is recorded at 5 Hz steps, at frequencies 5 to 30 Hz. "ERG recordings were made using a Ganzfeld sphere and a xenon strobe with a flash duration of 20 microseconds."

"flick-ten-yule"—see *phlyctenule*.

Flieringa scleral ring—applied to maintain the shape of the globe of the eye when vitreous is lost.

Flimm Fighter—percussor machine for patients with cystic fibrosis. Provides optimal postural drainage. See also *Vibracare*.

Flint Colon Injury Scale (FCIS)—a system of scoring abdominal trauma. A low FCIS correlates with less severe injuries. See also *PATI*.

flip angle—MRI term.

flipped meniscus sign—knee meniscal displacement identified on x-ray.

floaters—translucent specks of various sizes and shapes that float across the

floaters *(cont.)*
visual field; due to small bits of protein on cells floating in the vitreous.

flocculation—bentonite flocculation test for trichinosis.

Flocor (poloxamer 188)—used to improve blood flow in vascular occlusive disorders in the treatment of sickle cell patients with acute vaso-occlusive crisis. It may also be used to treat acute respiratory disorders and vascular disorders such as shock and stroke.

Flolan (epoprostenol)—used to treat primary pulmonary hypertension.

Flomax (tamsulosin HCl)—alpha blocker used for treating benign prostatic hypertrophy (BPH).

floppy—general term used to describe lack of muscle tone in extremities of newborns, due to hypoxia.

floppy guide wire—high-torque guide wire used in catheterization. See also *high-torque floppy guide wire*.

floral variant of follicular lymphoma (FFL)—normal lymph node structure altered in this type of lymphoma in such a way that, under the microscope, follicles are seen surrounded by atypical lymphocytes arranged in a scalloped pattern that resembles the petals of a flower.

Flo-Restors—devices for controlling backbleeding in microvascular anastomoses.

Florida pouch—a continent urinary reservoir using a detubularized right colonic segment as the urinary reservoir, thus allowing a large-capacity, low-pressure pouch.

FloSeal matrix hemostatic sealant—stops heavy bleeding during surgery.

flosequinan—used to treat congestive heart failure in patients who do not respond to other drugs such as diuretics or ACE inhibitors.

Flo-Stat fluid management system—used in outpatient endometrial resection/ablation (OPERA) procedures.

Flovent aerosol—an inhaled corticosteroid whose dose can be customized for the asthma patient.

Flovent Rotadisk (fluticasone propionate inhalation powder)—used for maintenance treatment of asthma for children as young as 4 years old. It is an inhaled powder corticosteroid asthma medication using a specially designed plastic device that is equipped with a dose counter to help with compliance and parental monitoring.

flow cytometry—a method to detect recurring bladder cancer by examining the DNA of urothelial cell sediment in urine specimens. It is thought to be more accurate than urine cytology.

flow effect artifact (MRI)—distortions caused by blood flow or cerebrospinal fluid (CSF) flow appearing as abnormal signal intensity within a vessel or CSF space, a band of noise across the image, or a spatially misregistered signal. Gating (timing of images) is helpful.

Flowers mandibular glove—a chin prosthesis developed by Dr. Robert Flowers.

FlowGun—suction/irrigation for minimally invasive surgical procedures.

FloWire—a Doppler ultrasound medical device that measures blood flow impairment in blood vessels.

Flowtron DVT—a pump system used during and after surgery to prevent deep venous thrombosis.

flow volume loop—a term used in spirometry reports.

Floxin (ofloxacin)—quinolone antibiotic used in treatment of skin and soft tissue infections.

Floxin Otic (ofloxacin)—broad-spectrum antibiotic ear drops.

floxuridine—see *FUdR*.

Floyd classification of peripheral nerves.

FLT (fluorothymidine).

fluasterone—a synthetic version of dehydroepiandrosterone (DHEA). Potential uses include prevention or treatment of cancer, lupus erythematosus, rheumatoid arthritis, multiple sclerosis, as well as management of obesity and type 2 diabetes mellitus.

fluconazole (Diflucan)—an antifungal drug similar in its action to ketoconazole (Nizarol) and amphotericin B but with fewer side effects. Used for severe fungal infections, particularly candidiasis, in immunocompromised patients with AIDS, cancer, or organ transplants.

flucytosine (5-FC, Ancobon)—used to treat fungus infections in AIDS and other immunocompromised patients.

fluctuancy (adj. fluctuant)—refers to the tactile quality of confined fluid. The palpating fingers of the physician can displace this fluid and perhaps even set up waves in it, as in compressing a balloon filled with water. Palpation or manipulation of a cyst, mass, organ, or body cavity containing fluid causes a characteristic feeling to be transmitted to the fingers due to the wavelike shifting (fluctuation) of the fluid. Anything that displays the property of fluctuancy is said to be fluctuant.

Fludara (fludarabine).

fludarabine (fludarabine monophosphate, Fludara, FAMP)—a chemotherapy drug used to treat non-Hodgkin's lymphoma and chronic lymphocytic leukemia.

fluences—pulse energy densities in laser surgery.

Flu-Glow—a fluorescein-impregnated paper strip used to diagnose corneal abrasion or the presence of a foreign body in the eye. The strip is moistened with a sterile solution and placed on the conjunctiva of the lower lid. Any break in the corneal epithelium will permit the fluorescein to be absorbed, and the defect will appear as a bright green fluorescence under appropriate lighting. No defect, no glow. Cf. *Fluor-i-Strip*.

fluid-attenuated inversion recovery (FLAIR).

fluid output, insensible. See *insensible fluid output*.

Flumadine (rimantadine HCl)—antiviral agent used to prevent infections by influenza type A viruses.

flumazenil (Mazicon)—an antagonist drug that reverses the action of benzodiazepine sedatives. Used for reversal of surgical anesthesia (particularly after endoscopy) or overdose involving benzodiazepines (such as Valium).

flumecinol (Zixoryn)—used to treat hyperbilirubinemia in infants not responding to phototherapy.

FluMist—nasally administered flu vaccine.

flunisolide (Nasarel).

Fluogen—influenza virus vaccine, trivalent, types A and B.

FLU-OIA—rapid (15-minute) test for detection of influenza A and B.

Fluoratec—technetium-based imaging agent for diagnosis of Parkinson's disease and ADHD.

fluorescein angiography—evaluates the anatomic and physiologic states of blood vessels in the choroid and retina after intravenous injections of fluorescein dye.

fluorescein dye disappearance test (DDT)—evaluates patients with possible partial nasolacrimal outflow obstruction.

fluorescein uptake (Oph).

Fluorescence activated cell sorter (FACS)—an automated lab tool which separates individual cells in a sample by fluorescence and size.

fluorescence in-situ hybridization (FISH) **protocol**—a procedure in which a fluorescent microscope is used to visualize a section of tumor embedded in paraffin and stained to study the chromosome pattern.

fluorescence overlay antigen mapping (FOAM).

fluorescence spectroscopy—see *spectrofluorometry*.

fluorescent cytoprint assay—an in vitro chemosensitivity assay that dissociates malignant cells from stromal tissue to facilitate the selection of the most effective chemotherapy regimen.

fluorescent treponemal antibody absorption (FTA-ABS)—a test for syphilis.

Fluor-I-Strip—ophthalmic strips; corneal disclosing agent (fluorescein sodium).

FluoroCatcher digital last-image hold, designed to reduce patient and operator radiation exposure.

fluorodeoxyglucose (F 18)—a radioactive tracer used in a PET scan to evaluate heart function at rest. It is able to differentiate between ischemic and normal myocardium.

Fluoropassiv thin-wall carotid patch—thin-wall patch with reduced thrombogenicity for use in carotid artery repair.

FluoroPlus angiography—provides real-time subtraction images for immediate diagnosis; minimizes radiation exposure.

FluoroPlus Cardiac—real-time digital imaging for cardiac catheterization lab. Provides instant display of all injection cycles, allowing immediate decisions during interventional procedures.

FluoroPlus Roadmapper—provides instant display of high-quality diagnostic images, enabling filmless diagnosis and decisions during PTA and ERCP procedures.

fluoroquinolone—a class of broad-spectrum antibiotics, including ciprofloxacin (Cipro), norfloxacin (Noroxin), ofloxacin (Floxin), and enoxacin (Penetrex).

FluoroScan (no space)—a mini C-arm imaging system with high resolution, used for intraoperative imaging. This type of imaging is often referred to in podiatric surgical procedures.

fluoroscopic cystocolpoproctography —see *cystocolpoproctography*.

fluoroscopic diskectomy (Ortho).

fluoroscopic road-mapping technique —used in radiologic invasive vascular procedures.

fluorosilicone oil—a type of substitute for vitreous humor, this drug is used to float and help facilitate the removal of a dislocated intraocular lens.

fluorothymidine (FLT)—for patients with AIDS.

Fluoro Tip cannula—used in ERCP. Has a radiopaque distal tip for location on fluoroscopy.

fluoxetine (Prozac)—an antidepressant chemically unrelated to any others but as effective as tricyclic antidepressants.

flush—method of taking blood pressure in infants.

flush aortogram (Cardio).

fluticasone propionate (Cutivate).

Flutter device—hands-free chest percussion therapy device that provides positive expiratory pressure to patients with mucus-producing respiratory conditions. It is a small, hand-held, pipe-shaped device that allows patients to clear their own airways of accumulated mucus and is used by patients with respiratory diseases such as cystic fibrosis, bronchitis, and bronchiectasis.

fluvastatin (Lescol)—used once daily to treat hypercholesterolemia in patients whose cholesterol remains high despite compliance with dietary restrictions. It acts by blocking the synthesis of cholesterol in the liver.

fluvoxamine (Luvox)—a 5HT blocker that inhibits the reuptake of serotonin by nerve cells in the brain. This results in increased levels of active serotonin which produces a therapeutic action in treating depression and obsessive-compulsive disorders. It appears to be effective with bedtime dosing against major depression and obsessive-compulsive disorder and may have fewer side effects.

"flying spot" excimer laser system—designed to correct low to moderate nearsightedness and astigmatism. The small-beam laser pulses 55 times a second and is directed by an active corneal tracking device that scans eye position 4000 times a second, rapidly hopping from one side of the cornea to the other to allow for thermal relaxation of tissue.

FMAP (feeding mean arterial pressure).

fmoles/mg (femtomoles/mg)—a measurement used with estrogen and progesterone receptors to determine if a patient with breast cancer should be categorized as positive or negative. (Greater than 10 fmoles/mg is considered positive.)

fMRI (functional MRI).

FNAB (fine-needle aspiration biopsy).

FNA cytology (fine-needle aspiration).

FNH (focal nodular hyperplasia)—MRI term.

FNM (fluorouracil, Novantrone, methotrexate)—chemotherapy protocol for breast carcinoma.

FO (foot orthosis).

FOAM (fluorescence overlay antigen mapping)—a technique to evaluate bullous skin disorders.

foam cell (foamy histiocyte)—a cell which has a ground-glass-appearing cytoplasm due to accumulation of fat, glycogen, or other material.

foam dressing—generally made from a hydrophilic polyurethane foam. Some have adhesive tape surrounding an "island" of foam. Highly absorbent foams may allow less frequent dressing changes. Foams that absorb exudate and keep it off the wound can decrease maceration of surrounding tissue. Foam dressings are often used on heavily exudating wounds, deep-cavity wounds, and weeping ulcers. See *dressing*.

foam stability test; index—a determination of maturity of the fetal lungs, as demonstrated by the ability of pulmonary surfactant in the amniotic fluid to form a stable foam in ethanol after being vigorously shaken. Also called *shake test*.

foamy esophagus—radiographic feature of *Candida albicans* esophagitis, seen on double contrast esophagograph, particularly in patients with scleroderma. It is caused when numerous tiny bubbles intermingle with barium suspension along the top of the barium column, producing a layer of foam.

foamy macrophages—a term used thus in dictation: "Panbronchiolitis is characterized histologically by mononuclear cell inflammation of respiratory bronchioles and the presence of foamy macrophages in the bronchiolar lumina and adjacent alveoli."

FOB (fiberoptic bronchoscopy).

Fobi pouch—transected vertical gastric bypass with Silastic ring band and gastrostomy performed for severe obesity. Developed by Dr. Mathias A. L. ("Mal") Fobi, Bellflower, California.

FOBT (fecal occult blood test).

focal and diffuse lung texture analysis (Rad).

focal expansion technology—a means by which direct pressure is "focalized," e.g., applying pressure only to the site of blockage or disease, thereby treating the site of the disease while lessening risk of damage to the surrounding healthy arterial wall. This is the technology used in the FACT line of catheters.

"focality"—a coined term derived from *focal*. "No gross focality was noted on neurological exam."

focal nodular hyperplasia (FNH).

FocalSeal—a liquid sealant used to seal air leaks in patients undergoing lung volume reduction surgery.

FocalSeal-S—a surgical sealant used in neurosurgical procedures.

focal vestibulitis vulvae—see *vulvar vestibulitis syndrome*.

focal vulvitis—see *vulvar vestibulitis syndrome*.

focused heat technology—new method of nonsurgical minimally invasive tumor ablation using heat alone.

Foerster capsulotomy knife—used in plastic and reconstructive procedures on the breast to remove spherical contractures from the breast pocket during re-do breast implant procedures.

Foerster sponge forceps.

fog artifact (Radiol)—caused by radiation scatter.

Fogarty adherent clot catheter—used in removing clots or other material adherent to synthetic bypass grafts. Also, *Fogarty balloon biliary catheter*.

folinic acid rescue—see *leucovorin rescue*.

Follistim (follitropin beta)—recombinant follicle-stimulating hormone (FSH), used for the treatment of infertility.

Folstein's Mini-Mental Status Examination—a method of grading the cognitive state of patients. This is one of the tests administered to patients with symptoms suggestive of Alzheimer's disease.

fomivirsen (Vitravene)—a drug for the treatment of cytomegalovirus retinitis.

FONAR-360 MRI scanner—"open sky" MRI which is, from the

FONAR-360 *(cont.)*

patient's point of view, a full-size room with two circular structures projecting from the ceiling and floor. There are no structures between the patient and the walls of the scanner room in any direction.

Fontan modification of Norwood procedure—for hypoplastic left-sided heart syndrome. See *Norwood; Gill/ Jonas; Sade.*

Fontan procedure—anastomosis of the right atrial appendage to the pulmonary artery, to separate the left and right heart circulations in patients with levotransposition of the great vessels, single ventricle, atrial septal defect, coarctation of the aorta, and small left atrium.

foot drop—passive plantar flexion of the foot due to paralysis of dorsiflexor muscles.

foot pound—a unit of measurement related to work, i.e., stress placed upon the extremities.

FOP (fibrodysplasia ossificans progressiva).

Foradil (formoterol fumarate)—bronchodilator for treatment of asthma.

foramen of Luschka—opening at the side of the fourth ventricle of the brain communicating with the subarachnoid space.

foramen ovale (*not* O'Valley, although it sounds like that)—an opening in the sphenoid bone through which pass a branch of the trigeminal nerve and some blood vessels (foramen ovale basis cranii), and also an opening in the septum secundum of the heart of the fetus between the atria (foramen ovale cordis).

Force balloon dilatation catheter.

forced expiratory volume (FEV).

forced midexpiratory flow (FEF_{25-75}) —a measure of the rate at which the patient can expel air from the lungs. Flow is measured in liters per second during the median half of forced expiration—that is, from the time that 25% of total volume has been expelled to the time that 75% has been expelled. This study is more sensitive to mild airway obstruction than other tests of pulmonary function. "Spirometry obtained at this time reveals a normal examination, with the exception of the $FEF_{25-75\%}$ which is reduced to 50% of predicted. These findings are sometimes considered indicative of some degree of small airway disease."

forced oscillation technique (FOT)—a noninvasive test used to measure the limitation of air flow in the respiratory system.

forced vital capacity (FVC).

forceps—an instrument with a pair of blades and handles, used in surgery to grasp tissue, and also surgical sponges, etc. Why do we give this well-known term? Simply to emphasize that, even though the word ends in "s," it is a singular (as well as plural) form—"an instrument," and takes a plural verb. An example of incorrect use: "This was resected with a double action bone forcep." But grasping with a single blade would be like clapping with one hand or eating with one chopstick. So, "forceps" it is. Examples:
ACMI Martin endoscopy
Acufex straight and curved basket
alligator grasper/forceps
ASSI bipolar coagulating
Barraquer
bayonet bipolar

forceps *(cont.)*
   Bechert lens-holding
   Bonaccolto utility and splinter
   bone-cutting
   Brown-Adson tissue
   Castroviejo-Colibri
   DeJuan
   Dodick Nucleus Cracker
   Drews
   end-biting
   Englert
   Ernest-McDonald soft IOL folding
   Foerster sponge
   Fujinon biopsy
   Grieshaber manipulator
   Halsted hemostatic mosquito
   Hardy microbipolar
   Hartmann
   Hildebrandt uterine hemostatic
   Iselin
   Jacobson hemostatic
   Jaffee capsulorrhexis
   Jawz endomyocardial biopsy
   Kraff nucleus splitter
   Kraff-Utrata tear capsulotomy
   Lalonde delicate hook
   Laurer
   Livernois lens-holding
   Livernois-McDonald
   Llorente dissecting
   Max Fine tying
   Mazzariello-Caprini
   McKerman-Adson
   McKerman-Potts
   McPherson
   microbipolar
   MIC Thermal Option
   Moolgaoker
   Neville-Barnes
   Ogura tissue and cartilage
   Olympus FBK 13
   Peyman intraocular
   Pierse corneal
   Pierse tip

forceps *(cont.)*
   Pilling Weck Y-stent
   Puntenney
   Quadripolar cutting
   Quire mechanical finger
   Radial Jaw single-use biopsy
   ring
   Rowe disimpaction
   Russian
   Seitzinger tripolar cutting
   Sinskey
   spoon
   SureBite biopsy
   Therma Jaw (or Thermajaw) hot
     urologic
   Tischler cervical biopsy punch
   Twisk
   Utrata capsulorrhexis
   Vickers ring tip
   Walsham
   Yeoman uterine biopsy

Fordyce granules—an ectopic collection of sebaceous glands or choristomas in the oral cavity that requires no treatment and causes no untoward effects.

foregut—bronchi, stomach, and proximal portion of duodenum. See *midgut* and *hindgut*.

foreign material artifact (MRI and Radiol)—In MRI, small ferromagnetic objects, accidentally within the magnet bore, produce a scrambled image. These may include hearing aids, hairpins, buttons, paper clips, clothing with metal objects, such as zippers or buttons, cigarette lighters, political buttons, or make-up or hair coloring made with ferromagnetic substances, or metal objects within the body as a result of surgery or trauma. In plain film radiography, buttons, zippers, bra underwires, necklaces, earrings, metal mesh in a

foreign material artifact *(cont.)* toupee or wig, rings, watches, pens, tooth fillings, or results of surgery such as shunts and probes produce images difficult or impossible to interpret.

Forel—see *space of Forel.*

ForeRunner—automatic external defibrillator device.

Forma water-jacketed incubator—for use in in vitro fertilization. This incubator fosters an embryo's growth by recreating the body's optimal temperature, humidity, and pH level.

forme fruste—atypical form of disease.

formication—a sensation of insects crawling over the skin; most commonly seen in cocaine or amphetamine intoxication. Cf. *fornication.*

formin cells (GEMM-CFC).

fornication—sexual intercourse between unmarried people. Cf. *formication.*

Fortaz (ceftazidime)—cephalosporin antibiotic.

Fortical (salmon calcitonin)—injectable drug used in treatment of osteoporosis.

fortification spectrum—a jagged formation of bright lines, sometimes seen as an aura of migraine headache and in other conditions. See *scintillating scotoma.*

Fortovase (saquinavir)—a soft-gel version of the antiviral saquinavir, an HIV protease inhibitor.

49er brace—knee brace; probably first used by that football team.

Forvade (cidofovir topical gel)—a drug for the treatment of refractory herpes simplex virus infection in patients with AIDS.

Fosamax (alendronate sodium)—for treatment of glucocorticoid-induced osteoporosis in men and women. It is also used in the prevention and treatment of osteoporosis in postmenopausal women and the treatment of Paget's disease of bone.

foscarnet (Foscavir; trisodium phosphonoformate)—alternative to ganciclovir in treating cytomegalovirus in AIDS patients, it is also active against herpes and HIV.

Foscavir (foscarnet).

fosinopril (Monopril)—an ACE inhibitor, used in conjunction with diuretics, in treatment of congestive heart failure. See also *ramipril.*

fosphenytoin (Cerebyx)—used to treat patients with grand mal status epilepticus.

fossa (pl., fossae)—a depression, hollow, or channel. "The pain radiates into both tonsillar fossae."

FOT (forced oscillation technique).

fotemustine (S 10036)—a chemotherapy drug for advanced gastric carcinoma.

Fouchet's reagent ("foo-shay").

4-aminopyridine—relieves symptoms of multiple sclerosis.

4-aminosalicylic acid (Pamisyl, Rezipas)—used to treat ulcerative colitis in patients who are allergic to sulfasalazine.

fourchette (Fr., fork)—a fork-shaped object or area; usually refers to the frenulum labiorum pudendi. "At surgery a small amount of scar was seen at the posterior fourchette."

4-epi-Adriamycin (epirubicin).

four-flap Z-plasty—for thumb web deepening, in surgery for repair of syndactyly.

Fourier analysis of electrocardiogram
—in exercise-induced myocardial ischemia.

Fourier transform infrared spectroscopy—a technique used in forensic pathology to examine plastic, paint coating, automobile lenses, paper, etc., to determine manufacturer or origin. See *Fourier transform Raman spectroscopy*.

Fourier transform Raman spectroscopy—a technique used in forensic pathology to supply complementary or confirmatory information about a substance under investigation. Cf. *Fourier transform infrared spectroscopy*.

Fourneau 309 (suramin).

Fournier's gangrene—a polymicrobial necrotizing fasciitis of the perineal, perirectal, or genital area. Diagnosed by CT scan. Also, *Fournier's syndrome*.

four-view chest x-ray—PA and lateral, and both oblique views.

FOV (field of view)—MRI term.

fovea centralis retinae—a tiny pit in the center of the macula, composed of slim, elongated cones; it is the area of clearest vision.

foveal avascular zone (FAZ).

Fowler-Stephens orchiopexy (orchidopexy)—a staged laparoscopic procedure for locating undescended testicles and moving them to their normal position. Testicles not moved are at risk for developing cancer.

FPA (fibrinopeptide A).

FPG (fasting plasma glucose).

FPL (flexor pollicis longus).

fractionated stereotaxic radiation therapy—combines the advantages of conventional fractionation (where the total radiation a patient receives is divided into smaller dosages delivered at different times) with radiosurgery. See *stereotactic radiosurgery* (SRS).

Fractura Flex—elastic plaster of Paris bandage. In applying the bandage to form a cast, the bandage material is first moistened in water and then applied in bandage-fashion to the extremity, rubbing each layer of the bandage into the layer beneath it. The cast is said to set within four minutes.

fracture
Bennett's
blow-in
blow-out
boxer's
burst
Cedell
Chance
circumferential
closed
corner
diastatic
finger
fulcrum
Galeazzi radial
hangman's
Kapandji radial
LeFort I, II, III
Malgaigne's
march
pillion
ping-pong
ring
sacral insufficiency (SIF)
Salter I through VI
seat belt
SER-IV
zygomatic-malar complex (ZMC)

fragile X syndrome (refers to X chromosome)—a form of retardation that males may inherit from the maternal side of the family.

fragment-in-notch sign (Ortho)—used in association with meniscal displacement of knee joint.

Fragmin (dalteparin sodium)—a once-daily low-molecular-weight heparin injection. Used as prophylaxis against deep vein thrombosis in abdominal surgery patients. An anticoagulant used to coat the Cragg stent.

fraise, diamond—an instrument used in dermabrasion.

Framingham criteria for heart failure.

Franceschetti-type freeblade (Oph).

Francisella tularensis—organism that causes tularemia.

Frank-Starling law of the heart—the heart pumps out of the right atrium all the blood returned to it without letting any back up in the veins. Named for Otto Frank (German) and Ernest Henry Starling (British), physiologists who, in the early 20th century, formulated the concept upon which the law of muscle contraction is based. Also called *Frank-Starling principle*.

Frank vaginal construction—creation of a new vagina in patients with congenital vaginal aplasia, or in males having a sex change operation. Other techniques include McIndoe and Davydov. See also *colocolponeopoiesis*.

Franseen needle—used in stereotactic fine needle aspiration biopsy.

frappage—clapping with a cupped hand on the patient's chest and back to loosen pulmonary secretions so they can be coughed up or suctioned out. See *percussion, chest PT.*

FRC (functional residual [or reserve] capacity).

FreAmine—amino acid injection; a nutrient solution for burn patients.

freckled—spotted, speckled. "There was a major intrasellar component that was a typical soft, freckled gray adenoma."

FRED (fog reduction/elimination device)—used on endoscopic instruments.

free air (Radiol)—air or gas in a body cavity where it does not belong, usually after escape from the gastrointestinal tract. Cf. *air-fluid level.*

free beta test—a screening test that detects a specific protein marker for Down syndrome at 14-17 weeks of gestation.

Freedom arthritis support—protects and supports the arthritic hand to maintain joint alignment and mobility without bulkiness.

Freedom knife—a diamond knife blade used during intraocular surgery.

FreeDop—hands-free Doppler monitor for obstetrical use.

Freehand system (Neuro, Rehab)—a surgically implanted neuroprosthetic device that allows people with quadriplegia to regain use of a paralyzed hand. The implanted components work in tandem with an external controller using radio waves and electrical stimuli. Electrodes attached to paralyzed hand and forearm muscles receive the stimuli and cause the muscles to contract, providing the patient with a functional hand grasp.

free induction decay (FID)—MRI term.

free induction signal—MRI term.

Freeman cookie cutter areola marker—used in reduction mammoplasty.

Freeman femoral component with a Rotalok cup.

Freeman Punctum Plug—a small, bullet-shaped plug made of silicone that is inserted in the opening of the tear duct at the inner aspect of the lower eyelid. It prevents tears from being drained from the eye and is used to treat dry eyes.

free PSA (prostate-specific antigen)— Some PSA clings to protein in the blood; some floats freely. The free form of PSA is key to identifying who really needs a prostate biopsy.

free radicals—some oxygen molecules turn into free radicals which can cause damage and even cancer. Diets to lessen or eliminate free radicals exist.

Freer elevator (Oph, ENT).

Freestanding Tissue Retraction Bridge system—free-standing balloon dissection system to maintain the dissected operative working space without tissue retractors. In dictation, you may hear just the word *Bridge* used in reference to this system.

Freestyle aortic root bioprosthesis—a stentless porcine aortic heart valve replacement.

free thyroxine index (FTI).

free-tissue transfer (FTT)—used in major skull-base resections, with wide surgical excision of dura and skull-base structures that normally separate the intracranial and extracranial cavities.

free toe transfer—construction of a finger, often the thumb, by transplanting a toe to the hand.

free/total PSA (prostate-specific antigen) **index**—a test that can better distinguish between men who have benign prostatic hypertrophy and those who have prostatic carcinoma, when PSA levels are less than 10 ng/mL or lower.

Freezor cryocatheter—device used in cryoablation procedures for the treatment of cardiac arrhythmias.

Freiberg's disease—avascular necrosis of metatarsal head, treated with DuVries arthroplasty.

French-eye needle—the eye of the needle has a split, or spring, at the end with a little slot for the suture material to slip into, rather than the customary way, through the eye.

French scale—used for denoting size of catheters, sounds, and other tubular instruments, each unit being roughly equivalent to 0.33 mm in diameter.

frequency domain imaging (FDI)—in ultrasound.

fresh frozen plasma (FFP).

Freund's complete adjuvant (FCA)— a water-in-oil emulsion of antigen which, when injected, induces antibody formation. Cf. *Freund's incomplete adjuvant*.

Freund's incomplete adjuvant—water-in-oil emulsion of antigen, without mycobacteria. Cf. *Freund's complete adjuvant*.

FRF (filter replacement fluid).

fria—pelvic muscle-training aid for women with urinary incontinence.

friable—crumbly; easily broken up or damaged.

Frialoc transgingival threaded dental implant.

friction knot—see *surgeon's knot*.

Friedländer's bacillus—see *Klebsiella pneumoniae*.

Friedländer marker—used during corneal surgery. Types: arcuate; optical zone; transverse incision.

Friedman curves (Ob-Gyn)—when each determination of dilatation and station is made during labor, it is plotted on a graph. The patterns of changes in these parameters are referred to as Friedman curves or "labor curves."

Friedman Splint (trademark)—polypropylene hip abduction brace for treating hip dysplasia in toddlers up to $2^1/_2$ years of age.

Frigitronics probe—used in freeze-thaw cryotherapy.

Frisium (clobazam)—antianxiety drug.

frogleg view—a radiographic study of one or both hip joints for which the patient lies on his back with thighs maximally abducted and externally rotated and knees flexed so as to bring the soles of the feet together.

Frohse, arcade of—in the elbow. Sports medicine physicians have found that some windsurfers develop compression of the median interosseous nerve over the head of the radius in the arcade of Frohse.

Froment's sign—a simple test of ulnar nerve function. The patient puts the tips of his thumb and index finger together, and if the resulting circle is askew, this is a positive Froment's sign and points to ulnar nerve damage and loss of thumb adductor function.

fronds, sea—description of neovascularization seen on eye examination.

frondy—see *fronds*.

frontal irregular rhythmic delta activity (FIRDA)—in electroencephalogram.

frontal release sign (Neuro).

frost—see *synovial frost*.

froth—see *meibomian froth*.

frovatriptan—5HT 1B/1D agonist for the treatment of acute migraine.

frown incision (Oph)—a downward curved incision above the superior limbus of the eye, patented by Dr. Pallin. Much controversy and litigation exist over the right to patent an incision method.

frozen section (Path)—a technique by which tissue removed in an operation is quickly frozen and pathology identified (while the patient is still on the operating table) so that the surgeons will know what they are dealing with; this will then determine their options in proceeding with the operation. Cf. *paraffin section, permanent section*.

Frykman classification—of hand fractures.

FSAD (female sexual arousal disorder).

F-scan—with a combination of computer technology and a sensor pad in the patient's shoe, an orthotist uses the F-scan to identify high-pressure areas in the foot of a diabetic patient where a nonhealing wound is likely to start. Using this information, the orthotist can design a shoe insert that will shift the pressure to areas less likely to have tissue breakdown.

FSD (female sexual dysfunction).

FSD (Fletcher-Suit-Delclos).

FSE (fast spin echo)—MRI term.

FSE-T2 with fat suppression (MRI)—used to detect ligamentous abnormalities.

FSH (facioscapulohumeral) **muscular dystrophy**.

FSH (follicle-stimulating hormone).

FTA-ABS—fluorescent treponemal antibody absorption test for syphilis.

FTI (free thyroxine index). "The FTI was normal at 2.6, and all other

FTI *(cont.)*
thyroid function tests were within normal limits."

F to N (sounds like *F2N*)—finger-to-nose test.

ftorafur ("tor-a-fur")—a chemotherapeutic agent.

FTT (failure to thrive).

FTT (free-tissue transfer).

FUdR (5-fluorouracil deoxyribonucleoside)—halogenated thymidine analogue; a radiosensitizer. Cf. *BUdR, IUdR.*

fugue state ("fyug")—a period of days, weeks, or years, in which a person loses memory and takes flight from a painful or untenable situation and may start a new life, new job, new marriage, etc., without memory of the past.

Fuji AC2 storage phosphor computed radiology system—eliminates many artifacts noted with earlier CR systems.

Fuji FCR9000 computed radiology (CR) system.

Fujinon biopsy forceps—used in endoscopic biopsies.

Fujinon Sonoprobe system for endoscopic procedures.

Fujita snake retractor (Neuro).

Fukushima C-clamp (Neuro).

Fukushima cranial retraction system.

Fukushima-Giannotta instruments—includes curettes, dissectors, needle holders, and scissors for use in keyhole eye surgery.

FUL (functional urethral length).

fulcrum fracture—seat belt fracture. See *Chance fracture.*

full-bladder technique (Radiol)—ultrasound examination of the pelvic region performed while the subject's bladder is distended with urine. This is done to improve the recognition of the bladder outline, which cannot be distinguished adequately when the bladder is empty.

full colon—dictated punctuation indicating the need for a colon mark, as opposed to a semicolon.

full-column barium enema (Radiol)—barium enema examination in which the contrast medium is injected into the colon under full pressure by elevation of the barium reservoir to the maximum safe height.

Fuller shield—a rectal dressing.

full stop—dictated punctuation indicating the need for a period.

full-thickness skin graft (FTSG).

Functional Capacity Evaluation (FCE) (Rehab)—a comprehensive objective test of a person's ability to perform work-related tasks. Used for guidelines for physical restrictions and return-to-work suitability.

functional endoscopic sinus surgery (FESS).

Functional Intact Fibrinogen (FiF) **test**—a fibrinogen determination test in blood coagulation conditions, such as disseminated intravascular coagulation, cardiovascular disease, and primary fibrinolysis.

functional MRI (fMRI).

functional urethral length (FUL).

fundal height—the distance from the symphysis pubis to the top (dome or fundus) of the uterus. After the twentieth week of pregnancy, the fundal height in centimeters equals the number of weeks of pregnancy. If the fundal height increases more than this, it may indicate a multiple pregnancy or a fetus that is large for dates. "The fundal height is approximately 31 cm."

fundoplication
Belsey Mark IV
Collis-Nissen
Hill gastropexy
laparoscopic Nissen and Toupet
ligamentum teres cardiopexy
Nissen
Toupet hemifundoplication
fundus oculi—the posterior inner part of the eye as seen with the ophthalmoscope.
funduscopic—*not* fundoscopic.
fungemia—systemic fungal infection.
fungus—see *pathogen*.
funicular suture—used in interfascicular or grouped fascicular repair.
Funston's syndrome—congenital cervical rib.
furrier's lung disease—extrinsic allergic alveolitis caused by exposure to animal fur and hair dust.
fusion—coordination of images seen by both eyes into one image.
fusion inhibitors—a new class of drugs that works specifically on a virus to prevent it from fusing with the cell and prevent viral replication. Fusion inhibitors are said to have great promise as anti-HIV drugs. Also called *HIS fusion inhibitors*.
fusion protein—a biotechnologic product that targets malignant cells and some normal lymphocytes that contain interleukin-2 (IL-2) receptors, for treating patients with advanced or recurrent cutaneous T-cell lymphoma.
futile cycles—high levels of cytokines causing fat to be stored as triglycerides, instead of being available for energy. Thought to cause some of the weakness and wasting in HIV disease. Futile cycles also exist for glucose and protein metabolism.
Futura resectoscope sheath—used in transurethral resection and ablation procedures within the urethra, prostate, and bladder.
FUVAC (fluorouracil [5-FU], vinblastine, Adriamycin, cyclophosphamide) —chemotherapy protocol.
FVC (forced vital capacity).
FVL (flexible video laparoscope).
FyBron alginate wound dressing.

G, g

gabapentin—provides significant relief for postherpetic neuralgia, the aching, burning pain often suffered for years after attacks of shingles. An anticonvulsant also used to treat amyotrophic lateral sclerosis. See also *Neurontin*.

GABEB (generalized atrophic benign epidermolysis bullosa).

GABHS (group A beta-hemolytic streptococcus)—the pathogen causing pharyngitis, rheumatic fever, toxic strep syndrome, and cellulitis.

Gabitril (tiagabine)—add-on therapy for treatment of partial-seizure epilepsy.

gadolinium-enhanced T1-weighted images—MRI term.

gadolinium-enhanced subtracted MR angiography, 3-D—can detect graft complications such as occlusions, stenoses, and aneurysms.

gadolinium EOB-DTPA (Eovist).

gadolinium texaphyrin (Gd-Tex)—a radiation sensitizer. Texaphyrin is a synthetic molecule that captures and focuses medically useful forms of energy, such as x-rays.

Gadolite oral suspension—contrast agent that enhances delineation of the small bowel in MRI procedures.

gadoteridol (ProHance)—contrast medium used in MRI scans of the nervous system.

Gaffney joint—orthosis for ambulation in children with cerebral palsy and myelomeningocele. Made of stainless steel vacuformed into polypropylene in seven sizes for use in a hinged ankle joint.

gag reflex—contraction of the pharyngeal musculature in response to stimulation of the pharyngeal mucosa.

gait and station—a term used in the physical examination. *Gait* refers to the way a patient walks, and the pattern of it. *Station* is a test for coordination problems. When the patient stands with feet close together and the body sways, this is one sign of incoordination.

gait cycle—the series of movements of the leg and foot between one touch of the heel on the ground and the next time the same heel touches.

279

gait lock splint (GLS) **brace**—maintains the leg in extension when the patient is weightbearing, without worry about the knee giving way.

GAIT (great toe arthroplasty implant technique) **spacer**—augments the Keller arthroplasty for class 3 Regnauld-type degeneration of the first metatarsophalangeal joint.

galactography—a pre-excision x-ray study of women with spontaneous nipple discharge, using contrast medium to outline breast ducts.

galactose (Levovist)—ultrasound contrast medium for echocardiography.

Galand disc lens—a rigid one-piece intraocular lens made from PMMA (polymethyl methacrylate).

galanthamine—acetylcholinesterase inhibitor/nicotinic receptor modulator for use in the treatment of Alzheimer's patients.

Galardin (matrix metalloproteinase inhibitor)—drug for corneal ulcers.

Galeazzi fracture of radius.

Galeazzi's sign—indicates dislocation of hip. Lying supine, with the knees bent, if one knee is lower than the other, there is dislocation of the hip, or a shortened femur.

Galen—see *vein of Galen*.

Galileo intravasular radiotherapy system—automated treatment designed to reduce or minimize restenosis in coronary arteries.

Gallavardin phenomenon (Cardio).

galling—chafing of apposed skin surfaces, as in the groin; intertrigo.

gallium-arsenid (GaA) **laser**—often used in acupuncture.

gallium nitrate (Ganite)—prevents hypercalcemia in carcinoma patients.

gallium scan (Radiol)—the intravenously introduced ^{67}Ga localizes in areas of granulocyte concentration, such as in osteomyelitis, thus revealing hidden infections.

gallium-67 citrate or **gallium citrate Ga 67** (^{67}GA)—a radioactive contrast medium used in scintigraphy to detect a latent breast abscess.

gallop—see *summation gallop*.

GALOP syndrome (Neuro)—characterized by ataxia, positive Romberg test, and polyneuropathy.

G   gait disorder
A   autoantibody
L   late-age
O   onset
P   polyneuropathy

GALT (gut-associated lymphoid tissue).

galvanic body sway test (GBST)—detects retrolabyrinthine disorder of the vestibular system.

galvanic stimulation—see *high-voltage stimulation and iontophoresis*.

galvanic vestibular stimulation (GVR)—maneuver used to study the vestibular system.

Galveston metacarpal brace—to treat fractured second through fifth metacarpals.

Galveston Orientation and Amnesia Test (GOAT)—a neuropsychological test given to patients with cognitive deficiencies following brain injury.

Gambee suture ("gam-bay").

Gambro Lundia Minor—brand of artificial kidney (hemodialyzer), parallel plate type.

gamekeeper's thumb—instability of first metacarpophalangeal joint due to ligament tear.

game leg—impaired by injury or disease.

gamete intrafallopian transfer (GIFT).

Gamimune N (immunoglobulin)—for intravenous administration to treat

Gamimune N *(cont.)*
immunodeficiency symptoms in patients who are unable to produce enough IgG antibodies or who have AIDS.

gamma glutamyl transferase (GGT).

gamma-herpesvirus—a virus of the family *Gammaherpesvirinae*, which includes Epstein-Barr virus and HHV-8.

gamma hydroxybutrate (GHB)—an increasingly dangerous, illicitly marketed substance with numerous potential health hazards. It has been used illicitly as a growth hormone, a fat-burning drug, a body-building aid, and a sleeping potion. It is also also used as a "date-rape" drug. Common street names include GHB, Liquid E, Liquid X, and Scoop. Dangerous side effects are numerous, and the drug is often home-brewed.

Gamma Knife—not a knife, but a radiosurgical instrument used in radiation therapy. The gamma rays are fired with such accuracy that only the diseased cells are destroyed, leaving the adjacent healthy tissues intact. Thus, more radiation can be administered to the tumor if that is indicated. Cf. *roentgen knife.*

gammaphos—see *ethiofos.*

gamma-ribbon radiation therapy—used for reduction of restenosis in patients with reoccluded or narrowed coronary artery stents. A closed-end lumen catheter with a tiny ribbon containing 6, 10, or 14 seeds of ^{192}Ir is inserted into the stenosed vessel.

Gammar-PIV (pasteurized intravenous [human] immune globulin)—used for the treatment of primary immune deficiency in adolescents and children who are at an increased risk of infection.

Gammex RMI DAP meter—real-time dose area product (DAP) meter that continuously measures accumulated radiation dose throughout fluoroscopic examination.

Gamna-Gandy body of the spleen—organized focus of hemorrhage, caused by portal hypertension. Contains fibrous tissue, hemosiderin, and calcium. Also called *siderotic nodules* or *bodies.*

ganaxolone—neuroactive steroid compound used in the treatment of migraine headaches.

ganciclovir (Cytovene, DHPG)—for cytomegalovirus infection and CMV retinitis in AIDS patients.

ganglioglioma—a rare variety of tumor composed of ganglion cells and glial cells; prevalent in first three decades of life.

ganglioside GM1—a natural component of cells in the central nervous system. Has been found to allow damaged nerves to regrow. Along with the now-standard treatment of methylprednisolone following spinal cord injury, the use of ganglioside GM1 produces an increase in neurologic function one year status post injury.

Ganite (gallium nitrate)—bone resorption inhibitor for hypercalcemia of malignancy.

gantry angulation—in CT-guided percutaneous biopsies.

Ganzfeld sphere (Oph).

Garcin's syndrome—unilateral paralysis of all or most of the cranial nerves due to a tumor at the base of the skull or in the nasopharynx. Called also *half base syndrome.*

Garden's classification of femoral neck fractures—uses the degree of dislocation as the criterion, which seems to be more accurate in terms of prognosis than Pauwel's classification. Cf. *Pauwel's classification.*

Gardner chair—used as an operating table, with the patient in the sitting position, in neurological surgery.

Gardnerella vaginalis—newer name for the bacterium formerly called *Haemophilus vaginalis.* Normal vaginal flora, but thought perhaps to be the cause of vaginitis infections.

Garin-Bujadoux-Bannwarth syndrome —see *Lyme lymphocytic meningoradiculitis.*

Garrett dilator—used in kidney transplant surgery.

GAS (group A streptococcus).

gas-bloat syndrome—complication of Nissen fundoplication for gastroesophageal reflux.

gas chromatography—an analytic technique with many applications in medicine, particularly in screening serum and urine for poisons and drugs of abuse.

gas density line (Radiol)—a linear band of maximal radiolucency, representing or appearing to represent a narrow zone of air or gas on x-ray.

gas-forming liver abscess.

gas-forming organism in bowel wall.

Gastaut's syndrome—HEE syndrome (hemiconvulsion, hemiplegia, and epilepsy).

gastric antral vascular ectasia (GAVE). See *watermelon stomach.*

gastric neobladder procedure—uses a wedge of stomach in bladder replacement surgery.

Gastrimmune (gemcitabine)—vaccine for stomach cancer. It has potential for treatment of other cancers of the gastrointestinal system.

gastrinoma—hormonally active tumor of pancreas or stomach.

Gastroccult—lab test for gastric occult blood as well as pH.

gastrocnemius reflex. Cf. *Achilles reflex and ankle jerk.*

gastroenterostomy—see *operation.*

gastroesophageal reflux (Radiol)—on upper GI series, abnormal backflow of material from the stomach into the lower esophagus.

gastroesophageal reflux disease (GERD).

Gastrografin (meglumine diatrizoate) —a radiopaque medium used in examination of the upper GI tract.

gastrointestinal cross—intentional ingestion of a metallic foreign body. Inmates reportedly have swallowed such objects to create an emergency surgical condition.

GastroMark (ferumoxsil)—oral contrast agent used for upper GI tract imaging.

gastroplasty—see *operation.*

gastrostomy—see *operation.*

Gastrozepine (pirenzepine HCl)—drug used to treat peptic ulcer disease.

gatch—from height of setting of Gatch bed, as "45° gatch."

Gatch bed.

gated blood (pool) **cardiac wall motion study**—a radionuclide study.

gated view (in multiple gated acquisition scan, or MUGA)—an image obtained by a technique synchronized with motions of the heart to eliminate blurring.

gating—timing of images (MRI term). See *electrocardiographic gating, MUGA, spirometric gating.*

gauge (noun)—standard measure, as of wire or needle diameter; (verb)—to find the exact measurement of. See *Dacomed snap gauge; mercury-in-Silastic strain gauge; Preston pinch gauge*. Cf. *gouge*.

gauss ("gowse")—see *tesla* (MRI).

gaussian ("gow'-zee-en") **mode profile laser beam**—MRI term.

Gauss' sign—the marked degree of mobility of the uterus, seen in the early weeks of pregnancy.

Gautier ureteroscope.

GAVE (gastric antral vascular ectasia). See *watermelon stomach*.

Gaynor-Hart position—positioning the patient for an axial radiographic projection of the carpal tunnel. See *carpal tunnel syndrome*.

Gazayerli endoscopic retractor—lifting device used in conjunction with CO_2 insufflation in laparoscopic procedures. A retractor with three prongs in the closed position is inserted into the abdomen and the prongs then splayed out in a fan or triangular shape. The fan retractor is then elevated by a powered mechanical arm, thus creating an enlarged laparoscopic cavity, avoiding the tenting of the cavity that occurs with other lifting schemes. Two "fans" attached to a cross-bar may be inserted into the abdomen and lifted by a single arm for obese patients.

gaze—see *disconjugate gaze*.

G banding—technique of chromosome staining.

GBC-590—a carbohydrate lectin inhibitor, which is a new class of anticancer drugs that specifically interfere with cellular interactions. This drug is currently being tested in patients with pancreatic carcinoma and may also be indicated for cancers of the colon, liver, and prostate.

GBST (galvanic body sway test).

GCA (giant cell arteritis).

G-CFC (granulocyte colony-forming cells).

G-CSF (granulocyte colony-stimulating factor, filgrastim)—a naturally occurring growth factor produced by epithelial cells and monocytes that acts on the bone marrow to increase the production of neutrophils. Used in chemotherapy and in treating bone marrow depression in AIDS patients. See *filgrastim*. Cf. *GM-CSF*.

GCT (germ cell tumor) of the central nervous system.

GDC (Guglielmi Detachable Coil).

Gd-DTPA (gadolinium diethylenetriamine-penta-acetate)—a contrast medium used in MRI scans.

GDNF (glial cell-derived neurotrophic factor).

GEA (gastroepiploic artery) **graft**—used instead of saphenous veins in coronary artery bypass surgery.

Geenan cytology brush.

Geenan Endotorque guide wire—used for cannulation of tortuous or strictured biliary ducts.

gegenhalten ("gay'-gen-hal-ten")—seen in cerebral cortical disorders, when the patient involuntarily resists passive movement. "Gegenhalten increase in tone is present and noticeable during the examination."

gelatin compression boot—used in the treatment of venous ulcer and stasis dermatitis. Works on the principle of even pressure on the veins, protecting them from further trauma. See *Unna boot*.

gelatin-resorcin-formalin glue—a tissue glue used instead of staples or sutures to repair dissected tissues.

gelatin sponge slurry—used like Gelfoam in arterial embolization.

gelbe cell—a cell in the mucosa of the gastrointestinal tract. Cf. *helle cell.*

Gelfoam—a purified gelatin product the body tissues will absorb. Used for hemostasis in surgery, and also used, in some forms, for treatment of gastric ulcer.

Gelfoam cookie. "A Gelfoam cookie was placed over the craniotomy." See *Gelfoam.*

Gellhorn pessary—a reduction device used to correct bladder prolapse.

Gelocast—a cast material.

Gelocast Unna boot compression dressing or wrap.

gel pads—used on the operating table to prevent or relieve pressure on shoulders, chest, or knees during surgery.

gemcitabine HCl (Gemzar)—a chemotherapy drug used to treat advanced gastric adenocarcinoma or malignant melanoma. It is the drug of choice for treating advanced or metastatic pancreatic cancer, replacing 5-FU.

Gemcor (gemfibrozil)—lipid-regulating agent that decreases serum triglycerides and VLDL (very low-density lipoprotein) cholesterol and increases HDL cholesterol.

Gem DR—implantable defibrillator that provides dual chamber pacing according to circulatory needs of the patient as well as detection and discrimination of ventricular and atrial tachyarrhythmia.

Gemini paired helical wire basket—used for ureteral stone retrieval in laparoscopic procedures.

gemistocytes—swollen astrocytes, either reactive or part of tumor.

GEMM-CFC (granulocyte, erythrocyte, monocyte, megakaryocyte colony-forming cells).

GEM-Premier analyzer—a 150-sample testing cartridge that can be used over a seven-day period, analyzing seven critical values from a single blood sample.

GEMSS (glaucoma, lens ectopia, microspherophakia, stiffness of the joints, and shortness) **syndrome.**

gemtuzumab ozogamicin—see *Mylotarg.*

Gemzar—see *gemcitabine HCl.*

gene and **oncogene**—see also *tumor marker* and *tumor suppressor gene.*

APC (adenomatous polyposis coli) tumor suppressor

Bcl-2 oncogene

BRCA1 (breast cancer one)

BRCA2 (breast cancer two)

c-erb B-2 oncogene

DCC (deleted in colon carcinoma) tumor suppressor

env

gag

HER-2-neu oncogene

MCC (mutated in colorectal carcinoma)

MLH_1

MSH_2

nef

NF1 (neurofibromatosis) tumor suppressor

NF2 (neurofibromatosis) tumor suppressor

p22 phox

p53

pol

PTEN

RB1 (retinoblastoma) tumor suppressor

rev

tat

TP53 (p53) tumor suppressor

VHL (von Hippel-Lindau) tumor suppressor

gene *(cont.)*
vif
von Hippel-Lindau (VHL)
vpr
vpu
WT1 (Wilms tumor) tumor
  suppressor
GeneAmp PCR (polymerase chain reaction) **test**—detects early HIV infection and also childhood leukemia
(chronic myeloid and acute lymphocytic). It is said to be one thousand
times more sensitive than previous
leukemia tests and weeks faster. See
polymerase chain reaction.
GeneChip system—see *Affymetrix
GeneChip system.*
genes in colorectal carcinoma—identified as DCC (deleted in colorectal
CA), APC (adenopolyposis coli),
and MCC (mutated in colorectal
CA). These do not follow the usual
naming methods of genes.
**Genentech biosynthetic human growth
hormone** (trade name, Protropin)—
produced by the DNA recombinant
method.
General Electric CT/T 8800 scanner
—analyzes stereotaxic data to obtain
X, Y, and Z coordinates for each
target lesion.
**generalized atrophic benign epider-
molysis bullosa** (GABEB)—a form
of nonlethal junctional epidermolysis
bullosa, characterized by generalized
blistering after birth, atrophic healing, and patchy bodywide atrophic
alopecia with onset in childhood.
generalized nephrographic (GNG)
phase imaging.
Generation 6—integrated radiotherapy
system that provides high-resolution
intensity modulated radiation therapy (IMRT) treatment for patients

with breast, head, neck, pancreatic,
and other cancers where precise
beam targeting and dose delivery
are needed.
GenESA System—combines a drug
and computer-controlled drug administration system for use in the
diagnosis of coronary artery disease
in conjunction with electrocardiography, echocardiography, and radionuclide imaging for patients who
cannot exercise adequately.
Genesis arthroplasty hardware.
Genesis 2000—a carbon dioxide laser
used in "laser tooth whitening."
**genetically modified or transgenic
pigs**—bred for the expression of a
human complement-regulatory protein to limit rejection in xenotransplantation.
geniculum—sharp, knee-like bend in a
structure or organ.
Genotropin (somatropin)—used to treat
children with growth hormone deficiency.
Gen-Probe—hybridization kit.
Gensini cardiac device.
GenStent biologic—gene-based therapeutic designed to help reduce
restenosis in patients following angioplasty or stent placement procedures.
gentamicin sulfate, liposomal (TLC-
G-65)—a drug for MAI infection in
AIDS patients.
Gentell alginate wound dressing.
Gentell foam wound dressing.
GentleLASE Plus—a laser system for
removal of hair and purpura-free
treatment of vascular lesions in large
leg veins.
GentlePeel skin exfoliation system—
removes old or damaged skin cells.
Gentle Touch—postoperative colostomy
appliance.

genuine stress incontinence (GSI).

Genutrain P3—active knee support for patellar realignment.

geographic tongue—a condition of the tongue in which irregular zones of redness appear and create an appearance somewhat like a map.

geophagia artifact (Radiol)—shows up radiologically as increased opacity in bowel and bands in fatty tissue. It is evidence of patients who eat dirt, paint, etc. Also *pica*.

Georgiade visor—halo fixation apparatus.

gepirone HCl—an antidepressant and anxiolytic similar to buspirone (Buspar), but chemically unrelated to benzodiazepines. General anxiety states are said to be improved with 2 to 3 weeks' treatment, with depressive symptoms improved faster.

GER (gastroesophageal reflux).

GERD (gastroesophageal reflux disease).

Gerdy's tubercle in the knee.

Geref (sermorelin acetate)—for growth hormone deficiency, anovulation, and AIDS-related weight loss.

Geristore—anhydrous nonacidic glass ionomer-based composite dental restorative.

Germanin (suramin)—antiparasitic.

germination tube—see *germ tube*.

germ tube test (brief form for *germination tube*)—a quick lab test to distinguish *Candida albicans* from other yeasts. "The patient had a yeast growing also, thought not to be *Candida albicans* by two-hour germ tube."

Gerstmann's syndrome—agraphia.

GE Senographe 2000D—fully digital mammography system.

gestodene (Minesse)—very low dose estrogen/progestin oral contraceptive.

Gey's solution—a fixative solution used with flexible bronchoscopy.

GFAP (glial fibrillary acidic protein)—a test for identifying some types of brain tumors.

GFR (glomerular filtration rate).

GFS Mark II inflatable penile prosthesis.

gfx (trademark) **coronary stent**.

GGT (gamma glutamyl transferase).

GGTP (gamma glutamyl transpeptidase)—a liver function test.

Ghajar guide—for intraventricular catheter placement. Used in trauma, in reduction of intracranial pressure; for placement of shunts in hydrocephalus; for placement of pharmacologic agents directly into cerebral ventricles.

GHB (gamma hydroxybutyrate)—drug used to treat narcolepsy and other sleep disorders.

Gherini-Kauffman endo-otoprobe—a type of laser probe used in ear surgery.

GHLs (glenohumeral ligaments).

Ghon complex—a peripheral calcified granuloma and lymph node in the lung, diagnostic of old tuberculous infection.

ghost vessels—in the cornea.

GHz (gigahertz).

Giampapa suturing technique—plastic surgical technique developed by Dr. Vincent C. Giampapa. It treats sagging neck and jaw muscles by tightening the underlying platysma muscle.

Giannestras step-down procedure—to lengthen post-traumatic shortness of the metatarsals.

Gianotti-Crosti syndrome—papular acrodermatitis of childhood.

giant anorectal condyloma acuminatum—giant anal wart caused by human papillomaviruses, and often oncogenic human papillomaviruses, with over 30% case rate of malignant transformation.

giant cell arteritis (GCA)—a systemic disease of unknown etiology; characterized by vasculitis in branches of the carotid artery, with narrowed vascular lumen and thickened intima. The artery may be occluded by thrombosis. This may be an immune-mediated abnormality. See *von Willebrand factor*.

Gianturco expandable (self-expanding) **metallic biliary stent**; **prosthesis**—a metal stent used to treat biliary and esophageal strictures; its wires are crisscrossed in a Z pattern. Also called *Z stent*.

Gianturco-Roehm—bird's nest vena cava filter.

Gianturco-Roubin flexible coil stent—an intracoronary stent used after a failed or suboptimal PTCA. Also used in hepatic revascularization.

Gianturco-Rösch Z-stent—an esophageal stent with an impermeable polyethylene film, inside and outside, to deter tumor ingrowth and seal fistulae.

Gianturco wool-tufted wire coil—used in embolization treatment of arteriovenous fistulae or pseudoaneurysms.

Giardia lamblia—a protozoan parasite virulent in AIDS patients. Can be transmitted in drinking water and through sexual contact.

GIA stapler—transects and staples. (GIA, gastrointestinal anastomosis.)

gibbous deformity—humped, humpbacked, protruding. Cf. *gibbus*.

Gibbs phenomenon (MRI term)—"ripples" parallel to sharp edges separating areas of different densities. See also *edge ringing artifact* and *truncation band artifact*.

gibbus (noun)—a hump. Cf. *gibbous*.

Gibson inner ear shunt—used to reduce inner ear pressure in patients suffering from Ménière's disease.

giddy headache—an old lay name for a headache preceded by vertigo.

Giebel blade plate—used in supratubular (or tubercular) wedge osteotomy.

GIFT (gamete intrafallopian transfer).

gift-wrap suture technique—the anatomic structure is wrapped on four sides with suture, and tied off at the top, resembling a gift-wrapped package.

gigahertz ("gig'-uh-herts") (GHz)—unit of frequency that equals 1 billion hertz (cycles per second); 10^9 Hz.

Gigli saw ("gee-lee," "jig-gly," or "gig-lee").

GIK (glucose, insulin, and potassium)—given to patients within 24 hours of experiencing heart attack symptoms. When administered, it is said the death rate from heart attack falls by half.

Gilles de la Tourette's syndrome—see *Tourette syndrome*.

Gillette joint—orthosis for ambulation in children with cerebral palsy and myelomeningocele. Made of rubber vacuformed into polypropylene to provide a plantar-flexion stop and free dorsiflexion.

Gilliam's suspension of the uterus.

Gillies elevation—procedure for fractured zygoma.

Gillies horizontal dermal suture.

Gill/Jonas modification of Norwood procedure—for hypoplastic left-

Gill/Jonas *(cont.)*
sided heart syndrome. See *Fontan; Sade.*

Gilvernet ("Jheel-vehr-nay") **retractor**.

gimpy—pejorative term for a lower extremity in which pain, spasm, or deformity causes a limp.

Gingrass and Messer pins—used in sagittal split ramus osteotomy.

Girard Fragmatome—a fragmentation probe used in cataract extraction.

Girdlestone-Taylor procedure (Ortho).

Gitelman syndrome—variant of hypokalemic-hypomagnesemic tubular disorder with hypocalciuria.

GITS (gastrointestinal therapeutic system)—a drug-delivery system that protects the GI tract.

gitter cell—not to be confused with *glitter cell.*

Gittes urethral suspension procedure (Dr. Ruben F. Gittes).

glabellar tap (Neuro)—a test for brain damage. With the extended index finger, the examiner taps the patient's forehead in the midline at the level of the supraorbital ridges. The patient blinks. This maneuver is then repeated. Normally the patient, knowing what is happening, does not again blink. However, a patient with certain central nervous system pathology blinks every time the glabella is tapped. A positive glabellar tap after infancy is a sign of brain damage.

Glandosane—flavored synthetic saliva to relieve dry mouth symptoms.

glandular atypia—atypical glandular cells of undetermined significance.

Glasgow Coma Scale (GCS)—assesses the prognosis of patients with head injuries by describing the patient's level of consciousness. It is divided into three parts:
Eyes open:
  spontaneously
  to speech
  to pain
  do not open
Best verbal response:
  oriented
  confused
  inappropriate words
  incomprehensible sounds
  no verbal response
Best motor response:
  obeys commands
  localizes pain
  flexion to pain
  extension to pain
  no motor response
Each of the parameters is scored on a scale of 1 through 5. The total of the values added together indicates the patient's level of consciousness. Normal would be 14 or 15; 7 or less would be considered coma. A score of 3 would be considered brain death (but is not conclusive). See *EMV grading.*

Glasgow Outcome Scale
Good recovery
Moderate disability
Severe disability
Permanent vegetative state
Death

glass eye artifact (Radiol)—appears on x-ray because of inadequate history given to radiologist.

Glassman clamp—used in thoracoscopy for compression and repositioning of the lung to facilitate stapling technique.

Glassman stone extractor—for removal of impacted common duct stones.

glaucoma—a disease characterized by increased intraocular pressure and impaired vision, ranging from slight abnormalities to absolute blindness.

Glaucoma Wick—for long-term treatment of glaucoma.

glaukomflecken—yeast-shaped opacities that form following acute glaucoma attack.

Gleason score—for carcinoma of the prostate: a grading for prognosis, on a scale of 1 through 5, from well differentiated to poorly differentiated. The test is done twice, in different areas, and the results added together. A score of 10, for example, would give a grave prognosis.

Glenn anastomosis procedure—in hypoplastic left heart syndrome.

Gliadel wafer (polifeprosan 20 with carmustine)—a biodegradable polymer implant used in the treatment of malignant glioma. Implanted in the cavity created when a brain tumor is removed, the Gliadel wafer slowly dissolves and releases carmustine to the tumor site. Since the carmustine is targeted directly to the tumor site, the total dose given via the Gliadel wafer is less than the dose that would be needed intravenously. See *Biodel, Septacin.*

glial cell-derived neurotrophic factor (GDNF).

glial fibrillary acidic protein (GFAP) —a test for identifying some types of brain tumors.

GliaSite—radiation therapy system implanted in the brain during the surgical procedure conducted to remove a tumor. The device is later filled with a liquid radiation source that places a high dose of radiation directly into the tissue most likely to contain residual cancer cells.

glide—a surgical instrument for intracapsular cataract extraction when the lens is subluxated.

Glidewire—trade name of a coated, kink-resistant guide wire used in endourology procedures. Also, Microvasive Glidewire. The generic *guide wire* is two words, *Glidewire* is one. See also *long taper/stiff shaft Glidewire.* Cf. *guide wire.*

glioblastoma multiforme—malignant tumor usually occurring in the cerebrum of adults.

Glisson's capsule—connective tissue covering of the liver.

glitter cell—not to be confused with *gitter cell.*

Global total shoulder arthroplasty.

globus hystericus—the sensation of having a lump in the throat, sometimes accompanied by choking, due to emotional upset. See also *globus pharyngis.*

globus pallidus—basal ganglia.

globus pharyngis—sensation of having a lump in the throat, often associated with esophageal motility disorder or stress (called *globus hystericus*).

glomerular filtration rate (GFR).

glomerulonephritis, acute poststreptococcal (APSGN).

glomus tumor—rare benign vascular tumor composed of a mass of arteriovenous anastomoses with a rich nerve supply and surrounded by special muscle cells known as glomus cells. Seventy-five percent of such tumors occur in the hand. Intraosseous (within bone) are rare.

glomus vagale—paraganglioma of the vagus nerve. Also called *glomus intravagale* or *nonchromaffin paraganglioma.*

GLS (gait lock splint) **brace.**

glucagon for injection (rDNA origin)— a recombinant form of glucagon to be used for the treatment of severe hypoglycemia in patients with diabetes and for diagnostic procedures involving the GI system. The recombinant form of glucagon will replace the animal-source glucagon product.

Glucometer DEX blood glucose monitor—a self-monitoring blood glucose system that allows diabetics the ability to test 10 times in a row through a self-calibrating 10-test cartridge.

Glucometer II—a home glucose monitoring system.

Glucophage (metformin hydrochloride) —a drug that lowers blood glucose without stimulating insulin secretion. Used to treat non-insulin-dependent diabetes mellitus (NIDDM).

Gluco-Protein—a self-test for glycated protein for use by patients with diabetes.

glucose, insulin, and potassium (GIK).

GlucoWatch—bloodless glucose monitor, worn like a wristwatch, and measuring glucose automatically through intact skin every 30 minutes, 24 hours a day.

glue—see *adhesive*.

glue ear—a term for middle ear effusion in which the secretions are glue-like.

glue-footed gait—an ataxic gait in which the patient seems unable to lift either foot from the floor.

glutaraldehyde cross-linked collagen injections—used to treat urinary incontinence in women. The material is biocompatible, biodegradable, sterile, nonpyrogenic, purified bovine dermal collagen which is cross-linked with the glutaraldehyde and dispersed in saline. The substance completely degrades in 9 to 19 months, resulting in the need for repeat injections to sustain efficacy.

glutaraldehyde-tanned bovine collagen tubes—for vascular xenografts or heterografts.

glutaraldehyde-tanned porcine heart valve—xenograft or heterograft.

gluteal bonnet—gluteus maximus and minimus.

Glutose—convenient, single-dose tube of oral glucose for quick treatment of hypoglycemia.

glycolic acid—a topical chemical agent used to induce facial skin peeling, and remove fine wrinkles, sun damage, actinic keratoses, or seborrheic keratoses. A 50-70% solution is left on the skin for 3-8 minutes, depending on the fairness and sensitivity of the patient's skin. This treatment is repeated four more times over one month.

glycol methacrylate—an embedding medium for pathology specimens.

Glycosal diabetes test—rapid doctors' office test to assist in the identification and management of diabetes.

glycosylated hemoglobin—an assay of diabetic control; glucose stays attached to the red cell for the life of the cell and can be measured.

Glylorin (monolaurin)—used for treatment of nonbullous congenital ichthyosiform erythroderma.

Glynase Pres Tab (glyburide)—an oral antidiabetic drug, also marketed as DiaBeta and Micronase.

Glypressin (terlipressin)—for treating bleeding esophageal ulcers.

Glyset (miglitol)—used to treat type 2 diabetes.

GM-CSF (granulocyte/macrophage colony-stimulating factor)—also regramostim, sargramostim, molgramostim).

GMS stain (Gomori, or Grocott, methenamine silver)—a stain used to establish the diagnosis of *Pneumocystis carinii* pneumonia.

GNG (generalized nephrographic) **phase imaging**—used on CT scan to detect acute renal infection.

GnRH (gonadotropin-releasing hormone). See *LHRH* (luteinizing hormone-releasing hormone).

GOAT (Galveston Orientation and Amnesia Test).

Goeckerman regimen—treatment for psoriasis including application of tar and tar-based medications, shampoos with tar, and two types of light treatment (shortwave ultraviolet light in increasing doses daily, and quartz light in increasing doses).

Goetz cardiac device.

goiter—see *lithiumogenic goiter.*

Golaski graft—a knitted Dacron graft used during carotid endarterectomy and carotid-subclavian artery bypass.

Golay coil—MRI term.

Goldenhar syndrome—oculoauriculovertebral dysplasia. A congenital anomaly involving the eye, ear, vertebrae, and mandible, temporal and zygomatic bones, and the muscles used in facial expression and mastication.

Goldman cardiac risk index score—a clinical scoring system used to predict cardiac morbidity.

Goldmann applanation tonometer—used to measure intraocular pressure.

Goldmann lens—a three-mirror contact lens used in photocoagulation

procedures for detached retina, or in lattice degeneration.

Goldman procedure—a nasal tip reconstructive technique.

Gold Probe bipolar hemostasis catheter.

Goldstein Microspike approximator clamp (Urol)—a clamp with tiny spikes on its surface to aid in gripping the vas deferens to assist in anastomosis during vasovasostomy.

Golgi complex—a collection of vesicles in the cell cytoplasm where products of cell metabolism are placed into vacuoles for excretion.

Goligher retractor—modification of the Berkeley-Bonney self-retaining 3-blade abdominal retractor for use in abdominal surgery.

GoLytely (polyethylene glycol-electrolyte solution)—gastrointestinal lavage prep for improved visualization in bowel examination.

Gomori (or Grocott) **methenamine silver** (GMS)—a stain used to establish the diagnosis of *Pneumocystis carinii* pneumonia.

gonadorelin acetate (Lutrepulse)—used to induce ovulation in women with amenorrhea resulting from dysfunction of the hypothalamus. Cf. *goserelin acetate.*

gonadotropin-releasing hormone (GnRH). See *goserelin acetate.*

Gonal-F (follitropin alfa for injection)—a recombinant follicle stimulating hormone used in treatment of infertility.

gonial angle—of the mandible.

gonioscope—an optical instrument for direct visualization of the anterior chamber through the use of a goniolens; e.g., Sussman gonioscope.

Gonzales blood group—a blood group character (antigen Goa) for which the antibody was reported in a mother (Mrs. Gonzales) of a newborn infant with erythroblastosis fetalis. This is an antibody apparently found only in individuals who are of African-American parentage, and it is distinct from all previously classified blood group systems.

Goodale-Lubin cardiac device.

Goodell's sign—softening of the cervix because of an increased blood supply, an early clue to pregnancy.

Goodenough test—a draw-a-man test to estimate intelligence. The name of the test does not refer to the performance; it is named for Florence Goodenough.

GoodKnight 418A, 418G, 418P—home care CPAP system for treatment of patients suffering from obstructive sleep apnea.

Gordon-Sweet staining—used to determine the growth pattern of tumors (follicular or follicular and diffuse).

Gore cast liner—waterproof cast liner that breathes.

gore pattern—created by cutting the surface of a sphere along longitudinal lines to change the radius of curvature. See *Hendel correction of scaphocephaly*.

Gore Smoother Crucial Tool—used as a trial graft and replacement tool in cruciate replacement operations.

Gore-Tex—nonabsorbable surgical suture and a graft material; also used for many other purposes. Examples:
bifurcated vascular graft
cardiovascular patch
catheter
knee prosthesis
limb

Gore-Tex *(cont.)*
shunt
soft tissue patch
stretch vascular graft
surgical membrane
tapered vascular graft
vascular graft

Gore-Tex FEP-Ringed vascular graft.

Gore-Tex nasal implant—used to augment the nasal dorsum or base in the rhinoplasty procedure.

Gore-Tex SAM (subcutaneous augmentation material) **facial implants** (Plas Surg)—made of expanded polytetrafluoroethylene (PTFE) that is reinforced with fluorinated ethylene propylene to make a rigid, but soft, material that is easy to carve or shape. It is easier to shape than non-reinforced PTFE, and its structure permits cellular ingrowth and incorporation of connective tissue.

Gore-Tex strips—used in plastic surgery as implants to augment soft tissue in facial contouring.

GOS (Glasgow Outcome Scale).

goserelin acetate (Zoladex)—a synthetic version of the naturally occurring gonadotropin-releasing female hormone. It is used to treat advanced prostate cancer which thrives in the presence of the male hormone androgen, to treat endometriosis, and to induce ovulation in women. Cf. *gonadorelin acetate*.

Gosling pulsatility index.

Gosset—see *spiral band of Gosset*.

gossypiboma (cotton)—a term applied to a laparotomy pad left in at previous surgery and recovered by laparoscopy.

Gottschalk Nasostat—a rubber cannula used to stop epistaxis (nosebleed).

Gott shunt—used in liver transplantation.

gouge—(noun) a hollow chisel used for cutting or removing bone or cartilage; (verb) to scoop out, as with a gouge. Cf. *gauge.*

Gould electromagnetic flowmeter—records arterial blood flow rates.

Gould polygraph—device for measuring gastric motility.

Goulian mammoplasty.

Gowers' maneuver—patients with weakness may find it necessary to "climb" up their legs with their hands, to rise from a sitting position.

Gowers sign—classical sign of Duchenne muscular dystrophy; also called *tripoding.*

GPC (giant papillary conjunctivitis).

gp41, gp120, gp160—parts of the envelope of the HIV virus, under study in development of possible AIDS vaccine.

GPI$_b$ (glycoprotein I$_b$)—a platelet membrane receptor.

GPMAL (obstetrical history): gravida, para, multiple births, abortions, live births.

gp120—an AIDS vaccine.

graciloplasty—see *dynamic graciloplasty.*

grade—see *classification.*

gradient coil—MRI term.

gradient magnetic field—MRI term.

gradient-recalled echo (GRE)—MRI term.

graft, graft material (see also *flap* and *graft, skin*)

AlloDerm processed tissue

AlloMatrix injectable putty bone graft substitute

AneuRx stent

aortofemoral bypass (AFBG)

Apligraf (graftskin)

graft *(cont.)*

Aria coronary artery bypass

autologous fat

BAGF (brachioaxillary bridge graft fistula)

Bard Composix mesh

Bard Sperma-Tex preshaped mesh

Bard Visilex mesh

batten

Biobrane/HF

Biograft bovine heterograft

BioPolyMeric

bone graft substitute—CHAG

BonePlast

Bonfiglio

bovine heterograft

brachiosubclavian bridge

BSGF (brachiosubclavian bridge graft fistula)

CABG (coronary artery bypass)

Calcitite

Capset (calcium sulfate) bone graft barrier

carbon fiber synthetic ligament

Carbo-Seal

cavum conchal cartilage

CHAG (coralline hydroxyapatite Goniopora)

Collagraft bone graft matrix

Cotton cartilage

Cragg endoluminal

cultured epithelial autograft

cymba conchal cartilage

Cymetra tissue replacement material

Dacron synthetic ligament material

Dardik Biograft

delayed xenograft rejection (DXR)

denatured homograft

Dermagraft human-based dermal replacement

Dermagraft-TC (transitional covering)

Diastat vascular access

discordant cellular xenograft

graft *(cont.)*
    discordant organ xenograft
    Distaflo bypass
    doubled semitendinosus and
        gracilis autograft (DST&G)
    DTAFA (descending thoracic aorta-
        to-femoral artery) bypass
    DualMesh biomaterial
    DuraGen
    Durapatite
    E-CABG (endoscopic coronary
        artery bypass graft)
    Edwards woven Teflon aortic
        bifurcation
    endovascular stent
    epidural blood patch
    flap
    Fluoropassiv thin-wall carotid patch
    full-thickness skin
    GEA (gastroepiploic artery)
    glutaraldehyde-tanned bovine
        collagen tubes
    glutaraldehyde-tanned porcine
        heart valve
    Golaski
    Gore-Tex
    Gore-Tex FEP-Ringed vascular
    Gore-Tex stretch vascular
    Gore-Tex tapered vascular
    Grafton DBM (demineralized bone
        matrix) bone
    Graftpatch
    Hapset bone graft plaster
    Healos synthetic bone-grafting
        material
    Hedrocel bone substitute material
    Hemashield
    heterografts, bovine and porcine
    human meniscal allograft
    hydroxyapatitite
    IEA (inferior epigastric artery)
    IMA (inferior mammary artery)
    infrarenal aortobifemoral bypass
    inlay

graft *(cont.)*
    InterGard Knitted collagen coated
    Interpore
    Ionescu-Shiley pericardial xenograft
    ITA (internal thoracic artery)
    Kimura cartilage
    LIMA (left internal mammary
        artery)
    Marlex synthetic
    Martius
    MD-111 bone allograft
    Meadox Microvel arterial
    Microknit vascular
    mitral valve homograft
    MycroMesh biomaterial
    myocutaneous
    Ne-Osteo bone morphogenic protein
        (BMP)
    Nicoll
    onlay
    Paritene mesh
    PepGen P-15 (peptide-enhanced
        bone graft)
    Perma-Flow coronary bypass
    PermaMesh
    Perma-Seal dialysis access
    PFTE (polyfluorotetraethylene)
    pigskin
    porcine xenograft
    portacaval H
    postage-stamp type skin
    ProOsteon 500 bone implant
    Proplast
    PTFE (polytetrafluoroethylene)
    pulmonary autograft (PA)
    Pyrost
    Rapidgraft arterial vessel substitute
    Sauvage
    sentinel skin paddle
    seromuscular intestinal patch
    skin
    Solvang
    Sperma-Tex preshaped mesh
    spreader

graft *(cont.)*
stem cell autograft
Sure-Closure skin-stretching system
Surgipro prolene mesh
SurgiSis sling/mesh
sutured in place, shield-shaped tip
Synergraft
Thiersch
Thoralon biomaterial
TransCyte skin substitute
transplanted stamp
Trelex mesh
Unigraft bone graft material
Unilab Surgibone
Vascu-Guard bovine pericardial
    surgical patch
vascularized fibula
Vascutek
Vectra vascular access (VAG)
Venaflow vascular
Weaveknit vascular
Wesolowski vascular
Wolfe
XenoDerm
xenograft
Zenith AAA (abdominal aortic
    aneurysm) endovascular
Zenotech

GraftAssist vein and graft holder—
reduces the chance of narrowing at
the anastomosis site.

GraftCyte—a gauze wound dressing
containing copper peptide. It is used
particularly in hair restoration procedures.

Grafton DBM (demineralized bone
matrix) **bone graft**. Also, Grafton
DBM gel, putty, and flex strips.

Graftpatch—used in general surgical
procedures to reinforce soft tissue.

graft, skin
split thickness—.010 to .035 inch
    thick

graft, skin *(cont.)*
full thickness—greater than .035
    inch thick
free graft—does not have its own
    blood supply; gets blood from
    capillary ingrowth from under-
    lying tissue
pedicle—gets its blood supply from
    subcutaneous vessels that came
    with the pedicle portion of the
    graft

Graftskin—a manufactured human skin
product used to treat chronic wounds
that do not respond well to traditional treatment.

graft versus host disease (GVHD)—
caused by reaction to an allograft,
from marrow transplant, etc. Following is the GVHD grading system
(written as clinical grade 1, etc.):

1 Mild skin rash (generally
   maculopapular). No gastrointestinal or liver function
   abnormalities.
2 Moderately severe skin rash.
   Mild gastrointestinal symptoms.
   Slight increase in bilirubin and
   perhaps also in liver enzymes.
3 Moderately severe skin rash,
   gastrointestinal symptoms, and
   liver function abnormalities.
4 Severe peeling and flaking of
   the skin, severe gastrointestinal
   symptoms, and liver function
   abnormalities.

graft versus host reaction—see *graft
versus host disease.*

Graham plication—an omental patch
sutured over a perforated ulcer site.

Graham Steell heart murmur (no
hyphen).

gram-negative organisms—*Haemophilus, Neisseria, Pseudomonas.* See
Gram's stain; gram-positive.

gram-positive organisms—*Clostridium, Corynebacterium, Staphylococcus, Streptococcus.* See *Gram's stain; gram-negative organisms.*

Gram's stain (named for Hans Christian Joachim Gram)—a stain using the bacterial property of stain retention or loss to help in classification and subsequent treatment. The smears are fixed to a slide by heat and stained with a solution of crystal violet, which stains all bacteria. An iodine solution then fixes the dye to the gram-positive organisms. The specimen is decolorized by washing with a mixture of acetone and alcohol, and then counterstained with a dye of another color (usually safranin). Gram-positive organisms retain the original purple stain; gram-negative organisms, however, turn pink (if safranin was used). Note: Capitalize *Gram's stain*, but lowercase *gram-negative* and *gram-positive.* See *gram-negative; gram-positive.*

GraNee needle (Riza-Ribe grasper needle)—single-use device used in laparoscopic surgical procedures for grasping free ends of a suture ligature for intracorporeal or extracorporeal tying.

granisetron HCl (Kytril)—antiemetic for prevention of acute chemotherapy-induced nausea and vomiting.

Granocyte (lenograstim)—said to speed the recovery of white blood cells, when given to lymphoma patients after they have been reinfused with mobilized peripheral blood progenitor stem cells.

granulocyte colony-stimulating factor —see *G-CSF.*

granulocyte/macrophage colony-stimulating factor (GM-CSF)—a naturally occurring growth factor which stimulates myeloid progenitor cells in the bone marrow to divide and differentiate into granulocytes and macrophages. Also stimulates mature granulocytes and macrophages to higher levels of migration towards pathogens, phagocytosis, and cytotoxic activity, thus enhancing the effectiveness of the immune system. Used in chemotherapy and in conjunction with AZT in treatment of AIDS. See *sargramostim.* Cf. *G-CSF.*

granulocyte transfusions—may have a greater effect on survival rates compared to use of broad-spectrum antibiotics in neutropenic patients with cancer.

granuloma—see *pyogenic granuloma* (granuloma pyogenicum).

granuloma gravidarum—gingival pyogenic granuloma of pregnancy.

granulomatous mastitis—a very rare lesion somewhat similar to duct ectasia, except that it is always peripheral and confined to the breast lobule. See *duct ectasia.*

graphesthesia—relates to the perception and identification of letters or numbers written on the skin with a blunt object.

graphospasm—writer's cramp.

grasp reflex—the reflex of an infant who will automatically grasp a finger placed against the palmar surface of its hand.

GRASS (gradient recalled acquisition in a steady state)—technique for cardiac MRI test.

gravida—the number of pregnancies a woman has had: *gravida 4*, having been pregnant 4 times; *gravida 5, para 3, ab 2,* five pregnancies, three live births, two abortions or miscarriages. See also *GPMAL; para.*

Gravindex—relatively sensitive pregnancy test used in physician offices.

gray (Gy)—the International System unit of absorbed dose, equal to the energy imparted by ionizing radiation to a mass of matter corresponding to 1 joule per kilogram. Used in radiotherapy. See *joule*.

Gray bone drill—developed by Frank B. Gray, M.D.

gray line—in the eye.

Grayson's ligament in hand—it keeps the skin sleeve from twisting around the bones of the digit. You may hear this referred to in operative procedures for Dupuytren's contracture. See also *Cleland's ligament*; they are *not* synonymous.

GRE (gradient-recalled echo)—used in the phrase, "three-dimensional GRE MR imaging of TFC (triangular fibrocartilage) tears and triangular fibrocartilage complex (TFCC)."

great vessels—on chest x-ray, the major vascular trunks entering and leaving the heart: the superior and inferior venae cavae, the pulmonary arteries and veins, and the aorta.

Greenfield IVC filter—a permanent inferior vena cava filter, placed via the right jugular vein into the inferior vena cava to filter out emboli that might otherwise reach the lung.

Greenwald cutting loop—used with Storz resectoscope.

Greenwald flexible endoscopic electrodes.

Greig cephalopolysyndactyly syndrome—a relatively rare condition in which fingers, toes, or other body parts are completely or partially webbed, with craniosynostosis sometimes present. It is caused by a chromosomal translocation thought to involve chromosome 7.

grenz ray—long wave irradiation; used in treatment of localized neurodermatitis and in lichen simplex chronicus; a low-energy x-ray.

Greulich and Pyle, bone age—for measurement of bone age and for staging skeletal maturation. Also referred to as *G & P*.

GRFoma—a rare pancreatic endocrine tumor.

Grice-Green procedure—to correct hindfoot valgus deformity.

Grieshaber manipulator—multi-function instrument used in vitreous surgery. It has a light source, a suction forceps, and a coagulator.

Griesinger's sign—swelling and pain in the neck on rotation, easily mistaken for meningitis, but in this case due to thrombophlebitis of the mastoid emissary vein.

Grinfeld cannula—a triple-lumen cannula that accommodates cardioplegia, arterial return, and aortic clamping during coronary artery bypass surgery.

Gripper needle.

grip tester—see *Jamar*.

Grocott (or Gomori) **methenamine silver (GMS) stain**. See *Gomori*.

Grollman catheter.

Groningen voice prosthesis.

Groshong catheter—used in central venous lines for administration of intravenous chemotherapeutic agents.

gross description (Path)—description of tissue as it appears to the unaided eye prior to fixation and paraffin embedding.

Grosse and Kempf locking nail system—femoral and tibial nails. There are two types: static locking (com-

Grosse and Kempf *(cont.)*
plete locking) and dynamic locking (partial locking). Stabilizes and controls fragment rotation and maintains desired bone length.

ground-glass cells—pathology as seen in chronic hepatitis B.

group A beta-hemolytic streptococcus (GABHS)—the pathogen that causes pharyngitis, rheumatic fever, toxic strep syndrome, and cellulitis. See *streptococcal A infection*.

Grover's disease—temporary skin disorder that consists of small, firm, raised red lesions on the skin. Small blisters containing a watery liquid are present, which tend to group and have a swollen red border around them. Its cause is unknown but is thought to be related to trauma to sun-damaged skin, and it occurs mainly in men over the age of 40.

Gruentzig—see *Grüntzig*.

grunting—involuntary noise made by newborns with respiratory distress to try to keep lungs adequately inflated.

Grüntzig (Gruentzig) **balloon catheter** —used in percutaneous transluminal dilatation and angioplasty. (An umlaut is required over the "u" in *Grüntzig*; if an umlaut is not available on the keyboard, the spelling is *Gruentzig*.)

GSI (genuine stress incontinence).

G6PD (glucose-6-phosphate dehydrogenase)—X-linked enzyme. Used as a cell marker to study possible origin of different neoplastic disorders.

G-suit—an external counterpressure device used to control hemorrhage; provides tamponade of pelvic fracture-induced hemorrhage.

GTD (gestational trophoblastic disease).

GTS great toe system—two-piece implant designed to provide anatomic movement for the first metatarsophalangeal joint.

GII (Generation II) **unloader knee brace**—provides symptomatic relief of pain caused by unicompartmental degenerative joint disease or osteoarthritis.

guaiac test of occult blood in the stool (blood in too small an amount to be detected by naked-eye observation). "Stool is guaiac negative." See also *fecal occult blood test*; *Hemoccult Sensa*; *Hemoccult II*; and *occult blood*.

Guardsman femoral screw—interference screw and delivery system used in endoscopic femoral fixation and orthopedic procedures where graft protection is required. Also used in knee arthroscopy.

Guardwire angioplasty system—seals one end of a bypass graft with a balloon to prevent debris from floating downstream into the coronary artery. A second balloon inflated at the site of blockage presses material that caused the blockage against the vessel wall within the bypass to restore blood flow to the heart. A low-pressure vacuum aspiration catheter then draws out remaining debris from inside the vessel.

Gudden's atrophy—retrograde degeneration of the thalamus after cortical lesions. Named for German neurologist, Bernhard Aloys von Gudden. Also, *Gudden's commissure, Gudden's tract, nucleus of Gudden*.

Gudden's tract—mammillotegmental tract in the brain.

Guepar II hinged knee prosthesis.

guerney—see *gurney*.

Guglielmi Detachable Coil (GDC)—used to treat intracranial aneurysms that are considered inoperable or at high-risk for surgery. The GDC is delivered to the aneurysm site by a microcatheter. The coil fills the aneurysm, isolating it from the circulation.

Guibor Silastic tube—used in surgery of the lacrimal system.

Guidant Multi-Link Tetra coronary stent system.

Guidant's TRIAD three-electrode energy defibrillation system (Cardio)—said to reduce the amount of energy needed for defibrillation.

guide wire (see also *Glidewire*)
   ACS Hi-Torque Balance Middleweight
   Athlete coronary
   Extra Sport coronary
   FasTrac
   floppy
   Geenan Endotorque
   HPC
   Lumina
   Lunderquist
   Magnum
   Microvasive Glidewire
   Mustang steerable
   QuickSilver hydrophilic-coated
   Radiofocus Glidewire
   ROTACS
   Silk
   steerable guide wire system
   Terumo
   WaveWire

Guilford brace.

Guillain-Barré syndrome—acute idiopathic polyneuritis, an acute, rapidly progressive nerve inflammation, with weakness of the muscles of the legs, then weakness in the arms and face, and may also affect the muscles of respiration. It appears to be self-limiting in 90 to 95% of patients, with complete recovery, but it can result in flaccid quadriplegia or respiratory failure. Also called *infectious polyneuritis, Landry-Guillain-Barré-Strohl syndrome, Landry-Guillain syndrome,* and *Landry's paralysis.*

Gullstrand's slit lamp—see *biomicroscope.*

gull-wing incision—a midcolumellar transverse incision that looks like the drawings of birds we all did in grade school. Used in nasal tip reconstructive surgery.

gum sculpting—grafting procedure in which sections of gum in one area of the mouth are inserted into a receded area. This produces teeth that appear even in length.

Gunderson conjunctival flap.

Gunn crossing sign (Cardio).

GunSlinger shoulder orthosis—for correct positioning and immobilization of the shoulder and arm following surgery.

gurney (guerney)—high wheeled cot for moving patients.

Gusberg hysterectomy clamp—with Kapp-Beck serrations.

Gustilo-Kyle cementless total hip arthroplasty.

gut-associated lymphoid tissue (GALT).

gut-hormone profile—a pattern of hormone release that may help to distinguish celiac disease from other abdominal problems.

Guttmann subtalar arthrodesis.

Guyon's canal—anatomical landmark in operative procedures designed to reduce ulnar nerve compression which occurs as the ulnar nerve

Guyon's canal *(cont.)*
passes behind the medial epicondyle, between the heads of the flexor carpi ulnaris, or along Guyon's canal from the pisiform bone to the hook of the hamate.

guy sutures *(not* Guy)—a steadying or guiding suture, to prevent movement.

GVAX—a cancer vaccine.

GVHD (graft-versus-host disease) (or reaction). See *graft-versus-host disease*.

GVR (galvanic vestibular stimulation).

GVR (growth velocity ratio).

gymnast's wrist—ulnar pain, ulnar variance of several millimeters, prominence of the ulnar head with either full or limited range of motion. These findings are due to repetitive compression of the bones of the forearm during handstands and other gymnastic maneuvers. The bones of the wrist may show abnormalities in the growth plates.

Gynecare Verascope hysteroscopy system—fiberoptic technology for diagnostic and operative hysteroscopy procedures.

Gypsona—a rapid-setting cast material.

gyromagnetic ratio—MRI term.

Gyroscan ACS NT MRI scanner.

gyrus—a folding in the surface (cortex) of the cerebrum.

Gyrus endourology system—uses PlasmaKinetic radiofrequency energy delivery for minimally invasive endoscopic treatment of urethral obstructions in men secondary to an enlarged prostate.

H, h

HA (hydroxyapatite)—coating for load-bearing implants.

HAART (highly active antiretroviral therapy)—used for patients with AIDS.

HAB (Histoacryl Blue).

habenula ("hah-ben´u-lah")—a small protuberance at the dorsal and posterior edge of the third ventricle, adjacent to the pineal body. It is part of the epithalamus.

Habitrol—see *Nicoderm*.

HACEK—an acronym for a group of gram-negative bacilli, including *Haemophilus aphrophilus* (and other *Haemophilus* species), *Actinobacillus actinomycetemcomitans, Cardiobacterium hominis, Eikenella corrodens,* and *Kingella kingae*, which are usually associated with infectious endocarditis, but can also occur with other infections.

H-Ae interval (retrograde conduction) —in electrophysiologic studies of supraventricular tachycardia.

Haemonetics Cell Saver—collects a patient's blood for retransfusion at the end of an operative procedure.

Haemonetics V-50—used to reduce volume and deplete red cells in harvested bone marrow.

Haemophilus ducreyi—the cause of soft chancres or chancroids on the genitalia of humans. Also called *Ducrey's bacillus*.

Haemophilus vaginalis—see *Gardnerella vaginalis*.

Hafnia alvei—new name of *Enterobacter hafnia*, associated with enteritis.

Hageman factor—factor XII of blood coagulation factors.

Haglund's deformity—causes traumatic inflammation of Achilles tendon and bursa.

HAI (hepatic arterial infusion).

Haid Universal bone plate system—titanium, MRI-compatible plate and screw system for treating fracture traumas, postlaminectomy instability, and degenerative spinal disease.

hairy-cell leukemia (HCL)—first described in 1958. On electron micrographs, the cells have projections radiating from their walls.

Hakim-Cordis pump—used in neurological surgery procedures.

Halban culdoplasty.

Halbrecht's syndrome—ABO erythroblastosis.

Halcion (triazolam)—hypnotic for insomnia.

Haldol (haloperidol).

Halfan (halofantrine HCl)—antimalarial.

half and half nails—a dull-white proximal half of the fingernails meets a reddish-brown distal half. A sign of possible renal disease that may precede symptoms of renal disease.

half base syndrome—see *Garcin's syndrome.*

half-dose enhanced MRI with MT (magnetization transfer). Cf. *standard-dose enhanced conventional MR imaging.*

half-Fourier acquisition single-shot turbo spin-echo (HASTE)—technique for MRU (magnetic resonance urography).

half-hitch—the simplest knot that can be tied in the two ends of a single looped strand; the first half of a square knot. Used in surgery.

half-moon mark artifact—see *kink artifact.*

Halifax interlaminar clamp system—provides stabilization of the posterior cervical spine with placement from C1 through C7 at multiple levels.

Hall dermatome—an oscillating blade type.

Haller's layer—the vascular layer of the choroid of the eye.

Hallpike caloric stimulation test (ENT) —see *caloric testing of vestibular function.*

Hallpike-Dix maneuver—a maneuver in which the direction of the vertical component of nystagmus is observed in patients with benign paroxysmal positional vertigo affecting the posterior canal.

Hallpike test—see *Dix-Hallpike test.*

hallucinosis—pathological entity characterized by hallucination. Types: alcoholic and drug-induced.

hallux abductovalgus—the deformity which causes the great toe to be abducted and everted (abductovalgus) and usually is corrected surgically with a bunionectomy.

Hall valve—a prosthetic heart valve by Medtronic.

Hall valvulotome—used to disrupt the valves in a vein and make the valve leaflets incompetent. This allows the vein to be used in distal saphenous vein bypass procedures.

halobetasol propionate (Ultravate)—a topical corticosteroid.

halofantrine HCl (Halfan)—antimalarial developed by the U.S. Army for multi-drug-resistant malaria. Cure rates of 83% to 100% have been shown in strains resistant to chloroquine (Aralen) and sulfonamide/pyrimethamine (Fansidar). It is not effective as prophylaxis.

halofuginone—specific inhibitor of collagen type I synthesis, used for treatment of scleroderma.

haloperidol (Haldol)—a common antipsychotic drug now prescribed for patients with Alzheimer's disease. It is producing significant improvement in symptoms of aggressiveness and behavioral problems.

halo test—a bedside test for cerebrospinal fluid rhinorrhea. In this test, a drop of bloody fluid from the nose is placed on a cloth surface. If present, the CSF will diffuse in a radial pattern along with the blood; however, the CSF will migrate farther

halo test *(cont.)*
than the blood, forming a "halo" effect.

halo traction—see *cervical support.*

HALS (hand-assisted laparoscopic surgery).

Halstead-Wepman Aphasia Screening Test.

Halsted hemostatic mosquito forceps (straight/curved).

Halsted inguinal herniorrhaphy (*not* Halstead).

HAMA (human antimurine antibody) **response**.

Hamman-Rich syndrome—diffuse interstitial pulmonary fibrosis.

Hamman's sign—a sign of pneumopericardium, an acute medical emergency. The physician hears a loud clicking or crunching sound in time with the heart beat.

Hammer mini-tubular external fixation system.

hammer toe—clawlike flexion contracture of the second and distal phalanges.

hammer toe repair—see *DuVries hammer toe repair.*

Hampton's hump—a pleurally based, triangular lung infiltrate.

Hamus wrist arthroplasty.

Hancke/Vilmann biopsy handle instrument—consisting of a steel needle with stylet, metal spiral sheath, and an aluminum biopsy handle. Used for gastrointestinal endoscopy.

Hancock M.O. bioprosthesis—a tissue valve for the small aortic root; used instead of a porcine valve.

Hancock M.O. II bioprosthesis porcine valve.

Hancock II tissue valve—porcine prosthetic heart valve indicated for both aortic valve and mitral valve replacement. Special features include a stent and a scalloped sewing ring to facilitate placement and implantation.

H&E stain (hematoxylin and eosin).

"H&H"—slang for hemoglobin and hematocrit.

hand—see *Myobock hand* and *Utah artificial arm.*

Handages—specially designed dressings for the burned hand that are shaped like a glove and feature a Velcro opening on the back for easy application and removal. The bandage gloves consist of three layers, including a breathable transparent film barrier that protects the wound from contamination, an absorbent middle layer, and a nonadherent wound contact layer. Handages can be removed without soaking. Because they do not adhere to the wound, changing them is not as painful as traditional bandages are.

hand-assisted laparoscopic surgery (HALS)—combines advantages of open surgery with minimal invasiveness and rapid recovery of laparoscopy; ideally suited to remove malignant kidney tumors and to repair renal, ureteral, and bladder abnormalities. Provides for minimally invasive kidney donation, reducing recovery time for donors (17 vs. 60 days) and a kidney that has suffered a minimal period of interrupted blood flow.

hand movements (HM).

Hands Free knee retractor system.

hand surgery graft—see *flap.*

hang-back technique—ophthalmic surgical method for performing bimedial rectus recession for correction of strabismus and exotropia. May also be called *anchored hang-back* or *adjustable hang-back technique.*

Hanger ComfortFlex—socket system that combines with a computerized knee prosthesis, allowing an amputee to have maximum control and command over the lower limb.

hanging panniculus—see *apron*.

hangman's fracture—sometimes the result of injury to the neck in motorcycle or automobile accidents, in which there is rupture of the anterior and posterior longitudinal ligaments, leading to anterior luxation of C2 over C3, with crushing of the intervertebral disk.

Hank's balanced salt solution (HBSS) —used in bone marrow transplantation.

Hansel's stain—used in microscopic examination of eosinophils.

Hantavirus pulmonary syndrome (HPS)—identified in 1993 in an outbreak in the American Southwest. The virus was named for the Hantaan River of Korea in 1978. HPS is caused by the Sin Nombre virus (SNV) and transmitted by rodents.

Ha-1A—a human monoclonal antibody found to be effective against gram-negative sepsis (a virulent and deadly multisystem disease caused by the endotoxins released in the bloodstream by gram-negative bacteria). Ha-1A binds to the endotoxins, inactivating them. See *Centoxin*.

HAP (hepatic arterial-dominant phase) **images** (CT scan).

Hapset—HA (hydroxyapatite) bone graft plaster also used for periodontal defects and tooth extraction sites. The plaster itself absorbs, leaving only an HA scaffold for bony ingrowth.

haptens—the little loops on implant cataract lens through which the sutures are passed to keep the lens in place. Used interchangeably with *haptics*.

haptics—see *haptens*.

HAR (hyperacute rejection).

Hardy-Sella punch—a small punch used to create an osteotomy in the lacrimal fossa.

Harmonic Scalpel—see *UltraCision ultrasonic knife*.

Harpoon suture anchor.

Harrell Y stent—Y-shaped stent with posts for short-term management of airway obstructions.

Harrington retractor (Ortho)—called "sweetheart," probably because the tip of the blade is somewhat heart-shaped. Used in acetabular fracture repair.

Harrington rod—used to correct scoliosis.

Harris-Galante porous-coated femoral component.

Harrison's groove—a horizontal groove along the lower thorax; seen in children with rickets, or in people who have had rickets.

Harrison-Nicolle polypropylene pegs —used in hand surgery.

Hartmann hemostatic mosquito forceps (straight/curved).

Hartmann's solution (Ringer's lactate) —a physiologic salt solution.

Hartzler ACX-II or RX-014 balloon catheter.

Hartzler Micro II balloon—used in coronary angioplasty.

Harvard Criteria for Brain Death— including unreceptivity and unresponsiveness, total unawareness to externally applied stimuli and inner need, and complete unresponsiveness, in addition to:

Harvard criteria *(cont.)*

No movements or breathing—no spontaneous muscular movements or spontaneous respirations or response to stimuli such as pain, touch, sound, or light for at least one hour. After a patient has been on a mechanical respirator, the total absence of spontaneous breathing may be established by turning off the respirator for three minutes and observing for any effort by the patient to breathe spontaneously.

No reflexes—fixed and dilated pupils that do not respond to a direct source of light, and absence of ocular movement, blinking, swallowing, yawning, vocalization, and corneal and pharyngeal reflexes.

Harvard pump—an infusion device which continually injects medication at a preset rate.

Harvard 2 dual syringe pump—a multiple syringe infusion pump that can deliver two drug agents simul taneously and alert clinicians to blockages in infusion lines.

harvest—to remove tissue or organs from a donor for transplantation; to take skin, bone, or cartilage from the patient for an autologous graft. See also *evisceration*, *recovery*, *stem-cell marrow harvesting*, *total abdominal evisceration*.

Harvey hospital prognostic nutritional index.

Hasson blunt-end cannula—used in laparoscopic procedures.

Hasson graspers—used in endoscopic procedures.

Hasson open laparoscopy cannula.

Hasson SAC (stable access cannula)—for use in laparoscopic procedures.

Hasson trocar—used in laparoscopic procedures.

HASTE (half-Fourier acquisition single-shot turbo spin-echo)—MRI term.

Hastings frame—frame attached to the operating table to keep the patient in a flexed knee-chest position for surgery on the spine. Cf. *Andrews spinal frame/table*.

HAT (hepatic artery thrombosis).

Hauser procedure—medial transplantation of the patellar tendon insertion, with reefing of the vastus medialis.

HAV (hepatitis A virus).

Haverhill fever (also, *ratbite fever*)—named for Haverhill, Massachusetts, where the first epidemic of this disease occurred. It is usually transmitted by the bite of an infected rat, but occasionally by the bite of infected dog, cat, or squirrel. The responsible organism is *Streptobacillus moniliformis*. The symptoms include high fever; enlarged regional lymph nodes; red, painful, and swollen joints; and there may also be a rash and back pain. Responds to treatment with antibiotics.

haversian canal—a microscopic feature of bone.

Havrix—inactivated hepatitis A vaccine for people at increased risk of hepatitis A infection (e.g., travelers, military personnel, persons engaging in high-risk sexual activity, employees of child day-care centers).

Hawkeye suture needle—used arthroscopically for soft tissue repair and anchoring.

Hawkins breast localization needle, with FlexStrand cable—used for marking nonpalpable lesions. These

Hawkins *(cont.)*
needles are designated I, II, and III. Number III can be used to inject dye, or for aspiration. They come in 5, 7.5, 10, and 12.5 cm lengths.

Hays retractor—used in hand surgery.

HbAg, HB Ag ("H-bag")—hepatitis B antigen.

HBcAb—hepatitis B core antibody (not to be confused with HBcAg, which is hepatitis B core antigen).

HBeAb—hepatitis B "e" antibody .

HBeAg—the soluble "e" antigen in hepatitis B antigen.

HBIG (hepatitis B immune globulin).

HBsAb—hepatitis B surface antibody.

HBsAg—hepatitis B surface antigen.

H₂ blockers—a class of drugs that block H_2 receptors in the stomach to stop release of histamine that stimulates gastric acid secretion; e.g., cimetidine (Tagamet) and ranitidine (Zantac).

HBSS (Hank's balanced salt solution).

HBV (hepatitis B virus).

HC—see 4-*HC*.

H-CAP (hexamethylmelamine, cyclophosphamide, Adriamycin, and Platinol)—chemotherapy protocol for ovarian carcinoma.

HCC (hepatocellular carcinoma).

hCFHrp (human complement factor H-related protein).

hCG, HCG (human chorionic gonadotropin).

HCT, HCTZ (hydrochlorothiazide)—a diuretic.

HD (hemodialysis).

HDI 1000—software-based, all-digital ultrasound system that can perform routine ultrasound as well as color imaging and tissue-specific imaging. It is equipped to provide Internet/Intranet access to digital images stored in the system's memory. Also, HDI 5000.

HD II (or 2) **total hip prosthesis**.

HDL (high-density lipoprotein)—the so-called "good" cholesterol that protects from arteriosclerosis and heart attacks. HDL levels are high in those who exercise, run, walk, etc., and HDL is thought to reduce the risks of heart disease. Cf. *LDL.*

HDL-C (high-density lipoprotein cholesterol).

HDPEB (high-dose PEB protocol)—chemotherapy protocol.

HDRA (histoculture drug response assay)—a cancer test.

HDRV (human diploid cell strain rabies vaccine)—rabies vaccine. Cf. *RDRV.*

HD-VAC (high-dose [methotrexate], vinblastine, Adriamycin, cisplatin)—chemotherapy protocol.

Healey revision acetabular component.

Healon (sodium hyaluronate, Amvisc) —a viscoelastic preparation used to protect eye tissues and cells during intraocular lens implantation.

Healon GV—a solution that gently separates tissues and maintains a deep anterior chamber during capsulorrhexis. *GV* stands for *greater viscosity*, said to be an improvement in the solution over original Healon.

Healon Yellow—Healon with added fluorescein; used for visualization of the eye.

Healos—synthetic bone-grafting material for use in spinal fusions.

HealthShield antimicrobial mediastinal wound drainage catheter.

heart and hand syndrome—Holt-Oram atriodigital dysplasia.

HeartCard—a cardiac event recorder the size of a credit card. When the patient experiences cardiac symp-

HeartCard *(cont.)*
toms, the HeartCard is placed directly on the chest and it records and stores EKG information that can be transmitted over the telephone to the hospital or doctor's office.

Heart Laser for TMR (transmyocardial revascularization)—used to drill 1 mm channels in the myocardium of the left chamber of the heart in order to get in fresh blood.

HeartMate—air-driven implantable left ventricular assist system (LVAS) utilized in patients awaiting heart transplant whose damaged or diseased heart is unable to function adequately on its own. It is implanted alongside the natural heart and takes over the pumping function of the left ventricle.

HeartMate vented electric LVAS (left ventricular assist system)—portable LVAS, consisting of a blood pump implanted in the abdominal area, connected by a cable through the skin to a small external computer worn at the waist. The computer can be powered by a base unit that is plugged into the wall or by batteries worn at the waist or under the arms.

Heartport Port-Access system—used with less invasive heart valve replacement and repair.

HeartSaver VAD—an artificial heart that is remotely powered and monitored.

Heartscan heart attack prediction test—ultrafast CT scanner used to identify narrowed coronary vessels. It is said to be greater than 95% effective in ruling out obstructive coronary artery disease.

Heartstream ForeRunner automatic external defibrillator.

HearTwave EP—measures Microvolt T-wave alternans in patients undergoing electrophysiology testing.

heater probe thermocoagulation—an alternative treatment to injection therapy for bleeding peptic ulcers.

HeatProbe—trade name of a water irrigation/lavage device.

heat shock protein 72 (HSP-72)—induction of this material may prevent neutrophil-mediated human endothelial cell necrosis.

heave and lift—often used interchangeably; a diffuse lifting impulse along the left sternal heart border with each heartbeat.

heavy-chain deposition—rare malignant neoplasms, indistinguishable from light-chain deposition by clinical features but detectable by using heavy-chain antibodies in biopsy studies, sometimes occurring in patients with renal symptoms associated with myeloma. Cf. *light chain deposition.*

heavy ion irradiation—helium is usually used for this therapy.

heavy-metal screening—lab test for poisoning from heavy metallic elements such as arsenic, iron, lead, and mercury. *Heavy* refers to the atomic weight, not to the physical weight of the metal.

hedgehog molecule—used to generate brain tissue for treatment of Alzheimer's and Parkinson's diseases.

Hedrocel—open-cell tantalum metal structure with the appearance of cancellous bone. Unlike existing bone substitutes, it can be formed or machined into complex shapes. It is distinguished from current porous materials by its uniformity and structural continuity, as well as by its

Hedrocel *(cont.)*
strength, toughness, and resistance to fatigue failure.

HEE—see *Gastaut syndrome.*

heelstick hematocrit—blood obtained from the heel of infants for hematocrit test.

heel-to-shin test—a test of cerebellar function. The patient is asked, while in the supine position, to place the heel of one foot on the knee of the other leg, and then to "run" the heel down the shin. This test is done bilaterally and provides an assessment of the patient's cerebellar function, as indicated by the smoothness and coordination with which it is performed.

Heffington lumbar seat spinal surgery frame—a table on which the patient is placed, kneeling on a little shelf extending out from the end, with the chest flat on the table. This position helps to decrease epidural venous bleeding.

Heimlich maneuver—a technique for removing foreign matter from the trachea of a choking victim.

Heineke-Mikulicz pyloroplasty.

Heinz body—seen in unstable hemoglobin disease (a congenital hemolytic anemia).

Heister valve—redundant cystic duct mucosal folds, which cause a valve-like obstruction of the cystic duct.

HeLa cells—cells from the first continuously cultured strain of human malignant tissue derived from the cervical carcinoma of Henrietta Lacks in Baltimore in 1951.

helical CT—see *spiral CT.* Cf. *electron-beam CT technology.*

Helicide—bismuth-based capsule containing colloidal bismuth subcitrate, metronidazole, and tetracycline for eradication of *Helicobacter pylori.*

Helicobacter hepaticus (H. hepaticus)—a species of bacterium related to *H. pylori.*

Helicobacter pylori (H. pylori) (formerly classified as *Campylobacter pylori*)—believed to be the cause for up to 90% of duodenal ulcers and 80% of stomach ulcers, and now recently found to be associated with non-Hodgkin's lymphoma of the stomach. No cause for the association can as yet be proved.

***Helicobacter pylori* breath test**—used to confirm the presence of *Helicobacter pylori* prior to treating a peptic ulcer with antibiotics. A dose of urea labeled with the radionuclide carbon-14 is given orally. The breath test indirectly measures urease activity. Urease, an enzyme produced by the bacteria, acts on urea to produce ammonia which can be measured in the breath. See *Helicobacter pylori, C-urea breath excretion test.*

Helidac (bismuth subsalicylate, metronidazole, and tetracycline)—used in combination with H_2 antagonist to treat patients with acute duodenal ulcer associated with *H. pylori.*

Helios diagnostic imaging systems.

Helioseal—titanium dioxide particles suspended in polymer containing a photoinitiator that cures under illumination with a blue light. Used as a diffuser with lasers.

heliotrope infraorbital discoloration—purplish discoloration under the eye (*not* ecchymosis).

Helisal rapid blood test—a minimally invasive whole-blood test to detect the presence of antibodies to *Helicobacter pylori (H. pylori)* bacteria.

Helistat—absorbable collagen hemostatic sponge.

Helitene—absorbable collagen hemostatic agent, in fibrillar form.

helium-neon laser—see *HeNe laser*.

Helivax—vaccine for *Helicobacter pylori*.

heliX knot pusher—for extracorporeal knot tying during laparoscopic surgery.

helle cell—a cell in the mucosa of the gastrointestinal tract. Cf. *gelbe cell*.

Heller-Belsey operation—for achalasia of esophagus.

Heller-Dor procedure—laparoscopic surgical procedure for treatment of esophageal achalasia (swallowing difficulty) by reducing the resistance of the esophageal sphincter.

Heller esophagomyotomy—minimally invasive surgery.

Heller-Nissen operation—for achalasia of the esophagus.

HELLP syndrome—a manifestation of preeclampsia. *HELLP* is an acronym for hemolysis, elevated liver enzymes, and low platelets.

helmet-molding therapy—cranial orthotic therapy following endoscopic strip craniectomy to manipulate cranial growth so that normocephaly will be attained. It is used for 3 to 4 months postoperatively.

Helmholtz coil—MRI term.

heloma durum—a callosity on the hand or the foot.

heloma molle—a soft corn.

helper cell—also called helper/inducer cell and T-4 cell; these are the lymphocytes that the AIDS virus specifically attacks and converts into a tool for making additional virus, and this is done much more quickly than with other viruses.

helper/suppressor cell ratio—this ratio changes in AIDS and the change is diagnostic. It may be dictated as the ratio of T-helper to T-suppressor cells or of T-4 to T-8 cells, or you may hear that "the ratio of OKT4 to OKT8 is less than 1.0," OKT4 and OKT8 being monoclonal antibodies to T-4 and T-8. What all of these references are describing is the disappearance of functioning T-4 helper cells.

Hemabate (carboprost tromethamine) —prostaglandin instilled into the uterus to initiate labor or to abort a fetus.

Hemaflex PTCA sheath with obturator—collagen hemostat specifically designed to stop blood flow from vessels in cardiovascular surgery, as it is easy to wrap around vessels. Placed percutaneously in the femoral artery in PTCA. Cf. *Hemaquet*.

hemangioma
choroidal
circumscribed choroidal (CCH)
diffuse choroidal (DCH)

hemangiopericytoma—a rare vascular neoplasm, usually benign.

Hemaquet PTCA sheath with obturator—see *Hemaflex*.

Hemaseel HMN—biological tissue glue for control of bleeding during surgical and orthopedic procedures.

Hemashield—a woven vascular graft enhanced with collagen which promotes intimal development and may reduce thrombogenicity. Used to replace diseased segments of the aorta or iliac arteries.

HemAssist—hemoglobin therapeutic, or "blood substitute," derived from human hemoglobin. It has potential applications in trauma, multiple

HemAssist *(cont.)*
organ failure, stroke, heart attack, and other conditions that would benefit from its oxygen-carrying properties.

HemaStrip-HIV 1/2—whole blood test for HIV 1 and 2.

Hemasure r/LS red blood cell filtration system—designed to reduce leukocytes in donated blood. Leukocytes can transmit a number of bacteria and viruses and cause reactions in patients receiving blood transfusions.

hematoma—see *DTICH* (delayed traumatic intracerebral hematoma).

hematometrocolpos—progressive accumulation of menstrual blood in the uterus due to obstruction of the genital tract.

hematopoiesis—the body's mechanism for replacing cells.

hematopoietic progenitor clonogenic assay—assesses bone marrow viability.

hematopoietic stem cell (HSC)—progenitor cell responsible for the formation of all circulating blood cells in the human body. Used as a transplant to restore bone marrow, WBCs, and platelets after chemotherapy.

hematoporphyrin derivative (HpD)—given intravenously, this photosensitizing agent is absorbed only by malignant cells which can then be destroyed by laser surgery.

hemicallotasis—surgical procedure for arthritic knees.

hemi-Fontan procedure—involves an atriopulmonary patch that directs superior vena caval blood flow into both pulmonary arteries and the inferior vena caval flow into the ventricle. Atrial conduction may be affected by the atrial suture lines with resulting arrhythmia. The procedure is performed to repair certain congenital heart defects.

Hemi Sling—designed to reduce shoulder subluxation.

Hemoccult Sensa—enhanced system for detecting hidden blood in stool. It is said to be easier to read than the standard Hemoccult test.

Hemoccult II—a test for fecal occult blood.

Hemochron high-dose thrombin time (HiTT)—a whole-blood assay for monitoring high-dose heparin anticoagulation. Used in monitoring coagulation time following coronary artery bypass procedures.

Hemoclip—a ligating clip; it comes in titanium and also in tantalum.

HemoCue photometer—for a quick office test for hemoglobin determination done on a drop of blood.

Hemo-Dial—dialysate additives.

hemodialyzer—apparatus used in the hemodialysis of kidney patients to remove toxic elements. There are three types of hemodialyzers: the coil, the hollow fiber, and the parallel plate.

hemofiltration—a technique by which waste products of hemodialysis are removed from the blood along with plasma water by rapid ultrafiltration, and then the blood is reconstituted with a solution, either before or after hemodialysis. The technique appears to reduce side effects of dialysis and seems to assure better tolerance of fluid removal, particularly in patients with high vascular instability. See *CAVH*.

Hemolink—a hemoglobin replacement product, or red blood cell substitute, for use in blood transfusions.

Hem-o-lok—polymer ligating clip.

hemolytic uremic syndrome (HUS) — a complication of the pathogen *E. coli* 0157:H7, occurring mostly in children and resulting in acute renal failure. Successful treatment depends on strict attention to fluid and electrolyte balance.

Hemopad—absorbable collagen hemostat, which comes as nonwoven pads that can be cut, folded, or wrapped around a bleeding site. It can be peeled away easily, but any remaining bits are soon absorbed.

hemophilia A—factor VIII deficiency (classical hemophilia).

hemophilia B—factor IX deficiency. See *Christmas disease*.

Hemophilus—see *Haemophilus*. With a lowercase "h," may refer generically to any bacterium of the genus *Haemophilus*. Also used for the Hemophilus B conjugate vaccine. If you are typing genus and species in a report, you should use the Latin spelling.

Hemopump—a temporary external pump which completely supports circulation, used in the treatment of cardiogenic shock. This device is an improvement over the intra-aortic balloon pump which provides only 25% circulatory assistance.

Hemopure (hemoglobin glutamer-250 [bovine])—hemoglobin-based oxygen therapeutic, designed to improve tissue oxygenation and prevent tissue damage in ischemic conditions relating to hemorrhagic shock, brain hypoxia, and heart attack.

hemostatic eraser (Oph)—used for pinpoint hemostasis in anterior and posterior segment surgery.

hemostatic material—see *collagen*.

Hemotene—absorbable collagen hemostat to control bleeding during surgery when sutures are not practical.

Hemotherapies liver dialysis unit—liver-assist technology used for treatment of patients with liver disease or liver impairment due to hepatitis, cirrhosis, overdose, drug toxicity, aggressive drug therapies, or other causes.

Hendel correction of scaphocephaly—uses a gore pattern to alter the shape of individual sections of the skull by changing the radius of curvature.

HeNe (**helium-neon**) **laser** (Oph)—has a visible low power red beam and is often used in conjunction with the carbon dioxide (CO_2) laser. The advantage of the HeNe is that the beam is visible and the surgeon can see its location.

Henning meniscal retractors—used in knee surgery.

Henning system—technique for arthroscopic meniscal repair. Also, *Henning instruments*.

Henoch-Schönlein—also *Schönlein-Henoch purpura*.

Hensen's cells—in the organ of Corti.

Hepamed-coated Wiktor stent—see *Wiktor stent*.

heparin—see *beef-lung heparin*.

heparinized CeeOn intraocular lens.

heparin lock—an intermittent infusion reservoir; permits periodic infusion of drugs without continuous fluid infusion. A heparin solution injected into the reservoir between infusions will keep the I.V. patent without the necessity of a continuous fluid drip. Although the heparin lock was first

heparin lock *(cont.)*
used for administration of heparin, it is also used for transfusion therapy and in the administration of a number of drugs, including chemotherapeutic agents and antibiotics.

HepatAmine—a nutrient solution for patients with liver disease.

hepatic arterial-dominant phase (HAP) images (CT scan).

hepatic arterial infusion (HAI) **chemotherapy**—high-dose chemotherapy performed under hepatic venous isolation by direct hemoperfusion (HVI-DHP). The hepatic vein is isolated by double balloon technique with an occlusion catheter and balloon catheter. This procedure allows higher doses than standard systemic chemotherapy in nonresectable hepatic carcinoma. Standard hepatic arterial infusion that does not occlude the hepatic vein from the systemic circulation is dose-limited due to systemic side effects of chemotherapy.

hepatic artery thrombosis (HAT).

hepatic resection—treatment for metastatic neuroendocrine cancers.

hepatic segmentectomy—a therapeutic approach for small hepatocellular carcinomas and in patients with chronic liver disease and impaired liver function.

hepatic venous isolation by direct hemoperfusion (HVI-DHP)—see *hepatic arterial infusion chemotherapy.*

hepatic venous web disease (in Budd-Chiari syndrome).

hepatic web dilation—to establish hepatic vein outflow (in hepatic venous web disease).

hepatitides ("heh-puh-tih´-tih-dees")—plural form of *hepatitis.*

hepatitis—inflammation of the liver caused by viral and bacterial infection and parasitic infestation. See related entries: *hepatitis A, B, C, D, E, F, NANB hepatitis, peliosis hepatitis.*

hepatitis A (infectious hepatitis)—an acute, self-limited infection, generally causing mild symptoms. The virus is transmitted chiefly by the fecal-oral route.

hepatitis B (serum hepatitis)—a more severe infection which, in some cases, becomes chronic and is transmitted chiefly via the bloodstream and also by sexual contact. After recovery some patients become carriers.

hepatitis B antigen (HbAg).

hepatitis C—the major cause of posttransfusion hepatitis, typically causing a mild clinical illness but becoming chronic in at least half of all cases. Formerly called *non-A, non-B hepatitis.*

hepatitis D—occurs only in persons previously infected with hepatitis B, although it is due to a distinct virus. Also called *delta hepatitis.*

hepatitis E—occurs chiefly in the tropics. Resembles hepatitis A in that it is transmitted by the fecal-oral route and does not become chronic or lead to a carrier state, but has a much higher mortality.

hepatitis F—the newer name for non-A, non-B, non-C hepatitis.

hepatization—transformation into a liver-like mass, as the solidified state of the lung in lobar pneumonia.

hepatobiliary scintigraphy—used in children to assess liver disease.

hepatocellular carcinoma (HCC)

hepatofugal flow—flowing away from the liver. "Angiography for esophageal varices was done and revealed hepatofugal flow."

hepatojugular reflux—swelling of the jugular vein caused by applying pressure over the liver. This swelling indicates right heart insufficiency.

hepatopancreatoduodenectomy.

hepatopetal flow—flowing toward the liver. "Angiography for esophageal varices was done and revealed hepatopetal flow."

"hep lock"—medical slang for *heparin lock*. See *heparin lock*.

Heprofile ELISA (enzyme-linked immunosorbent assay)—lab test for hepatitis B.

Heptalac—lactulose solution used as ammonia detoxification.

Heptavax-B—trade name for hepatitis B vaccine.

Heptazyme—for the treatment of patients infected with hepatitis C virus. Heptazyme is a ribozyme designed to selectively destroy hepatitis C virus RNA.

Heptodin (lamivudine)—for the treatment of hepatitis B.

herald patch—a single lesion that is seen before the eruption of pityriasis rosea.

Herbert bone screw.

Herbert classification—a method of describing fractures of the scaphoid bone, one of the carpal bones of the wrist. Screw fixation of a scaphoid fracture is generally preferred over conservative therapy and may involve the use of a Herbert screw.

Herbert-Whipple bone screw—used for reduction and compression of small bone and intra-articular fractures.

HercepTest—HER2 protein expression system for the guidance of breast cancer therapy.

Herceptin (trastuzumab)—anti-HER2 humanized monoclonal antibody, designed to block a protein receptor called HER2 that is produced in excess amounts in some women with breast cancer.

Herculon suture—synthetic material.

Herellea vaginicola—included in the genus of gram-negative coccobacilli *Acinetobacter*.

Hering, nerve of—carotid sinus nerve.

Heritage Panel—a patented genetic screening test, currently available only to high-risk Ashkenazim Jews affected with breast or ovarian cancer or who are related to a known mutation carrier. It can detect hereditary breast and ovarian cancers in the BRCA1 and BRCA2 genes.

Herp-Check—antibody test for herpes simplex virus which provides results in four hours, rather than up to seven days, as before.

herpesencephalitis (one word).

herpes simplex virus (HSV)—can disseminate in AIDS.

herpesvirus (one word).

herpes whitlow—herpesvirus infection, occurring in hospital workers and dentists, that can be transmitted through contact with the patient's oral mucous membrane or saliva. It involves the folds of tissue around the fingernail and consists of pyogenic and vesicular paronychia. Related terms: *paronychia, felon*.

herpes zoster virus (HZV)—can disseminate in AIDS.

Herplex Liquifilm (idoxuridine).

HER-2-neu—an oncogene that is a potential prognostic marker for breast cancer.

hertz (Hz)—a unit of frequency, equal to one cycle per second; measurement used in audiograms.

Hespan (hetastarch)—plasma volume expander; used in treatment of shock (cheaper than albumin).

hetastarch (Hespan) **plasma volume expander**.

heterografts, bovine and porcine—used as valves in cardiac surgery; they are specially prepared so they are not rejected as foreign bodies.

Hewlett-Packard ear oximeter—used to record oxygen saturation continuously. See *ear oximeter*. (Note: *Hewlett-Packard* has a hyphen.)

Hewlett-Packard phased-array imaging system—MRI term.

hexagonal keratotomy surgery—includes an intracorneal implant (Kerato-Gel) made from lidofilcon A.

Hexalen (altretamine)—oral drug used in treatment of bronchogenic carcinoma and advanced ovarian cancer.

Hexcelite—intermediate phase casting and thermoplastic light mesh immersed briefly in 80°C water and then wrapped around the extremity to be casted; hardens quickly.

Hexcel total condylar knee system—femoral and tibial components, and patellar dome.

Hex-Fix—a fracture fixation system.

hexoprenaline sulfate (Delaprem)—used to arrest uterine contractions during premature labor, in the same way as ritod rine (Yutopar) and terbutaline (Bricanyl), but with fewer side effects.

Hextend—physiologically balanced blood plasma volume expander for treatment of hypovolemia.

Heyer-Schulte tissue expander.

HFCWO (high-frequency chest wall oscillation)—see *ABI Vest Airway Clearance System* and *ThAIRapy Vest*.

HF infrared laser.

H5N1 virus—strain of influenza A originating in birds (usually poultry) and believed to be responsible for flu deaths in Hong Kong in 1997. Investigations are being conducted to determine how the virus is transmitted from avians to humans.

"H. flu"—slang for *Haemophilus influenzae*.

H-447—used in the treatment of various cancers that over-express EGF-R (epidermal growth factor receptor).

HFU (high-intensity focused ultrasound).

HGD (high-grade dysplasia).

HGE (human granulocytic ehrlichiosis).

hGH (human growth hormone)—see *Protropin*.

HGSIL (high-grade squamous intraepithelial lesion)—corresponds to Pap smear changes that were formerly called moderate and severe dysplasia or CIN 2 and CIN 3.

HHH or **triple-H** (hypertensive hypervolemic hemodilution) **therapy** after subarachnoid hemorrhage.

HHV-8 (human herpesvirus-8).

HIAA—see *5-HIAA* (hydroxyindoleacetic acid).

Hib (*Haemophilus influenzae* type b)—a conjugate vaccine.

Hib or **HIB** (pronounced "hib") (*Haemophilus influenzae* type B) **disease**—a leading cause of bacterial meningitis.

Hibiclens, Hibistat, Hibitane tincture (chlorhexidine gluconate)—antiseptic, antimicrobial skin cleansers.

HIB polysaccharide vaccine—used to treat HIB disease in children. See *HIB disease*.

Hickman catheter—indwelling right atrial catheter used in treatment of patients receiving bone marrow transplants and those whose medical care requires frequent access to their circulation, e.g., drawing blood, administering blood, for total parenteral nutrition. Also used for withdrawing blood for plasmapheresis and for central venous pressure monitoring. Its use eliminates the need for frequent venipuncture.

HIDA ("high-dah") (**h**epato**i**mino**di**acetic **a**cid) **scan**—a technetium scan. Also given as TcHIDA, or technetium-HIDA, for biliary tract imaging. See *PIPIDA*.

Hieshima coaxial catheter—used in some interventional procedures in radiology.

HIFU (high-intensity focused ultrasound).

Higgins technique for ureterointestinal anastomosis.

high-density linear array—term used in B-scan, Doppler, and color Doppler imaging. See *B-scan*.

high-density lipoprotein (HDL).

high-density lipoprotein–cholesterol (HDL-C).

high-energy lasers, hot lasers—used to make surgical incisions or destroy tumors.

higher integrative functions (HIF).

Highet and Sander criteria of Mackinnon and Dellon, modified—for measuring sensory recovery following nerve repair.

Highet and Sander criteria of Zachary and Holmes, modified—for measuring motor recovery following nerve reconstruction.

high field strength scanner—MRI device using a static magnetic field of maximal intensity.

high-frequency jet ventilation (Pulm)—the delivery of very small tidal volumes at extremely rapid rates (150 to 900 breaths per minute), allowing significant reduction in mean airway pressure and possible reduced risk of barotrauma. Volumes delivered are smaller than the physiologic dead space. May be related to bronchopleural fistulas and major volume-losing pneumothoraces when used in children with parenchymal lung disease. A similar technique is called *high-frequency oscillatory ventilation*.

high-frequency oscillatory ventilation—see *high-frequency jet ventilation*.

high-grade squamous intraepithelial lesion (HSIL).

high-intensity focused ultrasound (HFU, HIFU)—used to treat benign prostatic hypertrophy. Administered via transrectal probe.

highly active antiretroviral therapy (HAART).

high myope—one who has a high degree of myopia (nearsightedness).

high-osmolar media (Radiol)—controversial use of high-osmolar (or ionic) versus low-osmolar (or nonionic) contrast media. The media lower in osmolality are much more expensive but are thought to be less dangerous to some patients, particularly cardiac, asthmatic, or allergic patients.

high-resolution computed tomography (HRCT).

high-resolution multileaf collimator—computerized mechanical device that uses individually controlled leaves or fingers to sculpt a radiation beam to the shape of a tumor when delivering intensity modulated radiotherapy treatments in radiation oncology.

high-resolution storage phosphor managing—reportedly may replace conventional chest radiography in detection of subtle interstitial lung diseases.

High-Risk Hybrid Capture II HPV test—DNA-based technology designed to detect the 13 key types of human papillomavirus that cause cervical cancer.

high-speed rotational atherectomy (RA)—percutaneous procedure for treatment of coronary stenoses by plaque abrasion. It is an alternative to PTCA for complex lesions, especially those with extensive calcification.

high-voltage pulsed galvanic stimulator—controls pain and increases circulation following injury or surgery.

high-voltage stimulation (HVS)—delivers electrical energy to deep tissues without damage to superficial tissues. Is believed to relieve pain and accelerate wound healing. Similar to TENS. May be incorrectly referred to as *galvanic stimulation*.

Hildebrandt uterine hemostatic forceps—has a split in the jaws of the forceps that permits suturing with the forceps in place and then removing the forceps without disturbing the sutures.

Hilgenreiner line—between the inferior edges of the triradiate cartilage and the line tangential to the medial ossified edge of the proximal metaphysis of the femur.

Hilger facial nerve stimulator—used for clinical evaluation of the facial nerve, clinical testing of muscle tissue viability, and for nerve identification and testing during surgery.

Hill cluster harvest technique—micrograft technique.

Hill repair—for esophageal reflux.

Hill-Sachs lesion; **deformity** (Ortho).

HIM (health information management) —formerly known as *medical record management*.

hindgut—distal colon and rectum. See *foregut* and *midgut*.

hip arthrodesis—with the cobra head plate and pelvic osteotomy.

HIPciser abduction splint—for use as a hip abduction splint and an isometric exercise device.

hip dysplasia measurements in cerebral palsy
AA (acetabular anteversion)
AAI (axial acetabular index)
AD/FHD (ratio of acetabular depth to femoral head diameter)
AI (acetabular index)
CEA (center-edge angle) of Wiberg
FA (femoral anteversion)
MI (migration index
NSA (neck-shaft angle) of femur
SMAI (superior-medial acetabular index)

Hi-Per cardiac device.

HipNav process—a computer-assisted hip navigation system used in hip replacement surgery to improve accuracy when implanting a replacement for the acetabulum.

hip spica cast—used after surgery for correction of congenital hip dysplasia.

hippocampus (Greek *hippokampos*, sea horse)—area of cortex in bottom of inferior (temporal) horn of the lateral ventricle; it has the appearance of a seahorse, thus the name.

Hippocrates manipulation—for anterior dislocation of the shoulder joint. The physician exerts traction on the patient's arm and at the same time places his heel (with the shoe removed first!) in the patient's axilla

Hippocrates manipulation *(cont.)*
to give countertraction, thus forcing the head of the humerus from beneath the acromion.

hippocratic wreath—seen in men with male pattern baldness, the rim of hair surrounding the bald area. Cf. *male pattern baldness.*

Hirano bodies—structural changes revealed by pathological examination of brains of Alzheimer's disease victims. Also, *Hirano inclusion body.*

Hirschberg measurement of esotropia.

Hirschsprung's disease—congenital megacolon (giant colon).

hirudin (recombinant desulfatohirudin) —naturally occurring anticoagulant or thrombin inhibitor derived from leeches.

Hirulog (bivalirudin)—a direct thrombin inhibitor that is said to be better than heparin at opening blood vessels of patients suffering heart attacks.

HIS fusion inhibitors—a new class of drugs that works specifically on a virus to prevent it from fusing with the cell and prevent viral replication. Fusion inhibitors are said to have great promise as anti-HIV drugs. Also called *fusion inhibitors.*

Hismanal (astemizole)—antihistamine, for nasal congestion.

HiSonic—an ultrasonic bone conduction hearing device placed behind the ear on the mastoid bone. Allows profoundly deaf patients to perceive sounds.

Hi Speed Pulse Lavage—for debridement of bone surfaces during knee and hip replacements.

His-Purkinje conduction ("hiss pur-kin´gee") (Cardio)—as in bundle of His and Purkinje fibers.

Histoacryl Blue (HAB)—tissue adhesive used in closure of incisions and lacerations.

Histoacryl glue (cyanoacrylate)—a tissue adhesive used to seal some perforating-type corneal wounds as may be seen in stromal herpetic keratitis. Also used to close incisions in blepharoplasty procedures.

histoculture drug response assay (HDRA)—to detect certain cancers.

Histofreezer cryosurgical wart treatment—cryotherapy device for the treatment of benign skin lesions: verruca vulgaris, verruca plantaris, human papillomavirus, acrochordon, molluscum contagiosum, seborrheic keratosis, verruca plana, actinic keratoses, and lentigo.

Histoplasma—the fungus which causes histoplasmosis. Disseminated histoplasmosis was recently added to the growing list of once very rare (in disseminated form) infections which are now often seen in AIDS.

Histoplasma capsulatum—pathogen associated with sinusitis in AIDS patients.

Histoplasma capsulatum **polysaccharide antigen** (HPA)—detection of HPA, a rapid method for detecting histoplasmosis.

Histussin D (hydrocodone bitartrate/ pseudoephedrine hydrochloride)— antitussive-decongestant liquid for symptomatic relief of cough accompanying upper respiratory tract congestion.

HI titer (hemagglutination inhibition)— a rubella screening test.

Hitzelberger's sign (Derm).

HIV (human immunodeficiency virus) —the official name for the AIDS virus, changed because of the

HIV *(cont.)*
unwieldiness of the earlier terms and the debate over who discovered the virus first. HIV is a retrovirus, of the cytopathic lentivirus group.

HIV AC-le—potential AIDS vaccine by Bristol-Myers.

HIVAGEN—lab test for HIV.

HIV antibody—antibodies to the virus thought to lead to AIDS. Most AIDS tests are tests for the HIV antibody. Some very sophisticated ones test for part of the virus itself, such as the p24 antigen test, which is widely used in some areas.

HIV-associated thrombocytopenia—treated with high-dose intravenous immune globulin therapy.

HIV classification for children—the Centers for Disease Control and Prevention classification for HIV-infected or exposed children is as follows:
P0: Asymptomatic infants to 15 months of age in whom definitive HIV infection has not been diagnosed.
P1: Asymptomatic infants and children regardless of age in whom HIV infection has been established by HIV p24 antigen or HIV culture with or without laboratory evidence of immunodeficiency.
P2: Symptomatic HIV-infected child. Includes subgroups A-F based on disease manifestations.

HIV disease—infection with the HIV virus, as shown by p24 antigen or HIV antibody test. HIV disease itself is not AIDS. Whether all cases go on to full-blown AIDS is not known at this time.

HIV encephalitis—see *AIDS dementia complex.*

Hivid (zalcitabine).

HIV-1E—a virus subtype prevalent in Thailand, that grows much more efficiently in the cells that line the vagina than subtypes prevalent in the U.S. and elsewhere. May explain the rapid spread of AIDS among heterosexuals in Southeast Asia.

HIV phenotype test—still a research tool and not yet available through private physicians. Can detect which variants of the virus a patient has and whether the nonsyncytium inducing (NSI) variant has mutated to the more dangerous SI variant. See *NSI, SI.*

HKAFO (hip-knee-ankle-foot orthosis) —ambulation aid for children with cerebral palsy and myelomeningocele. Orthosis is in three forms: parapodium, reciprocating gait, and swivel walker.

HK-Cardiosol—used in heart transplant procedures.

HLA (human lymphocyte antigen)—a designation used in tissue typing for organ transplants.

HLA-A—see locus of HLA.

HLA-DR (histocompatibility antigen-DR)—a marker protein for the development of coronary artery disease in heart transplant patients. See also *ICAM-1.*

HLA-DR4—a genetic marker that has a correlation to the severity of the rheumatoid arthritis process in a patient.

HLHS (hypoplastic left heart syndrome).

HM (hand movements) (Oph).

HMFG1 (human milk fat globule 1)—injection antibody therapy for adjuvant treatment of ovarian cancer.

HMG (human menopausal gonadotropin)—used in treatment of some types of infertility.

HMG-CoA reductase inhibitors—a class of drugs used to decrease hypercholesterolemia and hypertriglyceridemia. Examples: simvastatin (Zocor) and pravastatin (Pravachol).

hMSCs (human mesenchymal stem cells).

HNP (herniated nucleus pulposus).

hockey-stick appearance of catheter tip (Cardio).

HOCM (hypertrophic obstructive cardiomyopathy).

Hoehn and Yahr scale—for Parkinson's disease staging.

Hoehne's sign (Ob-Gyn)—failure to respond to oxytocic drugs, a sign of uterine rupture.

Hoek-Bowen cement removal system by Micro-Aire.

Hoffa's tendon shortening—a procedure in which gathering stitches are run up a portion of the tendon, and then the suture is tightened to the appropriate length.

Hoffman and Mohr procedure—technique for repair of unicoronal cranial synostosis.

Hoffman-Clayton procedure—podiatric procedure to treat rheumatoid arthritis.

Hoffmann external fixation device—developed by Swiss surgeon Raoul Hoffmann.

Hoffmann mini-lengthening fixation device.

Hoffmann reflex—twitching of the thumb when the middle finger is snapped, one of the signs of upper neuron damage. Named for Johann Hoffmann, German neurologist.

Hofmeister gastroenterostomy.

Hohmann retractor (Ortho)—used in acetabular fracture repair. Also, *Mini-Hohmann.*

Hohn central venous catheter, single- and double-lumen.

Holdrinet method—calculates the fraction of bone marrow nucleated cells that come from peripheral blood.

Holinger anterior commissure laryngoscope.

Holladay formula (Oph)—a formula for calculating the depth of the anterior chamber of the eye.

Hollande's solution—used as a fixative for some types of pathology specimens.

Hollenhorst plaques—yellow-orange cholesterol plaques which, when seen on examination of the optic fundi, indicate the presence of atherosclerosis. "His optic fundi were closely inspected and were benign for Hollenhorst plaques, for papilledema and hemorrhage."

holmium laser—a pulsed noncontact laser similar to a carbon dioxide laser in that its wavelength is absorbed by water-containing tissues. It can operate in a fluid (liquid) medium and it can coagulate bleeding vessels. It can also resect and vaporize tough cartilaginous tissues.

holmium:YAG (yttrium-argon-garnet) **laser**—a laser used in endoscopic laser cholecystectomy and in angioplasty. Also known as *Ho:YAG.*

Hologic QDR 1000W—dual energy x-ray absorptiometry scanner.

Holt-Oram atriodigital dysplasia—heart and hand syndrome.

HOM (high-osmolar media) (Radiol). See *ionic contrast media.* Cf. *LOM, nonionic contrast media.*

Homans' sign—forced dorsiflexion of the foot causes discomfort behind the knee in thrombosis in the leg.

home ambulatory inotropic therapy—allows patients awaiting heart transplants to leave the hospital and enjoy a more normal lifestyle at home. The patients self-administer a regimen of medications through a tunneled subclavian Silastic catheter, using a syringe pump and syringe driver. Medication regimen is directed at maintaining hemodynamics and includes ACE inhibitors, digoxin, vasodilators, and amiodarone.

HomeChoice Pro with PD Link—home-based dialysis treatment with advanced computer technology to communicate therapy data to clinicians via data card or modem. The system allows clinicians to monitor patient data on a daily basis so that they can adjust prescriptions and identify potential problems between clinic visits.

home O$_2$ (oxygen)—as in "The patient was discharged on home O$_2$." In dictation it sounds like "homo-2."

Homer-Wright pseudorosette (Neuro).

Homer-Wright rosette—sometimes seen on histologic examination of medulloblastomas.

HomeTrak Plus—compact cardiac event recorder about the size of a pager, designed for cardiac patients with transient symptoms that cannot be captured via standard Holter monitor or 12-lead EKG.

HomMed Monitoring System—patient-friendly, cost-effective method of monitoring congestive heart failure patients from their homes.

homocysteine—an amino acid not in foods but produced in the body; it is said to cause as much fat deposit on arterial walls as cholesterol does. Homocysteine is produced by methionine, another amino acid, which is in foods. Vegetarian diets are low in methionine, which may be one reason vegetarians have low rates of heart attacks. Homocysteine may also be related to repeated early miscarriages.

homogeneous gene assay system—uses a fluorescent technique with bound probes to isolate and amplify the nucleotides (segment of DNA or RNA) of interest in a specimen. See *polymerase chain reaction.*

homograft—see *denatured homograft.*

Honan balloon—used in phakoemulsification of cataracts. "After ascertaining adequate akinesia and anesthesia, and after the Honan balloon was set at 30 mmHg for 15 minutes, the left face was prepared and draped in the usual sterile ophthalmic fashion."

Honan manometer—used in lowering intraocular pressure.

H1 receptors—histamine receptors in the respiratory tract which are blocked by antihistamines.

honeycomb mucosa—seen in the jejunum of patients with celiac disease.

honk, precordial—an abnormal heart sound.

hood O$_2$—humidified oxygen administered in a clear hard plastic container encasing the baby's head with an opening for the neck. Due to small air leaks around the neck it can attain only about 40% oxygen concentration.

Hood stoma stent—a device that utilizes a valve to allow a patient with a tracheostomy to speak without first having to put a finger over the stoma.

hook-fist positioning—postoperative exercise for tendon repair.

Hoover sign—for unilateral leg paralysis in suspected hysteria. The physician allows the patient to think he is testing the unaffected leg, but places a hand underneath the heel of the "paralyzed" leg. When the good leg is raised, an individual with normal muscle strength will be unable to refrain from pressing down on the bed with the heel of the other leg. Lack of such pressure indicates organic paresis.

Hopkins 70° rigid telescope—used in laryngoscopy.

hordeolum—acute inflammation of a sebaceous gland of the eyelid. See *sty (stye)*.

Horizon AutoAdjust CPAP system—a respiratory care product designed to provide patients suffering from obstructive sleep apnea (OSA) with relief through nightly therapy.

horizontal adduction test—see *cross-chest adduction test*.

Hormodendrum—an inhalant antigen.

hormone
Biotropin (human growth hormone)
follicle-stimulating (FSH)
Genentech biosynthetic human
gonadotropin-releasing (GnRH)
growth (Protropin)
human growth (Biotropin)
Humatrope human growth
hypothalamic luteinizing hormone-
   releasing
Innofem (estradiol tablets)
Leuprolide
long-acting thyroid-stimulating
   (LATS)
luteinizing hormone-releasing
   (LHRH)
parathyroid (parathormone)

hormone *(cont.)*
placental growth (PGH)
Protropin human growth
secretin

Horn endo-otoprobe—a laser probe used in ear surgery.

Hoskins nylon suture laser lens (Oph) —used to cut subconjunctival nylon sutures in postoperative situations such as trabeculectomies, sutures in cataract wounds causing astigmatism, and flap sutures that are too tight to permit filtration. This is a noninvasive procedure.

HOT (hypertension optimal treatment).

Hot and Cold Sensory System—designed to enhance upper extremity prostheses. It contains a fingertip temperature probe in the prosthetic hand. The temperature readings are sent to circuitry inside the prosthesis and then to a pair of corresponding electrodes that touch the patient's residual limb. The electrodes become warm or cool depending on the voltages received, and the patient registers the sensation of hot or cold in the prosthesis.

Hot/Ice Cold Therapy Cooler—portable cold therapy device for outpatient or home treatment. It delivers continuous cold therapy needed after orthopedic procedures such as foot, ankle, or knee surgery.

Hot/Ice System III—for controlled cold therapy following orthopedic procedures.

hot potato voice—hollow voice caused by edema or paralysis of the soft palate; most commonly observed in severe pharyngitis or peritonsillar abscess.

Hotsy Cautery—a disposable surgical cautery.

Houget's maneuver—used in inguinal hernia repair.

Hough ("huff") **hoe**—elevator with an angled tip and handle.

Hounsfield unit—density measurement indicative of calcium (on CT scan).

House and Pulec otic-periotic shunt—for treatment of progressive endolymphatic hydrops (Ménière's disease).

House-Brackmann grading scale—for facial nerve function in paralysis due to Wegener's granulomatosis. "This patient's facial nerve function at this time would be considered to be House-Brackmann grade 3."

Housecall—transtelephonic monitoring system that uses a telephone to download diagnostic data and programmed parameters from an implanted cardioverter-defibrillator.

housemaid's knee—older term for *prepatellar bursitis*, seen in patients who repeatedly traumatize the bursa by kneeling.

Houston Halo—to treat cervical spine disorders.

Howell biopsy aspiration needle.

Howmedica Universal compression screw (Ortho)—available in cancellous and cortical thread types.

Ho:YAG (holmium:yttrium-argon-garnet) **laser**.

Ho:YAG LTK (noncontact holmium: YAG laser thermal keratoplasty)—technique for correction of low hyperopia.

HPA (*Histoplasma capsulatum* polysaccharide antigen).

HPA (hypothalamic-pituitary-adrenal) **axis suppression**—a syndrome that occurs following systemic absorption of significant amounts of topically applied corticosteroids. This may occur from prolonged use or extensive use (over a large body area) of topical corticosteroids. Symptoms include Cushing's syndrome and elevated blood glucose levels.

HPCD (hemostatic puncture closure device)—used after interventional or diagnostic vascular procedures to seal the arteriotomy.

HPC guide wire—a flexible hydrophilic guide wire used to cannulate the biliary duct. Produces less trauma than other methods, in the presence of tight strictures.

Hp Chek—screening system for serological detection of *H. pylori* antibodies.

HpD (hematoporphyrin derivative).

Hpfast—an agar gel test for *Helicobacter pylori*.

HPMPC (cidofovir)—drug given parenterally for cytomegalovirus infection in AIDS. Although not an oral drug, it might be more effective than ganciclovir, the current drug also given parenterally.

HPRC (hereditary papillary renal cancer) **syndrome**—hereditary familial cancer syndrome.

HPS (hematoxylin, phloxine, and safranin)—histochemical stains.

HP (Hewlett-Packard) **SONOS 5500** ultrasound imaging system.

HPV (human papillomavirus).

HRARE (hybrid rapid acquisition with relaxation enhancement)—MR imaging to evaluate small bowel involvement in Crohn's disease. Cf. *HASTE*.

HRCT (high-resolution computed tomography).

H reflex study—electromyography, given in milliseconds (msec). Through an electrically induced spi-

H reflex study *(cont.)*
nal reflex, a determination can be made as to the presence of unilateral S1 radiculopathy.

HRL (Hardy-Rand-Littler) **screening plates**—test charts composed of dots of different colors. Geometric figures can be seen among the dots. The charts are used to test color vision.

HRS (hepatorenal syndrome).

HRT (hormone replacement therapy) **patch**—for treatment of vasomotor symptoms related to menopause.

Hruby lens ("ruby")—slit-lamp biomicroscopy.

HSC (hematopoietic stem cell).

HSC (Hospital for Sick Children) **Scale**—a scale used to measure pain experienced by patients undergoing Ilizarov limb-lengthening procedures. Measures pain for an extended period. Cf. *APPT.*

HSIL (high-grade squamous intraepithelial lesion).

H-SLAP (human stromelysin aggregated proteoglycan)—an ELISA diagnostic test to evaluate stromelysin inhibitors that degrade cartilage, leading to osteoarthritis and rheumatoid arthritis.

HSP-72 (heat shock protein 72).

HSSG (hysterosalpingosonography).

HS-tk gene therapy—for treatment of malignant brain tumors in children.

HSV (herpesvirus; herpes simplex virus).

HTLV-I retrovirus (human T-cell leukemia/lymphoma virus).

HTLV-III (human T-cell lymphotropic virus).

HT receptor blockers—see *5-HT receptor blockers.*

HTR-MFI implants—onlay facial augmentation implants for aesthetic facial surgery for augmentation of malar, paranasal, premaxillary, ramus, and chin regions.

H-TRON insulin pump.

Hubbard hydrotherapy tank—treatment for psoriasis.

Huber needle—a specially designed needle for use with ports. The sharply angled bevel leaves a line-like tear (in the rubber-covered entry site) which self-seals easily. Comes in straight or 90° angle design, the latter being used for continuous infusion because it will lie flat when taped to the skin.

Hudson-Stahli line—a linear subepithelial deposit of iron pigment on the surface of the cornea.

"huff" hoe—see *Hough hoe.*

Hughston knee evaluation (or score) —divides the patient's clinical performance into three categories: subjective, functional, and objective, yielding a combined score.

Hughston view—x-ray view of the flexed knee to demonstrate subluxation of the patella or fracture of the femoral condyle.

Hulka tenaculum.

Humalog (insulin lispro)—a long-acting insulin of recombinant DNA origin for injection.

Humalog Mix 75/25 Pen—75% insulin lispro protamine suspension, 25% insulin lispro injection (rDNA origin); first premixed insulin containing a rapid-acting insulin. Helps patients control blood glucose levels more easily throughout the day, at mealtime, between meals, and at nighttime.

human chorionic gonadotropin (hCG or HCG).

human diploid cell strain rabies vaccine (HDRV).

human fibroblast growth factor-I (FGF-I)—genetically engineered human protein that can induce growth of new blood vessels when injected into diseased heart tissue. A dense capillary network appears around the site of injection and brings about an increase in blood supply through the newly formed functional vessels.

Human Genome Project—cooperative international project to map the entirety of human DNA, including all 23 chromosomes and an estimated 100,000 genes.

human granulocytic ehrlichiosis (HGE)—a tick-borne disease, with some fatalities reported.

human growth hormone (hGH).

human herpesvirus 6 (HHV-6)—one of the most widespread members of the family of human herpesviruses, infecting up to 90% of most populations during infancy. Primary infection is either asymptomatic or manifests itself as a febrile illness that may include exanthem subitum. While severe or fatal complications are rare in immunocompetent patients, the virus poses an additional health risk for immunodeficient patients, particularly those who have undergone organ or bone marrow transplants or who are HIV seropositive.

human immunodeficiency virus (HIV).

human insulin—see *Humulin*. Cf. *semisynthetic human insulin*.

human lymphocyte antigen (HLA).

human mammary tumor virus (HMTV)—primitive retrovirus identified in human breast cancer tissues.

human meniscal allograft—used in knee surgery to repair large, complex tears of the meniscus, reestablishing normal load-bearing at the knee and delaying degenerative changes that follow total meniscectomy. The allografts are securely fixed by implantable bone anchors.

human menopausal gonadotropin (HMG).

human mesenchymal stem cells (hMSCs).

human papillomavirus (HPV)—cause of genital warts, a sexually transmitted disease and a risk factor for cancer of the cervix.

human parvovirus B19 (HPV B19)—the virus that causes erythema infectiosum (fifth disease), a common mild febrile exanthem of children. Less often it causes chronic anemia, neutropenia, myocarditis, vasculitis, or encephalitis, particularly in immunodeficient persons or pregnant women.

human serum-albumin (^{99m}Tc-GSA).

human stromelysin aggregated proteoglycan (H-SLAP).

human T-cell lymphotropic virus (HTLV-III)—name given to the virus isolated by Robert Gallo, the American researcher who thought he was the first to isolate the AIDS virus. The researchers at the Pasteur Institute in Paris were actually the first by a considerable margin. HIV (human immunodeficiency virus, now the official name for the AIDS virus), is one of the lentiviruses. See *HIV*.

Humatrix Microclysmic gel—wound filling material.

Humatrope (somatropin)—a human growth hormone, manufactured by recombinant DNA technology. It is used in treating children with growth hormone deficiencies. See *Protropin*.

HumatroPen—reusable growth hormone delivery device for administration of Humatrope as treatment for growth hormone deficiency and short stature associated with Turner syndrome.

Humegon (menotropin)—an ovulation stimulant for women, spermatogenesis stimulant for men; administered intramuscularly.

humeral—pertaining to the humerus bone. Cf. *humoral, humorous.*

humerus—the long arm bone between the shoulder joint and the elbow joint. Cf. *humeral, humoral, humorous.*

HumidAire heated humidifier.

HUMI uterine manipulator/injector.

Hummer—a powered microdebrider designed originally for temporomandibular joint surgery. It is also now used as a sinus surgery instrument. It consists of a power unit, a foot-switch pedal, a handpiece, and a disposable blade.

Hummingbird wand—used for ablation and excision of soft tissue in well-defined channels or submucosally in ENT procedures.

humoral—pertaining to the immunity provided by antibodies in the blood. Cf. *humeral, humorous.*

humorous—funny or witty in character. Cf. *humerus.*

hump—see *diaphragmatic hump.*

Humulin—a human insulin (of recombinant DNA origin).

Humulin 70/30, Humulin R, and **Humalog Pens**—prefilled disposable insulin delivery devices that hold 300 units of insulin and fit in pocket or purse. A dose knob can be dialed backward or forward in single-unit increments.

Hunner's interstitial cystitis (*not* Hunter)—a severe, chronic inflammation of mucosa and muscularis of the urinary bladder, associated with ulcers of the bladder. Also, *Hunner's ulcer.*

Hunner's ulcer (Urol)—see *Hunner's interstitial cystitis.*

Hunt and Hess neurological classification—to predict the prognosis in patients with subarachnoid hemorrhage and intracranial aneurysms, grades 1-4.

Hunter's canal (canalis adductorius)—contains the femoral vessels and saphenous nerve.

Hunter-Sessions balloon—used in inferior vena cava to intercept a venous embolus.

Hunter tendon rod insertion—a treatment for deep venous insufficiency (DVI) of the lower extremities which causes symptoms of chronic edema and pain because the valves in the veins of the lower leg are incompetent. An incision is made at the back of the leg in the popliteal fossa. The Hunter tendon rod (made of Dacron) is sewn to the gracilis tendon at the side of the leg, woven through the popliteal artery and vein deep inside the leg, sutured to the biceps tendon on the other side of the leg, and drawn up snugly as a sling. This device then acts as a substitute valve by periodically occluding the popliteal vein as it passes tightly across it. When the patient stands or sits, the popliteal vein remains unoccluded. However, when the knee is actively flexed and the gracilis and biceps muscles retract, the popliteal vein is occluded to prevent venous reflux and venous stasis in the leg.

Hunter *(cont.)*
    Results are said to be superior to those obtained with other techniques.

Hunt-Lawrence pouch—a modification of the Roux-en-Y esophagojejunostomy reconstruction after total gastrectomy for carcinoma. This pouch is constructed to replace the gastric reservoir (removed in the Roux-en-Y procedure), to relieve symptoms of feelings of fullness, nausea, vomiting, dumping, and abdominal discomfort.

Hürthle cell neoplasm.

Hurwitz dialysis catheter.

HUS (hemolytic uremic syndrome).

Hutchinson's teeth—older term for one of the manifestations of congenital syphilis, now rare; the teeth are broad at the base and the biting surface is narrow and notched. Also, *hutchinsonian molars.*

HVI-DHP (hepatic venous isolation by direct hemoperfusion).

HVO (hallux valgus orthosis) **splint in a bag**—a forefoot splint used to treat hallux valgus either pre- or postoperatively. The splint is placed in a bag, and boiling water is added to make it moldable for custom fitting.

HVS (high-voltage stimulation).

HVS (hyperventilation syndrome).

Hyalgan (hyaluronic acid)—intra-articular injection for osteoarthritis and temporomandibular joint syndrome.

hyaloid corpuscle—see *Mittendorf's dot.*

Hyams grading system (or criteria)—for esthesioneuroblastoma.

Hybrid Capture cytomegalovirus DNA test—provides clinicians with a cost-effective and timely aid for diagnosing CMV infection in solid organ transplant, bone marrow transplant, and HIV-positive/AIDS patients.

Hybrid Capture II—DNA-based test to detect the human papillomavirus.

hybridoma—fusion of an antibody-producing cell with an immortalized cell, resulting in an immortalized hybrid cell capable of generating antibodies.

Hybritech Tandem PSA ratio (free PSA/total PSA) (PSA, prostate-specific antigen)—a test to distinguish between prostate cancer and other conditions that are non-cancerous but involve an enlarged prostate.

Hycamptin (topotecan).

hyCare G hydrogel dressing.

Hycor rheumatoid factor (RF) IgA ELISA autoimmune test—for early diagnosis of rheumatoid arthritis.

hyCure collagen hemostatic wound dressing.

Hydrasorb foam wound dressing.

hydrazine sulfate—a drug to promote weight gain and appetite in patients with incurable colorectal carcinoma.

Hydrea (hydroxyurea)—reduces the number of sickle-cell crises by half, and the incidence of chest pain and fever associated with sickle cell disease. Though not a cure, hydroxyurea is the first effective treatment for sickle cell disease. Also approved as treatment for polycythemia vera (excess red blood cells), melanoma, ovarian carcinoma, and myelocytic leukemia.

HydroBlade keratome—Microjet device used to produce hinged corneal flaps and to alter the shape of the cornea for vision correction.

HydroBrush keratome—used in the debridement of epithelium from the cornea.

Hydrocol—see *hydrocolloid dressing material.*

Hydrocollator—a silica gel pack used in applying localized heat. The silica gel is encased in a canvas bag. The pack is immersed in water and heated to 140 to 160°F. The pack is then wrapped in several layers of terry cloth before applying to the area to be heated. The pack maintains its heat for approximately 20 to 30 minutes, which gives it an advantage over the hot water bottle.

hydrocolloid dressing (Hydrocol)—combines absorbent colloid materials with adhesive elastomers for application to wounds with light to moderate exudate. Most hydrocolloid dressings react with wound exudate to form gel-like coverings that protect the wound bed and maintain a moist wound environment. Hydrocolloid is available in occlusive and wafer-type dressings, as well as in powder and paste forms. See also *dressing.*

hydrofiber dressings.

HydroFlex—arthroscopy irrigating system.

hydrogel dressing—wound gel that helps create or maintain a moist wound environment. Some hydrogels provide absorption, desloughing, and debriding of necrotic and fibrotic tissue. See *dressing.*

hydrogel sheet—cross-linked polymer gels in sheet form for wound dressing. These materials help create or maintain a moist wound environment and may also provide absorption, desloughing, and debridement of necrotic and fibrotic tissue. See *dressing.*

hydrography, MR—see *MR hydrography.*

Hydrolyser microcatheter—used in thrombectomy systems to negotiate tortuous arterial curves.

Hydromer—coated bipolar coagulation probe.

Hydromer Aquatrix II—hydrogel technology for biosurgery applications. It is based on chitosan, a structural analog to hyaluronic acid derived from chitin, a natural biopolymer, and polyvinylpyrrolidone (PVP), a synthetic polymer.

Hydron Burn Bandage.

hydrophilic—water-loving. Used in medicine to refer to stains. Cf. *lipophilic*, fat-loving.

hydrophilic semipermeable absorbent polyurethane foam dressing (Surg)—provides a moist wound environment with a petrolatum gauze dressing for donor sites. It is said to produce less initial patient donor site discomfort and to produce more complete donor site healing by postoperative day 14.

Hydro-Splint II—used to immobilize fractures of upper or lower extremities. It is not only a splint, but also a cold (or warm) compress, and provides soft tissue compression for chronic or acute swelling.

HydroSurg laparoscopic irrigator.

HydroThermAblator—system to treat excessive uterine bleeding.

Hydroview intraocular lens—implant for correction of vision following cataract extraction procedures.

hydroxyapatite (or *hydroxylapatite*) (HA)—dense ceramic material manufactured from coral found in the ocean. It is porous, like human bone. Used as an adjunct to bone grafting in cranial defects, to restore normal contour. In ophthalmology, it can be formed into a sphere and used as an

hydroxyapatite *(cont.)*
ocular implant after enucleation of the eye. Also, *Biomatrix ocular implant, Durapatite, Interpore.*

hydroxyindoleacetic acid (5-HIAA).

hydroxylapatite—see *hydroxyapatite.*

hydroxyurea (Hydrea).

HyFil hydrogel dressing.

Hyfrecator—a desiccator-fulgurator-coagulator.

hygroma—a fluid-filled cystic mass, often seen in the necks of children.

Hylaform (hylan polymer)—viscoelastic gel for correction of facial wrinkles and depressed scars.

Hylagel-Nuro—viscoelastic gel for the reduction of postoperative scarring and adhesions secondary to lumbar surgery. It is administered via injection of the spinal area immediately following surgery.

Hylashield and **Hylashield Nite** (hylan A)—provides an elastoviscous shield and protects the surface of the eye from noxious environmental conditions.

Hylasine—viscoelastic gel device injected into anatomical compartments of the sinus during and following sinus surgery in order to coat surgically altered tissue, control intraoperative and postoperative bleeding, reduce postsurgical scarring and adhesions, minimize patient discomfort, and shorten postoperative rehabilitation time.

hymenal ring (*not* hymeneal, as it is often mispronounced).

Hypafix—nonwoven tape with a low-allergy adhesive used to hold dressings in place.

hyper-, prefix meaning *excessive, above, beyond.* Cf. *hypo-.*

hyperacute rejection (HAR)—graft rejection immediately after transplantation.

hyperbaric chambers—increasingly seen in hospital inventories because of oxygen's capacity to aid healing. Trainers for major sports teams also have the chambers on hand for athletes, and celebrities are touting them as age-defying devices.

hyperbaric oxygen therapy—high-pressure therapy used in treatment of cyanide poisoning, exceptionally high blood loss anemia, decompression sickness, and as adjunctive therapy in osteomyelitis, radiation injury, acute cerebral edema, and injury to the head and spinal cord. Also used as adjunctive therapy in the treatment of rhinocerebral mucormycosis. The fungi, when they infect immunosuppressed patients, can be highly invasive, causing a rapidly progressive infection.

hyperesthesia of the vulva—see *vulvar vestibulitis syndrome.*

Hypergel hydrogel dressing.

hypericin (VIMRxyn)—antiviral drug used to treat patients with HIV and AIDS.

Hyperion LTK (laser thermal keratoplasty)—holmium laser-based system for the performance of laser thermal keratoplasty.

hyperlipoproteinemia (HLP).

hyperopia—farsightedness.

hyperoxia—used for treating carbon monoxide poisoning, chronic nonhealing ulcers, acute traumatic and chronically ischemic wounds, and refractory osteomyelitis.

hyperprosody—excessive variation in voice features such as pitch, loudness, tempo, intonation, as occurs in

hyperprosody *(cont.)*
manic patients. In patients with Broca's aphasia, hyperprosody manifests as their using the very few words at their disposal to convey to the utmost their attitudes and emotions. Cf. *dysprody*.

hyperreninemia—a condition of elevated levels of renin in the blood, which may lead to aldosteronism and hypertension.

hypertelorism—abnormally increased distance between two organs, as in Crouzon's disease.

hypertension optimal treatment (HOT)—a five-year study begun in 1992 to determine precisely how far high blood pressure should be lowered to minimize cardiovascular morbidity and mortality. It also examines the effects of adding low doses of aspirin to the antihypertensive regimen. The HOT study involves patients from 26 countries on four continents and includes both male and female hypertensives.

hypertension standard—changed from 140/80 to 135/85, resulting in many more patients requiring medication.

hyperthermia, whole body—used in the therapy regimen of patients with certain types of tumors, some bone metastases, and Ewing's sarcoma. These cancer cells are particularly sensitive to heat; therefore, heat increases the effectiveness of chemotherapy and radiotherapy. When the patient's body is heated to 108°F after irradiation, the cancer cells cannot readily repair themselves. When the patient is given hyperthermia before chemotherapy is introduced, the cancer cells are more susceptible to the effects of chemotherapy agents.

hypertrophic cardiomyopathy (HCMP).

hypertrophic obstructive cardiomyopathy (HOCM).

hypertrophy, asymmetric septal (ASH).

hypertylosis of the palms—callosities.

hypesthesia—diminished sensitivity to stimulation, feeling, sensation or perception. Also, *hypoesthesia*.

hypnosis, focused open neurosensory induction of—a self-hypnotic method using vision, hearing, and kinesthetic sensations.

hypnotic—a drug used to induce sleep.

hypo-, prefix meaning *deficient, decrease, under, beneath, below*. Cf. *hyper-*.

hypoaeration (Radiol)—on chest x-ray, abnormal reduction in the amount of air in lung tissue.

hypoattenuating—coined word applied to CT scan findings of low attenuation.

hypoechoic ("hi-po-e-ko´-ic")—a term used in ultrasonography, when only few echoes are given off as the ultrasound waves bounce off structures or tissues at which they are directed. "The patient had a hypoechoic area in the right lobe of the prostate."

hypokinesis—abnormal reduction of mobility or motility; reduced contractile movement in one or both cardiac ventricles.

hypophysis—pituitary gland (hypophysis cerebri); pharyngeal hypophysis (a mass in the wall of the pharynx similar in appearance to the hypophysis). Cf. *apophysis, epiphysis, hypothesis*.

hypoplastic left heart syndrome (HLHS).

hypopyon—a complication associated with postoperative corneal graft infection.

hypothalamic-pituitary-adrenal axis (HPA).

hypothalamus—the portion of the brain that controls the autonomic mechanism.

hypothermia blanket—used for cooling patients to 28 to 30°C for open heart and brain surgery; reduces normal oxygen requirements.

hypothesis—a theory that appears to explain certain phenomena and is used as the basis of experimentation and reasoning to prove the theory. Cf. *apophysis, epiphysis, hypophysis.*

hysterectomy—see *CASH Semm hysterectomy.*

hysterosonography—the infusion of saline into the uterus through a catheter while a transvaginal ultrasound is performed. This procedure is used to identify lesions undetected by endometrial biopsy.

hysterosalpingosonography (HSSG)—a diagnostic ultrasound technique used to assess uterine cavity defects and patency of the fallopian tubes.

Hy-Tape—waterproof, medicated tape safe for direct use on skin and especially used by ostomy patients.

Hytrin (terazosin).

Hyzaar (losartan potassium HCl)—angiotensin II blockade, with the addition of a diuretic. Treatment for hypertension.

HZA (hermizona) **assay**—for the evaluation of sperm binding to the zona pellucida, with high predictive value for in vitro fertilization.

HZV (herpes zoster virus).

I, i

IABC (intra-aortic balloon counterpulsation).

IABP (intra-aortic balloon pump).

Ialo photocoagulation—of the whole retina.

Iamin Gel wound dressing—a hydrogel dressing used in the management of various types of wounds, including skin abrasions, first and second degree burns, diabetic and venous stasis ulcers, pressure sores, and surgical incisions.

I&D (incision and drainage). Cf. *IND*.

I&O, I/O (intake and output)—intake of liquid (intravenous, per mouth, per tube) and output (urine, tube, drain) plus insensible output, in a 24-hour period. Measured in cubic centimeters or milliliters. "The patient's I&O was monitored." See *INO; insensible output*.

iatrogenic illness—caused (inadvertently) by a physician. Cf. *nosocomial*.

IBD (inflammatory bowel disease).

I-B1 radiolabeled antibody—injection to deliver high doses of radiation to tumors.

ibopamine—dilates the arteries and acts as a diuretic.

ibotenic acid—one of the poisons from the deadly mushroom *Amanita muscaria*.

ibuprofen—antiarthritic, nonsteroidal anti-inflammatory drug (NSAID), and analgesic. It may be used in treating patent ductus arteriosus and cystic fibrosis.

ibutilide fumarate (Corvert).

ICA (intracranial aneurysm).

ICAM-1 (intercellular adhesions molecule-1)—a marker protein for the development of coronary artery disease in heart transplant patients.

ICCE (intracapsular cataract extraction).

ICD (implantable cardioverter-defibrillator). See *AICD*.

ICE (ifosfamide [with mesna rescue], carboplatin, etoposide)—chemotherapy protocol for small cell lung carcinoma, and Hodgkin's and non-Hodgkin's lymphomas.

ICE (intracardiac echocardiography).

ice cream headache—a sensation of sudden head pain upon biting into very cold ice cream.

ICE disorders—immunoglobulin-complexed enzyme disorders.

IceSeeds—see *SeedNet System.*

ICE syndrome—iridocorneal-endothelial syndrome.

ICEUS (intracaval endovascular ultrasonography).

ICG (iodocyanine green) **fluorescein angiography**—used to evaluate patients with multifocal choroiditis and macular holes.

ICIT (infrared coagulation of the inferior turbinate).

ICL (idiopathic CD4+ lymphocytopenia).

ICL (implantable contact lens)—refractive lens that is implanted over the natural lens of the eye for correction of myopia and hyperopia.

ICLH apparatus (Ortho)—by Imperial College, London Hospital.

i.com Comfort Shield—preservative-free viscoelastic ophthalmic solution for the treatment of dry eyes.

ICP catheter (intracranial pressure)—used with Tele-Sensor monitor after brain surgery. See *Cosman ICP Tele-Sensor.*

ICR (intrastromal corneal ring) or **KeraVision ICR**—an implant composed of two thin, transparent half-rings made of polymer material that are inserted into the periphery of the cornea, reshaping the clear tissue of the eye, to correct myopia. The procedure, which requires no cutting or removal of tissue, is designed to be a permanent implant, though it may be removed and replaced as vision changes.

ICS—intracellular-like, calcium bearing crystalloid solution. See *cardioplegic solution.*

ICSI (intracytoplasmic sperm injection).

ictal fear—an aura of anxiety or fear preceding temporal lobe seizures in some patients. May be more or less intense, with some patients reporting only uneasiness or nervousness and others intense fear and horror.

Idamycin (idarubicin).

idarubicin (Idamycin)—one of the special antibiotics (derived from the fungus-like bacterium *Streptomyces*) used as a chemotherapy agent for treatment of acute myeloid leukemia in adults.

IDEA (Inventory for Déjà Vu Experiences Assessment)—prolonged or frequent episodes of déjà vu have clinical significance in patients with complex partial seizures and psychotic relapses.

Ideal (trademark) **cardiac device.**

ideation (noun)—the process of forming ideas or images. "He has no suicidal or homicidal ideation."

idée fixe ("ee-day'-feeks")—an obsessively fixed idea.

idiojunctional rhythm, junctional or nodal rhythm—a phenomenon in which the AV node becomes the pacemaker for the heart. When effective electrical impulses are no longer generated by the sinoatrial (SA) node, the atrioventricular (AV) node (located near the junction of atria and ventricles) becomes the pacemaker for the heart.

idiopathic CD4+ lymphocytopenia (ICL)—name given by the Centers for Disease Control and Prevention for controversial cases where pa-

idiopathic *(cont.)*
tients seem to have AIDS-like symptoms in the absence of HIV.

idiopathic hypertrophic subaortic stenosis (IHSS).

idiopathic thrombocytopenic purpura (ITP).

idiosyncratic asthma—asthma characterized by the following factors: (1) the person has no history of allergic diseases, (2) symptoms usually begin after age 30, (3) it is difficult to distinguish from chronic bronchitis, and (4) attacks often begin with minor respiratory symptoms.

IDIS angiography system (intraoperative digital subtraction).

idoxuridine (IDU)—for nonparenchymatous sarcomas.

IDSS (internal decompression for spinal stenosis).

IEA (inferior epigastric artery) **graft**—may be used instead of saphenous veins in coronary artery bypass.

IECRT (intraoperative endoscopic Congo red test).

I/E ratio (inspiratory/expiratory ratio)—as in "Lungs: Normal I/E ratio, and no rales, rhonchi, or wheezes."

I-FABP (intestinal fatty acid-binding protein), **human serum.**

IFA test—indirect fluorescent antibody test for *Legionella pneumophila*. See also *DFA*.

I-Flow nerve block infusion kit—for the continuous infusion of local anesthesia as a regional nerve block for pain management before and after orthopedic and general surgical procedures.

IFN-A (interferon alfa).

IFT (interferential current therapy).

IGF-BP3 complex (SomatoKine).

IGF-1 (insulin-like growth factor 1)—women under 50 with high blood levels of this factor appear to have a greater risk for breast cancer. However, for postmenopausal women, there is no association between IGF-1 and breast cancer risk.

IgG, platelet-associated (PAIgG).

IgG 2A monoclonal antibody (Immu-RAIT-LL2)—labeled with iodine 131; a drug used to treat B-cell lymphoma and leukemias.

Iglesias fiberoptic resectoscope.

IgM-RF antibody (rheumatoid factor).

I-HAST (In-Home Alzheimer's Screening Test).

IHSS (idiopathic hypertrophic subaortic stenosis). Now called *ASH* (asymmetric septal hypertrophy).

IL-1—see *interleukin-1*.

IL-2—see *interleukin-2*.

IL-3—see *interleukin-3*.

IL4-PE (interleukin-4-*Pseudomonas* exotoxin fusion protein)—blood-cell-derived growth factor that is being investigated for treatment of malignant brain tumors.

IL-4R—an immune system protein, manufactured by Immunex Corporation, that stops allergic responses.

IL-10 (interleukin-10).

IL-11 (interleukin-11).

ILA stapler—has three interchangeable heads and a long handle, giving access to deep operative sites.

ileal conduit (*not* ileoconduit or ileo conduit)—a segment of ileum formed into a new bladder in patients who have undergone total cystectomy. The ends of the ureters are then anastomosed to the new ileal "bladder." See also *reservoir*.

ileal neobladder—see *W-stapled urinary reservoir*.

ileocystoplasty—see *operation*.

ileosigmoid knot—condition where loops of ileum wrap around the base of a redundant sigmoid loop. The closed proximal loops of the ileum become congested and gangrenous within a few hours. Surgical intervention is required. Also known as *compound volvulus*.

ileostomy—see *operation*.

ilepcimide—an anticonvulsant used to treat generalized tonic-clonic seizures resistant to other drugs.

ILE-SORB absorbent gel—introduced into ileostomy pouch to transform liquid into semi-solid gel in order to keep pouch contents away from stoma, reduce sloshing and pouch noise, and provide easier emptying.

ileum—the part of the small intestine located between the jejunum and the large intestine. Cf. *ilium*.

ileus—small-bowel obstruction due to failure of peristalsis.

iliopsoas test—for an inflammatory process. On abdominal examination, if pain is elicited when the patient flexes his thigh against pressure of the examiner's hand, there is an inflammatory process in contact with the iliopsoas muscle.

ilium—the superior portion of the hip bone. Cf. *ileum*.

Ilizarov limb lengthening procedure ("eh-liz´-a-rov").

Ilizarov system—instruments used to facilitate limb lengthening, fracture fixation, and nonunion of long bones.

illicit—unlawful, improper, not permitted, as "The patient denies use of illicit drugs." Cf. *elicit*.

Illi intracranial pressure monitoring and fixation device—for ICP monitoring in children and adolescents in pediatric neurotraumatology, hydrocephalus, and craniofacial surgery. Designed by Dr. O. E. Illi, it has two movable components compressing the skull from inside and outside and is fully compatible with a range of fiberoptic or pneumatic transducer systems.

illness, food-borne (FBI).

Illumen-8 guiding catheter.

Illumina PROSeries—laparoscopy system.

illusion—an unreal or misleading image or perception, as "He was suffering from the illusion that there were insects crawling over him." Cf. *allusion, elusion*.

ILUS catheter (intraluminal ultrasound) (GI).

IMA (internal mammary artery) **graft**. Also, inferior mesenteric artery.

IMA (inferior mesenteric artery) **retractor**—used in cardiac bypass.

IMAB (internal mammary artery bypass).

image acquisition time—MRI term.

ImageChecker—computer-aided detection system for mammography.

image-guided surgery—using a robotic microscope (SergiScope) and a surgical digitizer (The Viewing Wand).

Imagent GI (perflubron)—oral contrast agent for MRI and x-ray imaging.

Imagent US—imaging agent for cardiac ultrasound procedures.

imaging agent—see *medication*; *radioisotope; technetium*.

Imagyn microlaparoscope (Oph)—a very small laparoscope used in eye surgery.

Imatron Ultrafast CT scanner—uses electron beam technology. It is used for general purpose CT scanning, as well as for noninvasive diagnosis of coronary artery disease.

Imdur (isosorbide mononitrate)—the trade name for a once-a-day therapy to prevent angina.

IMED infusion device—for intravenous fluids.

IMEX scleral implants—solid silicone, sponge silicone, and Miragel buckling components. See *Miragel*; *implant*.

imidazotetrazines—a new class of drugs that works by damaging DNA in cancer cells, causing them to self-destruct. Noncancerous cells are not harmed and, unlike most cancer treatments, it can filter through the brain's protective barrier.

Imitrex (sumatriptan succinate)—trade name for a vascular serotonin agonist drug used to treat migraine headaches and cluster headaches. It is available in an injectable form, a film-coated tablet, and a nasal spray. The spray is often found to work faster than the tablet. The manufacturer (Glaxo) offers an autoinjector so that patients may medicate themselves as migraines occur. Unlike other migraine drugs which must be taken at the beginning of the migraine to be effective, Imitrex is said to relieve symptoms of pain, vomiting, and sensitivity to light and sound no matter when it is administered. For some patients, relief from pain lasts for only three hours, before the headache returns.

immersion foot—the third stage of trauma due to exposure to cold; first stage—frostbite; second stage—trench foot.

imminent—about to occur in the near future; immediately threatening. Cf. *eminence*.

Immix bioabsorbable implant—bioabsorbable tissue scaffolds for regeneration and repair of bone and cartilage defects.

immobilize—prevent from moving. Cf. *mobilize*.

ImmTher (disaccharide tripeptide)—immunostimulant for pulmonary and hepatic metastases of colorectal adenocarcinoma and osteosarcoma.

immune globulin—see *antibody molecules*.

immune system modulator (Imreg-1).

immunobead assay—measurement of platelet-associated and plasma auto-antibody. Also, a test to check for sperm antibodies.

ImmunoCard STAT! Rotavirus—a one-step test that can detect rotavirus, using a stool specimen.

ImmunoCyt—a noninvasive diagnostic test that uses a urine sample for the detection of superficial bladder cancer.

immunofixation in agar (Agar-IF)—of blood serum.

immunoisolating microreactors—implantable cell systems, or microreactors, containing living cells that produce a therapeutic molecule, e.g., insulin. The cells are encapsulated and injected into the body where they release the needed substance. Under study are microreactor treatments for hemophilia, Huntington's chorea, Parkinson's disease, Alzheimer's disease, cancer, and AIDS.

immunoliposomes—a combination of liposomes (small synthetic particles used to carry potent anticancer drugs) and antibodies that can recognize and bind to cancer cells. Immunoliposomes can selectively

immunoliposomes *(cont.)*
target and kill cancer cells while avoiding normal cells.

immunomodulation—manipulation of donor tissue antigens prior to transplantation to deter host rejection; may allow long-term cellular transplant survival without immunosuppression.

immunoperoxidase stain (Lab)—"Immunoperoxidase stains were performed in formalin-fixed, paraffin-embedded sections, using the peroxidase-antiperoxidase technique."

immunoproliferative small intestinal disease (IPSID)—also known as *small intestinal malignant lymphoma* or *Mediterranean lymphoma*, most prevalent in developing countries.

immunoreactive parathyroid hormone (iPTH) (lowercase *i*).

immunoscintigraphy—a study using technetium 99m-labeled antigranulocyte antibodies, when echocardiographic findings are equivocal. May also be used to monitor antibiotic therapy and to detect melanoma.

immunosuppressant cocktail—a combination drug in which several immunosuppressant drugs are given together.

immunosuppressive therapy (IST).

ImmuRAID (CEA-Tc 99m)—used in antibody imaging. See *RAID*.

ImmuRAIT-LL2 (IgG 2A monoclonal antibody; iodine ^{131}I murine MAb IgG 2A to B cell)—treatment for B-cell leukemia and lymphoma.

Imount instruments (Ortho)—used in total knee replacement.

Impact enteral formula—for advanced nutritional support.

Impact total hip system.

impactor—see *vertebral body impactor*.

IMP-Capello arm support—provides stability and access to the patient's arm to monitor I.V., blood pressure. (IMP stands for Innovative Medical Products.)

impedance plethysmography (IPG)—a noninvasive test to determine the presence and degree of deep vein obstruction in venous thrombosis. It evaluates patency of the veins by measuring venous volume changes.

impingement—contact or pressure, generally abnormal, between two structures.

impingement sign—produces pain in rotator cuff tendinopathy and tear.

implant—consisting of metal orthopedic implants used mainly for total joint replacement, Silastic silicone rubber implants used in plastic surgery, and silicone orthopedic implants used for hand and foot; also, breast, dental, ear, and eye implants. Examples:
Acticon neosphincter
anterior chamber acrylic
Arenberg-Denver inner-ear valve
Avanta joint skeletal
Baerveldt glaucoma
Biocell RTV saline-filled breast
Biocoral
Biodel
Bio-eye
Biomatrix ocular
Bionx SmartNail bioresorbable
Bio-Oss
bioresorbable
Branemark endosteal
Clarion multi-strategy cochlear
cochlear
Codere orbital floor
collagen meniscus implant (CMI)
Compliant pre-stress bone

implant *(cont.)*
 Contigen Bard cochlear
 Contigen collagen continent
 Contigen glutaraldehyde
   cross-linked collagen
 Contour Profile anatomically shaped
   silicone breast
 double plate Molteno
 Durapapite
 expanded polytetrafluoroethylene
   (ePTFE) facial
 Frialoc transgingival threaded
 Gliadel wafer
 Gore-Tex facial contouring strips
 Gore-Tex nasal
 Gore-Tex SAM facial
 Graftpatch
 GTS great toe system
 Heyer-Schulte
 HTR-MFI
 Hydroview intraocular lens
 hydroxyapatite (HA)
 ICL (implantable contact lens)
 ICR (intrastromal corneal ring)
 IMEX scleral
 Immix bioabsorbable
 IMZ endosteal
 Intacs
 Integral Omniloc
 Interpore
 intracorneal (Kerato-Gel)
 islet cell
 K-Centrum anterior spinal fixation
   system
 Kerato-Gel (intracorneal)
 KeraVision ICR
 Kinetik great toe
 Krupin-Denver eye valve
 LARSI (lumbar anterior-root
   stimulator implant)
 Macroplastique continent
 McCutchen
 McGhan facial
 methylmethacrylate, beads of

implant *(cont.)*
 Mini-Med continuous glucose
   sensor
 Miragel
 Natural-Knee system
 Nexus
 NovaGold breast
 NovaSaline inflatable saline breast
 Optimed glaucoma pressure
   regulator
 Osteonics-HA coated
 PhacoFlex II SI-30NB
 PharmaSeed palladium-103 seeds
 ProOsteon Implant 500
 radioactive seed implants
 Restore dental
 SAM (subcutaneous augmentation
   material)
 Septacin
 silicone
 SmartNail (Bionx SmartNail)
 SoftForm facial
 STAAR Toric implantable contact
   lens
 STOP (selective tubal occlusion
   procedure) permanent contra-
   ception device
 Suspend sling
 System•S soft skeletal
 TheraSeed
 Trilucent breast
 Unilab Surgibone
 Vitrasert intraocular
implantable cardioverter-defibrillator
   —see *AICD*.
implantable contact lens (ICL)—
   refractive lens that is implanted over
   the natural lens of the eye for correction of myopia and hyperopia.
implantation response—reperfusion
   injury of the postischemic lungs, as
   seen in lung or heart and lung transplant patients. It resolves within 3 to
   5 days. If a pathologic pulmonary

implantation *(cont.)*
process following lung transplantation takes longer to resolve, another process is probably responsible.

Implast bone cement.

Import vascular access port with Bio-Glide—features new hydrophilic properties on the catheter component of the access port.

impossible meningioma—physicians' term for a meningioma just anterior to the optic foramen; it is very difficult to detect by visualizing tests. The physician needs a high index of suspicion.

Impress Softpatch—incontinence care product from UroMed.

impulse, apical—MRI term.

Imreg-1, Imreg-2 (immune system modulator)—for treating AIDS and Kaposi's sarcoma.

I-MRI (interventional MRI).

IMRT (intensity modulated radiation therapy)—uses a 3-D computerized imaging system to deliver highly focused radiation beams to tumor targets.

ImuLyme—a vaccine for the prevention of Lyme disease.

Imuthiol (diethyldithiocarbamate)—a drug for treatment of AIDS.

IMV (intermittent mandatory ventilation).

IMZ endosteal implants (ENT).

inactivation technique, psoralen.

inamrinone—new name for *amrinone*, cardiotonic medication. The name was officially changed because of medication errors due to similarity with *amiodarone*.

INCA (infant nasal cannulae assembly) —an oxygen delivery system consisting of nasal prongs and flexible oxygen tubing connected by fasteners to a knit cap on the infant's head.

incentive spirometer—a device into which you blow, to measure the volume of air taken into the lungs. It registers on a vertical cylindrical plastic meter that works much like one of those games you see at county fairs, where you hit a metal plate with a heavy hammer and the plate goes up and rings a bell and you get a prize. When a nurse was asked what the prize is with the spirometer, she replied: "The prize is that you don't get pneumonia."

Incert—a bioabsorbable, implantable sponge designed to prevent post-surgical tissue adhesions. Placed over the surgical site and surrounding tissues and organs, it provides a physical barrier to prevent internal tissue surfaces from sticking together.

In Charge diabetes control system—handheld monitor for personal use. It performs both a rapid glucose test and a test for glycated protein.

incidence—in medicine, the number of new cases of a disease that occur in a given population in a certain period of time. Cf. *incidents*.

"incidentaloma"—a coined word for a finding on sonography of a nodule that is unrelated to a palpable mass.

incidents—events, happenings, occurrences. Cf. *incidence*.

incipient—just beginning to appear; initial or early stage.

incision—a cut or a wound made by a sharp instrument. Cf. *excision*.
Types of incisions include:
bayonet-type
Bevan
Bruser's skin
Cherney
chevron
clamshell
cross-tunneling

incision *(cont.)*
  cruciate
  curvilinear
  frown
  gull-wing
  intercartilaginous
  Kocher collar (thyroidectomy)
  LaRoque herniorrhaphy
  lazy H
  lazy Z
  minilaparotomy
  muscle-splitting
  relaxing
  Rethi
  Rockey-Davis
  scoring
  smiling
  Wilde
  Y
  Yorke-Mason

incisura dextra of Gans—deep groove on the inferior surface of the liver near the bed of the gallbladder.

inclusion body—see *body.*

Incomplete Sentence Blank Test (ISB) —mental status examination.

increment—amount by which a dose or value is increased, as "Steroids were increased in weekly increments of 5 mg to a maximum dose of 25 mg."

IND (investigational new drug)—a drug which may be used in clinical testing by licensed researchers with the permission of the FDA, but not yet approved by the FDA for marketing. Cf. *I&D.*

independent beam steering, electronic —a feature of advanced ultrasound units that allows the sonographer or clinician to separately manipulate B-scan, color flow, and pulsed-wave Doppler in real time. This makes it possible to keep a constant perpendicular angle of the beam with an

artery in vascular examinations and maximize the arterial interface to obtain the best images.

Indermil—topical tissue adhesive used in wound closure.

index—see also *test.*
  amniotic fluid (AFI)
  apnea/hypopnea (AHI)
  Broders'
  Dermatology Index of Disease Severity (DIDS)
  fetal-pelvic
  Fick cardiac
  foam stability
  free/total PSA
  FTI (free thyroxine)
  Gosling pulsatility
  Gravindex
  Growth Potential Realization
  Harvey hospital prognostic nutritional
  Insall-Salvati
  Mengert's pelvimetry
  Penetrating Abdominal Trauma Index (PATI)
  penile-brachial pressure (PBPI)
  prognostic nutritional (PNI)
  PSA (prostate-specific antigen)
  PSA free/total
  Quetelet's BMI
  short increment sensitivity (SISI)
  umbilical coiling

Indiana pouch—an ileocolic continent urinary diversion used in patients who require cystectomy for carcinoma or trauma, or patients who have a neurogenic bladder, bladder dysfunction, or congenital anomaly. Other procedures for continent urinary diversion: Camey ileocystoplasty, Kock pouch, Mainz pouch urinary reservoir, and Mitrofanoff.

Indiclor—an indium 111 (^{111}In) radioimaging agent used with OncoScint

Indiclor *(cont.)*
CR/OV to identify location and extent of colorectal and ovarian cancers.

Indigo LaserOptic treatment system —for the treatment of symptoms of benign prostatic hyperplasia. The Indigo system combines fiberoptics with diode laser fiber technology. Using direct visualization, a surgeon employs a diode laser to quickly destroy a precise area of the prostate by interstitial laser coagulation.

indinavir (Crixivan)—a protease inhibitor used as an anti-HIV drug.

indirect fluorescent antibody test (IFA).

indirect laser ophthalmoscope—used for treatment of ROP (retinopathy of prematurity).

indium (In-111) **pentetreotide** (Octreo-Scan)—imaging agent used as a somatostatin receptor to facilitate neuroendocrine tumor localization.

indium-111-labeled human nonspecific immunoglobulin G (^{111}In-IgG) —a radiopharmaceutical for imaging focal inflammation in febrile granulocytopenic patients.

indium 111 scintigraphy scan (^{111}In).

indocyanine green angiography—provides new ways of looking at optic nerve, choroidal, and retinal blood flow, when combined with color Doppler and digital image acquisition and analysis.

indocyanine green dye—for detection of intracardial shunt.

inducer cell—a name for the T-4 helper lymphocyte, the specific target of the AIDS virus; also called *helper/ inducer cell*; it plays an important role in activating other parts of the immune system.

indurated plantar keratoma (IPK).

Inerpan—a special dressing for burn patients that requires less frequent changing. This decreases pain for the patient and allows the donor site to heal more completely.

In-Exsufflator—cough machine that assists patients in removal of bronchial secretions.

in extremis—at the point of death.

Infanrix vaccine—an acellular vaccine containing diphtheria and tetanus toxoids. In clinical studies it has been proven to work as effectively as, and with fewer complications than, whole-cell vaccines.

Infant Flow nasal CPAP system.

In-Fast—a bone screw system used in transvaginal cystourethropexy and sling procedures.

Infasurf (calfactant)—natural surfactant obtained from a saline lavage of cows' lungs. Used to treat the lack of surfactant causing respiratory distress syndrome (RSD) disease in premature infants.

Infergen (interferon alfacon-1)—a bioengineered drug used for the treatment of chronic hepatitis C viral (HCV) infection.

inferior mesenteric artery (IMA).

infibulation (also referred to as "pharaonic circumcision")—the most extreme form of female genital mutilation consisting of removal of clitoris, adjacent labia (majora and minora), and joining of scraped sides of the vulva across the vagina, where they are secured with thorns or sewn with catgut or thread. A small opening is left to allow passage of urine and menstrual blood. Area is cut open to allow intercourse on the wedding night and closed again afterward to ensure marital fidelity.

infibulation *(cont.)*
See also *clitoridectomy* and *Sunna circumcision.*

Infiniti catheter (Cardio).

Infinity hip system—modular hip replacement implant.

InFix interbody fusion system—standalone lumbar fusion device that is inserted through an anterior approach. Height, width, and lordotic angle can be independently adjusted during implantation to match patient anatomy.

inflamed (one *m*, unlike *inflammation*, *inflammatory*).

inflammation—classic signs of inflammation are rubor (redness), calor (heat), dolor (pain), tumor (swelling), and loss of function.

infliximab—monoclonal antibody for patients with moderate to severe Crohn's disease. See *Remicade.*

influenza vaccine—may be administered as a nasal spray offering protection against flu. It has the ability to immediately block the growth of influenza viruses that cause disease, in addition to, and apart from, its ability to induce antibody formation. It is an attenuated live influenza virus but one which can block the growth of other influenza viruses. Other vaccines against the flu require two weeks to adequately stimulate the body's antibody defenses to produce immunity; this flu vaccine provides almost instantaneous protection—a real plus when a flu epidemic strikes. Of note, influenza is still the sixth leading cause of death in this country.

Inform—a HER-2/neu gene-based test for breast cancer recurrence. Using the original breast cancer tissue sample, the Inform test identifies the presence or absence of increased copies of the HER-2/neu gene. This indicates whether breast cancer is likely to recur.

infra-, prefix meaning under, beneath, below. Cf. *inter-, intra-, inner-.*

infranate—material that settles to the bottom of a liquid. Cf. *supernate.*

infrared coagulation of the inferior turbinate (ICIT)—provides relief of nasal obstruction.

infrarenal aortobifemoral bypass graft—procedure for aortoiliofemoral reconstruction in atherosclerotic occlusive disease.

Infumorph—solution of morphine sulfate given by the intrathecal or epidural route.

Infusaid—an implantable drug infusion pump.

InfusaSleeve II catheter—designed for coronary drug delivery, using "over-the-balloon" technology to track over a standard angioplasty balloon catheter.

Infuse-a-port—implantable vascular access system. Used for administration of chemotherapeutic agent via cephalic vein (or possibly other veins).

infusion—the slow therapeutic introduction of fluid other than blood into a vein. Cf. *effusion.*

Ingram regimen for psoriasis—similar to Goeckerman regimen. See *Goeckerman regimen.*

inhalant antigens (major outdoor allergens), including the fungi:
Alternaria
Cladosporium
Hormodendrum

inhaler—see *device; medication.*

injection technique—an alternative method to use on a thigh tourniquet

injection *(cont.)*
for creation of a bloodless field in operations for anterior cruciate ligament reconstruction. The injection technique uses lidocaine and epinephrine with bupivacaine. As these operations are lengthy, the tourniquet must be applied for long periods of time, which can cause muscular, vascular, and systemic problems postoperatively, and which puts pressure on the surgeon to rush, once the tourniquet is inflated.

injector—see *HUMI uterine.*

InjecTx—customized cystoscope which shrinks prostate tissue by injecting purified alcohol, killing prostate cells without painful swelling. The prostate then shrinks as the body eliminates the cells.

Injex—single-use disposable needle-free injector.

Injury Severity Scale (ISS)—a system used to describe multiple trauma injuries.

ink-potassium hydroxide test—"Ink-potassium hydroxide preparation of corneal scrapings showed *Acanthamoeba* cysts in the corneal stroma." India (writing) ink is used in this test. The principle involved is similar to that of the Schiller test for cancer of the cervix—a negative stain. The ink is not absorbed by *Acanthamoeba* cysts, and they appear as light structures on a dark background of the ink. Cf. *onlay graft.* See *Schiller test.*

inlay graft—a bone graft, not to be confused with onlay graft. Both are used in craniofacial surgery. Skin can also be used as an inlay graft.

InnerVasc—sheath for percutaneous vascular access in cardiology, radiology, neuroradiology, and critical care.

Innofem (estradiol tablets)—hormone replacement therapy.

Innohep (tinzaparin sodium)—a low-molecular-weight heparin for the prevention and treatment of deep venous thrombosis.

Innova home therapy system—for urinary incontinence.

InnovaTome microkeratome device—used by refractive surgeons in ophthalmology to perform LASIK (laser in situ keratomileusis).

Innovator Holter system (Cardio).

INO (intranuclear ophthalmoplegia). Cf. *I&O.*

INOmax (nitric oxide) **for inhalation**—a pulmonary vasodilator for use in term and near-term newborns suffering from hypoxic respiratory failure.

inosine pranobex (Isoprinosine)—investigational immunomodulating agent for AIDS. Studies show it enhances host defenses to slow the progress of AIDS prodrome to fully developed AIDS. Trials in other viral and immune system disorders have shown no efficacy.

inotropic therapy—medication regimen designed to preserve hemodynamics in patients with cardiomyopathy who are awaiting cardiac transplantation. See *home ambulatory inotropic therapy.*

Inoue balloon techniques.

INRO surgical nails—used for nail bed injuries. These prosthetic nails protect the nail bed and prevent adhesion of the eponychial fold to the nail bed. Note: You may want to capitalize all the letters (as the manufacturer does), or simply the first letter.

Insall-Burstein II system—total knee replacement.

Insall-Salvati index—ratio of the length of the patellar tendon to the length of the patella.

insensible fluid output—fluid loss that cannot be measured, such as by respiration and through the skin, without visible perspiration, as differentiated from measurable fluid output such as urine.

insidious—gradual or subtle development.

in situ—in the natural or normal place; confined to the site of origin without invasion of neighboring tissues, e.g., carcinoma in situ.

Inspiron—small inspiratory training device to strengthen the muscles used in breathing.

inspissated—a thickened or dried out secretion within a duct or cavity.

Instat—collagen absorbable hemostatic agent. Cf. *INSTAT MCH.*

INSTAT MCH (microfibrillar hemostat)—used as an aid in hemostasis when bleeding cannot be controlled by usual methods, or when the bleeding site cannot be reached. It looks something like building insulating material. It can be removed in this form if necessary; in contact with blood, it becomes a gelatinous mass which can be removed in that state. It is absorbable and, if indicated, may be left in situ, although the long-term effect is not known. Not recommended in urology, neurosurgery, or orthopedic surgery.

InstaTrak—a device that provides intraoperative localization during endoscopic sinus surgery.

InStent—developer of self-expanding and balloon-expandable stents used in a variety of medical therapies.

InStent CarotidCoil stent—resists compression after placement in the neck arteries to maintain blood flow to the brain.

in-stent restenosis—reduced by application of coronary radiation therapy with a gamma source (beta emitter 90-Yttrium).

instill—administration of a liquid, drop by drop. Do not confuse with *install*, although some dictators use these words interchangeably.

instrument—see type of instrument, e.g., clamp, forceps.

Insuflon—indwelling device for delivering insulin. It consists of a small needle inserted subcutaneously and allowed to remain in place for up to one week. The needle is connected to a small catheter which is easily accessible on the surface of the skin. The patient injects the insulin dose into the catheter. Insuflon eliminates multiple injections for patients whose diabetes requires one or more shots each day.

insulin-like growth factor I—developed as an outgrowth of research by Genentech on Protropin (human growth hormone). It has an insulin-like chemical structure but is actually being studied for its ability to preserve and restore muscle mass in patients with AIDS. The etiology of body wasting from AIDS is not understood, and it is thought that this drug, also known as somatomedin C, could be useful because of its protein-sparing attributes.

insulinotardic—when insulin comes out too slowly and in insufficient quantity.

insulinotropin—a naturally occurring peptide hormone which stimulates

insulinotropin *(cont.)*
insulin release in response to increase in blood sugar levels.

insulin resistance syndrome—a condition that may lead to type 2 diabetes and also may predispose patients to coronary heart disease. Exercise can play an important role in preventing and treating the syndrome.

InSurg—laparoscopic stone baskets, used for common bile duct stone retrieval during intraoperative cholangiograms: Segura CBD basket, Pursuer CBD basket; these come in 2, 4 and 3.0 French sizes, Helical, and the Mini-Helical basket which comes in 1.9 French.

InSync—a multisite cardiac stimulator implanted transvenously in patients suffering from heart failure. It is able to synchronize right and left sides of the heart.

Intacs—flexible micro-inserts that provide a nonlaser option for surgical correction of mild myopia. Intacs does not require cutting or removing tissue from the eye's central optic zone. It can be removed and exchanged for a new prescription if a person's vision changes because of age.

intake and output (I&O). See *I&O*.

Integra artificial skin—used in conjunction with the Dermal Regeneration Template. Together they are used for treatment of patients with life-threatening, full-thickness, or deep partial-thickness burns in situations where conventional autografts are not available or contraindicated due to the patient's condition.

Integral Omniloc implants—used for oral and maxillofacial surgery.

Integrated Wound Manager—Internet-based wound management technique including tools for digital photo documentation, wound measurement, advice, supply integration, and outcome-based data.

Integrilin (eptifibatide)—antithrombotic drug for unstable angina, acute coronary syndrome, myocardial infarction, and cardiac surgery.

Integris 3-D RA (rotational angiography)—provides reconstructed 3-D images of the patient's vascular morphology for use in planning neurointerventional surgical procedures.

Integrity AFx AutoCapture pacing system.

Integrity AFx pacemaker.

Intelligent Dressing—contains Acemannan Hydrogel to keep a wound at optimum moisture level, donating moisture to dry wounds and absorbing moisture from wounds that contain too much exudate.

intense pulsed light source (IPLS)—a pulsed photothermal device used to treat small leg varicosities.

intensifying screen artifacts (Radiol) —can include dust, hair on screen, rough handling of film when placing screen, static electricity, rivets in film carriers damaging screen, or warped cassette preventing film surface from being in direct contrast with screen.

intensity-modulated radiation therapy (IMRT).

Intensive Narcotic Detoxification—patented anesthesia-assisted one-day detox procedure for heroin addiction and dependencies on methadone, pain medications, and other opiates.

intentional transoperative hemodilution—a blood transfusion method.

intentional *(cont.)*

When a patient is prepared for surgery, up to 3 units of blood are taken from the patient and stored in regular blood donor bags. Blood expanders are then administered to the patient to restore the blood volume. Thus, during surgery, the patient loses only diluted blood. Then, near the end of the operative procedure, the previously removed blood is infused. This reduces the need for blood transfusion, with all its attendant risks.

inter-, a prefix meaning *between*. Cf. *intra-*.

Interax—a total knee system.

intercalary defect of the pollical ray —see *pouce flottant.*

intercartilaginous incision—used in rhinoplasties.

Interceed Adhesion Barrier—a pliable, biodegradable cellulose fabric that is used to prevent adhesions between tissues and organs following surgery, and specifically to prevent or reduce the possibility of pelvic adhesions. The knitted absorbable fabric becomes a gelatinous coating (over the organs just under the incision) which is absorbed in less than a month. Also known as *Interceed (TC7) Absorbable Adhesion Barrier.*

Intercept—oral fluid drug test.

interdigital clavus—a corn (clavus) between the fingers or toes, usually in the fourth interspace.

interferential current therapy—a method of pain relief which involves the application of alternating-current sine waves of differing frequencies via four electrodes applied in such a way as to generate a beat pulse in the area of interest. Interferential current may also be referred to as beat pulse or alternating modulation frequency. Studies have shown this therapy effective in relieving pain due to lateral epicondylitis, knee osteoarthritis, sprains, and jaw dysfunction.

interferential stimulator—controls pain and increases circulation following injury or surgery.

interferometer—see *Takata laser interferometer.*

interferon—glycoproteins produced by some cells in response to viral infections, which also seem to have antitumor properties. See *IL-2.*

interferon alfa-2a, recombinant (Roferon-A)—an antineoplastic used to treat hairy cell leukemia and Kaposi's sarcoma.

interferon alfa-2b *(not* alpha) (Intron A)—used in treating malignant melanoma, in conjunction with surgery, in patients who may have a possible recurrence of this cancer.

interferon alfa-n1 (Wellferon)—a drug used to treat Kaposi's sarcoma.

interferon alfa-n3 (Alferon LDO, Alferon N)—interferon that is not manufactured using recombinant DNA techniques but is derived from human WBCs. It is indicated for the treatment of genital warts (external condylomata acuminata) by intradermal injection. Alferon LDO is used to treat patients with AIDS.

interferon beta-1a (Avonex).

interferon beta, recombinant human (Betaseron)—used to treat CMV retinitis in AIDS patients. See *Betaseron.*

interferon, low-dose—see *low-dose interferon.*

Inter Fix—a titanium threaded spinal fusion cage for treatment of degenerative disk disease. The hollow, threaded cage is packed with small pieces of bone taken from another part of the body; the cage is then capped and implanted between adjacent vertebral structures.

Inter Fix RP (reduced profile) **threaded spinal fusion cage**—designed to be used in conjunction with the Inter Fix device. Both are cylindrical in shape, but the RP has a "C" cut out of one side that enables interlocking of the two devices, saving space while providing necessary vertebral support.

InterGard—knitted collagen coated grafts and patches.

Intergel adhesion prevention solution—used following laparotomy and laparoscopy.

interleukin-1 (IL-1), or **lymphocyte activating factor** (LAF)—a monokine released (in vitro) by cultured macrophages. It may affect the systemic response to inflammation by inducing fever and by stimulating the release of acute-phase reactants.

interleukin-1b—a urinary marker used to distinguish between bacterial and interstitial cystitis.

interleukin-2 (IL-2)—can produce focal entrapment of the median nerve at the wrist (carpal tunnel syndrome, CTS), which abates shortly after infusion. IL-2 mediates the inflammatory response and can cause interstitial edema, which likely causes CTS to develop.

interleukin-2 PEG (polyethylene glycol-interleukin-2)—a cytokine used to treat AIDS. Also called *PEG-interleukin-2.*

interleukin-2, recombinant (IL-2) (Proleukin, teceleukin, aldesleukin)—a drug used as intravenous therapy for patients with metastatic renal cell carcinoma. Although not seen as a cure, it can shrink tumors in some patients. The side effects, however, can be quite severe, are felt by almost all patients, and can include death.

interleukin-3, recombinant human (IL-3)—a drug used to treat HIV-positive patients.

interleukin-4—hormone-like substance produced by the body's white blood cells.

interleukin-6 (IL-6)—an inflammatory molecule that may be a sign of bacterial infection. Pregnant women who have high blood levels of this immune system molecule are at greater risk for premature delivery.

interleukin-10 (IL-10)—an anti-inflammatory cytokine produced by macrophages and lymphocytes that modulates inflammatory response. It has potential application in intestinal inflammatory diseases.

interleukin-11 (IL-11)—bioengineered product that reduces need for frequent platelet transfusion following high-dose chemotherapy.

intermittent exotropia—a common form of childhood strabismus that has a late onset. It may be treated with IM injections of botulinum toxin type A into the extraocular muscles, which is considered a safe, effective, and noninvasive drug alternative to surgical treatment of strabismus in adults.

intermittent mandatory ventilation (IMV)—used in weaning a patient from long-term ventilator use. While the patient remains on the ventilator, the number of mandatory breaths is

intermittent *(cont.)*
gradually reduced. In between the mandatory breaths, the system allows the patient to breathe independently. With this method, the muscles used in breathing are gradually strengthened until the patient can breathe independently.

internal mammary artery bypass (IMAB).

International Prostate Symptom Score (IPSS)—used extensively around the world to quantify the level of lower urinary tract symptoms in a standardized manner. The seven symptoms assessed include (1) the sensation of not having emptied the bladder completely after urination; (2) the urge to urinate again within two hours; (3) the urge to stop and start again several times during urination; (4) difficulty in postponing urination; (5) weak urinary stream; (6) the need to push or strain to begin urination; (7) the need to get up at night to urinate. The frequency of each symptom is quantified by the patient on a scale from 1 to 5, the maximum total score being 35. Patients with a total score of less than 7 are classified as having mild symptoms, whereas those with total scores of 8 to 19 and more than 20 have moderate and severe symptoms. Inconvenience caused by urinary symptoms is registered by a corresponding, almost identical questionnaire, which yields a separate score (called the "bother" score).

International System of Measuring Units (SI, the initials for Système International d'Unités in French, is used internationally). In the U.S., the American Medical Association and the College of American Pathologists are sponsoring its use. We are already using gray (Gy) as the unit of measuring absorbed radiation dose, equal to 100 rads; becquerel (Bq) as the unit of radioactivity; joule (J) as the unit of energy; hertz (Hz) as the unit of frequency equal to 1 cycle per second.

International 10-20 System—for placing electrodes on the scalp when performing electroencephalograms. The electrodes are placed in predetermined positions that are 10 to 20 percent of the distance between certain pairs of skull reference points.

Inter-Op acetabular prosthesis.

interpleural analgesia—a technique for providing pain management in patients with multiple rib fractures, or who have undergone thoracotomy. Interpleural analgesia provides prolonged analgesia and is administered via a percutaneously placed epidural catheter in the interpleural space (between the parietal pleura and the visceral pleura).

Interpore—a form of hydroxyapatite. See *hydroxyapatite*.

interrupted near-far, far-near sutures.

InterStim—a neurostimulation device designed for patients with urinary control problems. It sends mild electrical impulses to sacral nerves in the lower back that control bladder function, alleviating symptoms of urinary urge incontinence, urgency-frequency, and urinary retention. Based upon the electrical stimulation technology used for pacemakers.

interstitial cystitis (IC)—a chronic, progressive, and debilitating urinary bladder disease afflicting primarily women. Characterized by severe bladder and pelvic pain, and urinary frequency. See *Elmiron*.

interstitial markings—the radiographic appearance of lung tissue, as opposed to the appearance of air contained in the lung.

Inter-Vial drug delivery system—consists of a syringe that stores powdered medication in a standard vial and sterile diluent in a separate mechanically connected cartridge, enabling the user to mix wet and dry in one motion just prior to injection.

intestinal fatty acid-binding protein (I-FABP), **human serum**—a biochemical marker of erythrocyte origin. Establishes a useful diagnostic marker for acute ischemic disease of the small bowel.

in-the-bag implantation—implantation of an intraocular lens in the capsular bag.

"in the magnet"—said by radiologists, when they are working in the MRI unit. They say they're "in the magnet."

intra-, a prefix meaning *within*. Cf. *inter-*.

intra-aortic balloon counterpulsation (IABC).

intra-aortic balloon pumping (IABP)—effective for short-term support of cardiac patients. (Dictionaries retain a hyphen between the two *a*'s in *intra-abdominal*, *intra-aortic*, and *intra-atrial*, although some publications omit a hyphen.) Cf. *intra-atrial baffle*.

intra-aortic endovascular sonography—used in detecting aortic invasion by esophageal carcinoma.

intra-atrial baffle—used in repair of atrial septal defect.

Intrabeam intraoperative radiotherapy (IORT) **system**—uses a miniature x-ray source to deliver x-rays inside a tumor cavity.

intracardiac amobarbital sodium procedure—used to evaluate intractable epilepsy.

Intracath catheter.

intracaval endovascular ultrasonography (ICEUS)—a sonogram in which an intravascular ultrasonographic catheter is passed through the right femoral vein into the suprahepatic inferior vena cava under fluoroscopic guidance. From there it is gradually withdrawn, while recording cross-sectional ultrasonographic images. It is used for detecting intravascular tumor thrombi and is more diagnostic than conventional CT or cavography.

intracavernous injection test—a diagnostic procedure for impotence. The erectile response is observed following intracavernous administration of vasoactive agents with or without supplementary manual, vibratory, or audiovisual sexual stimulation. A positive test is a full and maintained erection.

Intracell—a device that treats myofascial trigger points due to repetitive strain injuries, cumulative trauma, overuse syndromes, or carpal tunnel syndrome. It is a nonmotorized device that can be operated by the patient. Moved over the affected area, it rolls, stretches, twists, and compresses the muscles, diffusing barrier trigger points and rehabilitating noncompliant muscles.

intracellular-like, calcium-bearing crystalloid solution (ICS).

Intrachol (choline chloride)—injectable used for treatment of choline deficiency in patients receiving TPN.

intracisternal tPA (tissue plasminogen activator)

IntraCoil—self-expanding nitinol stent for use in maintaining a patent lumen in the femoral and popliteal arteries of the leg in the treatment of peripheral vascular disease.

intracoronary artery radiation—procedure to reduce restenosis after angioplasty.

intracoronary Doppler flow wire—measures rate of blood flow through coronary arteries and assists clinicians in evaluating the severity of blockage and effectiveness of therapeutic treatment.

intracoronary ultrasonography—uses a mechanically rotated transducer contained within a monorail catheter to determine vessel diameter for selection of angioplasty balloon size. The catheter tip is delivered over a coronary guide wire, and automated pullback of the ultrasound device is performed. Images are recorded on videotape and then digitized into a computer.

intracranial pressure (ICP) **catheter**; **monitor**.

intracranial temperature monitoring —see *brain temperature monitoring*.

intracytoplasmic sperm injection (ICSI) (Ob-Gyn)—a technique used in couples with severe male factor infertility due to low or poor quality sperm. Cumulus-corona cells are enzymatically removed from the oocytes, and a single sperm is microscopically injected into each oocyte, all of which are then transferred into the uterine cavity 72 hours after ICSI.

intradiscal electrothermal (IDET) **annuloplasty**—minimally invasive procedure for the treatment of severe low back pain secondary to degenerative disk disease.

IntraDop—intraoperative Doppler probe used for blood vessel identification during laparoscopic surgery.

IntraDose-CDDP injectable gel—used to treat head and neck cancers and accessible tumors.

IntraDose gel—consists of purified bovine collagen, cisplatin, and epinephrine. Injection directly into breast cancer tumors has resulted in shrinkage of a significant percentage of tumors. It also shows promise for treatment of colorectal cancer metastatic to liver.

intraepidermal blistering diseases (pemphigus)—skin diseases characterized by detachment of epidermal keratinocytes, commonly referred to as acantholysis. Forms include:
bullous pemphigoid (BP)
cicatricial pemphigoid (CP)
epidermolysis bullosa acquisita (EBA)
herpes gestationis (HG)
linear IgA bullous dermatosis (LABD)
paraneoplastic pemphigus (PNP)
pemphigus foliaceus (PF)
pemphigus vulgaris (PV)

intrahepatic cholangioenterostomy (of 2 to 5 intrahepatic ducts)—a procedure using a Roux-en-Y loop and internal stents across the anastomosis. Involves pancreatogastrostomy, gastrojejunostomy in an end-to-end manner, and cholangiojejunostomy.

intralesional therapy—used for treatment of benign hemangiomas in children and adults. With the patient under general anesthesia, a laser

intralesional *(cont.)*
fiber is threaded into the lesion, allowing laser energy to pulsate into the tumor.

intralocular—within the locules of a structure. Cf. *intraocular.*

intraluminal brachytherapy (with or without endoluminal laser treatment) —used in treatment of non-small cell lung carcinoma (or cancer).

intramural duodenal hematoma after blunt abdominal trauma—treated by conservative therapy, with bowel rest and parenteral nutrition; it resolves spontaneously.

Intran—disposable intrauterine pressure measurement catheter.

intranuclear ophthalmoplegia (INO).

intraocular—within the eye. Cf. *intralocular.*

intraocular pressure (IOP)—the pressure of aqueous humor within the eye, as measured with a tonometer. IOP above 20 or 21 indicates the presence of glaucoma.

Intra–Op autotransfusion—a system for collecting and reinfusing autologous blood during surgery.

intraoperative autologous transfusion (IOAT).

intraoperative cholangiography (IOC).

intraoperative digital subtraction angiography (IDIS system).

intraoperative endoscopic Congo red test (IECRT)—used to assess completeness of vagotomy.

intraoperative high dose rate (IOHDR) **brachytherapy**—placement of radioactive material inside, or close to, a tumor during a surgical procedure.

intraoperative hippocampal cooling—a procedure during epileptic surgery in which iced liquid is irrigated into the temporal horn of the lateral ventricle until the hippocampus is "cooled." May be useful in determining the risk of postoperative memory disorder among patients who had epileptic surgery.

intraoperative lymphatic mapping—injection of radiocolloid and blue dye to identify sentinel nodes in the axilla of a patient with breast cancer.

intraoperative radiation therapy (IORT)—removal or debulking of tumor mass, followed by direct irradiation of site with electron beam radiation.

intraoperative radiolymphoscintigraphy—combined with blue dye mapping during lymphadenectomy for melanoma.

intraoperative transmyocardial revascularization (ITMR).

intraoperative ultrasonography (IOUS) —biliary exploration during a laparoscopic cholecystectomy.

intraosseous glomus tumor—see *glomus tumor.*

intraosseous pneumatocyst, cervical spine (Rad)—a finding on x-ray that mimics susceptibility artifacts from metallic hardware within the vertebral body.

intraperitoneal hyperthermic chemotherapy (IPHC).

intraperitoneal hyperthermic perfusion (IPHP).

intraperitoneal onlay mesh (IPOM)—laparoscopic hernia repair technique for small- to moderate-sized indirect hernias.

intraportal endovascular ultrasonography (IPEUS)—a high-frequency, high-resolution, intravascular ultrasound catheter is inserted into the portal vein. The catheter is then withdrawn slowly for sequential

intraportal *(cont.)*
observation of the cross-sectional images, providing precise information about the portal vein walls and any existing tumors.

intraretinal microangiopathy (IRMA).

intraretinal microvascular abnormalities (IRMA).

IntraSite gel—a sterile hydrogel for treatment of dry wounds and wounds with slough by creating and maintaining an optimal moist environment.

IntraStent DoubleStrut biliary endoprosthesis—balloon-expandable stainless steel stent used to open and support obstructed lumina or vessels. Investigation is currently being done to determine the safety and effectiveness of this stent in the iliac artery, the main artery supplying blood to the lower extremity.

intrastromal photorefractive keratectomy (IPRK).

intrauterine growth retardation (IUGR).

intrauterine pregnancy (IUP).

intravascular MRI—experimental catheter-based MRI technique used to identify components of coronary artery plaques and assess their potential for rupture which may result in heart attack or stroke.

intravascular oxygenator (IVOX)—artificial lung designed for temporary use in patients whose respiratory failure is caused by infection or trauma. It consists of a number of very thin 24-inch hollow tubes which are inserted together through the femoral vein into the vena cava. The tubes are then connected to a catheter which supplies oxygen. The oxygen diffuses through the tubes into the bloodstream. The IVOX helps reduce demands on the patient's lungs temporarily until they can again function fully.

intravascular red light therapy (IRLT)—uses a diode laser source to reduce neointimal hyperplasia and avoid restenosis following balloon-induced injury and coronary stenting.

intravascular signal intensity in MR angiography.

intravascular ultrasound (IVUS).

intravenous drug abuse (IVDA).

intravenous fluorescein angiography (IVFA).

intravenous pyelogram (IVP) or **intravenous urogram** (IVU)—evaluation of the urinary system by introduction of contrast material into a vein, and by x-ray films observing the concentration of the contrast material in the renal pelves, renal calices, ureters, and urinary bladder. The procedure demonstrates the presence of tumors, stones, or structural abnormalities.

Intrel II spinal cord stimulation system—to control chronic pain.

Intrepid PTCA catheter (percutaneous transluminal coronary angioplasty).

intrinsic sphincter deficiency—urethral cause of urinary incontinence.

Introl bladder neck support prosthesis—used in urinary stress incontinence. When placed in the vagina, the flexible, ring-shaped prosthesis elevates the urethrovesical junction to its normal position. It can be used as a temporary alternative to surgery, or a permanent one if surgery is not a choice. This is also a good indication if surgery would bring a permanent solution.

Intron A (interferon alfa-2b, recombinant)—an injection used as adjuvant therapy to surgery in treating malignant melanoma. Also used to treat chronic viral hepatitis B and C, malignant melanoma, hairy cell leukemia, AIDS-related Kaposi's sarcoma, and condylomata acuminata.

intubation—see *CAGEIN*.

invasive procedure—defined by the Centers for Disease Control and Prevention as surgical entry into tissues, cavities, or organs, or repair of major traumatic injuries associated with any of the following: 1) an operating or delivery room, emergency department or outpatient setting, including both physicians' and dentists' offices; 2) cardiac catheterization and angiographic procedures; 3) a vaginal or cesarean delivery or other invasive obstetric procedure during which bleeding may occur; or 4) the manipulation, cutting, or removal of any oral or perioral tissues, including tooth structure, during which bleeding occurs or the potential for bleeding exists.

inventory—see *test*.

Inversine (mecamylamine HCl)—antihypertensive.

inversion-ligation appendectomy—the appendix is inverted or intussuscepted using a blunt probe with a tie (ligature) placed around the base of the inverted appendix; principally used on children.

inversion-recovery technique—MRI term.

inversion time (TI)—MRI term.

inverted schneiderian papilloma—see *schneiderian papilloma, inverted*.

inverted U-pouch ileal reservoir—a technique for conversion of straight ileoanal pull-through used in surgical treatment of ulcerative colitis.

Invicorp—used in intracavernous injections for treatment of erectile dysfunction. It's a combination of a vasoactive intestinal polypeptide and phentolamine.

Invirase (saquinavir) **capsules**—HIV protease inhibitor used in combination therapy with nucleoside analogs, e.g., ZDV (zidovudine), ddC (dideoxyinosine, zalcitabine) as treatment for AIDS.

in vitro (L., in glass)—in the laboratory in glass dishes. Cell growth can be observed in vitro in scientific investigation in the laboratory. Cf. *in vivo*. See *GIFT; LAK; ZIFT*.

in vitro fertilization (IVF)—used for women with blocked fallopian tubes, to achieve pregnancy. The woman's eggs are placed in a dish with sperm from either her husband or a donor. The embryos are then placed into the uterus. Success also varies widely by age group. See *GIFT; ZIFT*.

in vivo (L., vivus, living)—within the living body. Cf. *in vitro*.

in vivo optical spectroscopy (INVOS)—uses low-intensity visible and near-infrared light to quantify various characteristics of human blood and tissue.

INVOS (in vivo optical spectroscopy).

INVOS cerebral oximeter—noninvasive monitoring system that continuously measures changes in the blood oxygen level in the adult brain.

INVOS 2100—an early warning test for breast cancer, using optical spectroscopy to detect growths before mammography.

INVOS 3100 (and **3100A**) **cerebral oximeter**—monitors regional blood

INVOS *(cont.)*
oxygen saturation (rSO_2) in microvascular structures of the brain by noninvasive means.

INX stainless steel stent—used for treatment of occluded and tortuous vessels deep in the brain secondary to atherosclerotic disease. The neurovascular stent is used to improve blood flow in areas of the brain where surgery is not possible and when medical therapy has failed.

IOAT (intraoperative autologous transfusion).

Ioban antimicrobial incise drape (*not* loban)—an iodine drape used in surgery.

IOCM (isosmolar contrast medium).

Iodamoeba buetschlii—intestinal protozoan parasite.

iodinated contrast medium—contains iodine rather than a metallic salt and is used in angiography, intravenous pyelography, oral cholecystography, and other studies.

iodine-131-MIBG, iodine-123-MIBG (I-131-MIBG, I-123-MIBG; ^{131}I-MIBG, ^{123}I-MIBG)—radioactive imaging agents used in CT scan and scintigram to demonstrate the primary tumor of neuroblastoma and metastasis. ^{131}I-MIBG (metaiodobenzylguanidine) theoretically has the possibility of delivering to the primary and metastatic sites of neuroblastoma a fatal dose of radiation, doses easily tolerated by the whole body. Synthetic MIBG is a guanethidine derivative similar to norepinephrine.

iodocyanine green (ICG) **fluorescein angiography**—see *ICG*.

Iodoflex absorptive dressing.

iodoform gauze.

iodophor—an iodine compound used in preoperative skin preparation and postoperative skin closure for protection against infection by controlling skin bacteria. Cf. *iodoform gauze*.

iodophor-impregnated adhesive drape.

Iodosorb absorptive dressing.

IOHDR (intraoperative high dose rate).

IOL (intraocular lens).

Iolab Slimfit lens—a three-piece intraocular lens made of PMMA; it has flexible haptics.

I/1 size test object—roman numeral I relates to luminescence, I to V; arabic numeral 1 relates to size in millimeters, 1 to 5.

I 131 and I 132—radioactive iodine with atomic weights of 131 and 132. Also written ^{131}I, [132]I.

Ionescu-Shiley pericardial xenograft; valve.

Ionescu tri-leaflet valve (Cardio).

ionic contrast media (Radiol)—also known as *high-osmolar media*, HOM; the singular is *medium*, which is often misdictated. Relatively inexpensive contrast agents can cause lethal allergic reactions in some patients and are illegal in several countries. Cf. *LOM, nonionic contrast media*.

ionized magnesium injection—given to patients with low serum ionized magnesium to relieve migraine headache pain, with complete reduction of head pain in 15 minutes, and no recurrence in 24 hours.

iontophoresis—a way to administer narcotics for pain relief, using galvanic current to drive charged particles into or through a biologic membrane. Weak solutions of both

iontophoresis *(cont.)*
water- and lipid-soluble drugs may be iontophoresed, including anesthetics, antibiotics, corticosteroids, and salicylates. Not to be confused with *electrophoresis*.

IOP (intraocular pressure)

iopamidol injection—intravascular contrast medium used in angiography, excretory urography, and contrast-enhanced computed tomography (CECT). It is the generic equivalent of Isovue 300 and Isovue 370.

iopentol—a nonionic contrast medium.

iophendylate (Ethodian)—a diagnostic aid and radiopaque medium.

Iopidine (apraclonidine ophthalmic solution)—used to reduce intraocular pressure.

IORT (intraoperative radiation therapy).

Iowa trumpet—guiding instrument used in the administration of a pudendal block.

ioxilan (Oxilan) contrast medium.

IPAA (ileal pouch-anal anastomosis).

IPAP (inspiratory positive airway pressure).

IPEUS (intraportal endovascular ultrasonography).

IPG (impedance plethysmography).

IPHC (intraperitoneal hyperthermic chemotherapy).

IPHP (intraperitoneal hyperthermic perfusion).

IPK (indurated plantar keratoma).

I-Plant brachytherapy seeds—radioactive ^{125}I seed (small encapsulated radiation sources approximately half the size of a grain of rice) used for primary brachytherapy treatment of early-stage prostate cancer.

IPLS (intense pulsed light source).

IPOL poliovirus vaccine—enhanced, inactivated polio vaccine recently licensed by the FDA for expanded use. This is in contrast to the live virus oral polio vaccine that causes 8 to 10 cases of polio each year.

IPOM (intraperitoneal onlay mesh).

IPP (inflatable penile prosthesis).

IPRK (intrastromal photorefractive keratectomy).

iproplatin—an antineoplastic agent, a second-generation platinum compound, with fewer renal side effects than cisplatin (its parent drug).

IPSID (immunoproliferative small intestinal disease)—see *Mediterranean lymphoma*.

ipsilateral—on the same side.

IPSS (International Prostate Symptom Score)—also known as AUA-SI (American Urological Association Symptom Index). See *International Prostate Symptom Score*.

iPTH (immunoreactive parathyroid hormone) (yes, lowercase *i*).

iridectomy—excision of a portion of the iris, either surgically or through laser photocoagulation.

iridencleisis (*not* iridenclysis)—an operative procedure to reduce intraocular pressure. It creates a permanent drain which filters the aqueous from the anterior chamber to the subconjunctival tissue.

irides, plural of *iris*.

iridis—see *rubeosis iridis*.

iridium 192 (^{192}Ir) (Iriditope)—a radioactive agent used in scans.

iridocorneal-endothelial syndrome (ICE).

irinotecan (Camptosar).

IRIS (Intensified Radiographic Imaging System)—used in STS lithotripsy system.

iris bombé ("bom-bay")—curving or swelling outward of the iris.

IRIS coronary stent—a tubular stent made of stainless steel.

iritis—an acute or chronic inflammation of the iris.

IRMA (intraretinal microangiopathy).

IRMA (intraretinal microvascular abnormalities).

irofulven—drug for treatment of ovarian cancer.

iron storage disease—see *bronze disease.*

irradiation—see *heavy ion irradiation.*

irregularly irregular cardiac rhythm—abnormal cardiac rhythm without any discernible pattern, beats occurring at random intervals.

Irrijet DS—system for debridement and irrigation of wounds.

IRS (impaired regeneration syndrome).

ISAtx247—an immunosuppressive drug used for prevention of organ rejection after transplantation and for treatment of autoimmune diseases such as arthritis and psoriasis.

iscador—an antiviral used to treat patients with AIDS. A derivative of mistletoe, a popular cancer remedy in Europe.

ISCs (irreversible sickled [red] cells).

ischemic penile gangrene—a disease in diabetics with end-stage atherosclerosis and renal disease.

ISD (intrinsic sphincter deficiency).

Iselin forceps (Plas Surg).

ISG (immune serum globulin).

Ishihara plates—test for color vision.

ISI laparoscopic instruments.

island of Reil—structure in the brain.

islet cell (*not* eyelet)—the cells that compose the islets of Langerhans in the pancreas.

islet cell antibodies (ICA)—a screening test for persons at high risk for developing type 1 insulin-dependent diabetes mellitus. High levels of ICA indicate that the person's immune system is attacking the insulin-secreting islets of Langerhans in the pancreas.

islet cell implant—technique of injecting islet cells from a cadaver into the portal vein of patients with diabetes. The islet cells migrate to the pancreas, where they begin to produce insulin.

Isletest and **Isletest-ICA**—kit that detects islet cell autoantibodies. It is used to identify individuals at high risk of developing type 1 diabetes several years before actual onset of the disease.

Ismo (isosorbide mononitrate)—used to prevent anginal attacks.

isobutyl 2-cyanoacrylate (IBC)—a tissue adhesive used to occlude an unresectable aortic aneurysm after axillofemoral grafting. Also, bucrylate.

Isocam SPECT imaging system.

isoechoic ("i-so-eh-ko´-ic")—refers to the even distribution of echoes in ultrasonography as the ultrasound waves bounce off structures or tissue. "The seminal vesicles were small and isoechoic."

isoenzymes—see *CPK isoenzymes.*

isoflurane—used with oxygen for anesthesia. "When IV lines were in place, the anesthesiologist continued anesthesia induction with oxygen, air, and isoflurane."

Isola spinal instrumentation system. The connectors and hooks have a patented V-groove which allows force to be applied to all four sides of the rod, creating additional gripping force, making this system more stable than other systems in which

Isola *(cont.)*
force can be applied from only two directions.

isolated heat perfusion of an extremity—therapy for malignant melanoma of the extremities. The vessels of the extremity are cannulated and the cannulae attached to the cardiopulmonary bypass machine. The temperature of the limb is elevated and perfusion carried out with melphalan included in the perfusate. The limb temperature may be elevated to about 40°C. The extremity vessels are washed out and perfused with fresh blood.

Isolex system—extracts and purifies stem cells for reinfusion into cancer patients to rebuild their immune systems after high-dose chemotherapy.

isoniazid—bactericidal; primary tuberculostatic.

Isoprinosine (inosine pranobex)—antiviral and immune-modulating drug recently found to be effective in treatment of patients with chronic fatigue syndrome.

isosmolar contrast medium (IOCM).

isosorbide mononitrate (Imdur, Ismo)—used in the treatment of angina.

Isospora—the protozoan parasite causing isosporiasis, which can cause an unusually virulent diarrhea in AIDS patients.

isosulfan blue (Lymphazurin).

isotopic cisternography—a test used to determine the presence of normal pressure hydrocephalus.

isotretinoin (13-cis-retinoic acid, Accutane)—chemotherapy drug for mycosis fungoides and cutaneous T-cell lymphoma. Also commonly known as a dermatology drug for severe recalcitrant cystic acne.

isovaleric acidemia—an inborn error of metabolism in which there is marked elevation in the isovaleric acid levels in the serum because of an inability to metabolize protein-rich foods. Manifested by severe metabolic acidosis and coma, slight intention tremor, slight psychomotor retardation, retinal vessel tortuosity, nonspecific mottling of the retina, and a locker room odor of the body, urine, and breath of patients with this entity. Also called *locker room syndrome.*

Isovorin (L-leucovorin).

Isovue (iopamidol, injectable)—a nonionic contrast agent used in digital subtraction angiography and in other special radiological procedures. Varieties include Isovue series (128, 200, 300, 370), parenteral injection; Isovue-M series (200, 300), intrathecal injection.

isoxicam (Maxicam)—a nonsteroidal anti-inflammatory drug said to be effective in the treatment of rheumatoid arthritis and degenerative joint disease.

isradipine (DynaCirc)—calcium channel blocker used to treat hypertension. Relaxes the smooth muscle of blood vessels to lower blood pressure.

ISS (Injury Severity Scale).

Isshiki thyroplasty type I (ITTI)—a procedure to treat unilateral vocal cord paralysis. It uses a Silastic implant placed in a window of the thyroid ala between the inner and outer perichondrium causing lateral compression of the vocal cord.

IST (immunosuppressive therapy).

i-STAT system—a handheld analyzer that performs a panel of critical

i-STAT system *(cont.)*
blood tests at patient's bedside or in emergency departments.

it's, its—the first a contraction, the second a pronoun. How to use *it's* and *its* correctly seems to present problems for many people; I see them misused all too often. Put as simply as I can, *it's* is a contraction of *it is*; use of the apostrophe indicates that a letter has been omitted. Its meaning changes when the apostrophe is omitted; *it's* then the possessive form, *its.* It might be helpful, when you use the word *it's*, to read the sentence aloud and substitute *it is*; you will then hear whether the sentence says what you mean to say.

ITA (internal thoracic artery) **graft** (also called *internal mammary artery*)—the use of an artery from the chest rather than the leg in heart bypass surgery. One end of an artery near the collarbone is stitched into the downstream end of the cardiac artery clogged by disease. As a result, blood pumped out of the heart through the aorta is detoured into the cardiac muscle. See *IEA and GEA.*

ITC balloon catheter—inserted through the carotid artery. This radiopaque catheter has a silicon balloon that is inflated to temporarily occlude a cerebral artery during operations for aneurysms, arteriovenous malformations, or tumors. (ITC stands for Interventional Therapeutics Corporation.)

ITE (in-the-ear) **hearing aid**—*ITE*, not the translation, is typed in medical reports.

iteration—the process by which multiple computerized images converge to make an increasingly accurate image.

ITP (idiopathic thrombocytopenic purpura).

itraconazole (Sporanox)—an antifungal used to treat histoplasmosis, blastomycosis, aspergillosis, and cryptococcal meningitis in AIDS patients.

Itrel 3 spinal cord stimulation system—a pulse generator implanted surgically in the abdominal area to control angina pain. The implanted system delivers mild electrical stimulation to the spinal cord to override pain signals to the brain.

IttI (Isshiki thyroplasty, type I).

IUdR (idoxuridine, iododeoxyuridine)—halogenated thymidine analogue, a radiosensitizer. Cf. *BUdR, FUdR.*

IUGR (intrauterine growth retardation).

IUP (intrauterine pregnancy).

IVAC electronic thermometer.

IVAC volumetric infusion pump—a positive pressure infusion device for delivery of intravenous solutions or drugs. IVAC is the manufacturer.

IVB (intraventricular block).

IVC (inferior vena cava).

IVDA (intravenous drug abuser).

I.V. (or **IV**) **drip**—intravenous administration of drugs in which the drug is mixed with the fluid in the I.V. bag or bottle and administered over several hours as the I.V. runs in slowly. Cf. *I.V. push.*

Ivemark's syndrome—splenic agenesis syndrome.

ivermectin (Stromectol)—antiparasitic.

IVF (in vitro fertilization).

IVFA (intravenous fluorescein angiography) (Oph).

IVH (intraventricular hemorrhage).

IVOX (intravascular oxygenator).

IVP (intravenous pyelogram).

I.V. (or **IV**) **piggyback**—see *piggyback.*

I.V. (or **IV**) **port**—see *port.*

I.V. (or **IV**) **push**—a method of administering drugs in which the entire dose of a drug is given intravenously by manually injecting it directly into a port in the I.V. line. The therapeutic effect is felt immediately. This method is often used in emergency situations. Cf. *I.V. drip*. See also *bolus*.

IVR (idioventricular rhythm).

IVUS (intravascular ultrasound) **catheter**—for viewing the interior of an artery or vein to determine the degree of stenosis or plaque formation.

Ivy bleeding time—the number of minutes it takes for a small incision in the skin (by puncture of the forearm), made with a lancet, to stop bleeding. Cf. *Duke bleeding time*.

IvyBlock—poison ivy, poison oak, and poison sumac skin protectant, available without a prescription.

Ixodes dammini—a species of tick, the carrier of Lyme disease.

Ixodes pacificus—western black-legged tick, implicated as a carrier in tularemia on the West Coast. Cf. *erythema migrans; Ixodes dammini; Lyme disease*.

J, j

JACE-STIM electrotherapy unit—
provides high-voltage, pulsed-current stimulation.

JACE W550—continuous passive motion wrist device.

jackknife position—The patient lies on his stomach with shoulders elevated and thighs at right angles to the abdomen. Used for rectal and coccygeal procedures. Also, *Kraske's position.*

Jackman orthogonal catheter (Cardio).

Jackson's epilepsy (possessive eponym), but *jacksonian* epilepsy, march, or seizure. Note: An adjective formed from an eponym is not capitalized.

jacksonian march—progression of a jacksonian seizure from one muscle group to adjacent areas or to a generalized motor seizure.

jacksonian seizure—focal seizure (also rolandic). Usually starts as a spasm in the face, a hand, or a foot, and then spreads to other muscles.

Jackson rod insertion technique—
used in spinal instrumentation procedures.

Jackson's sign—the wheezing produced by foreign bodies lodged in the bronchus or trachea, similar to that of asthma, audible without a stethoscope.

Jackson spinal surgery and imaging table—has the capability of rotating the patient 180° without the necessity of moving for repositioning.

Jackson-Weiss syndrome—craniostosis, broad big toes, tarsal-metatarsal conditions, and sometimes syndactyly. Caused by a mutation in the fibroblast growth factor receptor 2 (FGFR2).

jackstone calculus—a kidney stone shaped like the 6-pointed metal jacks that children play with.

Jacobson hemostatic forceps.

Jacobson's organ—an obscure structure in the nose of all mammals except porpoises, with its own nerve supply. It is thought to be important in chemoreception to pheromones.

Jacquemier's sign—the bluish-violet color seen in the vagina and cervix at 8 to 12 weeks of pregnancy. Also known as *Chadwick's sign.*

Jaeger eye chart—Findings on examination are given as *J* and a number, indicating the line on the chart with the smallest letters the patient can see.

Jaeger lid plate.

Jaffe-Campanacci syndrome—café au lait spots.

Jaffee capsulorrhexis forceps—forceps with blunt tips to hold the capsular bag and to tear a continuous curvilinear capsulorrhexis.

Jahnke anastomosis clamp.

Jako facial nerve monitor—for middle ear and mastoid surgery, enabling the surgeon to judge the depth of the nerve beneath the exposed tissue bed.

jamais vu (Fr., never seen)—the incorrect feeling that one has never seen or experienced a certain thing before, in contrast to déjà vu, already seen, the incorrect feeling that one has seen or experienced something before.

Jamar dynamometer—a device used to measure hand strength by calibrating the hand grip. Three readings are made for each hand, measured in pounds. Usually higher readings are seen on tests of the dominant hand, unless there has been an injury on that side. Also, *Jamar grip test*.

James fibers—in AV nodal area of the heart.

Jameson calipers—used to measure the lid crease in blepharoplasty.

Janeway lesions—erythematous macules that may be seen on the palms and soles in infective endocarditis.

Janus syndrome—see *Brett's syndrome*.

Jarit P.E.E.R. retractor—used in laparoscopic surgery.

Jarit Rotator—reusable instrument line for endoscopic surgical procedures.

Jatene arterial switch procedure and **valve** (*not* Jantene operation)—for correction of transposed great arteries in the neonate.

Jawz—endomyocardial biopsy forceps.

Jay seating system—for positioning patients.

Jedmed/DGH A-scan (Oph).

Jelco intravenous catheter.

jersey finger—an injury sustained to the finger of a football player when a gripped jersey is forced out of the tackler's hand.

Jerusalem syndrome—psychological phenomenon in which religious visitors to holy sites assume the identities of various biblical figures. Many stricken with this mental illness have no previous history of psychological problems; symptoms usually disappear within days of leaving the holy site that originally triggered the illness.

Jessner-Kanof lymphocytic infiltration of the skin—treated with thalidomide.

Jeter lag screws or position screws—in sagittal split ramus osteotomy.

jet lesion—usually an autopsy finding. A valvular or septal cardiac defect allows a strong jet of blood, over time, to produce an area of endocardial fibrosis or even an endocardial pocket.

Jevity isotonic liquid nutrition—for supplemental feeding tube nutritional support.

Jewel AF implantable defibrillator—all-in-one arrhythmia management device.

Jewett brace—used for spondylitis, spinal fusion, compression fractures.

Jewett's classification of bladder carcinoma:
O noninfiltrating (in situ)
A infiltrating submucosa
B invading muscle
C involvement of surrounding tissue
D distant involvement

J-FX bipolar head—prosthesis for use in cemented or uncemented hip surgery.

jittery—describes involuntary jerky muscle movements of extremities of babies with hypoglycemia or drug addiction.

JL4 catheter—Judkins left 4 cm curve catheter.

JL5 catheter—Judkins left 5 cm curve catheter.

J needle—named for its shape, it is a modification of the nonswaged fishhook needle used for hernia repair.

Jobst stockings (Vasc Surg).

Joe's hoe—a retractor, also known as the *Weinberg retractor*.

Joffroy's sign—absence of brow wrinkling in Graves' disease when the patient suddenly looks up.

Joint-Jack finger splint—provides steady, nonelastic force to correct flexion deformities of the fingers.

joint mice—loose fragments of cartilage or other material within the synovial capsule of a joint.

joint position sense (JPS).

joker—operating room slang for an instrument; in different services it could refer to different instruments.

Jonas modification of the Norwood procedure—for hypoplastic left-sided heart syndrome. See *Fontan; Gill/Jonas; Sade*.

Jones criteria, revised—used as a guide in the diagnosis of rheumatic fever. If there has been an earlier strep infection, the presence of one major and two minor manifestations, or of two major manifestations of the disease, makes the diagnosis of rheumatic fever likely. Minor manifestations include history of rheumatic fever or evidence of preexisting rheumatic heart disease, fever, arthralgias, abnormal erythrocyte sedimentation rate or C-reactive protein, or EKG changes. Major manifestations include subcutaneous nodules, carditis, chorea, polyarthritis, erythema marginatum.

Jonnson's maneuver—a modified Valsalva maneuver; produces maximal distention of the hypopharynx by holding the patient's nose and mouth closed while he makes forcible expiratory efforts. Note: Jonnson.

Joplin bunionectomy.

Josephs-Diamond-Blackfan syndrome —see *Blackfan-Diamond syndrome*.

joule ("jewel") (abbreviation, J)—unit of electric power, as in "The heart was defibrillated with a single shock of 40 joules." Named for J. P. Joule, an English physicist.

Joystick—used in laparoscopic surgery to retract the gallbladder.

J point—on an EKG tracing, the junction between the end of the QRS complex and the beginning of the ST segment.

JT1001—a prostate cancer vaccine.

Juberg-Marsidi syndrome—rare X-linked inherited disorder that affects males only and is apparent at birth or during the first few weeks of life. Affected children exhibit severe mental retardation, developmental delays, muscle weakness, diminished muscle tone, often delayed bone growth as well as growth retarda-

Juberg-Marsidi *(cont.)*
tion, hearing loss, microgenitalism, and/or abnormalities of the craniofacial area.

Judd repair—postoperative ventral hernia repair.

Judet ("joo-day") **grading classification**—a grading system (grades 1, 2, 3, 4a, 4b) for fractures of the epiphysis of the neck of the radius. The grade assigned correlates to the degree that the fracture fragment tilts as compared to its normal horizontal position.

Judet ("joo-day") **hip prosthesis**—a prosthesis which does not require the use of cement; the femoral and acetabular components are made to fit tightly.

Judkins 4 diagnostic catheter—used as a dilator in an artery.

Judkins selective coronary arteriography (*not* Judkin's). Also, *Dotter-Judkins technique*.

jugulodigastric nodes—deep cervical nodes in the area of the jugular trunk and the digastric muscle.

Juquitiba virus—a variation of hantavirus pulmonary syndrome found in Brazil.

juxtaposition—see *apposition*.

J-Vac closed wound drainage system—consists of a Blake silicone drain and a J-Vac suction reservoir.

JVP (jugular venous pressure).

J-wire—used in a procedure to support extracorporeal membrane oxygenation (ECMO) in infants with severe pulmonary insufficiency and pulmonary hypertension. "The chest tube catheter was then withdrawn, and we then used a J-wire which we passed down the jugular vein into the inferior vena cava. With this, we were able to slip the venous cannula over the J-wire into the right atrium, and the J-wire was then removed."

K, k

Kabikinase (streptokinase).

Kadian sustained-release morphine capsules—a single daily dosage, sustained-release morphine product developed for cancer pain relief.

Kadish staging of esthesioneuroblastoma (Neuro).

KAFO (knee-ankle-foot orthosis).

Kairos—rate-adaptive single and dual chamber pacemakers.

Kalginate alginate wound dressing.

kallikrein inhibitor unit (KIU).

kallikrein-kinin (KK) **system**—refers to possible mediator function in vasogenic brain edema.

Kaltostat—hydrofiber wound packing material which is highly absorbent.

Kambin and Gellman instrumentation—used in percutaneous lumbar diskectomy.

KAM Super Sucker—for arthroscopic surgery. Will accept particles of bone without clogging.

Kanavel brain-exploring cannula.

Kaneda (ka-nay′da) **device** (Kioshi Kaneda, M.D.)—anterior spine stabilizing system used in the treatment of burst fracture of the spine. See *Cotrel-Dubousset instrumentation*.

kangaroo care—used to treat premature infants (the name referring to kangaroos nurturing their helpless young in a pouch). With kangaroo care, a medically stable infant can be kept with the mother, lying on the mother's chest, skin to skin, rather than spending hours in an Isolette. This seems to result in fewer breathing problems and faster weight gain.

Kantor-Berci video laryngoscope—replaces the surgical microscope in laryngeal surgery, which has limited view in microsurgical operations on the larynx due to the laryngoscope spatula and its limited depth of focus. The Kantor-Berci instrument uses an endoscope connected to a video camera with a focus range from a few millimeters to infinity. The camera is connected to a video with better viewing and the ability for permanent documentation of findings.

Kao Lectrolyte—electrolyte replenisher used to treat dehydration in children.

Kapandji fracture of radius—a rare inferior dislocation of the distal radioulnar joint caused by spontaneous post-fracture epiphysiodesis of the radius.

Kapandji-Sauve technique—allows restoration of forearm deviation caused by a radioulnar joint dislocation in which the radius stopped growing and the ulna slowed but did not stop. The procedure provides maintenance of wrist stability and restores normal range of hand movement. Eponyms for the same procedure include *Baldwin Bowers, distal radioulnar joint repair, Milch, Moore-Darrach.*

Kaplan-Meier survival curves—used in the prognosis of cancer.

Kaplan PenduLaser 115—surgical laser system for skin resurfacing.

kaposiform hemangioendothelioma—a rare, aggressive vascular proliferation in children that is clinically and histologically distinct from hemangioma of infancy. It has no known association with the Kaposi's sarcoma related to HIV infection.

Kaposi's sarcoma (KS)—no longer considered to be one of the criteria included in the diagnosis of AIDS, but simply another of the opportunistic diseases a person with AIDS is likely to get.

Kappa 400 Series—the first of a new generation of pacemakers, featuring a unique integrated dual sensor combination (activity and minute ventilation) to provide patients with heart rate support regardless of activity level or exercise tolerance. The activity sensor is best for tracking low-level transient activities, while the minute-ventilation sensor increases heart rate at higher, sustained exertion levels.

Karapandzic flap—innervated musculocutaneous arterial lip and cheek flap used in lip reconstruction. It is named for Modrag Karapandzic.

karate chop phaco technique—for emulsification and removal of cataracts.

Karickhoff laser lens—used for panretinal photocoagulation.

Karl Storz Calcutript—for use with the Karl Storz ureteropyeloscope in upper urinary tract procedures.

Karl Storz flexible ureteropyeloscope—used to visualize the upper urinary tract and perform retrograde intrarenal surgery.

Karnofsky performance rating—used in selecting patients for chemotherapy for hepatic carcinoma.

Karnofsky rating scale of performance status of patients with malignant neoplasms.

100 normal, no complaint or evidence of disease
90 normal activity, with minor symptoms
80 normal activity, with effort, and some symptoms
70 cares for self, unable to do normal activity
60 requires occasional assistance
50 requires considerable assistance and care
40 disabled, requires special care and assistance
30 severely disabled; requires supportive measures
20 very sick
10 moribund

Karydakis procedure—operative technique for excision of pilonidal cyst and sinus with asymmetric flap advancement repair, developed by Dr. G. E. Karydakis.

karyotype—chromosomal composition, e.g., the human cell normally has 46 chromosomes in its karyotype.

Kasabach-Merritt syndrome—occurs in infants and is marked by giant hemangiomas of the skin and spleen associated with thrombocytopenic purpura and afibrinogenemia.

Kasai peritoneal venous shunt—for biliary atresia in infants, to deal with accumulated ascitic fluid.

Kaster mitral valve prosthesis. Also, *Hall-Kaster*.

Katena cannula—for hydrodissection and hydrodelineation of the lens nucleus.

KaVo reusable dental handpieces.

Kawasaki disease—mucocutaneous lymph node syndrome; usually occurs in infants and small children.

Kaycel towels—absorbent sterile towels used in the operating room as a drape. They have adhesive areas for sealing at the wound site and also for holding the drape in place.

Kaye tamponade balloon catheter—a method of controlling severe nephrostomy tract bleeding. Allows for continued drainage, which may be important if there is a perforation in the upper collecting system.

Kayser-Fleischer ring (Oph)—seen in the corneas of patients with Wilson's hepaticolenticular degeneration, a completely or partially pigmented ring which is green, and which encircles the cornea near the limbus.

Kazangia and Converse classification —for facial fractures involving the jaw.

Kazanjian midline forehead flap— used in nasal reconstruction procedures.

Kaznelson's syndrome—see *Blackfan-Diamond syndrome*.

K-Blade—disposable ophthalmic surgery and microsurgical blades, including keratome, slot, scleral, lamellar, miniature, and super-sharp blades.

K-Caps—protective caps to cover the sharp ends of Kirschner wires and similar types of fixation devices used in orthopedic and podiatric procedures.

KCD (kinestatic charge detector).

K-Centrum anterior spinal fixation system—implant for treatment of thoracolumbar instability secondary to burst fractures and tumors.

KCl—abbreviation for potassium chloride used for diuretic therapy. The trade drug Kay Ciel is one of many KCl drugs. When "KCl" is dictated, the abbreviation should be transcribed as dictated or translated as potassium chloride. A trade name should not be substituted for "KCl."

KDF-2.3 intrauterine catheter—trade name for catheter used for artificial insemination.

K diet, K+2 diet—low-fat, high-protein, low-carbohydrate ketogenic diets designed to provide dangerously obese children and adolescents with a rapid, healthy means of losing weight.

Kearns-Sayre syndrome—progressive ophthalmoplegia, with pigmentary retinopathy, ptosis, and heart block. Also, *Kearns-Sayre-Shy syndrome*— ophthalmoplegia plus oculocraniosomatic neuromuscular disease, mitochondrial cytopathy.

Kech and Kelly osteotomy—surgery for Haglund's foot deformity.

keel excision—an excision for diagnostic or therapeutic purposes in which the excised tissue is shaped like the keel of a boat. May be dictated in video-assisted thoracoscopy of lung.

Kegel exercises—to strengthen the pelvic/vaginal muscles, for control of stress incontinence.

k82 ImmunoCap—a blood test that can determine allergy to latex. The k82 Immunocap is combined with the patient's serum to measure the level of immunoglobulin E (IgE) antibodies to latex-specific proteins.

Keith's bundle—a bundle of fibers located in the right atrial wall of the heart, between the openings of the venae cavae. Also called *sinoatrial bundle*.

Keith-Wagener (K-W) classification of hypertensive retinopathy, roman numerals I through IV. (Not to be confused with *Kimmelstiel-Wilson disease*, also abbreviated *K-W*.)

Kelikian modified Z osteotomy.

Kell—blood antibody type; factor in agglutination. Also *Duffy, Kidd, Lewis, Lutheran*.

Kellan hydrodissection cannula—used for intraocular hydrodelineation and hydrodissection in cataract surgery.

Keller arthroplasty.

Keller bunionectomy.

Kelman phacoemulsification—used in cataract extraction.

kelvin (K). The kelvin is a unit of absolute temperature in the International System (SI) on a scale in which the zero point corresponds to absolute zero. When using the Kelvin scale, you do not use a degree sign—just the numerals followed by *K*. To convert temperatures from the Kelvin scale to the Celsius system, add

273.16. Named for Lord Kelvin, a British physicist. (Note that the unit *kelvin* is lowercase, and *Kelvin scale* is capitalized.)

Kempf internal screw fixation—used in sagittal split ramus osteotomy.

Ken nail—used in hip fracture repair.

Kent bundle—atrioventricular bundle in the heart. See *AV bundle*.

Keofeed feeding tube—used in nasogastric feeding.

Keppra (levetiracetam)—a drug for treatment of epileptic patients who experience partial-onset seizures.

keratectomy
IPRK (instromal photorefractive keratectomy)
PARK (photoastigmatic refractive keratectomy)
PRK (photorefractive keratectomy)
PTK (phototherapeutic keratectomy)

keratin—a highly insoluble protein (scleroprotein) in epidermis, hair, nails, and part of the teeth. Cf. *carotene, creatine, creatinine*.

keratinocyte growth factor (KGF)—an epithelial cell-specific mitogen.

keratin whorls (*not* whirls)—layers of squamous cells spiraled onto each other, producing a spherical body rich in the protein keratin.

keratitic precipitates; keratic precipitates; keratoprecipitates (KPs) (Oph).

keratitis, microbial—may be caused by extended-wear soft contact lenses, including disposable lenses.

keratoconus—a conical protrusion of the center of the cornea, without inflammation. Occurs most often in pubescent females.

keratome—see *Jaeger keratome*.

keratometer—see *Terry keratometer*.

keratomileusis, laser in situ (LASIK).

keratosis—production of keratin, producing a horny growth such as a wart or callosity. See *solar keratosis*.

KeraVision Intacs intracorneal ring —a tiny device consisting of two very small plastic arcs that are placed in the peripheral cornea, slightly stretching and flattening the cornea so that light rays are focused on the back of the eye, thereby correcting myopia, or nearsightedness. The implant is removable should a patient be dissatisfied or wish to take advantage of a future development in visual correction technology.

KeraVision ring—a tiny, insertable (and removable), clear polymer ring designed to replace glasses, contact lenses, and vision correction surgery techniques that permanently alter the eye's central optical zone.

Kerckring's folds—scalloped duodenal folds diagnostic for celiac disease.

kerfs—grooves or channels placed in bone grafts (e.g., in cranial synostosis surgical repair) to allow for bending or contouring of the graft.

Kerley's A (B or C) lines (*not* curly)— on chest x-ray: *A*, centrally located horizontal linear densities; *B*, horizontal linear densities in the bases of the lungs; *C*, fine linear shadows interlaced throughout the lung, giving a spiderweb appearance.

Kernohan grading—malignant astrocytoma of the spinal cord, given in roman numerals.

Kernohan notch—indentation and necrosis of the brain caused by pressure on the brain by the free edge of the tentorium cerebelli; this is sometimes associated with tentorial herniation.

ketanserin—a selective serotonin receptor antagonist which has antiarrhythmic effect.

ketoconazole (Nizoral)—an oral antifungal drug used with cyclosporine to decrease that drug's nephrotoxic effects after kidney transplant.

ketoprofen (Actron, Orudis, Oruvail) —a nonsteroidal anti-inflammatory drug.

ketorolac tromethamine (Acular, Toradol)—a nonsteroidal anti-inflammatory drug available in oral and injectable forms for treatment of severe acute pain. Also used to treat allergic conjunctivitis.

KetoSite—quantitative test to monitor the status of ketoacidosis.

ketotifen (Zaditen)—oral (non-inhalation) antiasthmatic used to prevent bronchial asthma attacks.

keyhole resection (ENT)—a surgical technique to decrease the width and length of the tongue in patients with congenital macroglossia, resulting in improved cosmesis and improved function of the oropharyngeal airway, with no change in speech and feeding.

keyhole surgery (Cardiol)—a surgical technique to treat patients with blocked coronary arteries. It is a minimally invasive heart bypass technique and uses only four Band-Aid-sized incisions.

Key-Med dilator.

Keystone last—used in management of hyperkeratotic lesions of the foot. See *last*.

KGF (keratinocyte growth factor).

kHz (kilohertz).

kick counts—a picture of the activity of the fetus. If there are enough kicks by the fetus, this is an indication of a healthy baby.

Kicker Pavlik harness—polypropylene hip abduction brace for treating hip dysplasia in toddlers up to $2^1/2$ years of age.

Kidd—blood antibody type; factor in agglutination. Also, *Duffy, Kell, Lewis, Lutheran.*

Kid-Kart—for children ages 1-10 with moderate to severe disabilities, and designed to be pushed by an attendant rather than self-propelled by the child.

Kidney Internal Splint/Stent (KISS) **catheter.** See *KISS.*

Kiel classification of non-Hodgkin's lymphoma.

Kienböck's lunatomalacia disease—refers to the lunate bone in the wrist. Thought to be caused by vascular interruption or by fracture of the lunate bone.

Kifa catheter.

Killian's dehiscence—a splitting open. "The Zenker's diverticulum is a herniation of pharyngeal mucosa through the weakened area of Killian's dehiscence just proximal to the cricopharyngeal muscle."

Killian-Lynch laryngoscope.

Killip classification—a classification of heart failure ranging from grade I (no failure) to grade IV (frank heart failure).

Killip wire—inserted to give the heart a shock during cardiac arrest.

kilohertz (kHz).

kilopascal (kPa)—a blood gas pressure measurement, equaling 1000 pascals; an SI unit of measurement.

Kimmelstiel-Wilson disease—not to be confused with Keith-Wagener, for both are often given as "K-W."

Kim-Ray Greenfield caval filter—a metallic filter inserted into the inferior vena cava for prevention of pulmonary embolism; transvenous insertion is the approach used. See also *Mobin-Uddin umbrella filter,* which is *not* synonymous.

Kimura cartilage graft—split-thickness costal cartilage graft for management of tracheal stenosis. Cartilage is an ideal material for this type of graft because it is semirigid and obtains its nutrients by diffusion and thus is not dependent on direct vascular supply.

Kinematic rotating hinge—knee prosthesis.

Kinerase (N[6]-furfuryladenine)—a skin cream used to help inhibit signs of aging. It is said to partially reverse the effects of photoaging without irritating the skin.

kinestatic charge detector (KCD)—a motion-compensated scanning device for computerized imaging of the breast. The primary difference between KCD and all other x-ray imaging methods is that KCD reduces the noise associated with the MR technology, and ultimately reduces the radiation dose required for a given signal-to-noise ratio.

KineTec hip CPM (continuous passive motion) **machine.**

Kinetik great toe implant—a total joint replacement for the first metatarsophalangeal joint.

Kinetin—used for treatment of aging- and photodamaged skin.

Kinetix instruments—including Surgenomic and AccuSharp endoscopic instruments used in carpal tunnel release.

KinetiX (capital *X*) **ventilation monitor**—handheld, compact monitor, used when single expired breath or maximum voluntary ventilation tests are needed.

King-Armstrong unit—measurement of alkaline phosphatase. Also *Bodansky unit, Bessey-Lowry unit.*

King cardiac device.

kink artifact (Radiol)—may be caused by rough handling of film. Static discharge, bending, or abrasion of film during processing can cause streaks or crescents which can resemble a fracture. This can be dangerous in the case of a skull film, causing an unnecessary admission to rule out fracture with other studies. Also, *crescent artifact, crinkle artifact, half-moon mark artifact, wrinkle artifact,* and *"pseudofracture."*

Kinsey atherectomy catheter.

Kinyoun stain—for acid-fast bacilli.

Kiricuta reconstructive breast operation.

Kirklin fence—area of mediastinal pleura used to retract the lung in thoracic surgery.

Kirschenbaum foot positioner—foot rest that positions leg in flexion, used in total knee surgery.

Kirsch laser welding technique—using a protein solder consisting of human albumins, hyaluronic acid, and indocyanine green dye.

Kirschner Medical Dimension—hip replacement system.

Kish urethral illuminated catheter set.

Ki-67—an immunophenotypic marker on the cells of patients with multiple myeloma; it is being evaluated for its correlation with relapses and overall survival.

KISS (Kidney Internal Splint/Stent)—a catheter believed to provide more reliable urinary drainage after pyeloplasty in children. The KISS catheter prevents occlusion because the segment of the tube draining the ureter/pelvis is constructed as a trough. The catheter is passed in a retrograde manner through the renal cortex using the trocar tip, and the trough is positioned in the pelvis-ureter. After pyeloplasty, the catheter drains externally for 24 hours, and after a week is clamped and removed.

kissing-type artifact (Radiol)—results when there are too many films in the processor tank, and some get unequal amounts of developer.

Kitano knot—used in laparoscopic procedures.

KIU (kallikrein inhibitor unit).

KJ (knee jerk).

Klagsbrun technique—to harvest chondrocytes which are used to provide a template for new cartilage formation in vivo.

Klaricid (clarithromycin)—antibiotic used for treatment of MAC (*Mycobacterium avium* complex) infection and eradication of *H. pylori*.

Klaron lotion (sodium sulfacetamide lotion) 10%—prescription acne medication developed for adult acne patients.

Klatskin needle—for liver biopsy.

Klatskin tumor—a tumor classification system.

Klebsiella oxytoca—newer name for *K. pneumoniae.*

Klebsiella pneumoniae, Friedländer's bacillus—a component of the normal flora of the oropharynx and GI tract in patients with functioning immune systems, but in AIDS it can cause a fatal sepsis.

kleeblattschädel (German)—cloverleaf skull.

Kleihauer-Betke test (K-B test)—used in assessing hemolysis.

Kleihauer test—of fetal-maternal hemoglobin.

Klein pump—used in liposuction.

Kleinsasser anterior commissure laryngoscope.

Klinefelter's XXY syndrome.

Kling—adhesive dressing.

Kling fluff rolls and sponges—all-purpose wound dressing.

Klintmalm clamp—used in liver transplantation surgery.

Klippel-Feil syndrome—congenital fusion of the cervical vertebrae.

Klonopin (clonazepam)—lyophilized wafers. The name was changed from Clonopin to Klonopin to avoid confusion with the medication *clonidine.*

KLS Centre-Drive screws—for application of rigid fixation devices.

knee—see *housemaid's knee.*

Kneed-It Kneeguard—for relief of minor knee pain associated with arthritis and tendinitis.

knee jerk (KJ).

Knee Signature System (KSS)—used to measure anterior tibial displacement and the angle of knee flexion. Manufactured by Acufex.

knife—see also *blade.*
A-K diamond
A-OK ShortCut
bladebreaker
Edgeahead phaco slit
Foerster capsulotomy
Freedom
Gamma radiosurgical
Harmonic Scalpel
Lebsche
Lorenz PC/TC scissors ultra-sharp
Neoflex bendable
NeoKnife electrosurgical instrument
Paufique
roentgen radiosurgical

knife *(cont.)*
ShortCut
sickle
Tiemann Meals tenolysis
UltraCision ultrasonic
Visitec circular
Visitec crescent
Visitec EdgeAhead phaco slit
Visitec stiletto

Knee Society Score—a measure of knee function. "Knee Society Score was greater than 80 after supracondylar varus osteotomy stabilized with a blade plate."

K9 Scooter—an alternative to crutches. It is steered with the knee, freeing up hands and arms.

Knodt rod—not easy to find in references unless you know it begins with a silent *K*; also may be erroneously heard as a *knot rod.*

Knuttsen bending roentgenograms.

Ko-Airan maneuver—a technique for controlling bleeding due to early division of the posterior cystic artery in laparoscopic cholecystectomy.

Koala intrauterine pressure catheter.

Kocher collar incision—used in thyroidectomy.

Kocher-Langenbeck—ilioinguinal approach in repair of acetabular fracture; it is the most frequently used posterior approach for this procedure.

Koch's node—see *sinoatrial node.*

Koch nucleus hydrolysis needle—used in cataract surgery.

Koch phaco manipulator/splitter—used in phacoemulsification to push and fracture the nucleus in cataract surgery.

Koch technique—a technique for intraocular lens insertion using a 4-5 mm incision and closure with the suture knots buried.

Kock nipple valve (Urol).

Kock ("coke") **pouch modified procedure**—to enable women who are postcystectomy to urinate through the rectum. The Kock pouch is connected to the kidneys via the ureters and then surgically attached to the sigmoid colon just above the rectum. Urine collects in the pouch and subsequently is eliminated through the rectum. Backflow is prevented by two valves. In a similar procedure for men, a Kock pouch is connected to the urethra, permitting normal elimination. Called *continent ileostomy, reservoir ileostomy.*

Koebner phenomenon (koebnerization) —psoriasis at the site of an injury.

Koenig MPJ implant and arthroplasty—two-component system for replacement of the first MPJ (metatarsophalangeal joint).

KoGENate—blood factor VIII product used in treating hemophilia A. It is produced through recombinant DNA rather than extracted from blood plasma by plasmapheresis.

KOH colpotomizer system—a device used in laparoscopic hysterectomy that provides improved visualization of anatomical landmarks.

Köhler lines—used to grade hip protrusion.

KOH mount (potassium hydroxide)—a test used in diagnosing cutaneous fungal disease. Scrapings are taken from the skin in the affected area. A few drops of 15 to 20% potassium hydroxide (KOH) are added to the scrapings on a slide. The slide is heated over a flame several times and can then be examined for fungal organisms.

koilocytotic—characteristic of a wart cell.

Kold Kap—plastic bag with a frozen gel, applied to scalp of patient undergoing chemotherapy to decrease hair loss. Also, *ChemoCap.*

Kollagen—purified bovine collagen derivative that promotes wound granulation.

König disease—osteochondritis dissecans (*not* dessicans) of the knee. Also, *Koenig.*

Kono procedure—patch enlargement of ascending aorta.

Konton catheter—used to position intra-aortic balloon pump.

Kontrast U—a radiopaque medium. May be used in myelography and also in x-raying the urinary tract.

Köper Knit—thin-wall carotid patch.

Koplik's spots—an indication of measles; tiny gray-white spots with a rim of erythema, appearing on the buccal mucosa before the skin rash of measles appears.

Korotkoff sounds—the sounds heard through the sphygmomanometer which, properly calibrated, indicate blood pressure. "The first and fifth phase Korotkoff sounds were taken as systolic and diastolic pressures, respectively."

Kostuik internal spine fixation system.

kPa (kilopascal)—a blood gas pressure measure, equaling 1000 pascals; an SI unit of measure.

KPs (keratoprecipitates, keratic precipitates, or keratitic precipitates)—large white keratic precipitates that resemble drops of solidified mutton fat; they are seen on corneal endothelium.

Krackow's point—orthopedic landmark in the knee.

Krackow suture—a suture technique used in ligament-tendon fixation,

Krackow suture *(cont.)*
particularly ACL reconstruction. Developed by Dr. K. A. Krackow.

Kraff nucleus splitter—fine forceps with serrated tips used to grasp and fracture the nucleus during cataract surgery.

Kraff-Utrata tear capsulotomy forceps—used to make the circular tear in the anterior capsule when performing capsulorrhexis.

Kraske's position in surgery—the jackknife position used for rectal and coccygeal procedures.

kraurosis vulvae—progressive atrophy of the vulva in postmenopausal women.

Kreiselman unit—apparatus used in resuscitation of newborn infants; provides oxygen, heat, suction, etc.

Kreuscher bunionectomy.

Krimsky measurement—of exotropia.

Kropp bladder neck reconstruction—to create bladder outlet competence.

Krukenberg's spindle—an opacity on the posterior surface of the cornea which is vertical, spindle-shaped, and brownish-red in color.

Krukenberg's tumor—carcinoma of the ovary, usually metastatic from cancer of the intestinal tract, stomach, or breast.

Krupin-Denver eye valve—surgically implanted for control of glaucoma (made by Storz).

Krupin valve with disc—for treatment of uncontrolled glaucoma. "In 1991 she underwent a Krupin valve with disc implant to the inferonasal quadrant."

Kruskal-Wallis test—for acoustic neuroma.

krypton (red) **laser photocoagulation**—used in treating choroidal neovascular membrane, and pigment epithelial detachment.

krypton, inhalation of—in positron scanning technique for measuring cerebral blood flow.

KS—see *Kaposi's sarcoma*.

KS 5 ACL brace—a functional brace designed to inhibit tibial translation.

KSHV (Kaposi sarcoma-associated herpesvirus).

K-Sponge—sterile hydrocellulose sponge used during ophthalmic or microvascular surgical procedures.

KTP (potassium-titanyl-phosphate) **laser** —used in laparoscopic laser cholecystectomy.

K-Tube—trade name for a silicone jejunostomy tube designed to facilitate easy surgical placement for use in enteral nutritional support in patients who are in bed or are ambulatory.

KUB (kidneys, ureters, and urinary bladder) (Radiol).

Kugelberg-Welander disease—juvenile hereditary motor neuron disease.

Kuhn-Bolger angled curette (ENT)—used in frontal sinus surgery.

L, l

LAAM (levomethadyl acetate hydrochloride)—used in treatment of heroin addicts. It has been shown to reduce heroin use by up to 90%.

LABA (laser-assisted balloon angioplasty).

Labbé ("lab-bay"), **vein of**.

label—to render a substance radioactive by incorporating a radionuclide in it; also, to cause a tissue or organ to take up radioactive material. Cf. *sensitize; tag*.

la belle indifférence—seen in certain patients with strokes or conversion disorders who show an inappropriate lack of concern about their disabilities.

labetalol—an antiadrenergic. "The patient began to have brief hypertensive episodes and received labetalol to stabilize his blood pressure."

labial (adj.)—(1) referring to the labia majora and labia minora, the fleshy structures in the genital area just anterior to the vagina (Gyn); (2) the surface of the incisor and canine teeth directly opposite the lips (Dental). Cf. *labile*.

labile—an adjective describing a condition or emotion easily or spontaneously changed; unstable. Examples: labile hypertension, labile affect.

labor—see *arrest of labor*; *stages of labor*.

labor curves—see *Friedman curves*.

labrum-ligament complex (LLC)—a structure involved in shoulder dislocations and instability of the shoulder joint.

Lachman test—used to determine the presence of a tear in the anterior cruciate ligament.

lacrimal scintigraphy (Oph).

lactamase—see *beta-lactamase*.

lactated Ringer's solution—a physiologic salt solution used for irrigation in surgery. *Lactated* does not refer to milk, but to lactic acid solution.

lactoferrin—a protein found in a number of human secretions (bile, saliva, milk, tears). It is an iron-binding protein and has been found to retard fungal and bacterial growth, possibly by depriving these organisms of iron.

Lactomer material—used for absorbable subcuticular skin staples.

Lactosorb—an advanced resorbable plating system used in correcting craniomaxillofacial deformities in infants and children.

lactulose solution—used as a laxative (Cronulac and Evalose) and as ammonia detoxification (Cephulac and Heptalac).

LAD (left anterior descending) **artery**.

LADARVision system—for treatment of myopia, with or without astigmatism, using LASIK.

Ladd's bands—tight peritoneal folds that pass over and across the second part of the duodenum, often seen associated with malrotation.

Ladd procedure—for correction of malrotation of the bowel (freeing up the duodenum and Ladd's bands, and bringing up the small bowel over to the right side of the abdomen and leaving the colon on the left side of the abdomen, thus broadening the base of the mesentery).

LADD (lacrimoauriculodentodigital) **syndrome**—genetic disorder characterized primarily by malformations of the upper limbs and inherited through an autosomal dominant trait. Other symptoms may include malformations in the lacrima, abnormalities of the teeth, small cupped ears, absent or underdeveloped salivary glands, hearing loss, abnormalities of the genitourinary system, and/or unusual skin ridge patterns.

Laerdal resuscitator—a right-angled nonrebreathing valve.

LAF (lymphocyte activating factor)—see *interleukin-1*.

Lafora body disease—the malignant form of Unverricht-Lundborg syndrome, a progressive myoclonus epilepsy associated with progressive dementia. See *Unverricht-Lundborg syndrome*.

LAG (lymphangiogram).

lagophthalmos—incomplete closure of the palpebral fissure when an attempt is made to shut the eyelids. May be caused by involvement of the facial nerve. It results in exposure and injury to the bulbar conjunctiva and cornea.

lag screw.

Laguna Negra virus—a variation of hantavirus pulmonary syndrome found in Paraguay.

Laing concentric hip cup.

LAIS laser—excimer laser for coronary angioplasty.

Laitinen CT guidance system and stereotactic head frame (Neuro).

LAK (lymphokine-activated killer) **cells** —cells capable of killing tumor cells in vitro. LAK cells are produced by incubation of peripheral blood lymphocytes with interleukin-2 for three days. Although LAK cells are capable of killing a great many autologous and allogenic tumor cells, they do not affect normal cells. LAK cells are used in treatment of gliomas and some other types of cancers, sometimes in combination with interleukin-2.

Lalonde delicate hook forceps— combines the advantages of needleholder jaws and overlapping skin hooks for two-handed closures. Used for skin closure in plastic surgery procedures.

LAL (*Limulus* amoebocyte lysate) **test** —gauges the presence of endotoxins

LAL *(cont.)*
such as *E. coli* by exposing the blood of horseshoe crabs (a limulus species) to the endotoxin, which causes the blood to clot. The amoebocytes in the crab blood are similar to human white blood cells. The cells are then spun in a centrifuge and intentionally ruptured to create a "lysate," the essence of the LAL test. The lysate is subsequently freeze-dried and looks like grains of salt. Pharmaceutical and medical device manufacturers use the LAL test to ensure that injectable products and invasive devices are endotoxin-free. Also known as *Bang's horseshoe-crab blood test.*

LAMA (laser-assisted microvascular anastomosis or laser-assisted micro-anastomosis).

Lambda (lanthanum carbonate)—an oral antihyperphosphatemia drug to treat high blood phosphate levels in patients with chronic kidney failure.

Lambda Plus PDL 1 and **Lambda Plus PDL 2 laser systems**—used to activate Photofrin in a two-step treatment system called photodynamic therapy for palliation of certain esophageal cancers.

lamellar body number density—an effective and inexpensive test for rapid identification of a fetus at high risk for respiratory distress syndrome. This test assesses fetal lung maturity by using an electronic cell counter.

Lamictal (lamotrigine)—an anticonvulsant used for seizure control.

laminaria (L., lamina, blade)—a sterile applicator made of kelp, used to dilate the cervix. See *Dilapan*; *Laminaria.*

Laminaria—a genus of seaweed (kelp). The dried *Laminaria digitata* is often used in induced abortion, since, as it absorbs fluids, it expands, thus dilating the cervix. See *Dilapan*; *laminaria.*

Lamisil (terbinafine)—a topical antifungal cream useful for treating athlete's foot, jock itch, and ringworm.

Lamisil DermGel—antifungal.

lamivudine—a drug used for patients with HIV; also reportedly effective in inhibiting replication of the hepatitis B virus.

lamivudine/AZT (Epivir/Retrovir)—combination of AIDS drugs.

lamotrigine (Lamictal)—an antiepileptic drug to be given to adults in addition to standard treatment when seizure control is inadequate.

Lamprene (clofazimine)—a drug used to treat leprosy, now used to treat MAC infection in AIDS patients.

lancinating pain—stabbing, piercing.

Landolt pituitary speculum.

Landolt ring—a device for testing vision. It is like a letter *C* with a very small opening. The opening is moved up, down, and to each side and is used to test vision in the same way as the E chart.

Landry-Guillain-Barré-Strohl syndrome—acute idiopathic polyneuritis. See *Guillain-Barré syndrome.*

Landry vein light venoscope—a fiberoptic illumination device. It has two arms, separated by a few inches, which, when pressed to the skin of the patient, transilluminate the skin and reveal the location of veins. It facilitates the visualization of veins which are deep seated or difficult to find so that an intravenous line can be quickly inserted.

Landsmeer's ligament—a deep fascial band in the hand. Reference is made to this structure in operative procedures for correction of Dupuytren's contracture.

Lane bone-holding clamp (Ortho).

Lange skin-fold calipers—used to measure fat in certain areas of the body in diet and weight assessment.

Lange tendon lengthening and repair.

lansoprazole (Prevacid).

Lanz—low-pressure cuff endotracheal tube.

lap—brief form for laparotomy. See *lap tape.*

"lap appy"—slang for laparoscopic appendectomy.

laparoscopic appendectomy—minimally invasive alternative, which cannot be performed if rupture or abscess is suspected. See *"lap appy."*

Laparofan—used in conjunction with Laparolift as an alternative to pneumoperitoneum produced by CO_2 gas insufflation.

LaparoLift system—an Airlift balloon retractor for use in gasless laparoscopy. It is a doughnut-shaped cushion inserted and inflated to allow free access to abdominal organs without requiring gas insufflation. It is an instrument for stone fragmentation in laparoscopic cholecystectomy.

LaparoSAC single-use obturator and cannula—used in laparoscopic surgery.

laparoscopically assisted vaginal hysterectomy (LAVH).

laparoscopically assisted colorectal resection—performed for colorectal carcinoma, both curative and palliative.

laparoscopic biopsy of liver—an alternative to open wedge biopsy of the liver.

laparoscopic bladder neck suture suspension procedure—anchors a suture in Cooper's ligament and transvaginally in the anterior vaginal wall to provide upper and lower suspension points.

laparoscopic Burch procedure.

laparoscopic cholecystectomy—laparoscopic gallbladder removal requiring only four small incisions, resulting in rapid recovery time. Acute inflammation may require conversion to the open procedure.

laparoscopic contact ultrasonography (LCU)—a viable alternative to intraoperative cholangiography. Used in the detection of ductal stones but less reliable in the disclosure of anomalous biliary anatomy.

laparoscopic Doppler probe—useful in identifying arteries during laparoscopic surgery.

laparoscopic Heller myotomy—used for surgical treatment of esophageal achalasia.

laparoscopic intracorporeal ultrasound (LICU)—used in place of cholangiography to examine biliary duct system.

laparoscopic laser-assisted autoaugmentation (Urol)—performed in children for neurogenic bladder dysfunction.

laparoscopic laser cholecystectomy (LLC)—laparoscopic gallbladder removal utilizing laser instead of electrocautery technique. See *"lap chole."*

laparoscopic lysis—a procedure for lysis of adhesions and placement of a periotoneal dialysis catheter.

laparoscopic Nissen and Toupet fundoplication—surgical treatment of complicated GERD (gastroesophageal reflux disease).

laparoscopic pelvic lymph node dissection and extraperitoneal pelvioscopy—operative staging procedures.

laparoscopic pneumodissection—dissection technique used in laparoscopic surgery that uses short bursts of high-pressure carbon dioxide as a dissection medium.

laparoscopic radical prostatectomy—performed on men with localized prostate cancer, low-volume tumors, and favorable pelvic anatomy. Surgeons performing this procedure are better able to visualize the prostatic apex and urethra, facilitating reconnection of the bladder neck to the urethra and offering the possibility of better postoperative continence.

laparoscopic surgeon's thumb—area of paresthesia in the distribution of the lateral digital nerve due to holding laparoscopic instruments for long periods. Generally resolves within hours, but sometimes takes days.

laparoscopic transcystic duct exploration—used to treat common bile duct stones and allows for open choledochotomy.

laparoscopic transcystic papillotomy—for endoscopic bile duct stone removal in laparoscopic cholecystectomy.

laparoscopic ultrasound (LUS).

laparoscopic urinary diversion procedure—for intestinal urinary conduit.

laparoscopic uterine nerve ablation (LUNA).

laparoscopy under local anesthesia (LULA).

Laparosonic coagulating shears for autograft harvesting.

laparotomy—see *second-look*.

Lap-Band adjustable gastric banding (LAGB) **system**—for the surgical treatment of morbid obesity. The device is placed laparoscopically in the upper abdomen to form a small gastric pouch and stoma. Increasing or decreasing the amount of saline within the band allows the size of the stoma to be adjusted.

"lap chole"—slang for laparoscopic cholecystectomy.

Laplacian mapping—see *body surface Laplacian mapping*.

lap Nissen (laparoscopic Nissen fundoplication)—may be done with esophageal lengthening variation for treatment of gastroesophageal reflux with short esophagus. (A short esophagus is the end result of severe, long-standing GE reflux.)

Lapro-Clip—ligating clip system.

Lap Sac—used to enclose larger organs or masses of resected tissue, which are then morselized for removal through a small laparoscopic incision. See *Pleatman sac*.

lap tape (pad or sponge)—a large laparotomy sponge used in major abdominal (laparotomy) surgery. A small one is called "appy" tape (for appendectomy). "The wound was packed with a moist lap tape."

LAP (leukocyte alkaline phosphatase) **test**—a test for chronic myelogenous leukemia. Result is given as a score, with normal being greater than 20.

LapTie—endoscopic knot-tying instrument.

Lapwall—trade name of a laparotomy sponge and wound protector.

LAR/CAA (low anterior resection in combination with coloanal anastomosis)—for primary rectal cancer.

large clothing artifact (Radiol)—caused by wrinkles in gowns that are too large, imitating calcified arteries on film. Also, rolled-up pants may have radiopaque objects such as stones in the folds, confusing the radiologists.

large loop excision of the transformation zone (LLETZ)—an alternative to colposcopically directed punch biopsy for diagnosing cervical intraepithelial neoplasia (CIN). It is also used as an alternative to the carbon dioxide laser in the treatment of CIN.

large skull-implant surgery—used to repair the skulls of persons who have undergone brain surgery or have suffered serious head trauma, including gunshot wounds. Previously, only defects 3 cm or smaller could be covered by traditional surgery.

Larmor equation; frequency—terms used in MRI.

LaRoque herniorrhaphy incision.

Larrey's hernia—a herniation through the subcostosternal space. More commonly known as a Morgagni hernia. Named for Dominic John Larrey, Napoleon's surgeon general, who described the surgical approach to the pericardial cavity through the anterior diaphragmatic defect.

LARS (laparoscopic antireflux surgery).

LARSI (lumbar anterior-root stimulator implants).

laryngeal framework surgery (LFS) (also called *thyroplasty* or *phonosurgery*)—a procedure to change or improve the voice.

laryngeal web (ENT)—a congenital anomaly, malformation; it can be either a thin membrane or a thick one, most often at the level of the vocal cords. This membrane compromises the airway and may require surgery.

laryngomalacia—treated by unilateral supraglottoplasty or epiglottoplasty.

laryngoplastic phonosurgery (ENT)—laryngeal framework surgery to treat voice disorders. Includes medialization laryngoplasty and the arytenoid adduction procedure for unilateral paralysis.

LAS (lymphadenopathy syndrome).

LASE (laser-assisted spinal endoscopy).

Lasègue's sign ("la-segz")—straight leg raising test. A positive Lasègue's sign is indicative of nerve root irritation or possible low back pathology.

laser (light amplification by stimulated emission of radiation)—used in many procedures for everything from brain surgery to cleaning out clogged arteries to disintegrating stones in the biliary duct and kidney. See individual entries:
AccuLase excimer
acupuncture
alexandrite (solid-state)
AlexLazr *or* AlexLAZR
Apex Plus excimer
ArF excimer
argon
argon/krypton
ArthroProbe
Aura desktop ENT
Aurora diode-based dental
Aurora diode soft-tissue
biocavity
Candela 405 nm pulsed dye
carbon dioxide (CO_2)

laser *(cont.)*
    Centauri Er:YAG dental
    CHRYS CO_2
    ClearView CO_2
    Coherent CO_2 surgical
    Coherent UltraPulse 5000C
    copper-vapor pulsed
    CorneaSparing LTK system
    coumarin pulsed dye
    CTE:YAG (CrTmEr:YAG)
    Derma K
    DermaLase
    Derma 20
    diode
    dye
    Eclipse TMR
    ELCA
    endoscopic
    Epic ophthalmic 3-in-1
    EpiLaser
    EpiTouch
    erbium:YAG (Er:YAG)
    ErCr:YAG
    excimer
    FeatherTouch CO_2
    Femtosecond laser keratome
    Fiberlase
    flashlamp-pulsed Nd:YAG
    flashlamp-pumped pulsed dye
    Flexlase 600
    "flying spot" excimer
    gallium-arsenid (GaA)
    Genesis 2000
    GentleLASE Plus
    Gherini-Kauffman endo-otoprobe
    Heart Laser (for transmyocardial
      revascularization)
    HF infrared
    high-energy
    holmium
    holmium:YAG (yttrium-argon-
      garnet)
    Horn endo-otoprobe
    hot

laser *(cont.)*
    Hyperion LTK
    Kaplan PenduLaser 115
    Kirsch
    krypton (red)
    KTP (potassium-titanyl-phosphate)
    LADARVision excimer
    LAIS excimer
    Lambda Plus PDL 1 and PDL 2
    laparoscopic
    Laser Lancet
    Lasermedic's Microlight 830
    LaserPen
    LaserSonics EndoBlade
    LaserSonics Nd-YAG Laser Blade
    LaserSonics SurgiBlade
    Laserthermia
    LaserTripter MDL 3000
    Lasertrolysis
    LaserTweezers
    LightSheer (and LightSheer SC)
      diode
    Lightstic 180 and Lightstic 360
    LPI (Laser Photonics, Inc.)
    LTK (laser thermal keratoplasty)
    LX 20
    Lyra
    Mainster retina
    Maloney endo-otoprobe
    Max FiberScan
    Microlase transpupillary diode
    Microprobe
    midinfrared
    Multi-Operatory Dentalaser (MOD)
    Nidek EC-5000 excimer
    NovaLine Litho-S DUV excimer
    NovaPulse CO_2
    Nuvolase 660
    OcuLight SL diode
    OLM (ophthalmic laser micro-
      endoscope)
    OmniPulse-MAX holmium
    Opmilas 144 Plus
    Opmilas CO_2

laser *(cont.)*
  OtoLam
  Pegasus Nd:YAG surgical
  PhotoPoint
  Polaris 1.32 Nd:YAG
  Prima
  Prostalase
  PulseMaster
  Pulsolith
  Q-switched neodymium:YAG
  Q-switched ruby
  RevitaLase erbium cosmetic
  ScleroLaser
  ScleroPlus
  ScleroPLUS HP
  Selecta 7000
  Sharplan SilkTouch flashscan
    surgical
  SilkLaser aesthetic carbon dioxide
  Silk Touch laser skin resurfacing
  Skinlight erbium YAG
  SoftLight
  Softscan
  Spectranetics laser sheath (SLS)
  SPTL-1b vascular lesion
  Surgilase Nd:YAG
  Surgilase 150
  THC (thulium, holmium,
    chromium):YAG
  Topaz CO_2
  TruPulse CO_2
  2040 erbium SilkLaser
  UltraFine erbium
  UltraPulse CO_2
  Urolase fiber
  Vbeam
  VersaLight
  VersaPulse holmium
  Versatome
  Visulas Nd:YAG
  VISX excimer laser
  VISX Star S2 excimer
  Vitesse Cos
  Xanar 20 Ambulase CO_2

laser *(cont.)*
  XeCl (xenon-chloride)
  YAG (yttrium-aluminum-garnet)
  YagLAZR *or* YagLazr
  Zeiss Visulas 690s
  Zyoptix

laser acupuncture—used to promote analgesia locally or systemically.

laser-assisted balloon angioplasty (LABA)—a thermal laser delivery system that creates a small channel in the artery (particularly the femoral artery), followed by balloon angioplasty to dilate the residual stenosis, thereby allowing sufficient blood flow for symptom relief.

laser-assisted microanastomosis or **laser-assisted microvascular anastomosis (LAMA)**—use of a laser instead of sutures to seal small vessels at anastomotic site.

laser-assisted spinal endoscopy (LASE)—a less invasive technique for automated percutaneous lumbar diskectomy. Laser fibers are inserted through 18 or 20 gauge needles for vaporization of lumbar disk material. Using the holmium:YAG (Ho:YAG) laser, a flexible cannula is inserted, through which a malleable and directable laser fiber is inserted under visual control via optical fibers also within the cannula. Constant irrigation through the same cannula keeps the disk space cool, decreasing the risk of thermal injury.

laser-assisted tissue welding technique—bladder augmentation or enterocystoplasty method.

laser-assisted uvulopalatoplasty (LAUP)—for treatment of snoring, but not sleep apnea. See *LAUP*.

laser biomicroscopy (Oph)—provides visualization and photographic rec-

laser biomicroscopy *(cont.)* ord of vitreoretinal structures at the macula.

laser correlational spectroscopy (LCS) —method for diagnosing malignant diseases by blood plasma analysis.

laser Doppler flowmetry (LDF)—noninvasive measure of cochlear blood flow through the intact otic capsule bone.

Laserflo blood perfusion monitor (BPM)—for evaluating or monitoring in situ microvascular circulation invasively or noninvasively.

laser image custom arthroplasty (LICA).

laser in situ keratomileusis (LASIK).

Laser Lancet—laser device for capillary blood draws for screening purposes. It eliminates the need for needle sticks, thereby making the procedure safer for patients and healthcare workers.

Lasermedic Microlight 830—a handheld, battery-operated, nonsurgical laser device that uses photo-biostimulation to treat carpal tunnel syndrome.

laser myringotomy—for treatment of serous otitis media. A small hole is created in the tympanic membrane (myringotomy) without the insertion of ventilation tubes. The opening allows for drainage and endoscopic evaluation of the middle ear space, which remains open for several weeks, followed by spontaneous and complete healing of the tympanic membrane. The procedure may be done in a physician's office under local anesthesia on patients age six years or older.

laser nucleotomy—a surgical technique for correction of a herniated disk.

Under local anesthesia, the Versa-Pulse holmium laser is inserted into the nucleus pulposus of the disk, and a portion of the disk vaporized.

LaserPen—handheld instrument used to stimulate muscles and nerves in acupuncture.

laser photoablation.

laser plume—the toxic by-product of laser and electrosurgical procedures, composed of chemicals, bacteria, and viruses.

laser sclerostomy (Oph)—use of the laser to produce an outflow channel in treatment of glaucoma.

LaserSonics EndoBlade—for laparoscopic use.

LaserSonics Nd:YAG LaserBlade scalpels.

LaserSonics SurgiBlade—for colposcopic procedures.

laser speckle—used to assess degree of night myopia. When light from a laser is reflected from a granular surface, a speckled pattern is seen; and when a patient with night myopia looks at this pattern and moves his head, the speckles seem to move, and move opposite to the direction of head movement if the eye is myopic at that distance. Correcting the refractive error with lenses will neutralize the pattern's movement.

laser stapedotomy (ENT)—the procedure of making a small opening by a laser into the footplate of the stapes (instead of removing the entire stapes) to correct deafness caused by otosclerosis.

laser thermal keratoplasty (LTK)—a laser treatment performed through the lens of a specially modified slit-lamp biomicroscope. With use of an

laser thermal *(cont.)*
infrared laser, the corneal collagen is changed from a double-helix conformation to a partly coiled state, resulting in contraction of the fibers and change in the curvature of the cornea.

Laserthermia—see *transurethral balloon Laserthermia prostatectomy.*

laser trabeculodissection (LTD)—glaucoma surgery ablation technique using a scanning excimer laser.

LaserTripter MDL 3000—provides precise destruction of calculi with least thermal effect.

Lasertrolysis—proprietary name for hair removal using the EpiLaser to heat and disable the hair follicle without causing harm to the surrounding skin.

LaserTweezers—for optical trapping. It uses the pressure of a laser to isolate particles or cells and move them.

laser uterosacral nerve ablation (LUNA).

laser welding—sutureless tissue welding using a diode laser and protein solder. Used with anastomoses of the blood vessel, bowel, ureter, and nerve.

Lasette laser finger perforator—used for sampling capillary blood for glucose and other blood chemistry readings. It is reportedly less painful to patients than needle sticks, but also eliminates accidental fingersticks and the possibility of cross-contamination from the patient.

Lash hysterectomy technique.

LASIK (laser in situ keratomileusis) (Oph)—a corneal procedure for vision correction. A flap of anterior corneal stroma is dissected, the deeper layers are partially ablated with the laser, and the hinged superficial flap is then replaced.

L-asparaginase (L-ASP, asparaginase) —used to treat acute lymphatic leukemia.

Lassa fever—a highly virulent disease found in some central and western African countries, named for Lassa, Nigeria, where it was first recognized.

last—a metal or plastic form shaped like the human foot and over which a shoe is shaped or repaired. See *bunion last* and *Keystone last.*

Latarjet, Andre, a French anatomist. See *nerve of Latarjet.* Also, *Latarjet's vein* (vena prepylorica).

Latarjet nerve—see *nerve of Latarjet.*

late luteal phase dysphoric disorder (LLPDD)—the most debilitating form of premenstrual syndrome.

lateral acetabular shelf operation (Ortho).

lateral crural steal (LCS)—a technique for nasal tip reconstruction that involves advancing (in essence, "stealing") the lateral crura onto the medial crura to project the nasal tip anteriorly.

lateral hypopharyngeal pouch (LHP).

lateral mamillary nucleus of Rose (Neuro).

lateral transverse thigh flap (LTTF).

latissimus dorsi myocutaneous flap—a method of breast reconstruction utilizing the latissimus dorsi muscle, and skin transferred from the back. It can be combined with a breast implant to produce a larger breast mound.

LATS (long-acting thyroid-stimulating) **hormone**.

lattice degeneration (retinal)—a sharply demarcated circumferential lesion

lattice degeneration *(cont.)* that is located at, or somewhat anterior to, the equator, characterized by an interconnecting network of fine white lines, and may be associated with numerous round, punched-out areas of retinal thinning or actual retinal holes. May lead to retinal detachment.

Latzko vesicovaginal fistula repair.

LAUP (laser-assisted uvulopalatoplasty) —alternative surgical procedure to UPPP (uvulopalatopharyngoplasty) for treating snoring. It is not recommended for obstructive sleep apnea due to unpredictable response.

Laurence-Moon-Biedl syndrome—hereditary syndrome characterized by obesity, retinitis pigmentosa, mental retardation, polydactyly and hypogonadism. Other abnormalties may include ataxia, dwarfism, heart defects, and ocular complications.

Laurer forceps.

Laurin x-ray view.

LAVH (laparoscopically assisted vaginal hysterectomy).

Lawrence Add-A-Cath—sharp-tipped, bevelled trocar and peel-off sheath for suprapubic insertion into the bladder.

Lazarus-Nelson technique—generally used for peritoneal lavage that may be adapted for creating a pneumoperitoneum for laparoscopy. Generally felt to be safer, especially in obese patients, than other blind methods for introducing pneumoperitoneum.

lazeroids—in cerebral hypoxia-ischemia.

LazerSmile—a tooth-whitening system for home use. It uses a light source embedded within a battery-operated toothbrush and clear, nonabrasive tooth-whitening gel.

lazy H incision.

lazy leukocyte syndrome (LLS).

lazy Z incision.

LBP (low back pain).

L-Cath peripherally inserted neonatal catheter.

LCD (liquor carbonis detergens).

LCF (left circumflex) **coronary artery**.

LCIS (lobular carcinoma in situ).

LCS (laser correlational spectroscopy).

LDF (laser Doppler flowmetry).

LDI-200—used in the treatment of refractory leukemia.

LDL (low-density lipoprotein).

LDL Direct—a test for LDL (low-density lipoprotein) using a process called *immunoseparation*. It does not require a triglyceride measurement and can be performed on nonfasting patients. In the past, tests were based on a mathematical equation using the results of total cholesterol, HDL, and triglycerides.

LDP-02—a humanized monoclonal antibody for the treatment of inflammatory bowel diseases.

LDR (labor, delivery, and recovery) **room**, where the expectant mother goes through labor, delivery, and recovery in the same room.

LDX System—see *Cholestech LDX System*.

leading bar—a device by which a surgeon can guide the tape or the thread to the outside of the abdomen, facilitating extracorporeal lifting of the round ligament and gallbladder for exposing Calot's triangle during laparoscopic surgery.

Leadbetter-Politano ureterovesicoplasty—submucosal tunnel technique.

lead line—a blue line which is observed on the gums in lead poisoning cases.

leather-bottle stomach—a kind of gastric carcinoma (also called *linitis plastica*). The tumor is hard (scirrhous) and the stomach wall becomes thick and rigid.

LeBag reservoir—an ileocolic urinary reservoir for urinary diversion in total cystectomy patients.

Leber's ("lay-berz") **disease**—hereditary optic atrophy occurring in young men between the ages of 20 and 30. The optic nerve degeneration is rapidly progressive, but finally stabilizes, and some vision remains.

Leber's miliary aneurysms (Oph).

Lebsche knife—a heavy knife with a curved end (to hook under the xiphoid process) and a T-shaped handle; used for splitting the sternum for quick entry into the thoracic cavity.

lecithin/sphingomyelin ratio—see *L/S ratio*.

LED (liposome-encapsulated doxorubicin)—see *Doxil*.

Leder stain (chloracetate esterase)—used in identifying granulocytic sarcoma by differentiating that entity from lymphoma, Ewing's sarcoma, embryonal rhabdomyosarcoma, and undifferentiated carcinoma.

LeDuc anastomosis—a method of ureteral reimplantation used in urinary diversion procedures.

LeDuc-Camey ileocystoplasty—antireflux implantation of the ureters, for patients with bladder cancer.

leech—see *mechanical leech*.

Leeds-Keio ligament prosthesis—an open-weave tube of polyester mesh that can be fixed to bone at each end with bone plugs. New ligament tissue forms along the scaffold of the mesh, providing a sound new ligament within two years.

LEEP (loop electrosurgical excision procedure).

leflunomide (Arava)—an inflammatory for rheumatoid arthritis and possible antirejection drug; antineoplastic.

LeFort I apertognathia repair.

LeFort II fracture—pyramidal fracture of the maxilla.

LeFort III fracture—craniofacial disjunction and transverse facial fracture.

LeFort urethral sound.

LeFort uterine prolapse repair.

left anterior descending (LAD) **artery.**

left circumflex (LCF) **coronary artery.**

left shift—see *shift to the left*.

left ventricular end diastolic pressure (LVEDP).

left ventricular outflow tract obstruction (LVOTO).

Legasus Sport CPM (continuous passive-motion) **device**—used for sports medicine rehabilitation.

Legionella pneumophila—gram-negative organism causing legionnaires' disease and Pontiac fever. Can be devastating in AIDS patients. Other species include:
L. bozemanae
L. dumoffii
L. feeleii
L. gormanii
L. jordanis
L. longbeachae (serogroups 1 and 2)
L. micdadei

legionnaires' disease—pulmonary form of legionellosis, resulting from infection with *Legionella pneumophila*. Called legionnaires' disease because of an outbreak at a 1976 convention of the American Legion in Phila-

legionnaires' disease *(cont.)*
delphia, when the causative agent was first identified. Patients with this disease have very high fevers, abdominal pain, headaches, and pneumonia. They may also have kidney, liver, and nervous system involvement. According to the CDC, legionellosis is spread with breathing water mists in air conditioner cooler towers, whirlpool spa and showers, but not from household or car air conditioner units.

Lehman cardiac device.

Leibinger miniplate system—see *E-Z Flap*.

Leibinger Profyle system—a titanium hand and small bone fragment fixation system. This is a plating system for rigid internal fixation of hand fractures.

Leishmania donovani—an opportunistic parasite found in the GI tract of patients with AIDS. It causes leishmaniasis.

Lejeune's syndrome—see *cri du chat*.

Lejour-type breast reduction, modified—breast reduction technique that utilizes a vertical scar. Reportedly, the result is a better breast shape with significantly reduced scars.

Leksell stereotaxic frame—used to place electrodes.

LeMaitre Glow 'N Tell tape—radiopaque tape with centimeter markings placed on the leg to pinpoint the site of saphenous branches.

lemon sign—concave deformity of the fetal frontal bones seen in association with spina bifida.

LENI (lower extremity noninvasive)—an acronym (usually plural) used to refer to patients checked for emboli in legs. "LENIs were positive."

Lennox-Gastaut syndrome—mixed seizure disorder.

Lenox Hill brace (*not* Lennox)—knee orthosis.

lens, lenses
AcrySof acrylic foldable intraocular
Adaptar contact
AMO Array IOL
Bagolini
Baron
CeeOn heparinized intraocular
Cilco Slant
Coburn equivonvex
Dulaney intraocular implant
etafilcon A
Galand disc
Goldmann
heparinized CeeOn intraocular
Hoskins nylon suture laser
Hruby ("ruby")
Hydroview intraocular
ICL (implantable contact lens)
IOL (intraocular)
Iolab Slimfit
Karickhoff laser
Leiske
Lieb–Guerry cataract implant
Mainster retina laser
MemoryLens intraocular
Monoflex
PC-IOL
Pearce Tripod implant cataract
PhacoFlex
PMMA (polymethylmethacrylate) contact
Prokop intraocular
RGP (rigid gas permeable) contact
Sauflon PW (lidofilcon B)
SeeQuence disposable
Sensar intraocular, The
Silsoft extended wear contact
SingleStitch PhacoFlex
SinuScope rigid rod
Slant

lens *(cont.)*
   Staar foldable IOL
   Staar implantable contact (ICL)
   STAAR Toric implantable contact
   T lens
   Toric intraocular
   Unfolder intraocular, The
   Volk Pan Retinal
   Volk QuadrAspheric fundus
   Volk SuperPupil NC (noncontact)
   Worst gonioprism contact
lenses, intraocular (IOL). Styles:
   anterior chamber IOL (secured in front of iris)
   iridocapsular/iris fixation lens or iris plane lens (sewn to iris)
   posterior chamber IOL (secured in back of iris)
lens lasso—for repositioning of dislocated posterior chamber intraocular lens.
lens-sparing external beam radiation therapy (LSRT)—treatment for patients with diffuse choroidal hemangiomas. Cf. *episcleral plaque brachytherapy.*
Lente insulin—insulin zinc suspension.
lenticular nuclear sclerosis.
lentinan—a drug used to treat patients with AIDS.
lentivirus—a retrovirus.
Leonard Arm (first assistant)—a pneumatic action support device for laparoscopy and endoscopy.
LEOPARD syndrome—acronym for multiple **l**entigines, **e**lectrocardiographic conduction abnormalities, **o**cular hypertelorism, **p**ulmonic stenosis, **a**bnormal genitalia, **r**etardation of growth, and sensorineural **d**efects.
Lepper-Trier formula—a formula for calculating the depth of the anterior chamber of the eye.

leptomeninges—inner two membranes covering the brain and spinal cord.
Leriche syndrome—intermittent claudication of the buttocks and inability to maintain an erection, due to insufficiency of the external iliac arteries.
Lermans-Means scratch—a systolic grating sound heard in the second left intercostal space during expiration in hypertension. It is due to friction between the pleural and pericardial surfaces. Also may refer to a rub heard at the left sternal edge in thyrotoxicosis, possibly due to increased blood flow.
LES (lesser esophageal sphincter).
Lesch-Nyhan syndrome—hereditary hyperuricemia.
Lescol (fluvastatin)—a cholesterol-lowering drug.
LES incompetence—lower esophageal sphincter incompetence, which can cause severe esophagitis.
lesion (see also *disease*)
   Antopol-Goldman
   bull's eye
   cyclops
   dendritic
   DREZ
   frondy
   herald patch
   high-grade squamous intraepithelial (HGSIL)
   Hill-Sachs
   Janeway
   jet
   Lynch and Crues type 2
   macro-orchidism
   phlyctenule
   pinguecula
   satellite
   shagreen
   SLAP
   squamous intraepithelial (SIL)

lesion *(cont.)*
synchronous airway lesions (SALs)
target (of Lyme disease)
LESP (lower esophageal sphincter pressure).
Lester Martin modification of the Duhamel procedure—a treatment for Hirschsprung's disease.
Letterer-Siwe disease—a fulminant disease with multisystem manifestations, including skin, bone, pulmonary, central nervous system and endocrine features, and hepatosplenomegaly.
lettering artifact (Radiol)—lettering or designs picked up on film from some Band-Aids or underwear marketed for children.
leucine aminopeptidase test.
leucine zipper—investigational chain of amino acids which "zips" up to half of the AIDS virus, preventing replication.
Leucomax (GM-CSF, molgramostim)—used to treat Kaposi's sarcoma, AIDS, and CMV retinitis.
leucovorin (Isovorin)—an isomer of leucovorin (Wellcovorin) used in combination with methotrexate to treat metastatic colorectal carcinoma. See *leucovorin rescue*.
leucovorin calcium injection—used for treatment of megaloblastic anemias due to folic acid deficiency.
leucovorin rescue—used to decrease the toxicity of folic acid antagonist chemotherapy drugs such as methotrexate and fluorouracil. It rescues normal cells, but not malignant cells, from the toxic effects of the chemotherapy. Also known as *citrovorum factor rescue* and *folinic acid rescue*.

leukanakmesis—arrest of maturation of white cell series.
leukemia
acute lymphoblastic (ALL)
acute lymphocytic (ALL)
acute monoblastic (AMOL)
acute myeloblastic (AML)
acute myelomonoblastic (AMMOL)
acute promyelocytic (APML)
Burkitt-type acute lymphoblastic
chronic lymphocytic (CLL)
chronic myelocytic (CML)
hairy-cell
monoblastic
null cell lymphoblastic
leukemia classification
FAB, M1 (myeloblastic, with no differentiation)
FAB, M2 (myeloblastic, with differentiation)
FAB, M3 (promyelocytic)
FAB, M5 (monocytic)
FAB, M6 (erythroleukemia)
leukemia inhibitory factor (LIF).
Leukine (GM-CSF, sargramostim)—used to counter the effects of chemotherapy in the treatment of acute myelogenous leukemia. Also, may be used as the first growth factor in mobilizing peripheral blood progenitor cells (PBPC) and after PBPC transplantation.
leukocyte alkaline phosphatase test (LAP).
leukocyte-poor red blood cells—red blood cells from which at least 70% of the leukocytes have been removed by a saline-washing process or by centrifuge. Used for patients who have had severe, febrile nonhemolytic reactions to blood transfusion. Also, *leuko-poor red cells*.
LeukoNet Filter—removes leukocytes from blood components.

leuko-poor red cells—see *leukocyte-poor red blood cells.*

LeukoScan (technetium Tc 99m sulesomab)—an infectious disease imaging agent.

Leukotrap RC (red cell) **storage system**—used to reduce transfusion reactions and HLA sensitization by removing the white cells prior to red cell storage.

leukovirus—an RNA virus causing leukemia and tumors.

leupeptin—used during microsurgical repair of peripheral nerves.

leuprolide acetate—a neoplastic administered through Atrigel drug delivery system over a 120-day period to patients with advanced prostate cancer. Leuprolide is a hormone that reduces testosterone levels to inhibit prostate tumor growth.

LeuTech—radiolabeled imaging agent for diagnosing equivocal appendicitis.

Leuvectin—a gene-based oncology product that may benefit patients with advanced metastatic renal cell carcinoma; also used in treatment of prostate cancer.

levamisole (Ergamisol)—chemotherapy agent that increases T-cell response and also that of other cellular components in the blood (including neutrophils, monocytes, and antibodies) responsible for destroying cancerous cells. Given intravenously in combination with fluorouracil (Adrucil, 5-FU), for treating Dukes' stage C cancer of the colon.

Levaquin (levofloxacin)—an antibiotic used for treating respiratory infections.

LeVeen peritoneal shunt—used in peritoneal venous shunt for portal venous drainage in Budd-Chiari syndrome.

levetiracetam—drug for treatment of epileptic patients who experience partial-onset seizures.

levobupivacaine—a long-acting local anesthetic.

levocabastine HCl (Livostin)—topical ophthalmic antihistamine for temporary relief of seasonal allergic conjunctivitis.

levonorgestrel (Norplant).

levothyroxine sodium (Levoxyl)—a drug used to treat hypothyroidism. Formerly Levoxine, but the name was changed to prevent confusion with a medication of a similar name.

Levovist (galactose)—ultrasound contrast medium for echocardiography.

Levoxyl (levothyroxine sodium) (formerly Levoxine)—thyroid replacement.

Levulan Kerastick—used to apply aminolevulinic acid to actinic keratoses. The application is followed 14 to 18 hours later by irradiation with the BLU-U source of blue light.

Levulan photodynamic therapy (PDT) —a topical solution for the treatment of precancerous actinic keratoses of the face and scalp. Also, used to treat cervical intraepithelial neoplasia (CIN).

Lewis blood antibody type—a factor in agglutination. Also *Duffy, Kell, Kidd, Lutheran.*

Lewis Pair-Pak needle—a needle with a double-armed suture used in intraocular surgery.

Lewis-Tanner procedure—a subtotal esophagectomy and reconstruction.

Lewis upper limb cardiovascular disease—a congenital disorder.

Lewy inclusion body—in Parkinson's disease.

Lewy suspension laryngoscope.

Lexer gouge (Ortho).

lexipafant (Zacutex)—medication used in the treatment of acute pancreatitis.

Lexirin—oral drug designed to inhibit effects of diarrhea encountered in cancer chemotherapy, radiotherapy for prostate cancer, and AIDS.

Leydig cells—endocrine cells of the testis, producing testosterone. When Leydig cells are found with Reinke crystals on testicular biopsy of pre-pubertal boys, they are indicative of precocious puberty.

Lezak's Malingering Test (Psych).

L-5HTP (L-5-hydroxytryptophan)—a drug for postanoxic intention myoclonus.

LFS (laryngeal framework surgery).

LFS (Li-Fraumeni syndrome).

LFTs (liver function tests).

LGD (low-grade dysplasia).

LGSIL (low-grade squamous intra-epithelial lesion)—the term for squa-mous cellular changes seen on Pap smear that were formerly called mild dysplasia or CIN 1, including cellular atypia characteristic of hu-man papillomavirus infection.

Lhermitte-Duclos disease (dysplastic gangliocytoma of the cerebellum). This uncommon condition is seen usually in young and middle-aged adults. It is a benign mass lesion of the cerebellum, probably hamarto-matous.

LHMT (low-range heparin management test)—measures lower doses of heparin and is used primarily in diagnostic and interventional cardiol-ogy procedures.

LHPs (lateral hypopharyngeal pouches) (Rad)—protrusions of the lateral hy-popharyngeal wall that appear in the intradeglutitive phase of swallowing and disappear in the same or post-deglutitive phase, as seen on radio-logical studies.

LHRH (luteinizing hormone-releasing hormone)—polypeptide hormone also known as *GnRH* (gonadotropin-re-leasing hormone). This hormone is used in research on contraception, including contraceptives to be taken by males. It has been used in treat-ment of precocious puberty, delayed puberty, cryptorchidism, endome-triosis, acute intermittent porphyria, and hormone-dependent tumors.

Liberty CMC thumb brace—a hand therapy product.

Liberty One splint—a one-size, ambi-dextrous wrist splint.

LICA (laser image custom arthro-plasty).

lichen planus—a skin disorder.

Lich-Gregoire repair—used in kidney transplant surgery.

Lich technique—for ureteral implanta-tion in transplantation surgery or neobladder construction following total cystectomy.

Lichtenstein hernia repair—tension-free technique consisting of a cir-cumferentially sutured onlay patch. Cf., *mesh plug hernioplasty*.

licostinel—used in treating a stroke.

LICU (laparoscopic intracorporeal ul-trasound).

Lidakol cream (n-docosanol)—used for treatment of oral herpes.

lid lag—abnormally sluggish movement of the upper eyelid over the eye in exophthalmos. Commonly seen in thyroid disease.

lid margin vascular dilation (brush marks) (Oph).

lidocaine (Xylocaine)—given intrave-nously to treat ventricular arrhyth-

lidocaine *(cont.)*
mias or injected as a local anesthetic. Also used topically during bowel surgery; it is applied to the cut edges of the colon to relax the colonic musculature, and allows the insertion of the EEA circular stapler for anastomosis.

Lidoderm (lidocaine patch 5%)—for treatment of pain associated with postherpetic neuralgia.

LidodexNS—combination of lidocaine and dextromethorphan, administered intranasally, to provide rapid and prolonged relief of acute migraine headaches.

lidofilcon A—a glucose-permeable hydrogel with an equilibrium water content of 68%. Used in an intracorneal implant (Kerato-Gel).

Lido Lift—simulates actual work functions, for testing and rehabilitation.

lie (noun)—the relative position of the long axis of a fetus with respect to that of the mother: longitudinal or transverse.

Lieb-Guerry cataract implant lens.

LIF (leukemia inhibitory factor).

LifeGuide System—handheld blood glucose monitor for use by diabetics.

LIFE-Lung fluorescence endoscopy system—allows identification of areas of abnormal fluoresence that may not be visible on white-light examination.

Life-Pack 5 cardiac monitor.

LifeSite hemodialysis access system—provides dialysis access through the use of a valve implanted below the skin. Reportedly minimizes the pain associated with insertion and removal of a standard dialysis fistula needle. The valve closes immediately after use, providing immediate hemostasis.

Lifestream coronary dilatation catheter.

L-IFN (human) (lymphoblastoid interferon).

Li-Fraumeni syndrome (LFS)—predisposes carriers of the syndrome to cancers including rhabdomyosarcoma, osteosarcoma, brain tumors, leukemia, adrenocortical carcinomas, and breast carcinoma.

LiftMate—patient transfer device.

lift-off test—an orthopedic test to assess partial versus full-thickness tear of subscapularis muscle.

Liftstation—simulates actual work functions, for testing and rehabilitation.

Ligaclip—used in minimally invasive procedures for surgical dissection.

ligament
glenohumeral (GHL)
posterior cruciate (PCL)

ligamentum teres cardiopexy—also called *esophageal sling procedure.* Entails complete mobilization of the ligamentum teres (round ligament), which is passed behind the esophagus and anchored to the lesser curvature of the stomach. This secures the lower esophageal sphincter in the abdomen. Intraoperative manometry is used to adjust the sphincter pressure. This procedure is done in an attempt to avoid the complications associated with total fundoplication.

ligand (L., to bind)—organic molecules (chemical "superglue") used to bond therapeutic agents to monoclonal antibodies.

ligase chain reaction—uses a thermostabile enzyme ligase to detect a known DNA or RNA sequence in a specimen. See *polymerase chain reaction.*

ligature—see *suture ligature.*

light-chain deposition—a disease process closely related to light-chain amyloidosis that can occur in patients with immunoproliferative disorders. Cf. *heavy-chain deposition*.

light reflection rheography—imaging procedure that detects deep vein thrombosis using near-infrared light. The light is beamed from diodes to a depth of 1-2 mm into the skin. In the absence of disease, dorsiflexion of the foot will empty the venous plexus of the calf, reduce the amount of light absorbed, and result in an increased signal. In chronic venous insufficiency, light absorption is reduced to 10-15 seconds. In deep vein thrombosis, light absorption is reduced to less than 10 seconds, showing significantly reduced venous emptying.

light reflex—constriction of the pupil in response to light striking the retina.

LightSheer and **LightSheer SC**—high-performance diode laser hair removal system.

Lightstic 180, Lightstic 360—fiberoptic lasers that diffuse the laser light laterally rather than out the end of the fiber. This reportedly allows physicians to heat and destroy diseased cells in a less invasive and therefore less costly procedure.

Light Talker—a computerized communication device (designed by Dr. Janice Light) which enables patients who are unable to speak (due to neurological or traumatic injuries) to convey messages. With a movement even as slight as raising an eyebrow, the patient can indicate a selection which is spoken by a speech synthesizer or printed out on paper.

LILI (low-intensity laser irradiation).

Liliequist membrane—located near the pituitary gland and stalk.

Lilliput—neonatal oxygenator for use in ECMO.

LILT (low-intensity laser therapy).

LIMA (left internal mammary artery) **graft**—used in coronary artery surgery. "He underwent quadruple coronary artery bypass grafting, including LIMA."

LIMA-Lift—used to provide a window into the chest cavity, allowing the surgeon to efficiently harvest the left internal mammary artery (LIMA) for use as a bypass conduit around the blocked area in MIDCAB, minimizing incisions.

LIMA-Loop—enables the surgeon to reach into the chest to help isolate the left internal mammary artery (LIMA) for harvest during MIDCAB.

limbal groove.

limb length discrepancy developmental causes
avascular necrosis of hip
hip dislocation
idiopathic
Klippel-Trenaunay-Weber syndrome
linear scleroderma
local tumor
melorheostosis
neuromuscular
osteomyelitis
slipped capital femoral epiphysis
talectomy
trauma

limbus corneae—the edge of the cornea where it joins the sclera.

Limitrol-DM—a fat-free chewable wafer form of the herb fenugreek (*Trigonella foenum-graecum*) that assists diabetic patients in achieving tight blood glucose control.

Limulus **amoebocyte lysate (LAL) test**—see *LAL test*.

LINAC or **linac radiosurgery** (Neuro) —a coined word or acronym referring to *linear accelerator*. It is written in all capitals in some medical journals and in lowercase letters in others. Its form as a word will probably follow the pattern of *laser* and *radar*, terms which came into the language as initialisms and quickly became accepted as acronyms.

Lindholm operating laryngoscope.

Lindorf lag screws or **position screws** —used in sagittal split ramus osteotomy.

Lindseth's modified technique—treatment of spinal deformity in patients with myelomeningocele with kyphectomy with wire fixation and posterior and anterior spinal fusion. In modification of Lindseth's technique, the wires are crisscrossed posteriorly, said to result in better stability at the osteotomy site.

Lindstrom arcuate incision marker (Oph).

linear accelerator (LINAC or linac) **radiosurgery**—*not* radiotherapy. A single exposure of multiple radiation beams is used to eradicate tumor tissue. Cf. *Gamma Knife*.

line imaging—MRI term.

line of Zahn—a phenomenon due to the layering of fibrin and blood cells in a clot.

line scanning—MRI term.

line width—MRI term.

linezolid—see *Zyvox*.

lingoscope—an endoscope (modified laryngoscope) used to facilitate visualization of the base of the tongue and excision of the lingual tonsils.

linguine sign—multiple wavy lines in the breast seen on MRI scan as the classic sign of silicone implant rupture.

linitis plastica—see *leather-bottle stomach*.

Link cementless reconstruction hip prosthesis.

Link Endo-Model rotational knee— total knee replacement prostheses.

Link Lubinus SP II—anatomically adapted total hip replacement system.

Link Stack Split splint—finger splint with a split down the middle, for ease of application and removal.

Linomide (roquinimex)—imunomodulator for HIV; may be used in bone marrow transplant for leukemia.

linopiridine—a compound with properties similar to 4-aminopyridine. It enhances release of ACh and other neurotransmitters, such as dopamine and serotonin.

Linvatec cannulated interference screw—used in knee arthroscopy.

Linvotec microdebrider (ENT)—power instrument used for sinonasal tract surgery.

LINX-EZ cardiac device.

lion jaw tenaculum (Ortho).

LIP (lymphocytic interstitial pneumonitis).

lipid-associated sialic acid—a nonspecific tumor-associated marker seen on serum assays for the presence of gynecological malignancies.

lipid storage disease—see *Fabry's disease*.

Lipiodol—an iodized poppy seed oil used as a myelographic contrast medium.

Lipitor (atorvastatin calcium)—HMG-CoA reductase inhibitor that reduces elevated LDL cholesterol and triglycerides.

lip lift—a plastic surgery procedure in which skin is removed at the base of the nostril, hiding the incision directly in the nasal sill. This procedure may or may not be performed as an adjunct to corner mouth lift. See *corner mouth lift.*

lipoid nephrosis—see *nil disease.*

Lipomel—therapeutic vaccine for malignant melanoma.

lipophilic—fat-loving, in reference to stains. Cf. *hydrophilic*, water-loving.

liposhaver—a handheld device with a sharp orifice and sharp edges that oscillates and takes rapid "bites" of tissue, which are then suctioned away. Originally designed for use in sinus surgery, the liposhaver is now being used to remove fat from the neck and chin without the trauma associated with liposuction. See *XPS Sculpture System.*

liposomal doxorubicin (Doxil).

liposome-encapsulated doxorubicin (LED)—said to produce fewer severe side effects than free doxorubicin and to have other advantages in the treatment of leukemia and many solid tumors.

liposomes, encapsulated—particles of water surrounded by a membrane of phospholipids. They hold (or encapsulate) certain drugs such as amphotericin B (to treat severe systemic fungal infections), doxorubicin (to treat various types of cancer), and TLC G-65 (an antibiotic to treat MAI infection), reducing drug toxicity and unwanted side effects.

Liposorber LA-15 System—a machine that removes LDL cholesterol by filtering all the blood in a patient's body. The blood slowly passes from a tube placed in one arm, through a machine which separates plasma from other cells, through the Liposorber which filters the "bad" cholesterol out of the plasma, and then is returned to the body via a tube in the patient's other arm. Used in patients with severe hypercholesterolemia uncontrolled by medicine or diet. The procedure is not a cure and must be repeated indefinitely.

LipoTECA—1% cream used to treat keloid scars.

Liprostin—liposomal treatment of critical limb ischemia, which occurs when circulation in limbs becomes so inadequate that there is danger of gangrene and subsequent amputation.

liquid crystal thermography (LCT).

Liquiderm liquid healing bandage—for treatment of minor cuts and abrasions. It creates a moist wound-healing environment and provides a barrier to infection.

Liquifilm—sterile ophthalmic solution.

LiquiVent—liquid intrapulmonary ventilating agent for treatment of acute respiratory failure in children.

LIS (lung injury score).

Lisch spots—nodules on the iris seen on slit lamp exam.

Liss CES device—see *cranial electrical stimulation.*

Listeria **meningitis**—often seen in neonates but also in the immunocompromised and the elderly.

Lister's tubercle—located in the wrist, near the posterior interosseous nerve.

listing gait—leaning toward one side when walking.

LiteNest portable seating system—for wheelchairs, chairs, or 3-wheel scooters.

lithium carbonate—sometimes used in AIDS treatment for anemia, instead of for its effect against bipolar psychiatric disorders; it has what used to be considered a side effect of raising the white blood cell count.

lithiumogenic goiter—caused by lithium therapy, which is used to treat bipolar affective disorders, major depression, and schizoaffective disorders.

Lithostar—a lithotriptor. With the Lithostar, the patient is treated on a table and requires no anesthesia. In earlier lithotripsy treatment, the patient was immersed in water, and the shock waves that disintegrated the stones were conducted through the water.

lithotripsy—ultrasonic lithotripsy, electrohydraulic lithotripsy, and laser lithotripsy. The medium used in laser lithotripsy is coumarin dye (*not* coumadin).

lithotripsy, extracorporeal shockwave—procedure for treating upper urinary tract stones. See *lithotriptor*.

lithotriptor (or *lithotripter*)—an extracorporeal stone-disintegrating machine. It generates shock waves that are focused on the kidney stones to break them up. The patient is immersed in water while the shock waves are generated. The disintegrated stones are then passed in the urine over a several-day period.
Calcutript lithotripter
DoLi S extracorporeal shock wave
Dornier gallstone lithotriptor
Lithostar lithotriptor
Modulith SL 20 lithotriptor
Piezolith-EPL (extracorporeal piezoelectric lithotriptor)
Swiss lithoclast

lithotrite—an instrument used to grasp and crush large stones occurring in the bladder.

litmus test—for acidity and alkalinity. Cf. *Titmus test*.

LITT (laser-induced thermotherapy).

Littleford/Spector introducer—allows the rapid and atraumatic insertion of one or more permanent pacemaker electrodes into the heart using a peel-away sheath in the subclavian vein. Also known as *subclavian peel-away sheath, permanent lead introducer*.

Little League elbow (also *pitcher's elbow*)—a condition that affects professional baseball players. It is now seen in children ages 7 to 15 years whose coaches and parents encourage more training time. Little League players are at greater risk than professionals because they overtrain when they throw, relax their elbows less quickly, and do not have the arm strength of older players.

littoral cell angioma—benign vascular tumor unique to the spleen. Patients present clinically with splenomegaly, thrombocytopenia, or anemia. In many cases the tumor is discovered incidentally during abdominal surgery performed for another reason.

Littre, glands of—glands in the distal urethra of the male where gonococcal infection usually begins.

"live flesh"—a term used by patients to describe their condition of having multiple fasciculations.

liver-directed ex vivo gene therapy—treatment for homozygous familial hypercholesterolemia.

liver flap—asterixis; a coarse flapping tremor of the hands, so called be-

liver flap *(cont.)*
cause it is often seen in hepatic failure.

liver function tests (LFTs).

Livernois lens-holding forceps—having thin jaws for use in insertion of thin soft intraocular lenses.

Livernois-McDonald forceps—for use in ophthalmic surgical procedures.

liver palms—intense redness of the hypothenar and thenar eminences, suggestive of cirrhosis of the liver on physical examination.

Liver Panel Plus 9—trade name for a reagent disc product that is designed to measure hepatic function.

liver span (the size of the liver)—the distance between the upper and lower limits of hepatic dullness, as determined by percussion. Normal range is 6 to 12 cm, depending upon the age, sex, and size of the patient.

Livewire TC ablation catheter—electrophysiologic catheter for diagnosis and treatment of supraventricular tachycardia.

Livostin (levocabastine HCl).

LJP-394—drug for treatment of lupus erythematosus.

LLC (labrum-ligament complex).

LLETZ (large loop excision of the transformation zone).

L-leucovorin—a drug used with the antibiotic Bactrim in treating AIDS patients who have *Pneumocystis carinii* pneumonia.

Llorente dissecting forceps—used with EndoMed laparoscopic systems.

Lloyd-Davies scissors.

LLPDD (late luteal phase dysphoric disorder).

LLS (lazy leukocyte syndrome).

LMA-Unique—a disposable laryngeal mask airway used in elective surgery and for emergency cases.

LM-427 (rifabutin, Mycobutin)—for prevention of *Mycobacterium avium* complex (MAC) in advanced HIV patients.

LMR (localized magnetic resonance)—MRI term.

loading dose—an initial dose of a medication, larger than the subsequent maintenance doses, given in order to achieve effective blood and tissue levels promptly.

loath (adj.)—reluctant, unwilling. "The patient is loath to undertake surgery at this time, so we will follow her closely for a while longer." Cf. *loathe*.

loathe (verb)—dislike intensely; hate; detest. Cf. *loath*.

localizing or **focal neurological signs**—indicate the location of a lesion to the neurologist. See *soft neurological signs*.

Lochol—over-the-counter plant pharmaceutical shown to have the potential of significantly reducing harmful levels of cholesterol and triglycerides, while improving the ratio of HDL to LDL in the blood stream.

Locilex topical cream (pexiganan acetate)—topical antibiotic therapy of infected diabetic ulcers, made from the skin of frogs.

Locke clamp—used in podiatric surgery to grasp the phalanx, metatarsal, or sesamoid.

locked-in syndrome—complete paralysis due to brain stem injury. The patient cannot communicate but is thought to remain fully conscious.

locker room syndrome—see *isovaleric acidemia*.

loculated effusion—on chest x-ray, a collection of fluid in the pleural space; its distribution is limited by

loculated effusion *(cont.)*
adjacent normal or abnormal structures.

locus of HLA (human leukocyte antigen)—used in tissue typing for transplants. Each HLA locus (A, B, C, D, or DR) contains multiple alleles. Some 19 alleles have thus far been identified at locus A, 20 at locus B, 8 at locus C, 10 at locus D, and 10 at locus DR. These are written HLA-C8, HLA-DR2, etc. (no subscript or superscript).

Lodine; Lodine XL (etodolac)—analgesic and anti-inflammatory drug.

lodoxamide tromethamine (Alomide) —for vernal keratoconjunctivitis. An ophthalmic mast cell stabilizer available, it inhibits hypersensitivity reactions in the eye, combining the anti-inflammatory action of a corticosteroid with the antiallergic action of an antihistamine.

Löffler's syndrome (also Loeffler)— chronic eosinophilic pneumonia.

logorrhea—extreme loquacity; a copious flow of talk, often incoherent.

loin pain hematuria syndrome (LPHS) —occurs mostly in women. Symptoms of LPHS include loin pain and hematuria, usually bilateral, and often accompanied by dysuria and low-grade fever. LPHS is difficult to diagnose because renal function is normal, urine cultures are negative, and IVPs and renal biopsies are negative. The true cause is unknown and the diagnosis is made by excluding other pathologies. The pain can become so severe that nerve blockade, nephrectomy, and even renal transplantation have been tried as treatments. Narcotics for pain relief remain the only effective therapy.

LOM (low-osmolar media) (Radiol). Cf. *HOM, ionic contrast media.* See *nonionic contrast media.*

Lone Star retractor—used to facilitate surgical access during a mucosal proctectomy and said to eliminate the need for anal dilatation and the use of a Gelpi retractor. Produced by Lone Star Medical Products of Houston, Texas, this self-retaining retractor encircles the anus and uses eight elastic holders, or stays, around the anal circumference (which gives the instrument a star-shaped appearance) to hold back all edges of the anal canal.

long-acting thyroid-stimulating hormone (LATS).

long-echo-train fast spin-echo sequence—MRI term.

longitudinal magnetization; relaxation—MRI terms.

longitudinal melanonychia—a mole-like lesion of the nail matrix that mimics the appearance of malignant melanoma. Excision is usually performed to rule out malignancy. It is rare and more common in non-Caucasians.

long taper/stiff shaft Glidewire—used in coronary artery imaging.

long-term nonprogressors—individuals with HIV who have had at least 10 years of seropositivity, without symptoms or T-cell depletion, in the absence of therapy.

long tract—the main spinal nerve fibers and their pathways connecting the spinal cord and the brain. See *long tract signs.*

long tract signs—seen in patients with upper neuron damage. Include the upgoing great toe on the Babinski, twitching of the thumb on the

long tract signs *(cont.)*
Hoffmann, and twitching of the chin on the palmomental test.

long TR/TE (also, *T2 weighted*)—MRI term. TR (repetition time); TE (echo time).

lonidamine—chemotherapy drug.

loop—oval, closed or nearly closed turn in a tube, suture, rope, or figure. Example: loop of bowel, sentinel loop. Cf. *loupe*.

loop electrosurgical excision procedure (LEEP)—used to treat precancerous lesions of the cervix, in addition to laser and cryosurgery techniques. A wire loop through which radio waves are conducted is used to excise cervical tissue. Both cryosurgery and laser surgery destroy the precancerous tissue, but LEEP allows cervical specimens to be excised and examined by the pathologist.

loopogram—ileostogram.

Looser's zones—in insufficiency fractures.

LoPro—right angle ArthroWand.

Lorabid (loracarbef).

loracarbef (Lorabid)—an antibiotic drug used to treat ENT, pulmonary, skin, and urinary tract infections.

LORAD StereoGuide stereotactic breast biopsy system.

loratadine (Claritin)—long-acting, nonsedating antihistamine, taken orally once a day.

Lorcet 10/650—an oral narcotic and analgesic combination of hydrocodone and acetaminophen used to treat moderate to severe pain.

Lord total hip prosthesis—uses no cement; instead, its rough surface stimulates growth of new bone in the medullary canal, and the growth of new cancellous bone incorporates the prosthesis into the structure of the limb. Also known as *madreporic hip*.

Lorentzian line—MRI term.

Lorenz PC/TC scissors ultrasharp knife (Surg).

Lortat-Jacob hepatic resection—used to gain initial vascular control prior to liver resection by ligating the hepatic artery, the portal vein, and the hepatic veins, followed by liver parenchymal transection.

losartan potassium HCl (Hyzaar).

Losec (omeprazole)—trade name which was changed to Prilosec to avoid confusion with Lasix. See *omeprazole*.

Lotemax (loteprednol etabonate ophthalmic suspension 0.5%)—an ophthalmic topical steroid.

Lotensin (benazepril).

Lotrel (amlodipine besylate)—once-a-day dosing for treatment of hypertension.

Lotronex (alosetron HCl)—developed specifically for treatment of symptoms of irritable bowel syndrome in women.

"lottery fantasy" syndrome—a form of psychological depression that can occur in lottery purchasers when they think they will win and don't.

Louis-Bar's syndrome—ataxia telangiectasia.

loupe ("loop")—convex lens in a short tube, used for magnifying or for concentrating light on an object. Used by ophthalmologists, microsurgeons, and jewelers. Cf. *loop*.

Lovaas program—behavior modification technique for the treatment of autism, based on the work of Ivar Lovaas.

Lovenox (enoxaparin)—a low molecular weight heparin. It is an injectable antithrombotic administered postoperatively in hip replacement surgery for prevention of deep vein thrombosis.

Lovibond's angle—the angle at which the fingernail meets the finger, normally less than 180°, but exceeding this in clubbing of the fingers.

Low-Beers projection (Radiol).

low-density lipoprotein (LDL)—the so-called "bad" cholesterol linked with arteriosclerosis and myocardial infarctions. This is a plasma protein which carries cholesterol through the blood. At high levels it increases risk of arteriosclerosis and heart attack. Cf. *high-density lipoprotein*.

low-dose interferon—a less costly and less toxic alternative to high-dose interferon. Interferon plays a critical role in immune system modulation. Low-dose interferon is used or under study in the treatment of AIDS, hepatitis, Sjögren's syndrome, lupus, and more.

low-dose screen-film technique—a radiographic technique designed to provide adequate imaging with less radiation than conventionally.

low-energy lasers (LELs)—used in sports medicine to promote healing and reduce pain associated with tendinitis, bursitis, tennis elbow, and other musculoskeletal injuries. May be used to stimulate cellular repair and treat wounds and soft tissue disorders, arthritis, and peripheral neuropathies. The infrared gallium arsenide and the visible helium-neon (HeNe) lasers are the most common LELs. Also called *cold, low-power*, or *soft lasers*, *low-intensity laser therapy*.

lower extremity noninvasive (LENI).

lower soft-tissue attenuation of the accordion sign (Rad)—represents marked thickening of the haustral folds due to intramural edema.

Lowe's syndrome—inborn error of metabolism resulting in mental retardation, cataracts and glaucoma, muscular dystrophy, and renal tubular defect for amino acids.

low-grade squamous intraepithelial lesion (LGSIL).

low-intensity laser therapy (LILT)—see *low-energy lasers*.

low-intensity pulsed ultrasound—found to promote fracture healing. This is the diagnostic range ultrasound, not the usual higher-frequency therapeutic ultrasound.

Lown-Ganong-Levine syndrome—a combination of short P-R interval and short QRS complex demonstrated by electrocardiography, and including paroxysmal tachycardia.

low-osmolar media—see *high-osmolar media*.

low-range heparin management test (LHMT).

low-resistance rolling seal spirometer.

low signal intensity—MRI term.

low-surface reactive bioglass—a bioceramic joint replacement material.

low-tension glaucoma (Oph)—occurs with a sudden increase in pressure in the eye, with resulting damage to the optic nerve.

low urethral pressure (LUP).

low-voltage microampere stimulation (LV-MS, microcurrent)—similar to TENS, considered experimental for the relief of pain.

Lp(a)—an apolipoprotein (cholesterol-carrying protein) that has been found to be a separate and distinct risk factor (besides total serum cholesterol

Lp(a) *(cont.)*
and triglycerides, smoking, hypertension) for premature atherosclerotic peripheral vascular disease. Lp(a) levels, measured by electroimmunoassay, greater than 30 mg/dL, are considered a risk factor.

LPI (Laser Photonics, Inc.) **laser system**—an excimer laser system for treatment of psoriasis.

LPPS (low-pressure plasma spray) **hydroxyapatite**—for cementless fixation.

LP 2307—potential therapy for malignant melanoma.

LR (length ratio)

LRT (living related transplant).

LRUT (locally made rapid urease test) —a test for detecting *Helicobacter pylori*, the pathogen that can cause duodenal ulcers.

LSA₂L₂—chemotherapy regimen used in treatment of nonlocalized non-Hodgkin's lymphoma in children.

LSIL (low-grade squamous intraepithelial lesion).

L/S ratio—a test on amniotic fluid (by amniocentesis) to determine the maturity of the fetal lungs. Lecithin and sphingomyelin are the two phospholipids which comprise surfactant. Low levels of surfactant contribute to hyaline membrane disease in premature infants. Cf. *lamellar body density count*.

LSRT (lens-sparing external beam radiation therapy).

LSU (Louisiana State University) **reciprocation-gait orthosis**—bracing device for use by paralytic patients or patients who would otherwise be confined to wheelchairs. It gives structural support to the trunk and lower extremities and consists of a system of cables and joint-locking devices.

LTD (laser trabeculodissection).

LTK (laser thermal keratoplasty).

Lubri-Flex stent—a hydrophilic-coated urologic stent with inner lumen hydrogel coating to ensure ease of placement over a guide wire.

lucent defect—abnormal zone of decreased resistance to x-rays.

LUCs (large undifferentiated cells)— may be dictated in the differential leukocyte count.

Ludlof's fleck—intercondylar notch line.

Ludwig's angina—infection of the deep tissues of the neck and floor of the mouth. The resultant swelling can push the tongue up and back, interfering with breathing. Edema of the glottis can occur and the process can be fatal before fluctuation or redness of the neck occurs. Antibiotics have made this a rare condition.

Luhr fixation system.

Lukes-Collins classification—of non-Hodgkin's lymphoma.

LULA (laparoscopy under local anesthesia).

lumbar anterior-root stimulator implant (LARSI)—a surgically placed device that stimulates the roots of the lower spinal nerves supplying the muscles of the leg. It is hoped the LARSI implant will enable some paraplegic patients to stand with support and walk short distances.

Lumina guide wire—coated guide wire with radiopaque gold markings.

Lumiscan 150 scanner.

Lumiwand—light used in eye examination.

LUNA (laparoscopic uterine nerve ablation)—procedure for treatment

LUNA (*cont.*)
of pelvic pain by disruption of the uterine nerves.

LUNA (laser uterosacral nerve ablation).

lunate prosthesis—for the lunate bone of the wrist, fashioned of acrylic cement.

Lund Browder burn diagram, modified—diagram of the anterior and posterior aspects of the human body, divided into segments; used in estimating the percentage of burned body tissue area. One of these diagrams is made at each surgery, to show the areas covered with skin, skin grafts, donor sites, biosynthetic grafts, or xenografts. These will provide a continuous picture of the progress of the coverage of the burn wounds. Note: No hyphen in *Lund Browder.*

Lunderquist guide wires (*not* Linderquist)—used with a Chiba needle for percutaneous stone manipulation, and in catheter cholangiography. Also, *Chiba needle, fine needle, Skinny needle.*

Lunderquist-Ring torque guide—used in catheter cholangiography, and in maintaining long-term percutaneous antegrade biliary drainage.

Lunelle (estradiol cypionate and medroxyprogesterone acetate)—a once-a-month injectable contraceptive.

lung volume reduction surgery (LVRS)—involves an innovative surgical stapling technique for removing emphysematous lung tissue, using bovine pericardium strips to reinforce surgical staple lines and thus prevent persistent air leaks along the staple lines.

lunula (pl., lunulae)—crescent-shaped light-colored area at the base of the fingernail. "Examination of the thumb reveals swelling and tenderness over the lunula and paronychial margin medially, with some pus seen under the nail."

LUP (low urethral pressure) (Urol).

lupus pernio—seen in sarcoidosis as violaceous, shiny patches on the skin of the face, fingers, and toes.

Luque rods and sublaminar wires—used in spinal fusion for scoliosis.

LUS (laparoscopic ultrasound).

Lusk instruments—for pediatric endoscopic sinus surgery.

Lustra (hydroquinone)—for treatment of ultraviolet-induced skin discolorations and hyperpigmentation associated with pregnancy, superficial trauma, the use of oral contraceptives, and hormone replacement therapy.

lutein—yellow pigment from the corpus luteum. Lutein change in the ovary is revealed by the amount of lutein remaining of an egg cell which secretes hormones to support a pregnancy.

luteinizing hormone-releasing hormone. See *LHRH, GnRH.*

Lutrepulse (gonadorelin acetate).

Lutrin—photosensitizer for photodynamic therapy of patients with recurrent breast cancer to the chest wall.

Luvox (fluvoxamine maleate)—used for treatment of depression and obsessive-compulsive disorders.

Luxiq (betamethasone valerate)—treatment for chronic dermatoses of the scalp.

Luxtec fiberoptic system—a fiberoptic light source for diagnostic and surgical visualization; used with arthroscopes and endoscopes.

luxury perfusion (Neuro)—abnormally increased flow of blood to an area of the brain, leading to swelling. Causes include trauma, nearby cerebral infarction, and epileptogenic focus.

LVAS (left ventricular assist system) **implantable pump**. See *HeartMate*; *Novacor*.

L-Vax—autologous therapeutic cancer vaccine for leukemia.

LVOTO (left ventricular outflow tract obstruction).

LVRS (lung volume reduction surgery).

LX 20 laser—used in skin rejuvenation procedures.

Lyme disease ("*lime*")—named for Old Lyme, Connecticut, where the disease, transmitted by the bite of the deer tick, was first recognized. The infectious agent is the spirochete, *Borrelia burgdorferi*. The first manifestations of Lyme disease are a skin rash at the site of the bite, chills, fever, flu-like symptoms, drowsiness, fatigue, joint swelling, headache, which responds to antibiotics. There may be a second stage of the disease, with cardiac irregularities, meningitis symptoms, and, rarely, paralysis. Third-stage symptoms are arthritis, and occasionally skin and neurologic manifestations.

Lyme lymphocytic meningoradiculitis —causes respiratory failure in patients with Lyme disease. Also called *Garin-Bujadoux-Bannwarth syndrome*.

LYMErix—recombinant protein vaccine against *Borrelia burgdorferi*, organism that causes Lyme disease.

lym-1 monoclonal antibody—labeled with iodine 131. Used to treat B-cell lymphoma.

lymphadenopathy syndrome (LAS)—considered by some to be a prodrome to development of AIDS.

lymphapheresis—removal of peripheral blood lymphocytes; used on an experimental basis as pretreatment in rejection of liver transplants.

Lymphazurin (isosulfan blue)—a diagnostic aid for lymphangiography.

Lymphedema Alert bracelet—worn by breast cancer survivors to protect them from receiving treatment to their affected arm or arms that could trigger onset of lymphedema. Treatments triggering the problem include blood pressure measurements, injections, blood draws, and chemotherapy.

lymphedema praecox—the classic form of primary lymphedema, seen mostly in young women in their early twenties.

lymph node location system of the neck—developed by the Memorial Sloan-Kettering Group:
Level I—submental group and submandibular group
Level II—upper jugular group
Level III—middle jugular group
Level IV—lower jugular group
Level V—posterior triangle group
Level VI—anterior compartment group

lymphoblastoid interferon, human (L-IFN)—potential treatment for hepatitis C cirrhosis.

LymphoCide—human antibody product for use in treatment of non-Hodgkin's lymphoma.

lymphocyte activating factor (LAF)—see *interleukin-1*.

lymphocytic choriomeningitis virus (LCMV)—arenavirus seen in intrauterine LCMV infection, causing

lymphocytic *(cont.)*
fetal or neonatal death, as well as hydrocephalus and chorioretinitis in infants. LCMV may be a frequent cause of central nervous system disease in newborns.

lymphocytic interstitial pneumonitis (LIP)—once a rare pulmonary disease and now seen more frequently in AIDS patients.

lymphogranuloma venereum (LGV) —caused by a strain of *Chlamydia*. Also called *fifth venereal disease*.

lymphokines—a group of substances produced by various stimulated cells of the immune system, which include interferons and interleukin-2. See *interleukin-2*.

lymphoscintigraphy—peritumor injection of filtered technetium sulfur colloid, followed by gamma camera scanning. It is used to document nodal basins at risk for metastatic breast cancer. Images are obtained of the breast, sternum, and axilla.

Lynch and Crues Type 2 lesion—seen in the knee on MRI scan when the subchondral plate is interrupted.

lyodura loop—used in colpopexy or colporrhaphy to fix a prolapsed vaginal vault to promontory cartilage.

LYOfoam dressing—its gas-permeable design reduces wound maceration. Also, *LYOfoam C* and *LYOfoam tracheostomy dressings*.

Lyo-Ject—a syringe used in the administration of injectable Cardizem.

lyophilized—freeze-dried, as in frozen corneal tissue used for lamellar keratoplasty.

LyP (lymphomatoid papulosis).

Lyra laser system—for treatment of leg veins. The extended pulse duration technology may be used for hair removal.

Lyrelle patch—for treatment of vasomotor symptoms related to menopause. See also *HRT patch*.

Lysholm knee score—a subjective evaluation system with eight categories: instability, pain, locking, swelling, support, limp, stairs, and squatting. Used in association with tests like Lachman, drawer, pivot-shift.

lyssa inclusion body (lowercase *l*)— found in rabies. Also, *Negri body*.

lytic lesion (or osteolytic)—a disease or abnormality resulting from or consisting of focal breakdown of bone, with reduction in density.

M, m

m (meta-stable)—in technetium, as in ^{99m}Tc or Tc 99m.

MAA (^{99m}Tc-MAA, macroaggregated albumin)—used in a technetium perfusion lung scan in nuclear medicine.

Maalox HRF (heartburn relief formula)—a specially formulated Maalox to relieve heartburn.

MAb, MoAB, MOAB (monoclonal antibody).

MAb-170—a monoclonal antibody for surgical detection of breast cancer.

MabThera (rituximab)—monoclonal antibody treatment for patients with non-Hodgkin's lymphoma.

MAC (methotrexate, actinomycin D, and cyclophosphamide)—chemotherapy protocol for metastatic gestational trophoblastic neoplasm.

MAC (Miami Acute Care) collar—for cervical support.

MAC (minimal alveolar concentration of an anesthetic agent).

MAC (monitored anesthesia care)—local infiltration.

Macewen's ("mak-u′enz") sign—written with lowercase first *e*. See *cracked pot sign*.

machinery murmur—a rumbling cardiac murmur, continuous through systole and diastole with only slight variation in pitch and intensity. It is heard in patent ductus arteriosus.

MACHO (methotrexate, asparaginase, cyclophosphamide, hydroxydaunomycin, Oncovin)—chemotherapy protocol.

MAC (*Mycobacterium avium* complex) infection—frequently seen in AIDS patients. Also called *Battey-avium complex*.

Mackay-Marg tonometer—measures intraocular pressure.

MacKinnon-Dellon Diskriminator—an instrument used to assess two-point discrimination.

Macritonin—peptide drug, salmon calcitonin, used in treatment of osteoporosis.

macro-, a prefix meaning large or abnormally big in size. Cf. *micro-*.

macrodacryocystography—see *digital subtraction macrodacryocystography.*

macrolides—a class of antibiotics similar in effectiveness to penicillin and erythromycin but with fewer side

macrolides *(cont.)* effects. Particularly effective against *Mycoplasma pneumoniae* and resistant strains of *Haemophilus influenzae.* Examples: clarithromycin (Biaxin) and troleandomycin (Tao).

macro-orchidism lesion (Urol).

macrophage colony-forming cells (M-CFC).

Macroplastique implant—placed between the midurethra and the bladder neck to resolve or diminish stress urinary incontinence by augmenting the function of the bladder neck sphincteric mechanism.

macroscopic magnetization vector.

Macrotec (technetium ^{99m}Tc medronate).

macula—a spot or area which can be distinguished by color or other characteristic from surrounding tissue; often refers to the macula retinae.

macular degeneration—see *"dry" age-related macular degeneration* and *"wet" age-related macular degeneration.*

macular fan; macular star—a fan- or star-shaped folding or pleating of the retina due to edema.

macular rash (Derm).

Madayag biopsy needle—used for fine-needle percutaneous aspiration/biopsy, percutaneous pancreatic aspiration biopsy, renal cystic puncture, and soft tissue biopsy.

mad cow disease—see *bovine spongiform encephalopathy.*

Maddacrawler—an adjustable tubular crawler frame with attached pad. It supports the abdomen of a child while the legs and arms are free to touch the floor and initiate movement. Assists crawling motions for children in therapy.

Madden technique—for repair of incisional hernia.

MADDOC (mechlorethamine, Adriamycin, dacarbazine, DDP [cisplatin], Oncovin, cyclophosphamide)—chemotherapy protocol for neuroblastoma.

Maddox rod test (Oph)—assesses the degree of muscle dysfunction.

Madigan prostatectomy—a procedure in which adenomatous tissue is removed from outside the urethra which is preserved intact, so that the urinary tract is not entered.

madreporic coral (Madrepora group, genus *Porites*)—a substitute for autologous bone in cranial reproduction, in bur holes, and even larger implants. A coral graft can be at least partially ossified, and with its use, incisions for harvesting rib or iliac crest grafts are unnecessary (thus obviating the pain and the risk of infection), and the operative procedure takes less time to perform. The coral is prepared for use by ultrasonic treatment and is then cut into cone-shaped plugs for bur holes, and in various-sized blocks which can be cut and shaped intraoperatively. See *Biocoral.*

madreporic hip prosthesis—see *Lord total hip prosthesis* and *madreporic coral.* Also called *madreporic trochanterodiaphysary support system.*

Madura foot—a rare fungal infection of the feet, seen in farm workers who work without shoes.

Maffucci's syndrome—characterized by enchondromatosis, hemangiomatosis, and malignant tumors.

MAFH (multicentric angiofollicular hyperplasia).

Magerl technique—for screw placement in lower cervical spine.

"magic angle" artifact (MRI)—noted to occur when curving structures such as tendons assume an angle of 55° to the bore of the magnet. Other views can confirm that the "lesion" seen is artifactual.

MagnaPod—pain relief magnets. The system features thin magnets that are said to increase blood circulation; they are marketed with elastic braces for application on arms, wrists, legs, and back.

MAGneedle controllers.

Magnes 2500 WH (whole head) **imager**.

Magnetic Controlled Suturing (MCS) (trademark).

magnetic field gradients (MFG).

magnetic resonance angiography (MRA)—gated inflow technique.

magnetic resonance cholangiography (MRC)—uses three-dimensional fast spin-echo technology. Used increasingly in neonates and infants to detect biliary atresia, congenital choledochal dilatation, and biliary complications in hepatic transplantation.

magnetic resonance cholangiography with HASTE (half-fourier acquisition single-shot turbo spin-echo).

magnetic resonance elastography (MRE)—combines sound waves with magnetic resonance imaging to noninvasively quantify and "visually feel" the hardness of tissues within a patient's body.

magnetic resonance imaging (MRI)—noninvasive radiologic procedure for imaging tissues of high fat and water content that cannot be seen with other radiologic techniques. An MRI image gives information about the chemical makeup of tissues, thus making it possible to distinguish normal, cancerous, atherosclerotic, and traumatized tissue masses in the image. It can measure vessel flow and does not involve ionizing radiation. Formerly called *nuclear magnetic resonance imaging* (NMR). For a quick-reference list of terms, see *MRI terms*.

magnetic resonance mammography (MRM)—useful in detecting silicone rupture, the need for biopsy for cancer, and in cancer staging.

magnetic resonance neurography (MRN).

magnetic resonance spectroscopy (MRS)—a noninvasive technique to study the body chemistry, using magnetism and radio waves, without radiation or needles. The patient is placed within a large circular magnet (as in magnetic resonance imaging), and radio waves are beamed toward the patient. The body's atoms are excited by these waves, and the radiofrequency of each chemical is interpreted by computer, which thus maps out the chemical components of each area. Chemical changes caused by heart attack or stroke can be detected quickly. The MRS may prove useful in studying changes in muscle of patients with multiple sclerosis and could lead to new forms of therapy.

magnetic resonance urography (MRU).

magnetic source imaging (MSI)—uses ultrasensitive antenna to detect the magnetic field in the human body and provides noninvasive information about neurological and cardiac functions. Also called *3-D MSI*.

magnetic stimulation—a treatment for nonunion of fractures in which electric, or magnetic, currents stimulate more rapid regrowth of bone in cases of failure of healing in fractures of long bones. A noninvasive means of treatment that may avoid the necessity of surgery and possible bone grafting. See *EBI bone healing system, OrthoGen/OsteoGen*.

Magnetic Surgery System—uses external magnetic fields to direct a magnet-tipped flexible catheter to a target within the brain along a specific route planned by the surgeon. The surgeon can thus map out a pathway that maneuvers around vital brain areas instead of going through them, in order to perform such procedures as tissue biopsy.

magnetic susceptibility artifact—an air-tissue interface, such as at the sella turcica or temporal bones, can produce a bright band or focal distortion.

magnetoencephalogram (MEG)—used in the diagnosis of epilepsy. MEG technique can record the location, depth, orientation, and polarity of magnetic spike field strength in epileptic patients.

Magnetom MRI system—open design that eases the anxiety often caused patients by a closed system. It permits kinematic joint studies and allows for visualization of blood flow and cardiac motion.

Magnevist (gadopentetate dimeglumine) —contrast medium for MRI.

Magnum guide wire—used in coronary angioplasty.

MAGPI (meatal advancement, glanuloplasty, penoscrotal junction meatotomy) **operation**—an acronym for a procedure to correct hypospadias. Pronounced "magpie," like the bird.

Ma-Griffith end-to-end anastomosis— repairs a lacerated Achilles tendon.

Magrina-Bookwalter vaginal retractor—provides exposure of the vagina for surgical procedures; it can expand for use in multiple surgical fields. See *Bookwalter retractor*.

Mahaim bundle in the heart—a term used in electrophysiologic studies of supraventricular tachycardia.

Maico Gamma programmable hearing aids.

Maico-MA 20 audiometer—used to perform bedside audiography.

MAI (*Mycobacterium avium-intracellulare*) **infection**—a TB variant once considered not to be a pathogen in humans, but now appearing as disseminated tuberculosis in AIDS patients. "The patient was referred for ongoing management of HIV-related issues, including MAI bacteremia." Cf. *MAC infection*.

main d'accoucheur ("obstetrician's hand")—the position in tetany that the hand assumes after a positive Trousseau's sign (carpopedal spasm). See *Trousseau's sign*.

main magnetic field inhomogeneity artifact (Radiol)—a hardware artifact in which poor shimming of the MRI magnet can produce distortions of image appearance. A square-appearing object can thus appear barrel-shaped, cushion-shaped, or trapezoidal.

Mainstay urologic soft tissue anchor.

Mainster retina laser lens—for panretinal photocoagulation and focal laser therapy.

maintain—to control or limit the effects of an illness or abnormal state with diet, medicine, or other means.

Mainz pouch urinary reservoir—a urinary pouch made from a combination of cecum and ileum. Pronounced "mintz" with a long *i*.

MAIPA (monoclonal-antibody-specific immobilization of platelet antigens) **assay**.

Makler insemination device—for intrauterine insemination.

MAK-6 (monoclonal anticytokeratin)—cocktail that identifies normal and malignant cells of epithelial origin to facilitate identification of poorly differentiated epithelial malignancies.

malacoplakia of kidney—rare granulomatous disorder of unknown etiology simulating malignancy.

maladie-de-Roger (Fr., "ro-zhay," Roger's disease)—congenital defect of the interventricular septum of the heart.

malaria—infectious febrile disease characterized by periodic paroxysms of fever, chills, and sweating. It is caused by four species of protozoa of the genus *Plasmodium* (*P. vivax, P. falciparum, P. malariae*, and *P. ovale*), parasitic in the red blood cells, and transmitted to the bloodstream of humans by the bite of Anopheles mosquitoes. Cf. *miliaria*.

Malassezia furfur **pustulosis**—nonfollicular pustulosis of the newborn, caused by a pathogenic yeast. Cf. *neonatal acne; sebaceous miliaria*.

Malbran approach—in transscleral fixation of intraocular lens.

Malcolm-Lynn C-RXF cervical retractor frame—a system of cervical retractors made of a carbon composite that is radiolucent rather than radiopaque as are standard metal retractors. These retractors are used during neurosurgical procedures that require intraoperative x-ray visualization of fixation devices.

male pattern baldness—characteristic thinning of hair along the temples, front, and back of the head in men. Also called *male pattern alopecia*. See also *hippocratic wreath*.

Malgaigne's fracture—bilateral vertical pelvic fracture.

malignant mixed tumor—see *carcinoma ex pleomorphic adenoma*.

Malis CMC-II bipolar coagulator—used with Malis irrigation forceps, and irrigation module, for irrigation, coagulation, and cutting.

malleable retractor (Surg).

Malleoloc anatomic ankle orthosis—used to prevent excessive inversion and eversion.

malleolus—the rounded lateral projections of the bone at the ankle. See *malleus*.

mallet toe—flexion contracture of the distal joints of the second, third, fourth, and fifth toes.

malleus—the outermost of the three small bones in the ear. Cf. *malleolus*.

malleus nipper—a surgical instrument used in ear surgery.

Mallinckrodt Laser-Flex tube—stainless steel, laser-resistant endotracheal tube.

Mallinckrodt sensor systems—for in vitro diagnostic blood gas and electrolyte evaluation.

Mallory-Azan stain—a special stain for collagen fiber.

Mallory-Head modular calcar system.

Mallory's PTAH (phosphotungstic acid-hematoxylin)—see *PTAH*.

Mallory-Weiss tear—a tear in the mucosa at the cardioesophageal junction, generally caused by retching or

Mallory-Weiss tear *(cont.)*
vomiting, resulting in upper GI bleed.

Malmstrom cup (Ob-Gyn)—attached to a vacuum source to facilitate vacuum-assisted vaginal deliveries.

Maloney endo-otoprobe—laser probe used in ear surgery.

malpighian corpuscles—urine-forming units in renal cortex of kidneys; aggregations of lymphoid tissue in white pulp of spleen.

MALT (mucosa-associated lymphoid tissue) **lymphoma** or **MALT tumor**. See *MALToma*.

MALToma—mucosa-associated lymphoid tissue lymphoma, a low-grade B-cell lymphoma.

mammaplasty—see *mammoplasty*.

mammastatin—a protein that controls abnormal cell growth in breast tissue. Found in healthy breast tissue but absent or reduced in breast cancer patients, mammastatin is being developed for use in the treatment of advanced-stage breast cancer.

mammography
contoured tilting compression
CT laser (CTLM)
step-oblique

mammoplasty—plastic augmentation or reduction reconstruction of the breast. Also spelled *mammaplasty*.

MammoSite RTS (radiation therapy system)—single-use catheter and radiation solution source used to deliver local radiation therapy to the tissue surrounding a resected malignant breast tumor. After the tumor is resected, the catheter is inserted into the tumor cavity before surgical closure. Once the patient has recovered from surgery, the radiation liquid (Iotrex) is delivered through the catheter to provide local radiation therapy directly to the tumor cavity. When the treatment is completed, the radiation source and catheter are removed.

Mammotest system—a breast biopsy system by Fischer Imaging that allows accurate localization of small breast lesions for placement of a core biopsy needle for histologic sampling.

Mammotome—a new handheld version of a minimally invasive breast biopsy device. It employs computer technology to replace open surgical procedures.

m-AMSA (amsacrine)—a drug used in treatment of acute adult leukemia.

Mancini plates—referred to in quantitation of immunoglobulins, as: "Mancini plates showed IgA 72 g/L, IgG 2.5 g/L."

Mandibular Excursiometer—for measuring mandibular excursion on the X and Y axis in the coronal plane during active opening during temporomandibular joint treatment.

mandrin, wire—a probe, stylet, or guide for a catheter. Examples:
coudé curve
Guyon-Benique curve
malleable tip
Van Buren curve

maneuver—see *operation*.

manic-depressive—see *bipolar affective illness*.

manifest refraction (Oph).

manipulated autologous structure (MAS) cells.

manofluorography (MFG)—simultaneous fluoroscopy and manometric evaluation of pharyngeal swallowing and dysphagia. The swallowing events (as seen by fluoroscopy) and

manofluorography *(cont.)*
the pressure generated during swallowing (manometry) are displayed simultaneously on a screen. See *deglutition mechanism, peristaltic wave.*

Mantoux test—an intradermal tuberculin test. Read at 48 to 72 hours after injection, induration of more than 10 mm in diameter at the injection site is considered positive.

MAP (mean arterial pressure).

maple bark stripper's disease—extrinsic allergic alveolitis caused by exposure to moldy maple bark.

maple leaf flap—used in gynecological reconstruction of vulvar deformities.

maple-syrup urine disease (MSUD)—caused by a defect in metabolism of the ketoacid analogs of leucine, isoleucine, and valine. The maple-syrup odor in the urine is caused by the presence of these compounds.

MAPs (microtubule-associated proteins).

Maquet ("muh-kay'") **technique**—advancement of the tibial tuberosity by elevation of the tibial crest.

Marathon guiding catheter—used during coronary angioplasty.

Marburg fever—Ebola-like hemorrhagic fever currently active in Africa. See also *Ebola virus.*

march fracture (not an eponym)—a fracture of the shaft of the second or third metatarsal bone without a history of injury.

Marchiafava-Bignami disease—uncommon demyelination of the corpus callosum.

Marcus Gunn syndrome ("jaw winking")—unilateral ptosis of the eyelid, with association of movements of the affected upper eyelid with those of the jaw. Named for Robert Marcus

Gunn, an English ophthalmologist. Note: There is no hyphen in the name.

Marie's ataxia—a hereditary disease of the nervous system.

marimastat—an oral antineoplastic taken to prevent tumors from metastasizing.

Marinol (dronarinol)—an antiemetic drug given with chemotherapy; also used to treat loss of appetite in AIDS patients. The active ingredient is derived from the marijuana plant.

marital—pertaining to marriage, as in "marital relationship" or "marital introitus." Cf. *martial.* These are often confused. It is, of course, entirely possible that both adjectives could apply to the same relationship.

marker—see also *gene marker; tumor marker; markers, refractive surgery.*
AFP (alpha-fetoprotein)
ALZ-50 (Alzheimer's disease)
Arrowsmith corneal
Berkeley optic zone
Bores radial
CA1-18 tumor
CA 15-3 tumor
CA 19-9 tumor
CA 72-4 tumor
cathepsin D
CEA (carcinoembryonic antigen)
chromosome tumor 14q
DNA polymerase-alpha
DSM
Freeman cookie cutter areola
Friedländer arcuate
Friedländer transverse incision
G6PD cell
HLA-DR4 genetic
Ki-67
Lindstrom arcuate incision
lipid-associated sialic acid
McDonald optic zone

marker *(cont.)*
   nicked free beta subunit of human chorionic gonadotropin
   Nordan-Ruiz trapezoidal
   P-glycoprotein gene
   PLAP serum
   PSA (prostate-specific antigen)
   sigmaS serum tumor
   Storz radial incision
   Thornton 360° arcuate
   tripe palm
   tumor

markers, refractive surgery (Oph):
   Arrowsmith corneal
   Berkeley optic zone
   Lindstrom arcuate incision
   Lindstrom small incision
   McDonald optic zone
   Nordan-Ruiz trapezoidal

Mark IV Moss—decompression-feeding catheter.

Markov chain Monte Carlo technique—a method of probability calculation rather than an imaging technique. You may hear this in the future as PACS workstations become more commonplace.

Marlex—synthetic graft material used in hernioplasties and in other abdominal surgery where the tissues need reinforcement.

Marlex methylmethacrylate sandwich.

Marlow Primus instrument collection—handles, shafts, and tips used for minimally invasive surgery.

Marogen (epoetin beta).

Marquest Respirgard II nebulizer—for aerosolized pentamidine.

MARS (Modular Acetabular Revision System) (trademark).

MARSA (methicillin-aminoglycoside-resistant *Staphylococcus aureus*)—a strain of *S. aureus* which is resistant to methicillin and the aminoglyco-side class of antibiotics (gentamicin, kanamycin, tobramycin). See *MRSA*.

Marshall and Tanner pubertal staging—see *Tanner Developmental Scale*.

Marshall's syndrome—a rare pediatric skin disease that is characterized by acquired, localized neutrophilic dermatitis, followed by loss of elastic tissue in the dermis and cutis laxa. The cause of this syndrome is unknown.

Mark VII cooling vest—worn by some patients with multiple sclerosis to decrease body temperature and temporarily alleviate symptoms of fatigue and poor coordination. The vest was originally designed for NASA astronauts and is attached via a cord to a battery-operated cooling unit.

Mark II Chandler retractor—used to retract soft tissue away from bone during hip and knee surgery.

Mark II Kodros radiolucent awl—used with image intensifier to locate holes in interlocking nails.

Mark II Sorrells—hip arthroplasty retraction system to expose the acetabulum.

Marsupial—an adjustable terrycloth belt with an attachable pouch, used by postmastectomy patients to free their hands from the dangling drains. The pouch-like product can also be used to help patients recovering from cardiac and orthopedic surgeries.

martial—pertaining to war or battle. Cf. *marital*.

Martius flap and fascial sling—used to cover a urethral repair and create a continent urethra.

Martius graft—used in urethral reconstruction.

Martius labial fat pad flap.

Martorell hypertensive ulcer.

Marx bridging plate system—low-profile system that minimizes soft tissue dehiscence on mandibular fixation.

Marx's classification of microtia.

Marx protocol—for treatment of osteoradionecrosis.

Maryland dissector.

MAS (manipulated autologous structure)—living human cells manipulated outside the body and returned to the patient for structural repair or reconstruction. See *Carticel.*

MAS (meconium aspiration syndrome).

Mascot indirect ophthalmoscope.

MASE (microsurgical extraction of sperm from epididymis).

Masimo SET (signal extraction technology)—pulse oximetry designed for accuracy during conditions of low perfusion, bright ambient light, and electrosurgical interference.

Masket technique—a technique for intraocular lens insertion using a 4-7 mm incision with closure involving multiple small, interlaced stitches with the suture knots buried.

mask facies—the expressionless appearance of the face seen in patients with Parkinson's disease.

masking technology—involves the treatment of the donor cells prior to transplantation to prevent T-cell activation. Alteration of initial T-cell recognition confers T-cell anergy and long-term acceptance of the graft.

Mason abdominotranssphincteric resection (Surg).

Mason vertical-banded gastroplasty.

mass effect—the radiographic appearance created by an abnormal mass in or adjacent to the area of study.

massive genital prolapse—mainly affects elderly women.

mass lesion—anything that occupies space within the body and is not normal tissue.

Masson's tumor—papillary endothelial hyperplasia (PEH); also, Masson's vegetant intravascular hemangioendothelioma, Masson's pseudoangiosarcoma, intravascular endothelial proliferation, and intravascular angiomatosis. Now you know why *PEH* seems to be the preferred term.

mast cell—a type of inflammatory cell which releases histamine and is important in allergic reactions.

Master Flow Pumpette—a disposable I.V. pump that maintains I.V. flow rate under changing conditions, i.e., bed height, patient position, and fluctuations in venous pressure.

Master's two-step test—a timed stress test in which the patient climbs and descends two 9-inch steps a given number of times; indicates the degree of decreased coronary artery blood flow and the consequent degree of ischemic heart disease.

MAST (military antishock treatment) **suit**—a pneumatic antishock garment that reverses the effect of shock on the body's blood distirbution by applying external counterpressure to the legs and abdomen. Also called *medical antishock trousers.* One company has trademarked the acronym *MAST.* See *DMAST.*

Masuka staging system, modified—for thymic carcinoma.

maternal blood clot patch therapy—a procedure in which maternal blood is given under ultrasonic guidance to produce a clot patch when amniocentesis is complicated by amniorrhea (escape of amniotic fluid).

maternal serum alpha fetoprotein (MSAFP)—screening performed to identify presence of twins, erroneously dated pregnancies, or fetal demise, and to identify fetal anomalies such as spina bifida and abdominal wall defects.

matricectomy ("may-tris-sec'tum-ee") —excision of nail matrix (nail plate) for chronic nail disease or deformity.

Matritech NMP22—a test kit for bladder cancer.

matrix metalloprotease inhibitor (MMPI)—used orally in cancer treatment. Matrix metalloproteases (MMPs) are natural body chemicals that break down material between cells to make room for new cellular growth. When produced or present at the wrong time, they can break down extracellular matrix that holds cells together, allowing growth of unhealthy tissue, such as cancer and rheumatoid arthritis, by contributing to three processes that lead to progression of cancer: invasion, metastasis, and angiogenesis. An oral MMPI can block these processes, while limiting damage resulting from broad suppression of MMPs. See *Galardin*.

Matroc femoral heads—used for long-term implantation. Utilizes Zyranox zirconia or Vitox alumina ceramic materials.

Matsner median episiotomy and repair.

Mattox maneuver—extensive mobilization of the left colon, left kidney, spleen and tail of the pancreas, and stomach, and reflecting these structures to the midline, in exposure of the suprarenal aorta. Used in treating patients with vascular injuries (hematoma or active hemorrhage) from penetrating abdominal wounds.

mature cataract—a cataract in which the lens is completely opaque or ripe for surgery.

maturity-onset diabetes of the young (MODY).

Mauriceau-Smellie-Veit maneuver— method of delivery of the aftercoming head, with the infant resting on the physician's forearm. Also, *Smellie-Veit, Smellie method, Mauriceau method*.

Maxalt (rizatriptan benzoate)—used to treat migraine headaches. It is said to provide significantly faster relief of pain than sumatriptan and better controls nausea and vomiting.

Maxamine (histamine dihydrochloride) —used in combination with interleukin-2 for treatment of stage IV malignant melanoma.

Maxaquin (lomefloxacin HCl)—an antibiotic taken once a day for three days to treat simple urinary tract infections and lower respiratory tract infections. It may also be used to treat chronic bacterial prostatitis.

MaxCast—fiberglass casting tape consisting of a knitted fiberglass fabric impregnated with a water-activated polyurethane resin. Cf. *Fractura Flex, Gypsona*.

Max FiberScan laser system.

Max Fine tying forceps (Oph)—Max Fine, M.D., ophthalmic surgeon.

Max Force catheter—balloon catheter used to dilate biliary stenosis.

Maxicam (isoxicam)—a nonsteroidal anti-inflammatory used for arthritis.

Maxilift Combi patient-lifting system.

Maxima Forté blood oxygenator.

Maxima II TENS unit—see *TENS*.

Maxim modular knee system.

maximum predicted heart rate (MPHR).

maximum urethral closure pressure (MUCP).

Maxon polyglyconate monofilament suture.

Maxorb alginate wound dressing.

May anatomical bone plates—used to repair proximal humeral fractures.

Mayday distal first metatarsal osteotomy for hallux valgus—a surgical modification of the spike osteotomy of the neck of the first metatarsal. It has the advantages of simplicity, no shortening of the first metatarsal, and no risk of dorsal displacement of the distal fragment.

Mayer-Rokitansky-Kuster-Hauser syndrome—congenital aplasia of the vagina and uterus in women with normal female phenotype and with anatomically and functionally normal ovaries.

Mayfield-Kees headholder (Neuro).

Mayfield three-pin skull clamp—used intraoperatively with a halo ring in cervical spine stabilization in cervical fractures.

Mayo Clinic system for primary biliary cirrhosis—a set of evaluation criteria to determine prognosis for patient survival.

Mayo culdoplasty—fixation of the vaginal vault to the sacrospinous ligament or to the uterosacral ligament.

Mayo-Gibbon heart-lung machine—artificial cardiopulmonary support in extracorporeal membrane oxygenation.

MAZE (m-AMSA, azacitidine, etoposide)—chemotherapy protocol used to treat acute myeloid leukemia.

maze procedure (Cardio)—used for ablation of refractory atrial fibrillation.

Open heart surgery is used to create a complex maze of incisions in the atrial myocardium, providing an electrical conduit to channel atrial impulses from the sinoatrial node to the atrioventricular node. The procedure is done to restore sinus rhythm, reduce the risk of thromboembolism, and improve hemodynamics.

Mazicon (flumazenil)—name changed to *Romazicon*, a benzodiazepine antagonist.

mazindol (Sanorex)—a drug used to treat Duchenne muscular dystrophy.

Mazzariello-Caprini forceps.

m-BACOD (methotrexate, bleomycin, Adriamycin, cyclophosphamide, oncovin, and dexamethasone)—a chemotherapy regimen.

M-BACOS (methotrexate, bleomycin, Adriamycin, cyclophosphamide, Oncovin, Solu-Medrol)—chemotherapy protocol for advanced lymphomas.

MB bands of CPK—the number relates to the amount of myocardial damage in myocardial infarction, or suspected myocardial infarction.

MBP (myelin basic protein) **assay**—a test on cerebrospinal fluid of patients with various kinds of tumors, including malignant tumors, using radioimmunoassay.

MBTS (modified Blalock-Taussig shunt).

mc, mCi (millicurie).

MC (multifocal choroiditis).

MCA (middle cerebral artery).

MCAG (multiple colloid adenomatous goiter).

MCC (*Mycobacterium* cell wall complex).

MCC (mutated in colon cancer) **gene**—seems to be involved with the regulation of growth in normal and

MCC gene *(cont.)*
cancer cells and may suggest a way in which a new class of chemotherapy drugs might be developed. Damage to four different genes has been linked to the development of colon cancer: the MCC gene on chromosome 5, the p53 gene, the DCC gene, and the RAS oncogene. See also *MSH₂ gene.*

McCain TMJ arthroscopic system—includes cannulas, trocars, probes, scissors, forceps, files, scalpels, curets, switching stick, and monopolar and bipolar cautery probes.

McCall modified posterior culdoplasty—see *culdoplasty.*

McCarey-Kaufman (M-K) medium—used to store excised cornea with scleral rim attached. This preserves the corneal endothelium for grafting purposes.

McCort's sign—one of the radiologic criteria of the presence of ascites.

McCoy facial Tri-Square (Plas Surg).

McCraw gracilis myocutaneous flap—for vaginal reconstruction.

McCune-Albright syndrome—triad of fibrous dysplasia of long bones and cranium, irregular café au lait spots, spurious episodes of precocious sexual development accompanied by ovarian follicular activity.

McCutchen implant—press-fit titanium femoral implant with longitudinal grooves that enhance rotational stability.

McCutchen SLT hip prosthesis.

McDonald bone plates—used in sagittal split ramus osteotomy.

McDonald optic zone marker (Oph).

McDonald procedure—cervical cerclage.

McDougal prostatectomy clamp—used for dissection of the dorsal vein complex during radical retropubic prostatectomy procedures.

M-CFC (macrophage colony-forming cells).

MCFSR (mean circumferential fiber-shortening rate) (Cardio).

McGaw volumetric pump—used for continuous nasogastric feedings.

McGee platinum/stainless steel piston—used in ear reconstruction.

McGhan facial implants (Plas Surg).

McGhan tissue expander (Plas Surg).

McGill pain questionnaire—method used in pain management programs to rate pain.

McGlamry elevator (*not* McClamary).

McIvor mouth gag—used in tonsillectomies.

McKenzie extension exercises (*not* MacKenzie).

McKernan-Adson forceps.

McKernan-Potts forceps.

McKinley EpM pump—designed for epidural infusion of analgesic pain medications.

McKrae strain—herpes simplex virus.

McLeod blood phenotype—reported in patients with chronic granulomatous disease.

McMurray's maneuver—to assess the knee for torn cartilage. To demonstrate, flex the knee and turn the foot out and feel knee cartilage; flex the knee and turn the foot in and feel knee cartilage. A clicking indicates a torn knee cartilage.

McMurray sign (Ortho).

McNaught keel—laryngeal prosthesis.

McNeill-Goldmann blepharostat (Oph)—a fixation ring.

McNemar's test—a test for the presence of ascites.

M-component—see *M-protein*.

McPherson forceps.

McRoberts maneuver—used in vaginal delivery to deliver the infant's shoulders.

MCS (Magnetic Controlled Suturing).

MCS (mesocaval shunt).

M-CSF (macrophage colony-stimulating factor).

MCT (Motor Control Test).

MCTC (metrizamide CT cisternogram) (Neuro).

MCTD (mixed connective tissue disease).

MCT (medium-chain triglyceride) **oil**—a source of extra calories, given in formula to premature infants.

MCV (methotrexate, cisplatin, vinblastine)—chemotherapy protocol used to treat bladder carcinoma.

MCV (molluscum contagiosum virus).

MDAC (multiple dose activated charcoal)—for drug overdose.

MDILO—portable electronic device that monitors the medication intake of patients using metered dose inhalers. It records the date, time, and quality of dispensing (patient shaking, dispensing, and inhaling of medication).

MDLO (metoclopramide, dexamethasone, lorazepam, ondansetron)—protocol of drugs to prevent vomiting in patients receiving cisplatin chemotherapy. Consists of a gastric stimulant, a steroid, an antianxiety agent, and a centrally acting antiemetic.

MD-111—bone dowel and interference screw allograft, machined from cortical bone.

MDR (multidrug resistance)—to chemotherapy agents.

MDR-TB (multidrug-resistant tuberculosis).

MDS (myelodysplastic syndrome).

MDX-240—used to treat HIV-infected patients.

MEA (multiple endocrine adenopathies, or abnormalities).

Meadox Microvel arterial graft material—double velour knitted Dacron.

meat wrapper's asthma—from inhalation of the isocyanate fumes caused by heat used in cutting and sealing plastic wrapping for meat.

Mebadin (dehydroemetine)—anti-infective for amebiasis and amebic dysentery.

mecamylamine HCl—antihypertensive.

mecamylamine HCl and nicotine—a transdermal patch for smoking cessation. While high doses of nicotine or mecamylamine produce side effects, smaller doses of the two used in combination counteract each other and are believed to produce no negative symptoms.

mecasermin (recombinant human insulin-like growth factor)—see *Myotrophin*.

mechanical leech—experimental device that performs essentially as a medicinal leech to relieve venous congestion following replantation procedures but without the increased possibility of infection via the medicinal leech's gut contents.

meclofenamate (Meclomen)—nonsteroidal anti-inflammatory drug.

meconium aspiration syndrome (MAS).

meconium stain—fecal material produced by the fetus, which stains the placenta and membranes when decreased oxygen is present.

Mectra Tissue Sample Retainer—for the collection of resected tissue during endoscopy or laparoscopy. See *Pleatman sac* and *Lap Sac*.

Medela breast pump—collects breast milk in presterilized plastic bags for refrigeration or freezing.

Medelec DMG 50 Teflon-coated monopolar electrodes—used in body plethysmography.

Medfusion 2001 syringe infusion pump.

Medgraphics body plethysmograph.

medial olivocochlear bundle (MOCB).

medial tibial stress syndrome (MTSS) —injuries such as shin splints that occur following continuing physical stress to the bones and muscles in the lower leg, inner aspect.

median sternotomy (*not* medium, medial, or mediosternotomy)—a midline incision into the sternum. See *mediastinotomy* and *mediastinum*.

mediastinotomy—incision into the mediastinum, an anterior mediastinotomy or cervical mediastinotomy, or a dorsal or posterior mediastinotomy. Cf. *median sternotomy*.

mediastinum—a group of tissues and organs separating the sternum in front and the vertebral column behind, containing the heart and large vessels, trachea, esophagus, thymus, lymph nodes, and other structures and tissues. It is divided into anterior, middle, posterior, and superior regions.

medical holography—an innovative, newly designed imaging technology that permits three-dimensional visualization of complex anatomic structures, the translucent images of which are amenable to viewer interaction. Because the images can be viewed from a variety of angles, this technology allows a surgeon to study surgical anatomy and topographical relationships in order to format planning and rehearsal of complex surgical procedures. The technology also provides an educational tool for surgical residents.

medicated urethral system for erection (MUSE) (alprostadil).

medication—a quick-reference list of pharmaceuticals defined in main entries throughout the book, including AIDS drugs, chemicals, chemotherapy drugs and protocols, classes of drugs, contrast media, investigational drugs, natural substances, prescription and over-the-counter drugs, monoclonal antibodies, radioisotopes, and solutions.

abacavir
Abbokinase (urokinase)
ABCD (amphotericin B colloid dispersion)
Abelcet
ABLC (amphotericin B lipid complex)
ABPP (bropirimine)
acarbose (Prandase)
Accolate (zafirlukast)
Accupril (quinapril)
Accuretic (quinapril HCl)
AccuSite injectable gel
Accutane/Rezulin cocktail
Accuzyme enzymatic debriding agent
acecainide (Napa)
ACE chemotherapy protocol
Acel-Imune vaccine
Acel-P
acemannan (Carrisyn)
acetaminophen
Aciphex (rabeprazole sodium)
ACOP chemotherapy protocol
acrivastine (Semprex-D)
AcryDerm hydrogel sheet
ActHIB (*H. influenzae* type B vaccine)

medication *(cont.)*
Actigall (ursodiol)
Action-II (pimagedine)
Actiq (oral transmucosal fentanyl
   citrate)
Actisite (tetracycline hydrochloride)
Activase (alteplase, recombinant
   t-PA)
activated charcoal
ACT MicroCoil
Actonel (risedronate)
Actos (pioglitazone HCl)
Actron (ketoprofen)
Acular (ketorolac tromethamine)
Acusyst-Xcell monoclonal antibody
acylfulvenes class
Adagen (pegademase bovine,
   PEG-ADA)
Adalat CC (nifedipine)
Adcon-L
Adcon-P
Adderall
ADE chemotherapy protocol
Adenocard
Adenoscan
Adept (icodextrin) solution
Adipex-P (phentermine HCl)
adrenergic antagonist
ADR-529
Advantage 24 (nonoxynol-9)
AeroBid (flunisolide)
AERx
Aflexa (glucosamine)
AFM chemotherapy protocol
Agenerase (amprenavir)
AG 1549 (now capravirine)
Aggrastat (tirofiban HCl)
aggregated human IgG (AHuG)
Aggrenox (extended-release
   dipyridamole/aspirin)
agonist drug
Agrelin (anagrelide)
AHG (antihemophilic globulin)
AIDSVAX B/B vaccine

medication *(cont.)*
AK-Con-A (AcuHist) eyedrops
Akne-mycin (erythromycin)
Alamast (pernirolast potassium)
albumin (^{99m}Tc-GSA)
Albunex ultrasound contrast
albuterol sulfate inhalation solution
   (Volmax)
Aldara cream 5%
aldesleukin (Proleukin)
Aldurazyme
alendronate (Fosamax)
Alesse oral contraceptive drug
Aleve (naproxen)
alfacalcidol
Alferon LDO (interferon alfa-n3)
Alferon N (interferon alfa-n3)
alglucerase (Ceredase)
Alibra (alprostadil/prazosin HCl)
AlitraQ nutritional formula
Alkeran (melphalan)
Allegra (fexofenadine HCl)
Allegra-D (fexofenadine HCl;
   pseudoephedrine HCl)
Allergan 211 (idoxuridine)
AlloDerm
allopurinol (Zyloprim)
Allovectin-7
all-trans retinoic acid (Vesanoid)
allylamine class of drugs
Alocril (nedocromil sodium
   ophthalmic solution 2%)
Aloe Vesta antifungal ointment
Alomide (lodoxamide trometha-
   mine)
Aloprim (allopurinol sodium)
alosetron
alpha-BSM (bone substitute
   material)
alpha Gal antibody
Alphagan (brimondine tartrate)
alpha interferon (interferon alfa,
   IFN-A)
Alpha Leukoferon

medication *(cont.)*
alpha$_1$-antitrypsin
AlphaNine
alpha$_1$-proteinase inhibitor
alpha-TGI (teroxirone)
alprostadil (Caverject, Edex, prostaglandin E1)
Alprox-TD vasodilator (alprostadil)
Alredase (tolrestat)
Alrex (loteprednol etabonate)
Altace (ramipril)
alteplase (Activase)
altretamine (Hexalen, Hexastat)
Altropane ^{123}I-based radioimaging agent
Amaryl (glimepiride)
Ambien (zolpidem tartrate)
AmBisome (liposomal amphotericin B)
Amdray (valspodar)
Amen (medroxyprogesterone)
Amerge (naratriptan)
amifostine (Ethyol, gammaphos)
amiloride (Midamor)
Amin-Aid enteral nutrition
aminobiphosphonates
aminoglutethimide (Cytadren)
aminopyridine (4-aminopyridine)
aminosalicylic acid (Paser)
aminosterols class of drugs
amiprilose HCl (Therafectin)
Amiscan
amlodipine (Norvasc)
amlodipine besylate (Lotrel)
amoxicillin/clavulanate (Augmentin)
ampakine CX-516
Amphotec (amphotericin B cholesteryl sulfate)
amphotericin B colloid dispersion (ABCD)
amphotericin B lipid complex (ABLC)
Ampligen (polyribonucleotide)
amprenavir

medication *(cont.)*
amrinone (former name of inamrinone)
Amsidyl (amsacrine)
anabaseine
Anadrol-50 (oxymetholone)
Anandron (nilutamide)
Anaprox (naproxen)
anastrozole (Arimidex)
ancrod (Viprinex)
Andractim (dihydrotestosterone gel)
Androderm testosterone transdermal skin patch
Androgel (testosterone)
Androsorb cream
Angiocidin
Angiocol
AngioMark MRI contrast agent
Angiomax (bivalirudin)
anistreplase (APSAC, Eminase)
Annamycin
Antabuse (disulfiram)
Antagon (ganirelix acetate injection)
antagonist drug
anthracenedione class of drugs
anti-CD11a humanized monoclonal antibody
anti-CD18 humanized antibody
Anticort
anti-D antibody (WinRho SD)
anti-EGF-receptor antibody for cancer
antihemophilic globulin (AHG)
anti-IgE humanized monoclonal antibody
anti-IL-8 antibody
antisense oligodeoxynucleotides (ODNs)
antithrombin III (ATnativ)
antithymocyte globulin (ATG)
antitussive class of drugs
anti-VEGF antibody
Antizol (fomepizole)
anxiolytic class of drugs

medication *(cont.)*
Anzemet (dolasetron mesylate)
AOPA chemotherapy protocol
AOPE chemotherapy protocol
APE chemotherapy protocol
Aphthasol (amlexanox oral paste
5%)
APO chemotherapy protocol
Apo E-4 (apolipoprotein E-4)
Apo-Etodolac (etodolac)
apomorphine
Apo-Zidovudine (zidovudine, AZT)
Apri (desogestrel and ethinyl
estradiol) tablets
aprotinin (Trasyol)
APSAC (anisoylated plasminogen
streptokinase activator complex;
anistreplase)
Aptosyn (exisulind)
aquaporin 1 protein
Aquatab C, Aquatab D,
and Aquatab DM
Arava (leflunomide)
arbutamine
Aredia (pamidronate disodium)
argatroban (Novastatin)
Aricept (donepezil HCl)
Arimidex (anastrozole)
aripiprazole
Aromasin (exemestane)
Arthrotec (diclofenac/misoprostol)
Arvin (ancrod)
arylcyclohexylamines
ASA (acetylsalicylic acid, aspirin)
Asacol (mesalamine)
A-SHAP chemotherapy protocol
AS-101
Astelin (azelastine) nasal spray
Astringedent topical hemostatic
solution
Atacand (candesartan cilexetil)
atevirdine
ATG (antithymocyte globulin)
A33 monoclonal antibody

medication *(cont.)*
ATnativ (antithrombin III)
atorvastatin
atovaquone (Mepron)
Atragen
Atridox
Atrigel
Atrisol aerosol
Atrovent (ipratropium bromide)
Augmentin (amoxicillin/clavulanate)
AuTolo Cure Process
Autoplex
Avakine (now Remicade)
Avandia (rosiglitazone maleate)
Avapro (irbesartan)
Avelox (moxifloxacin)
Avicidin
Avicine
Avitene
Avita
Avonex (interferon beta-1a)
Axokine
azacitidine (5-AZA)
azalide class of drugs
azathioprine (Imuran)
AzdU (azidouridine)
azelaic acid (Azelex)
azelastine (Astelin)
Azelex (azelaic acid)
azidothymidine (now zidovudine)
azidouridine (AzdU)
azithromycin (Zithromax)
azlocillin
Azmacort (triamcinolone acetonide)
azodicarbonamide
AZT (azidothymidine)
Aztec (zidovudine)
Azulfidine En-Tabs (sulfasalazine
delayed-release tablets)
bacillus Calmette-Guérin (BCG)
Bactrim (trimethoprim/
sulfamethoxazole)
Bactroban Cream (mupirocin
calcium 2%)

medication *(cont.)*
BalAsa (balsalazide disodium)
Baycol (cerivastatin sodium)
Baypress (nitrendipine)
BBVP-M chemotherapy protocol
BCX-34
BEAC chemotherapy protocol
becaplermin
beef-lung heparin
Belzer's solution
BEMP chemotherapy protocol
benazepril (Lotensin)
Benecol margarine
BeneFix
BeneJoint topical cream
benzodiazepine class of drugs
BEP chemotherapy protocol
bepridil (Vascor)
beractant (Survanta)
Berotec (fenoterol)
BES (balanced electrolyte solution)
besipirdine hydrochloride
beta-endorphin
beta interferon (Betaseron)
BetaKine (TGF-beta-2)
betamethasone mousse
Betapace (sotalol)
Betaseron (interferon beta-1b)
Betaxon (levobetaxolol HCl oph-
    thalmic suspension) eye drops
bethanidine
Betoptic S (betaxolol HCl)
bexarotene (Targretin)
Bexxar (iodine ^{131}I tositumomab)
Biafine RE (radiodermatitis
    emulsion)
Biafine WDE (wound dressing
    emulsion)
Biaxin (clarithromycin)
Bicarbolyte
BioByPass
Biodel (carmustine)
BioFIT Herbgels
Biofreeze with Ilex analgesic
    ointment

medication *(cont.)*
BioHy
Biolex wound cleanser
BioMend
Biotropin (human growth hormone)
BIP chemotherapy protocol
bisoprolol (Zebeta)
Blenoxane (bleomycin sulfate)
bleomycin sulfate (Blenoxane)
Bonefos (disodium clodronate
    tetrahydrate)
BOP chemotherapy protocol
Botox (botulinum toxin, type A)
botulinum toxin, type A (Botox;
    Ortholinum)
Bouin's solution
bovine superoxide (Orgotein)
BrachySeed
Bradycor
Breathe Right nasal strips
Bretschneider-HTK cardioplegic
    solution
Brevibloc (esmolol HCl)
Bricanyl (terbutaline sulfate)
brimonidine tartrate
bromocriptine-dopamine agonist
bromodeoxyuridine (BUdR,
    broxuridine)
bromontan
Brompton solution
Bronkosol (isoetharine HCl)
Brontex (codeine phosphate and
    guaifenesin)
bropirimine (ABPP)
Broxidine (broxuridine)
Broxine (broxuridine)
BSS (balanced salt solution)
BSS Plus
bucindolol
budesonide (Rhinocort)
BUdR (bromodeoxyuridine,
    broxuridine)
Bumex (bumetanide)
bupropion
Burow's solution

medication *(cont.)*
   Busulfex (busulfan)
   butenafine
   butorphanol tartrate (Stadol NS)
   butyl-DNJ (deoxynojirimycin)
   butyrylcholesterinase inhibitor
   CAB (combined androgen blockade)
   cabergoline (Dostinex)
   CAC chemotherapy protocol
   CAD chemotherapy protocol
   CAE chemotherapy protocol
   CAF chemotherapy protocol
   Cafcit (caffeine citrate)
   caffeine
   CAFTH chemotherapy protocol
   Calcijex
   calcipotriene (Dovonex)
   calcitonin (Miacalcin) nasal spray
   calcium acetate (PhosLo)
   calcium and magnesium-free
      Hanks' balanced salt solution
      (CMF-HBSS)
   calcium channel blockers
   calcium entry blockers
   CALF chemotherapy protocol
   CALF-E chemotherapy protocol
   calusterone
   Campath
   Camptosar (irinotecan)
   Cancell
   canstatin
   CAP chemotherapy protocol
   CAPPr chemotherapy protocol
   capravirine (formerly AG 1549)
   Caprogel (aminocaproic acid)
   Capset (calcium sulfate) bone graft
      barrier
   carbacephem class of drugs
   Carbatrol (carbamazepine
      sustained-release)
   Carbex (selegiline)
   carbovir
   Cardiolite (^{99m}Tc sestamibi)
   cardioplegic solution

medication *(cont.)*
   Cardiosol
   CardioTec or CardioTek
      (^{99m}Tc teboroxime)
   Cardizem CD (diltiazem HCl)
   Cardizem Lyo-Ject
   Cardizem Monovial
   Cardizem SR (diltiazem HCl)
   Cardura (doxazosin mesylate)
   Carlesta
   carmine dye (cochineal extract)
   carmustine wafer
   carprofen (Rimadyl)
   Carrisyn (acemannan)
   Carticel autologous cultured
      chondrocytes
   carvedilol (Coreg)
   Casodex (bicalutamide)
   Cataflam (diclofenac potassium)
   Catapres (clonidine)
   Catatrol (viloxazine)
   cathepsin D
   CAV chemotherapy protocol
   Caverject (prostaglandin E1,
      PGE1, alprostadil)
   Cavilon barrier ointment
   CBP-1011
   CC49 monoclonal antibody
   CD26 protease
   CD4-IgG
   CD4, recombinant soluble human
      (Receptin)
   CD5-T lymphocyte immunotoxin
   CD5+ monoclonal antibody
   CDA (chenodeoxycholic acid)
   CDE chemotherapy protocol
   Cd-texaphyrin
   CEAker
   CEA-Scan contrast medium
   CEA-Tc 99m (^{99m}Tc CEA)
   CEB chemotherapy protocol
   CECA chemotherapy protocol
   Cedax (ceftibuten)
   CEF chemotherapy protocol

medication *(cont.)*

cefmetazole (Zefazone)
cefpodoxime proxetil (Vantin)
cefprozil (Cefzil)
ceftibuten (Cedax)
Cefzil (cefprozil)
Celebrex (celecoxib)
Celexa (citalopram HBr)
celiprolol (Selecor)
CellCept (mycophenolate mofetil)
Celsior solution
CEM chemotherapy protocol
Cenestin (synthetic conjugated estrogen)
Centovir (C-58 monoclonal antibody)
Centoxin (nebacumab) (Ha-1A monoclonal antibody)
CEP chemotherapy protocol
cephalosporin class of drugs
Cephulac (lactulose)
Ceptaz (ceftazidime pentahydrate)
cerebrolysin (FPF 1070)
Cerebyx (fosphenytoin)
Ceredase (alglucerase)
Ceretec technetium 99m contrast imaging agent
Cerezyme
Cernevit-12 (multivitamin for infusion)
Cervidil (dinoprostone)
cesium chloride
cetiedil citrate
cetirizine (Reactine)
Cetrotide (cetrorelix for injection)
CharcoCaps homeopathic formula
Chemet (succimer)
ChemoCap
chemotherapy protocol
Chenix (chenodiol)
chenodiol (Chenix)
Chibroxin (norfloxacin)
Chirocaine (levobupivacaine)
chlorotrianisene (Tace)

medication *(cont.)*

ChlVPP chemotherapy protocol
CHOD chemotherapy protocol
Cholestagel (now Welchol)
Choletec (^{99m}Tc mebrofenin)
CHOP-BLEO chemotherapy protocol
CHOP chemotherapy protocol
CHOPE chemotherapy protocol
Chronulac
Chrysalin
cibenzoline succinate (now cifenline succinate)
cidofovir (HPMPC, Vistide)
cidofovir gel (Forvade)
cifenline succinate (Cipralan)
cilazapril (Inhibace)
Ciloxan (ciprofloxacin)
Cipralan (cifenline succinate)
Cipro (ciprofloxacin)
ciprofloxacin (Ciloxan, Cipro)
Cipro HC Otic suspension (ciprofloxacin hydrochloride/ hydrocortisone otic suspension)
cisapride (Propulsid)
cisatracurium besylate (Nimbex)
CISCA chemotherapy protocol
cisplatin (cis-platinum, Platinol)
cis-retinoic acid (isotretinoin)
citicoline
citrovorum rescue (leucovorin rescue)
cladribine (Leustatin)
clarithromycin (Biaxin)
Claritin (loratadine)
Cleocin (clindamycin phosphate) vaginal ovules
Climara estradiol transdermal system
clindamycin
Clindoxyl (clindamycin/benzoyl peroxide gel)
Clinoril (sulindac)
clobazam (Frisium)

medication *(cont.)*
  Clobetasol E Cream
  clofazimine (Lamprene)
  clonidine gel (Catapres)
  clostridial collagenase
  clotrimazole (Mycelex)
  clozapine (Clozaril)
  Clozaril (clozapine)
  CMF-HBSS
  CMFP chemotherapy protocol
  CMFPT chemotherapy protocol
  CMFPTH chemotherapy protocol
  CMFVP chemotherapy protocol
  CMH chemotherapy protocol
  CMOPP chemotherapy protocol
  CMV chemotherapy protocol
  Coagulin-B
  COAP chemotherapy protocol
  COF/COM chemotherapy protocol
  Colazide (balsalazide disodium)
  Cognex (tacrine)
  colchicine
  colfosceril palmitate (Exosurf
    Pediatric)
  collagenase (Santyl)
  collagen injection
  Collins' solution
  colloidal bismuth subcitrate
  colloid solution
  Colomed enema
  Colyte
  Combidex MRI contrast agent
  CombiPatch (estradiol/
    norethindrone acetate)
  Combivent (ipratropium
    bromide/albuterol sulfate)
  combretastatin A-4
  Compassia (dronabinol)
  compound Q (trichosanthin)
  Comprecin (enoxacin)
  COMT (catechol-O-methyltrans-
    verase)
  Comtan (entacapone)
  Comvax

medication *(cont.)*
  Concerta (methylphenidate HCl)
  conjugated estrogen and medroxy-
    progesterone (Prempro)
  ConXn (recombinant human
    relaxin H2)
  COPA plus cytokine interferon
  Copaxone (glatiramer acetate)
  COP-BLEO chemotherapy protocol
  COPE chemotherapy protocol
  copolymer-1 (COP 1)
  Cordarone (amiodarone hydro-
    chloride)
  Cordase (collagenase)
  Cordox (fructose-1,6-diphosphate)
  Coreg (carvedilol)
  Corvert (ibutilide fumarate)
  Cosmederm-7
  Cosopt
  Coumadin (warfarin)
  Covera-HS (verapamil)
  COX-2 inhibitors
  Cozaar (losartan potassium)
  CPB chemotherapy protocol
  CP-Cardiosol
  CPC chemotherapy protocol
  Crinone bioadhesive progesterone
    gel
  Crixivan (indinavir)
  cryoprecipitate
  Cryptaz (nitazoxanide)
  crystalloid solution
  CTCb chemotherapy protocol
  C225 EGFr antagonist
  Curosurf (poractant alpha)
    intratracheal suspension
  Curretab (medroxyprogesterone)
  Cutivate (fluticasone propionate)
  CVAD chemotherapy protocol
  CVD chemotherapy protocol
  CVP chemotherapy protocol
  CVPP chemotherapy protocol
  CVT-124
  cyclosporine (Sandimmune)

medication *(cont.)*

Cycrin (medroxyprogesterone)
CyHOP chemotherapy protocol
Cylexin
Cymetra
CYP3A4
Cystadane (betaine anhydrous)
Cystagon (cysteamine bitartrate)
Cytadren (aminoglutethimide)
cytarabine (Cytosar-U; ara-C)
CytoGam (cytomegalovirus
    immune globulin)
cytokine class of drugs
Cytolex
cytomegalovirus immune globulin
    (CytoGam)
CytoRich preservative
CytoTAb polyclonal antibody
Cytovene (ganciclovir)
dacliximab monoclonal antibody
    (Zenapax)
Dakin's solution
Dalgan (dezocine)
dalteparin sodium (Fragmin)
dapiprazole (Rev-Eyes)
dapsone
dapsone plus trimethoprim
    (DAP/TMP)
DAP/TMP (dapsone plus trimetho-
    prim)
DAT chemotherapy protocol
DaTSCAN imaging agent
DATVP chemotherapy protocol
daunorubicin HCl (Cerubidine)
daunorubicin, liposomal
    (Daunoxome)
DaunoXome (liposomal daunoru-
    bicin HCl)
DAVA (desacetyl vinblastine
    amide, vindesine sulfate)
Daypro (oxaprozin)
D-chiro-inositol
DDAVP (desmopressin acetate)
ddC (dideoxycytidine, Hivid,
    zalcitabine)

medication *(cont.)*

ddI (didanosine, dideoxyinosine,
    Videx)
DECAL chemotherapy protocol
defensins
dehydroemetine (Mebadin)
Delaprem (hexoprenaline sulfate)
Demadex (torsemide)
Demser (metyrosine)
Denavir (penciclovir)
deoxy-D-glucose
deoxynojirimycin (butyl-DNJ)
deoxyspergualin
Depacon (valproate sodium
    injection)
DepoAmikacin
DepoCyt
DepoMorphine
Depo-Provera (medroxyproges-
    terone)
Dermablend
Dermacea
Dermagraft-TC
Dermagran ointment
Derma-Smoothe/FS
Dermatop (prednicarbate)
desflurane (Suprane)
desloratadine
desmopressin acetate (Stimate)
    nasal spray
Desogen (progestin desogestrel,
    estrogen)
desogestrel
Detoxahol
Detrol (tolterodine tartrate)
dexamethasone
dexfenfluramine (Redux)
dexrazoxane (Zinecard)
dextran sulfate (Uendex)
Dey-Wash skin wound cleaner
dezocine (Dalgan)
d4T (didehydrodideoxythymidine,
    stavudine, Zerit)
DFV chemotherapy protocol
DHAC (dihydro-5-azacytidine)

medication *(cont.)*

DHAP chemotherapy protocol
DHE, DHE-45 (dihydroergotamine)
DHPG (dihydroxypropoxymethylguanine, ganciclovir)
DiaBeta (glyburide)
DiabKlenz wound cleanser
Diab II
Diacol
Diastat (diazepam solution)
diatrizoate
diaziquone (AZQ)
dibenzodiazepine class of drugs
dibromodulcitol (DBD, mitolactol)
diclofenac potassium (Cataflam)
diclofenac sodium (Voltaren)
didanosine (ddI, Videx)
didehydrodideoxythymidine (d4T,
stavudine)
dideoxycytidine (ddC, Hivid)
dideoxyinosine (ddI, didanosine,
Videx)
Didronel (etidronate)
diethyldithiocarbamate (Imuthiol)
Differin (adapalene) gel
DiffGAM
Diffistat-G polyclonal antibody
Diflucan (fluconazole)
diflunisal (Dolobid)
difluorodeoxycytidine (gemcitabine)
difluoromethylornithine (eflornithine)
Digibar 190 (barium sulfate for
suspension) imaging agent
Digibind (digoxin immune Fab)
Digidote (digoxin immune Fab)
digoxin immune Fab (Digibind,
Digidote)
dihydroergotamine (DHE-45)
Dilacor XR
Dilapan
dilevalol
Diltia XT

medication *(cont.)*

diltiazem (Tiazac)
dinoprostone (Prepidil) gel
Diovan (valsartan)
Dipentum (olsalazine)
dipyridamole (Persantine)
Dirame (propiram)
Ditropan XL (oxybutynin chloride)
DMARDs (disease-modifying
antirheumatic drugs)
DNJ (N-butyl-deoxynojirimycin)
docetaxel (Taxotere)
domperidone (Motilium)
Dopascan
dopexamine
Doral (quazepam)
dornase alfa (Pulmozyme)
Dostinex (cabergoline) tablets
dothiepin HCl (Prothiaden)
Dovonex (calcipotriene)
doxacurium chloride (Nuromax)
doxazosin mesylate (Cardura)
doxepin hydrochloride cream
(Zonalon)
Doxil (doxorubicin HCl liposome
injection)
DOX-SL (liposomal doxorubicin)
droloxifene
dronarinol (Marinol)
Droxia (hydroxyurea)
DSM (degradable starch micro-
spheres)
DST (donor-specific transfusion)
DTaP vaccine
DTC-101
DTIC-Dome (dacarbazine)
DTPA (diethylenetriamine-penta-
acetic acid or acetate)
DuoDerm hydroactive gel
Duodopa (levodopa/carbidopa)
Duraclon (clonidine hydrochloride)
Duract (bromfenac sodium
capsules)
Duragesic (fentanyl)

medication *(cont.)*
DuraPrep surgical solution
DuraScreen
Durasphere bulking agent
DVP chemotherapy protocol
Dynabac (dirithromycin)
Dynacin (minocycline)
DynaCirc (isradipine)
Dysport (*Clostridium* botulinum
toxin type A)
EAAT2 protein
Ebastel (ebastine)
ebastine (Ebastel)
eboxetine mesylate
echinomycin
EchoGen (perflenapent injectable
emulsion) contrast agent
Echovist (galactose)
ECMV chemotherapy protocol
E. coli L-asparaginase
EcoNail
Ecovia (remacemide)
ECS (extracellular-like, calcium-
free solution)
EDAM (10-EDAM)
EDAP chemotherapy protocol
Edex (alprostadil)
edible vaccines
Edronax tablets (reboxetine)
Effexor XR (venlafaxine HCl)
Efidac/24
E5 monoclonal antibody
eflornithine (Ornidyl)
EGCg (epigallocatechin gallate)
Elase enzymatic debriding agent
Eldepryl (selegiline)
Eldisine (vindesine sulfate)
ELF chemotherapy protocol
eliprodil
Ellence (epirubicin)
Elmiron (pentosanpolysulfate
sodium)
Eloxatin (oxaliplatin)

medication *(cont.)*
EMACO chemotherapy protocol
Emcyt (estramustine phosphate
sodium)
Emdogain
EMLA cream (lidocaine, prilo-
caine)
E-MVAC chemotherapy protocol
Enable (tenidap)
Enbrel (etanercept)
encainide (Enkaid)
encapsulated liposomes
Endosol
Endostatin
Engerix-B
enisoprost
Enkaid (encainide)
Enlon-Plus (atropine, edrophonium)
enoxacin (Comprecin, Penetrex)
enoxaparin (Lovenox)
Ensure Plus enteral nutrition
entacapone
Entero Vu (barium sulfate for
suspension) contrast medium
Entocort CR (budesonide)
Enzogenol
enzymatic debriding agents
Eovist (gadolinium EOB-DTPA)
contrast agent
epi-ADR, epi-Adriamycin
(epirubicin)
Epicel autologous skin cells
epidermal growth factor
epinephrine
epirubicin (EPI, epi-Adriamycin)
Epivir-HBV (lamivudine)
Epivir/Retrovir (lamivudine/
zidovudine)
EPO (synthetic erythropoietin)
EPOCH chemotherapy protocol
epoetin alfa (EPO)
epoetin beta (Marogen)
Epogen (epoetin alfa)

medication *(cont.)*
epoprostenol (Flolan)
epoxyeicosatrienoic acid
eprosartan mesylate (Teveten)
eptifibatide
Ergamisol (levamisole)
Ergoset tablets
ERT patch
Erwinase (*Erwinia* L-asparaginase)
Erwinia L-asparaginase
ERYC
Ery-Tab
erythropoietin, recombinant human
    (Eprex, Marogen)
ESAT-6 protein
Esclim estradiol transdermal system
esmolol HCl (Brevibloc)
esprolol plus sildenafil citrate
    (Viagra)
Essiac
Estalis estrogen/progesterone
    transdermal delivery system
estazolam (ProSom)
estramustine phosphate sodium
    (Emcyt)
estrogen
estropipate (Ortho-Est)
Estrostep (norethindrone acetate
    and ethinyl estradiol)
ethambutol (Myambutol)
ethinyl estradiol
Ethmozine (moricizine)
Ethodian (iophendylate)
Ethyol (amifostine)
etidronate (Didronel)
etodolac (Lodine)
etoglucid
etoposide (VePesid, VP-16)
Eucerin
Eulexin (flutamide)
Eulexin plus LHRH-A
Evacet liposome-encapsulated
    doxorubicin
EVA chemotherapy protocol
Evac-Q-Kwik

medication *(cont.)*
EVAL (ethylene vinyl alcohol)
Evalose
Evista (raloxifene hydrochloride)
Evoxac (cevimeline hydrochloride)
Exelon (rivastigmine tartrate)
Exidine (chlorhexidine gluconate)
Exorex
Exosurf Neonatal (colfosceril
    palmitate)
extracellular-like, calcium-free
    solution
FAC-M chemotherapy protocol
Factive (gemifloxacin)
FAM chemotherapy protocol
FAM-CF chemotherapy protocol
famciclovir (Famvir)
FAME chemotherapy protocol
FAMP (fludarabine monophos-
    phate)
FAMTX chemotherapy protocol
Famvir (famciclovir)
Fansidar (sulfadoxine-
    pyrimethamine)
FAP chemotherapy protocol
Fareston (toremifine citrate)
FCAP chemotherapy protocol
FCR 9501HQ imaging agent
FEC chemotherapy protocol
FED chemotherapy protocol
Felbatol (felbamate)
felodipine (Plendil)
Femara (letrozole) tablets
femhrt or FemHRT (norethindrone
    acetate and ethinyl estradiol)
FemPatch
Femprox
Femstat 3 (butoconazole nitrate)
    vaginal cream
fenoprofen (Nalfon)
fenoterol (Berotec)
fentanyl (Duragesic)
fentanyl citrate tablet (Oralet)
Feridex I.V. (ferumoxides) MRI
    contrast agent

medication *(cont.)*
  Ferrlecit (sodium ferric gluconate)
  Fertinex (urofollitropin)
  ferumoxsil (GastroMark)
  FIAC (fiacitabine)
  FIAU (fialuridine)
  Fiblast (trafermin)
  Fibrillex (NC-503)
  Fibrimage technetium imaging agent
  fibroblast growth factor (FGF)
  filgrastim (Neupogen)
  finasteride (Propecia; Proscar)
  5-alpha-reductase inhibitors
  5-ASA (mesalamine)
  5-AZA (azacitidine)
  5-fluorouracil (5-FU)
  5-FU (5-fluorouracil)
  566C80
  FK-565
  FLAC (5-fluorouracil, leucovorin, doxorubicin, cyclophosphamide)
  Flagyl ER
  FLAP chemotherapy protocol
  Flarex (fluorometholone acetate)
  FlashTab
  Flexeril
  Flolan (epoprostenol)
  Flomax (tamsulosin HCl)
  FloSeal matrix hemostatic sealant
  flosequinan
  Flovent aerosol
  Flovent Rotadisk (fluticasone propionate inhalation powder)
  Floxin (ofloxacin)
  Floxin Otic (ofloxacin)
  floxuridine (FUdR)
  FLT (fluorothymidine)
  fluasterone
  fluconazole (Diflucan)
  flucytosine (5-FC, Ancobon)
  Fludara (fludarabine)
  fludarabine (FAMP, Fludara)
  Flu-Glow
  Flumadine (rimantadine HCl)

medication *(cont.)*
  flumazenil (Mazicon)
  flumecinol (Zixoryn)
  FluMist flu vaccine
  flunisolide (Nasarel)
  Fluogen influenza virus vaccine
  Fluoratec technetium-based imaging agent
  Fluor-i-Strip
  fluorodeoxyglucose (FDG)
  fluoroquinolone class of drugs
  fluorosilicone oil
  fluorothymidine (FLT)
  fluoxetine (Prozac)
  fluticasone propionate (Cutivate)
  fluvastatin (Lescol)
  fluvoxamine (Luvox)
  FNM chemotherapy protocol
  FocalSeal liquid sealant
  Follistim (follitropin beta)
  fomivirsen (Vitravene)
  Foradil (formoterol fumarate)
  Fortaz (ceftazidime)
  Fortical (salmon calcitonin)
  Fortovase (squinavir)
  Forvade (cidofovir gel)
  Fosamax (alendronate sodium)
  foscarnet (Foscavir, trisodium phosphonoformate)
  Foscavir (foscarnet)
  fosinopril (Monopril)
  fosphenytoin (Cerebyx)
  fotemustine (S 10036)
  Fouchet's reagent
  4-aminopyridine
  4-aminosalicylic acid (Pamisyl, Rezipas)
  4-epi-Adriamycin (epirubicin)
  Fourneau 309 (suramin)
  Fragmin (dalteparin sodium)
  FreAmine nutrient solution
  Frisium (clobazam)
  frovatriptan
  ftorafur

medication *(cont.)*

FUdR (floxuridine, fluorodeoxy-
uridine)
fusion inhibitors
fusion protein
FUVAC chemotherapy protocol
gabapentin (Neurontin)
Gabitril (tiagabine)
gadolinium (Gd-DTPA)
gadolinium texaphyrin (Gd-Tex)
Gadolite oral contrast medium
gadoteridol (ProHance) contrast
medium
galactose (Echovist; Levovist)
galanthamine
Galardin (matrix metalloproteinase
inhibitor)
gallium nitrate (Ganite)
gallium-67 citrate (^{67}GA)
Gamimune N (immunoglobulin)
gamma hydroxybutyrate (GHB)
gamma interferon (IFN-G)
gammaphos (ethiofos)
Gammar-PIV (pasteurized
intravenous)
ganaxolone
ganciclovir (Cytovene, DHPG)
ganglioside GM1
Ganite (gallium nitrate)
Gastrimmune (gemcitabine) vaccine
Gastrografin (meglumine
GastroMark (ferumoxsil) oral
contrast agent
Gastrozepine (pirenzipine HCl)
GBC-590
G-CSF (granulocyte colony-
stimulating factor; filgrastim)
Gd-DTPA (gadolinium diethylenetriamine-penta-acetate)
GDNF (glial-cell-derived neurotrophic factor)
Gelfoam
gemcitabine (difluorodeoxycytidine)
gemcitabine HCl (Gemzar)

medication *(cont.)*

Gemzar (gemcitabine HCl)
Genoptic eye drops
Genotropin (somatropin)
gentamicin sulfate, liposomal
(TLC G-65)
gepirone HCl
Geref (sermorelin acetate)
Germanin (suramin)
gestodene (Minesse)
Gey's solution
GHB (gamma hydroxybutyrate)
GIK (glucose, insulin, and
potassium)
Glandosane
Glaucoma Wick
Gliadel (polifeprosan 20 with
carmustine)
glucagon for injection (rDNA
origin)
Glucarate ^{99m}Tc imaging agent
glucose, insulin, and potassium
(GIK)
glucuronate
Glutose
glycolic acid
Glylorin (monolaurin)
Glynase Pres Tab (glyburide)
Glypressin (terlipressin)
Glyset (miglitol)
GM-CSF (granulocyte/macrophage
colony-stimulating factor)
GM1 monosialotetrahexosyl-
ganglioside
GnRH (gonadotropin-releasing
hormone)
Goeckerman psoriasis regimen
GoLytely (polyethylene glycol-
electrolyte solution)
gonadorelin acetate (Lutrepulse)
Gonal-F (follitropin alfa for
injection)
gonatropin-releasing hormone
(GnRH)

medication *(cont.)*
 goserelin acetate (Zoladex)
 gp120 AIDS vaccine (AIDSVAX)
 Graftskin
 granisetron HCl (Kytril)
 Granocyte (lenograstim)
 GVAX cancer vaccine
 Habitrol (nicotine patch)
 Haemonetics V-50
 Halcion (triazolam)
 Haldol (haloperidol)
 Halfan (halofantrine HCl)
 halobetasol propionate (Ultravate)
 halofantrine HCl (Halfan)
 halofuginone
 haloperidol (Haldol)
 Ha-1A monoclonal antibody
 Hartmann's solution
 Havrix hepatitits A vaccine
 H-CAP chemotherapy protocol
 hCG or HCG (human chorionic
  gonadotropin)
 HCT, HCTZ (hydrochlorothiazide)
 HDPEG chemotherapy protocol
 HDRV (human diploid cell strain
  rabies vaccine)
 HD-VAC chemotherapy protocol
 Healon (sodium hyaluronate)
 Healon GV
 Healon Yellow
 heat shock protein 72 (HSP-72)
 Helicide
 Helidac (bismuth subsalicylate,
  metronidazole, and tetracycline)
 Helioseal
 Helistat
 Helivax vaccine
 Hemabate (carboprost trometha-
  mine)
 hematoporphyrin derivative (HpD)
 hemoglobin (SFHb)
 Hemolink blood replacement
  product
 Hemopure (hemoglobin
  glutamer-250 [bovine])

medication *(cont.)*
 HepatAmine solution
 Heptalac
 Heptavax-B vaccine
 Heptazyme
 Heptodin (lamivudine)
 Herceptin (trastuzumab)
 Herplex Liquifilm (idoxuridine)
 Hexalen (altretamine)
 hexoprenaline sulfate (Delaprem)
 Hextend plasma volume expander
 H-447
 Hibiclens
 Hibistat
 Hibitane tincture
 HIB polysaccharide vaccine
 Hib (*Haemophilus influenzae*
  type B) vaccine
 high-osmolar media (HOM)
 hirudin (recombinant desulfato-
  hirudin)
 Hirulog (bivalirudin)
 HIS fusion inhibitors
 Hismanal (astemizole)
 Histussin D (hydrocodone bitartrate/
  pseudoephedrine hydrochloride)
 Hivid (dideoxycytidine, ddC,
  zalcitabine)
 HK-Cardiosol
 HLA-DR (histocompatibility
  antigen-DR) marker protein
 HMFG1 (human milk fat globule 1)
 HMG (human menopausal
  gonadotropin)
 HMG-CoA reductase inhibitor
 Hollande's solution
 HpD (hepatoporphyrin derivative)
 HPMPC (cidofovir)
 HRT (hormone replacement
  therapy) patch
 Humalog (insulin lispro)
 Humalog Mix 75/25 Pen (insulin
  lispro protamine suspension,
  insulin lispro injection) (rDNA
  origin)

medication *(cont.)*
  human diploid cell strain rabies
  human growth hormone (hGH)
  human menopausal gonadotropin
    (HMG)
  Humatrope (somatropin)
  Humegon (menotropins)
  Humulin
  Hyalgan (hyaluronic acid)
  Hycamptin (topotecan)
  hydrazine sulfate (HDZ)
  Hydrea (hydroxyurea)
  hydroxyurea (Hydrea)
  Hylaform (hylan polymer)
    viscoelastic gel
  Hylagel-Nuro viscoelastic gel
  hylan polymer (Hylaform)
  Hylasine viscoelastic gel
  hypericin (VIMRxyn)
  Hytrin (terazosin)
  Hyzaar (losartan potassium HCl)
  I-B1 radiolabeled antibody
  ibopamine
  ibuprofen
  ICAM-1 (intercellular adhesions
    molecule-1)
  ICE chemotherapy protocol
  IceSeeds
  i.com Comfort Shield ophthalmic
    solution
  ICS solution
  Idamycin (idarubicin)
  idarubicin (Idamycin)
  idoxuridine (IDU)
  IDU (idoxuridine)
  IFN-A (interferon alfa)
  IGF-BP3 complex (SomatoKine)
  IGF-1 (insulin-like growth factor 1)
  IgG 2A monoclonal antibody
    (Immurait)
  IL4-PE (interleukin-4-pseudomonas
    exotoxin fusion protein)
  IL-10 (interleukin-10)
  IL-11 (interleukin-11)

medication *(cont.)*
  ilepcimide
  ILE-SORB absorbent gel
  Imagent GI (perflubron) contrast
    medium
  Imagent US contrast medium
  Imdur (isosorbide mononitrate)
  imidazole carboxamide
  imidazotetrazines class
  Imitrex (sumatriptan)
  ImmTher (disaccharide tripeptide)
  immune globulin (RespiGam)
  immunoisolating microreactors
  immunoliposomes
  immunomodulation
  immunosuppressant cocktail
  immunovar (Isoprinosine)
  ImmuRAID (CEA-^{99m}Tc)
  ImmuRAIT-LL2 (IgG 2A mono-
    clonal antibody)
  Impact enteral feeding
  Imreg-1, Imreg-2
  ImuLyme vaccine
  Imuthiol (diethyldithiocarbamate)
  inamrinone (new name for amri-
    none)
  IND (investigational new drug)
  indinavir (Crixivan)
  indium 111 (^{111}In)
  indium-111-labeled human
    nonspecific immunoglobulin G
    (^{111}In-IgG)
  Infanrix vaccine
  Infasurf (calfactant)
  Infergen (interferon alfacon-1)
  infliximab monoclonal antibody
  influenza vaccine
  Infumorph solution
  Ingram psoriasis regimen
  Inhibace (cilazapril)
  Innofem (estradiol tablets)
  Innohep (tinzaparin sodium)
  INOmax (nitric oxide) for inhalation
  inosine pranobex (Isoprinosine)

medication *(cont.)*
insulin
insulin-like growth factor I
  (somatomedin C)
insulin lispro (Humalog)
insulinotropin
Integrilin (eptifibatide)
interferon alfa-n1 (Wellferon)
interferon alfa-n3 (Alferon LDO,
  Alferon N)
interferon alfa-2a (Roferon-A)
interferon alfa-2b (Intron A)
interferon beta (Betaseron)
interferon beta-1a (Avonex)
Intergel adhesion prevention
  solution
interleukin-1 (IL-1)
interleukin-1b
interleukin-2 PEG
interleukin-2, recombinant (IL-2,
  Proleukin, teceleukin)
interleukin-3 (IL-3)
interleukin-4
interleukin-6 (IL-6)
interleukin-10 (IL-10)
interleukin-11 (IL-11)
Intrachol (choline chloride)
IntraDose-CDDP injectable gel
IntraDose gel
IntraSite gel
Intron A (interferon alfa-2b,
  recombinant)
Inversine (mecamylamine HCl)
Invicorp
Invirase (saquinavir)
IOCM (isosmolar contrast medium)
iodinated contrast medium
iodine 131 MIBG (^{131}I MIBG)
iododeoxyuridine
iodophor
ionic contrast medium
iopamidol intravascular contrast
  medium
Iopidine (apraclonidine ophthalamic
  solution)

medication *(cont.)*
iopentol
iophendylate (Ethodian)
ioxilan (Oxilan)
I-Plant radioactive ^{125}I seed
IPOL poliovirus vaccine
iproplatin
iridium (IR-192, ^{192}IR, Iriditope)
irinotecan (Camptosar)
irofulven
ISAtx247
iscador
Ismo (isosorbide mononitrate)
isobutyl 2-cyanoacrylate
isoflurane
isoniazid
Isoprinosine (inosine pranobex)
isosmolar contrast medium (IOCM)
isosorbide mononitrate (Imdur,
  Ismo)
isosulfan blue (Lymphazurin)
isotretinoin (Accutane)
Isovorin (L-leucovorin)
Isovue, Isovue M (iopamidol)
isoxicam (Maxicam)
isradipine (DynaCirc)
itraconazole (Sporanox)
IUdR (idoxuridine, Allergan)
ivermectin (Stromectol)
IvyBlock
Jevity isotonic liquid nutrition
JT1001 prostate cancer vaccine
Kabikinase (streptokinase)
Kadian sustained-release morphine
  capsules
Kao Lectrolyte
KCl (potassium chloride)
Keppra (levetiracetam)
ketamine
ketanserin
ketoconazole (Nizoral)
ketoprofen (Actron, Orudis,
  Oruvail, Orudis KT)
ketorolac tromethamine (Toradol)
ketotifen (Zaditen)

medication *(cont.)*
Kinerase (N[6]-furfuryladenine)
Kinetin
Klaricid (clarithromycin)
Klaron lotion (sodium sulfaetamide lotion)
Klonopin (clonazepam) lyophilized wafers
KoGENate blood factor VIII
Kold Kap
Kollagen
Kontrast U
Kytril (granisetron hydrochloride)
LAAM (L-alpha-acetyl-methadol)
LAAM (levomethadyl acetate hydrochloride)
labetalol
lactated Ringer's solution
lactulose solution
LAF (lymphocyte activating factor) (interleukin-1)
Lambda (lanthanum carbonate)
Lamictal (lamotrigine)
Lamisil (terbinafine HCl)
Lamisil DermGel gel (terbinafine)
lamivudine/AZT (Epivir/Retrovir)
lamotrigine (Lamictal)
Lamprene (clofazimine)
lansoprazole (Prevacid)
L-asparaginase (L-ASP)
LATS (long-acting thyroid stimulating) hormone
LDI-200
leflunomide (Arava)
Lente insulin
lentinan
Lescol (fluvastatin)
Leucomax (molgramostim, GM-CSF)
leucovorin (Isovorin, Wellcovorin)
Leukine (sargramostim, GM-CSF)
LeukoScan (technetium 99m sulesomab)
leuprolide acetate

medication *(cont.)*
LeuTech infection imaging agent
Leuvectin
levamisole (Ergamisol)
Levaquin (levofloxacin)
levetiracetam
levobupivacaine
levocabastine HCl (Livostin)
levonorgestrel (Norplant)
levothyroxine sodium (Levoxyl)
Levovist (galactose) ultrasound contrast agent
Levoxyl (levothyroxine sodium)
Levulan
lexipafant (Zacutex)
Lexirin
L-5HTP (L-5-hydroxytryptophan)
LHRH (luteinizing hormone-releasing hormone)
licostinel
Lidakol cream (n-docosanol)
Lidoderm (lidocaine patch 5%)
LidodexNS
Limitrol-DM
linezolid
Linomide (roquinimex)
linopiridine
Lipiodol
Lipitor (atorvastatin calcium)
Lipomel vaccine for malignant melanoma
liposomal doxorubicin (Doxil)
liposome encapsulated doxorubicin (LED)
LipoTECA cream
Liprostin
Liquifilm ophthalmic solution
Liqui-Vent or LiquiVent
lisinopril (Zestril) tablets
lithium carbonate
Livostin (levocabastine HCl)
LJP-394
L-leucovorin
LM-427 (Mycobutin, rifabutin)

medication *(cont.)*
Lochol
Locilex topical cream (pexiganan acetate)
Lodine; Lodine XL (etodolac)
lodoxamide tromethamine (Alomide)
long-acting thyroid stimulating (LATS) hormone
lonidamine
Lorabid (loracarbef)
loracarbef (Lorabid)
loratadine (Claritin)
Lorcet 10/650 (hydrocodone, acetaminophen)
losartan potassium HCl (Hyzaar)
Losec (omeprazole)
Lotemax (loteprednol etabonate ophthalmic suspension 0.5%)
Lotensin (benazepril)
Lotrel (amlodipine besylate)
Lotronex (alosetron HCl)
Lovenox (enoxaparin)
low-osmolar media (LOM)
LP 2307
LSA2L2 chemotherapy protocol
Lunelle (estradiol cypionate and medroxyprogesterone acetate)
Lupron (leuprolide)
Lustra (hydroquinone)
luteinizing hormone-releasing hormone (LHRH)
Lutrepulse (gonadorelin acetate)
Luvox (fluvoxamine maleate)
Luxiq (betamethasone valerate)
L-Vax leukemia vaccine
LYMErix recombinant protein vaccine
lym-1 monoclonal antibody
Lymphazurin (isosulfan blue)
lymphocyte activating factor (LAF, interleukin-1)
lymphokines (interleukin-2)
Lyrelle patch

medication *(cont.)*
Maalox HRF
MAb-170 monoclonal antibody
MabThera (rituximab) monoclonal antibody
MAC chemotherapy protocol
MACHO chemotherapy protocol
MACOP-B chemotherapy protocol
Macritonin
macrolide class of drugs
macromolecular
Macrotec (^{99m}Tc medronate)
MADDOC chemotherapy protocol
Magnevist (gadopentetate dimeglumine)
Magnevist Syringe
MAK-6 cocktail
mammastatin
m-AMSA (amsacrine)
manipulated autologous structure (MAS) cells
marimastat
Marinol (dronarinol)
Marogen (epoetin beta)
matrix metalloproteinase inhibitor (Galardin)
Maxalt (rizatriptan benzoate)
Maxamine (histamine dihydrochloride)
Maxaquin (lomefloxacin HCl)
Maxicam (isoxicam)
MAZE chemotherapy protocol
Mazicon (flumazenil)
mazindol (Sanorex)
M-BACOS chemotherapy protocol
m-BACOD (methotrexate, bleomycin, Adriamycin, cyclophosphamide, oncovin, and dexamethasone)
MCC (*Mycobacterium* cell wall complex)
McCarey-Kaufman medium
MCT oil
MCV chemotherapy protocol

medication *(cont.)*

MDAC (multiple dose activated charcoal)
MDLO chemotherapy protocol
MDX-240
Mebadin (dehydroemetine)
mecamylamine HCl
mecamylamine HCl and nicotine transdermal patch
mecasermin
medicinal botanicals
medroxyprogesterone (Amen, Curretab, Cycrin, Depo-Provera, Premphase, Prempro)
mefenamic acid (Ponstel)
mefloquine (Lariam; Mephaquin)
Megace (megestrol acetate)
megestrol acetate (Megace)
meglumine diatrizoate
Melacine
melphalan (Alkeran)
memantine
memapsin 2 protein-cutting enzyme, or protease
Memorial Sloan-Kettering protocol
Menorest (transdermal 17-beta-estradiol)
menotropins (Humegon)
Mentane (velnacrine)
Mentax (1% butenafine hydrochloride) cream
mercaptopurine (Purinethol)
Meridia (sibutramine HCl)
meropenem (Merrem)
Merrem (meropenem)
mesalamine (5-ASA, Asacol, Rowasa, Pentasa)
Mesalt
mesna (Mesnex)
Mesnex (mesna)
Metadate ER (extended-release methylphenidate)
metaiodobenzylguanidine (MIBG)
Metastron (strontium Sm 89)

medication *(cont.)*

methazolamide (Neptazane)
methionine-enkephalin
methisoprinol (inosiplex)
methotrexate (MTX, Mexate, Folex)
methoxsalen (Oxsoralen)
Methylin (methylphenidate)
methylphenidate (Methylin)
methyl tertiary butyl ether (MTBE)
metipranolol (OptiPranolol)
metoclopramide (Sensamide)
metoprolol succinate (Toprol XL)
metoprolol tartrate (Lopressor)
metrizamide
Metrodin (urofollitropin)
metyrosine (Demser)
Mevacor (lovastatin)
Mexate (methotrexate)
Mexitil (mexiletine)
Mezlin (mezlocillin sodium)
mezlocillin sodium (Mezlin)
MGBG
Miacalcin (calcitonin) nasal spray
MIBG (metaiodobenzylguanidine)
Micardis (telmisartan)
miconazole nitrate vaginal cream
MicroKlenz wound cleanser
Micronase (glyburide)
micronized fenofibrate (Tricor)
MigraSpray
midodrine HCl (ProAmatine)
Mifegyne (mifepristone)
mifepristone (Mifegyne)
Migra-Lieve
Migranal (dihydroergotamine mesylate) nasal spray
MiKasome
Millon's reagent
milrinone lactate (Primacor)
MINE chemotherapy protocol
Minesse (gestodene, progestin, and ethinyl estradiol)
Minnesota antilymphoblast globulin

medication *(cont.)*
minoxidil
Mirapex (pramipexole dihydro-
chloride tablets)
Mirena
mirtazapine (Remeron)
misoprostol
Mithracin (plicamycin)
mitolactol (dibromodulcitrol)
mitomycin (mitomycin-C, MTC,
Mutamycin)
mitoxantrone HCl (Novantrone)
Mivacron (mivacurium)
mivacurium (Mivacron)
MKC-442 for treatment of HIV
MMOPP chemotherapy protocol
MN rpg120 vaccine for AIDS
MOAB, MoAb, MAB (monoclonal
antibody)
Mobic (meloxicam)
modafinil (Provigil)
moexipril HCl (Univasc)
MOF chemotherapy protocol
Mogadon (nitrazepam)
molgramostim (Leucomax)
Monistat (miconazole nitrate)
monobactam class of drugs
Monodox (doxycycline)
Monoket (isosorbide mononitrate)
monolaurin (Glylorin)
Monopril (fosinopril)
Monsel's solution
Monurol (fosfomycin trometha-
mine)
MOPP chemotherapy protocol
Moranyl (suramin)
moricizine (Ethmozine)
Mother2Be skin products
Motilium (domperidone)
Motrin Migraine Pain (ibuprofen)
moxa (Chinese herb)
MSL-109 monoclonal antibody
MTBE (methyl tertiary butyl ether)
MTP (microsomal triglyceride
transfer protein)

medication *(cont.)*
MTP-PE (muramyl-tripeptide)
Multikine (interleukin; leukocyte)
mupirocin (Bactroban)
muromonab-CD3 monoclonal
antibody
MUSE (medicated urethral system
for erection) urethral supposi-
tory (alprostadil)
Mutamycin (mitomycin)
MVAC or M-VAC chemotherapy
protocol
M-Vax cancer vaccine
M.V.C.9+4
MVF chemotherapy protocol
M.V.I.-12
MVT chemotherapy protocol
Myambutol (ethambutol)
Mycobutin (rifabutin)
mycophenolate mofetil (CellCept)
myeloid progenitor inhibitory
factor-1 (MPIF-1)
Mylotarg (gemtuzumab ozogamicin;
CMA-676)
Myoscint (imciromab pentetate)
Myotrophin (mecasermin)
Myoview
M-Zole 3 Combination Pack
M-Zole 7 Dual Pack
Nabi-HB (hepatitis B immune
globulin [human])
Nabi-NicVAX nicotine vaccine
nabumetone (Relafen)
NAC (N-acetyl-L-cysteine)
N-acetyl-L-cysteine (NAC)
nafamostat mesilate
nafarelin (Synarel)
Naganol (suramin)
nalmefene HCl (Revex)
naltrexone hydrochloride
Nanox
naphthyalkalone class of drugs
Naphuride (suramin)
Naprelan (naproxen sodium)
Napron X (naproxen)

medication *(cont.)*

Naprosyn (naproxen)
naproxen (Aleve, Amaprox,
  Napron X, Naprelan, Naprosyn)
naproxen sodium (Naprelan)
Naropin (ropivacaine hydro-
  chloride)
Nasacort AQ (triamcinolone
  acetonide)
Nasarel (flunisolide)
Nascobal gel (cyanocobalamine)
Nasonex (mometasone furoate
  monohydrate) aqueous nasal
  spray
nateglinide
Natrecor (nesiritide)
Navelbine (vinorelbine tartrate)
N-butyl-deoxynojirimycin (DNJ)
nebacumab (Ha-1A monoclonal
  antibody)
NebuPent (aerosolized pentamidine)
nedocromil sodium (Tilade)
nefazodone (Serzone)
nelfinavir (Viracept)
Neocate
Neoral (cyclosporine for micro-
  emulsion)
Ne-Osteo
NeoTect (depreotide)
Neotrofin (AIT-082, leteprinim
  potassium)
Neovastat
NephrAmine solution
Nepro nutritional formula
Neumega (oprelvekin) (recombinant
  human interleukin-11)
nerve growth factor (NGF)
Neupogen (filgrastim)
Neuprex
NeuroCell-HD
NeuroCell-PD
Neurolite (technetium Tc 99m
  bicisate) contrast medium
Neurontin (gabapentin)

medication *(cont.)*

Neutralase (heparinase 1)
NeuTrexin (trimetrexate nevirapine)
  (BI-RG-587)
nevirapine (BIRG 0587)
Nexacryl
Nexium (esomeprazole magnesium)
NF-ATc proteins
Niaspan (niacin)
nicardipine hydrochloride
  (Cardene)
NicErase-SL (lobeline sulfate)
Nicoderm, Nicoderm CQ
Nicorette chewing gum
Nicorette inhaler
Nicotrol inhaler
NicVAX vaccine
Nilandron (nilutamide)
nilutamide (Anandron; Nilandron)
Nimbex (cisatracurium besylate)
nimodipine (Nimotop)
Nipent (pentostatin)
nisoldipine (Sular)
nitazoxanide (NTZ; Cryptaz)
nitrazepam (Mogadon)
nitrendipine (Baypress)
nitrogen-13 ammonia
nitroglycerin
Nitrol ointment
"nitro paste" (slang for nitro-
  glycerin ointment)
NitroQuick (nitroglycerin)
  sublingual tablets
Nizoral (ketoconazole)
N-methyl-D-aspartate (NMDA)
Nolvadex (tamoxifen citrate)
nonoxynol 9 (Advantage)
nonspecific immunoglobulin G
norastemizole
Norditropin SimpleXx (somatropin
  [rDNA origin] for injection)
Norelin
norfloxacin (Chibroxin, Noroxin)
Norian SRS (skeletal repair system)

medication *(cont.)*
Noritate (metronidazole) cream
Normiflo (low molecular weight
    heparin; ardeparin sodium
    injection)
Noroxin (norfloxacin)
Norplant (levonorgestrel)
Norvasc (amlodipine)
Norvir (ritonavir) capsules and
    oral solution
No Sting barrier film
Novantrone (mitoxantrone for
    injection concentrate)
Novapren
Novasome (nonoxynol-9)
Novastatin (argatroban)
NovoNorm (repaglinide)
NovoSeven (factor VIIa,
    recombinant)
NOX-100
NPH insulin
NSAIDs (nonsteroidal anti-inflam-
    matory drugs)
NTZ (nitazoxanide)
Nucletron
NuLytely solution
Nuromax (doxacurium chloride)
Nu-Trim
NutriMan TNT (*Tribulus terrestris*
    extract)
Nutropin (somatotropin)
Nutropin AQ (somatotropin)
Nutropin Depot (somatotropin)
Nuvance (interleukin-4 receptor)
Nyotran (nystatin liposomal)
Nystatin-LF (liposomal formula-
    tion)
Obecalp (placebo)
Obetrol
OCT medium
OctreoScan radiologic imaging
    agent (indium-111 pentetreotide)
octreotide (Sandostatin)
Ocufen (flurbiprofen sodium)

medication *(cont.)*
Ocuflox (ofloxacin)
OcuHist (AK-Con-A) eyedrops
Ocupress (carteolol HCl)
ofloxacin (Floxin, Ocuflox)
OKT3 monoclonal antibody
    (Orthoclone OKT3)
OKT4 monoclonal antibody
OKT8 monoclonal antibody
olanzapine (Zyprex)
oligozymes
olsalazine (Dipentum)
omeprazole (Prilosec)
Omnicef (cefdinir)
Omniflox (temafloxacin)
Omnipaque (iohexol) imaging agent
Omniscan (gadodiamide) contrast
    medium
OMS (oral morphine sulfate)
Oncaspar (pegaspargase)
Oncolym radiolabeled monoclonal
    antibody
Onconase
Oncophage cancer vaccine
OncoScint CR/OV (satumomab
    pendetide) contrast medium
OncoScint CR103 imaging agent
ondansetron (Zofran)
Ontak (denileukin diftitox)
Onyx liquid embolic system
OPPA chemotherapy protocol
OptiPranolol (metipranolol)
Optiray (ioversol)
Optisol
Optison ultrasound contrast agent
Optrin (motexafin lutetium; Lu-Tex)
Optro (recombinant human
    hemoglobin)
Oralease
Oralet lollipop (fentanyl citrate)
Oralex
Oralgen oral insulin
Oramorph SR (morphine sulfate)
orgotein

medication *(cont.)*
  orlistat (Xenical)
  Ornidyl (eflornithine)
  orphan drug
  Ortho-Cept (progesterone
    desogestrel, ethinyl estradiol)
  Orthoclone OKT3 monoclonal
    antibody
  OrthoDyn
  Ortho-Est (estropipate)
  Ortholinum (botulinum toxin,
    type F)
  Ortho-mune
  Ortho-Prefest (17[beta]-estradiol/
    norgestimate)
  Orthovisc
  Orudis (ketoprofen)
  Orudis KT (ketoprofen)
  Oruvail (ketoprofen, Orudis)
  OSCM (oil-soluble contrast
    medium)
  Osteogenics BoneSource
  Osteopatch
  Osteoset bone graft substitute
  OTC (over-the-counter) drugs
  OTFC (oral transmucosal fentanyl
    citrate)
  OvaRex MAb
  OvaRex vaccine
  O-Vax vaccine
  OvuStick
  oxandrolone (Oxandrin)
  Oxilan (ioxilan)
  oxothiazolidine carboxylate
    (Procysteine)
  Oxsoralen (methoxsalen)
  oxyazolidinones
  oxycodone and acetaminophen
    capsules
  oxycodone HCl (Roxicodone)
  Oxycontin (oxycodone HCl)
  Oxygent (perflubron emulsion)
  oxymetholone (Anadrol-50)
  oxyphenbutazone

medication *(cont.)*
  PAB-Esc-C chemotherapy protocol
  PACE chemotherapy protocol
  Pacis BCG
  pagoclone
  palladium 103 (Pd103, 103Pd)
  pamidronate disodium (Aredia)
  Panafil enzymatic debriding agent
  Panafil White ointment
  Pancrecarb MS-8 (pancrelipase)
  pancrelipase
  Pannaz
  Panretin (alitretinoin) 1% gel
  PANTA (polymyxin B, ampho-
    tericin B, nalidixic acid,
    trimethoprim, and azlocillin)
  pantoprazole (Pantozol)
  Pantozol (pantoprazole)
  papaverine topical gel
  Paraplatin (carboplatin)
  parathormone (PTH)
  parecoxib
  Parkland formula
  paroxetine (Paxil)
  PARP (ADP-ribose) polymerase
  Parsol 1789
  Paser (aminosalicylic acid)
  Patanol (olopatadine hydrochloride
    ophthalmic solution)
  PAVe chemotherapy protocol
  Paxene (paclitaxel)
  Paxil (paroxetine)
  PCE chemotherapy protocol
  PCP (phencyclidine)
  PC-SPES
  PCV chemotherapy protocol
  Pearl Omega
  PEG-ADA (pegademase bovine,
    Adagen, Imudon)
  pegademase bovine (PEG-ADA,
    Adagen)
  pegaspargase (Oncaspar)
  Pegasys (PEG-interferon alfa-2a)
  PEG-hemoglobin oxygen carrier

medication *(cont.)*

PEG-IL-2 (interleukin-2)
PEG-Intron
PEG-Intron A (interferon alfa-2b
conjugated polyethylene glycol)
PEG-LES
pegylated-liposomal doxorubicin
Pemoline C-IV
penciclovir (Denavir)
Penetrex (enoxacin)
penicilloylpolylysine (PPL,
Pre-Pan)
Penlac nail lacquer (ciclopirox)
Pennsaid topical lotion (diclofenac
potassium)
Pentam 300 (pentamidine isethion-
ate)
pentamidine isethionate (Pentam
300)
pentamidine isethionate, aerosolized
(NebuPent, Pneumopent)
Pentasa (mesalamine)
pentosan polysulfate sodium
(Elmiron)
peppermint oil
Peptamen isotonic elemental
Perative nutritional formula
Perceptin
perflubron
perfosfamide (Pergamid)
Pergamid (perfosfamide)
Peridex
Periostat
pertechnetate sodium (technetium)
P-glycoprotein
PharmaSeed palladium-103 seeds
phentolamine mesylate (Vasomax)
PHNO (4-propyl-9-hydroxy-
naphthoxazine)
phosphonoformate, trisodium
Photofrin (sterile porfimer sodium)
photosensitizing agent
PHRT chemotherapy protocol
phthalocyanine photosensitizing
agent

medication *(cont.)*

phycobiliproteins
PIA chemotherapy protocol
Pilostat (pilocarpine)
pimagedine HCl (Action-II)
pinacidil (Pindac)
Pindac (pinacidil)
pipecuronium (Arduan)
PIPIDA (N-para-isopropyl-aceta-
nilide-iminodiacetic acid)
pirarubicin
pirenzepine HCl (Gastrozepine)
piritrexim isethionate (BW 301U)
piroxicam (Feldene)
placebo (Obecalp)
placental growth hormone (PGH)
Plan B (levonorgestrel)
platelet-derived growth factor
Plasma-Lyte A pH 7.4
Plasma-Lyte 56
Plasma-Lyte 148
Plasma-Lyte R
Plavix (clopidogrel bisulfate)
pleconaril antiviral
Plendil (felodipine)
Pletal (cilostazol)
plicamycin (Mithracin)
PM-81 monoclonal antibody
PMPA
PMT (pyridoxyl-5-methyl tryptophan) imaging agent
P-MVAC chemotherapy protocol
PMX-F (polymixin B fibers)
pneumococcal conjugate vaccine
Pneumopent (aerosolized
pentamidine isethionate)
POCC chemotherapy protocol
Podiatrx-AF and Podiatrx-TFM
polyethylene glycol electrolyte
lavage solution (PEG-LES)
polyribonucleotide (Ampligen)
Polytrim ophthalmic solution
POMP chemotherapy protocol
porcine fetal lateral ganglionic
eminence (LGE) cells

medication *(cont.)*
   Portagen dietary powder
   Posicor (mibefradil)
   postoperative regimen for oral
     early feeding (PROEF)
   potassium iodide (SSKI)
   PPL (penicilloyl polylysine,
     Pre-Pen)
   pramipexole (Mirapex)
   pramlintide (Symlin)
   Prandase (acarbose)
   Prandin (repaglinide)
   Pravachol (pravastatin)
   PreCare Conceive nutritional
     supplement
   prednicarbate (Dermatop)
   prednimustine (Sterecyt)
   PremesisRx
   Premphase (medroxyprogesterone)
   Prempro (conjugated estrogen and
     medroxyprogesterone)
   Pre-Pen (penicilloyl polylysine)
   Prepidil (dinoprostone) gel
   Prepodyne solution
   Presaril (torsemide, Demedex)
   Preservex
   Prevacid (lansoprazole)
   Prevnar vaccine
   Priftin (rifapentine)
   Prilosec (omeprazole)
   Primacor (milrinone)
   primaquine phosphate
   Primsol solution (trimethoprim HCl
     oral solution)
   Prinzide (HCTZ, linisopril)
   PRL (prolactin)
   Pro-Air (procaterol)
   ProAmatine (midodrine HCl)
   Pro-Banthine (propantheline
     bromide)
   Procardia XL (nifedipine)
   procaterol (Pro-Air)
   Procrit (epoetin alfa)
   Proctozone P (pramoxine HCl) and
     Proctozone H (hydrocortisone)

medication *(cont.)*
   Procuren platelet-derived growth
     factor
   Procysteine (oxothiazolidine
     carboxylate)
   PROEF (postoperative regimen for
     oral early feeding)
   Prograf (tacrolimus)
   ProHance (gadoteridol) contrast
     medium
   ProLease encapsulated sustained-
     release growth hormone
   Proleukin (aldesleukin)
   ProMACE-CYTABOM chemo-
     therapy protocol
   ProMem (metrifonate)
   Promensil isoflavone-based dietary
     supplement
   Prometrium (progesterone,
     micronized)
   Promycin (porfiromycin)
   propafenone (Rythmol)
   propantheline bromide
     (Pro-Banthine)
   Propecia (finasteride)
   proprietary medicine
   Propulsid (cisapride)
   Proscar (finasteride)
   ProSol (amino acid injection)
   ProSom (estazolam)
   Prosorba
   prostaglandin E1 (PGE1)
   ProstaScint (CYT-356 radiolabeled
     with 111 indium chloride)
   ProstaSeed ^{125}I
   ProStep (nicotine)
   protease inhibitor
   Proteque SPS
   Prothiaden (dothiepin HCl)
   Protonix (pantoprazole)
   Protropin, Protropin II
   PRO 2000 Gel
   Provigil (modafinil)
   Provir
   Prozac (fluoxetine)

medication *(cont.)*

pseudoephedrine HCl/guaifenesin (Syn-Rx)

Pseudovent (guaifenesin/ pseudoephedrine HCl) capsules

psoralen

PTH (parathormone, parathyroid hormone)

P-32 (chromic phosphate, phosphorus 32)

Pulmicort Turbuhaler (budesonide)

Pulmo-Aide nebulizer

Pulmozyme (dornase alfa)

Puri-Clens wound cleanser

Purlytin (tin ethyl etiopurpurin)

PVA chemotherapy protocol

PVA (polyvinyl alcohol) particles

PVB chemotherapy protocol

PVDA chemotherapy protocol

PVP chemotherapy protocol

pycnogenol natural supplement

Pylorid (ranitidine bismuth citrate)

pyranocarboxylic acid class of drugs

pyridoxilated stroma-free hemoglobin (SFHb)

pyrimethamine (Daraprim)

Quadramet (samarium Sm 153 lexidronam)

quaternary ammonium chloride

quazepam (Doral)

quinacrine

quinapril (Accupril)

Quintessence

quinupristin; dalfopristin (Synercid)

Quixin (levofloxacin ophthalmic solution)

rAAT (recombinant alpha-1 antitrypsin)

RabAvert (human rabies vaccine)

rabies vaccine, Rhesus diploid cell strain (RDRV)

racemic fluoxetine (S-fluoxetine)

R-albuterol

medication *(cont.)*

raloxifene

ramipril (Altace)

ranolazine

Rapamune (sirolimus; formerly rapamycin)

RapiSeal patch

Raplon

Raxar (grepafloxacin HCl)

RBC-CD4

rCD4 (Receptin)

RDRV (Rhesus diploid cell strain rabies vaccine)

Reactine (cetirizine)

Rebetol (ribavirin)

Rebetron (ribavirin and interferon alfa-2b)

Rebif (recombinant interferon beta)

Receptin (CD4, recombinant soluble human)

recombinant alpha-1 antitrypsin

recombinant desulfatohirudin (hirudin)

recombinant human erythropoietin (rhEPO)

recombinant human granulocyte colony stimulating factor (r-met HuG-CSF)

recombinant human neutral endopeptidase (rNEP)

recombinant human relaxin (relaxin)

recombinant interferon beta (Rebif)

recombinant novel plasminogen activator (rNPA)

recombinant prourokinase

recombinant tissue plasminogen activator

Recombinate

Reductil (sibutramine)

Redux (dexfenfluramine)

ReFacto antihemophilic factor (recombinant)

Refinity skin products

medication *(cont.)*
Refludan (lepirudin rDNA) injection
Reglan (metoclopramide)
Regranex gel (becaplermin)
Regressin
Relafen (nabumetone)
relaxin (recombinant human
    relaxin)
Relenza (zanamivir)
ReLibra (testosterone gel)
Relpax (eletriptan)
remacemide
Remeron (mirtazapine)
Remicade (infliximab)
Reminyl (galantamine)
remnant-like particle (RLP)
    lipoprotein
remoxipride (Roxiam)
Remune (formerly HIV-1
    Immunogen)
Renacidin solution
Renagel (sevelamer HCl)
Renotec (^{99m}Tc iron-ascorbate-
    DTPA)
Renova (tretinoin emollient cream)
ReoPro (abciximab) monoclonal
    antibody
Repel
Repifermin (keratinocyte growth
    factor 2 [KGF-2])
Replens gel
Repliform
Requip (ropinirole HDl)
Rescula (unoprostone isopropyl
    ophthalmic solution) eye drops
RespiGam (immune globulin,
    Respivir)
Respirgard II nebulizer
Respivir (respiratory syncytial virus
    immune globulin) (RespiGam)
Resten-NG
Retavase (reteplase)
reticulose
Retin-A Micro (tretinoin gel)

medication *(cont.)*
Retrovir (zidovudine, AZT)
ReVele imaging agent
Reversionex (HE317)
Revex (nalmefene HCl)
Rev-Eyes (dapiprazole)
ReVia (naltrexone hydrochloride
    tablets)
RG 12915
RG-83894 AIDS vaccine
RG-201
r-gp160 vaccine
rHb1.1 (recombinant hemoglobin)
rhEPO or EPO (recombinant
    human erythropoietin)
rhIGF-1 (recombinant human
    insulin-like growth factor)
Rhinocort Aqua (budesonide) nasal
    spray
Rice-Lyte
riCitrasol (anticoagulant sodium
    citrate solution)
Ridaura (auranofin)
RIDD chemotherapy protocol
Rid Mousse (pyrethrum extract)
rifabutin (Mycobutin)
rifalazil
rifapentine (Priftin)
Rifater (rifampin, isoniazid, and
    pyrazinamide)
rifaximin
Rilutek (riluzole)
riluzole (Rilutek)
Rimadyl (carprofen)
rimantadine HCl (Flumadine)
rimexolone (Vexol)
Ringer's lactate
Risperdal (risperidone)
risperidone (Risperdal)
Ritalin (methylphenidate)
ritonavir (Norvir)
Rituxan (rituximab)
rituximab (Rituxan)
rivastigmine

medication *(cont.)*
Rizaben (tranilast)
RMP-7
rNEP (recombinant human neutral endopeptidase)
rNPA (recombinant novel plasminogen activator)
Robaxacet (methocarbamol and acetaminophen)
Rocephin IM (sterile ceftriazone sodium)
rofecoxib oral
Roferon-A (interferon alfa-2a)
Rogaine
rogletimide
Romazicon
ropinirole (Requip)
ropivacaine (Naropin)
roquinimex (Linomide)
Rotamune vaccine
RotaShield vaccine
Rowasa (mesalamine) enema
Roxiam (remoxipride)
Roxicodone (oxycodone HCl)
rt-PA (recombinant tissue plasminogen activator)
rubitecan (RFS2000)
RU-486 (Mifeprex)
Ryna-12 S (phenylephrine tannate/ pyrilamine tannate) suspension
Rythmol (propafenone HCl)
SAARD (slow-acting antirheumatic drug)
Sabril (vigabatrin)
Saf-Clens chronic wound cleanser
Saf-Gel for wound hydration
SA-IGIV (*Staphylococcus aureus* immune globulin intravenous [human])
Saizen
Salagen (pilocarpine hydrochloride)
Salix (sorbitol) lozenges
salmeterol xinafoate (Serevent)
samarium Sm 153 lexidronam (Quadramet)

medication *(cont.)*
Sandostatin (octreotide)
Sandostatin LAR Depot (ocreotide acetate for injectable suspension)
Sanorex (mazindol)
Santyl (collagenase)
saquinavir (Fortovase; Invirase)
sargramostim (Leukine)
satumonab pendetide (OncoScint CR/OV)
Savvy vaginal gel
sCD4 (soluble CD4, recombinant)
sCD4-PE40
Schlesinger's solution
Sclerosol (sterile aerosol talc)
SD Plasma
seabuckthorn seed oil
Seasonale oral contraceptive
SeaSorb alginate wound dressing
secretin polypeptide
Segard (afelimomab)
SelCID
Selecor (celiprolol)
selective estrogen receptor modulator (SERM) class of drugs
selegilene
selenium-75 (^{75}Se)
Semprex-D (acrivastine)
Sensamide (metoclopramide)
SEPA/ibuprofen gel
SEPA/minoxidil
Sepracoat coating solution
Seprafilm (sodium hyaluronate and carboxymethylcellulose)
Septra (TMP-SMZ, SMZ-TMP)
Serenoa repens extract (Permixon)
Serevent (salmeterol xinafoate)
SERM (selective estrogen receptor modulator)
sermorelin acetate (Geref)
Seroquel (quetiapine fumarate)
Serostim (somatoprin of rDNA origin)
serotonin type-3 receptor antagonist drug class

medication *(cont.)*
 SERPACWA (Skin Exposure
  Reduction Paste Against
  Chemical Warfare Agents)
 sertindole
 sertraline (Zoloft)
 Serzone (nefazodone)
 sestamibi (^{99m}Tc sestamibi,
  Cardiolite)
 sevelamer HCl (Renagel)
 17-1A monoclonal antibody SFHb
  (pyridoxilated stroma-free
  hemoglobin)
 sevoflurane (Ultane)
 S-fluoxetine (racemic fluoxetine)
 Shade UVAGuard
 Shohl's solution
 Shur-Clens wound cleanser
 sibrafiban
 Simdax (levosimendan)
 Simulect (basiliximab)
 simvastatin (Zocor)
 Singulair (montelukast)
 sitostanol ester margarine
 sivelestat
 6-AN protocol
 Skelid (tiludronate disodium)
 Skinvisible hypoallergenic hand
  lotion
 Sleeping Buddha sedative
 Slo-phyllin Gyrocaps (theophylline)
 SMF chemotherapy protocol
 SMZ/TMP (sulfamethoxazole and
  trimethoprim, Bactrim, Septra)
 SnET2 (tin ethyl etiopurpurin)
 Sn-protoporphyrin
 Sodium Sulamyd (sulfacetamide
  sodium)
 sodium tetradecyl sulfate (Sotradecol)
 Solagé ("so-la-JAY") (mequinol;
  tretinoin)
 Solarese (diclofenac gel)
 SoloSite wound gel
 SomatoKine (IGF-BP3 complex)

medication *(cont.)*
 somatropin (Nutropin)
 somatuline
 Somavert (pegvisomant for
  injection)
 Sonata (zaleplon)
 Sonazoid ultrasound contrast agent
 Soothe-N-Seal
 sorbitol (Salix) lozenges
 Soriatane (acitretin)
 sotalol (Betapace)
 Sotradecol (sodium tetradecyl
  sulfate)
 sparfloxacin (Zagam)
 Spectracef (cefditoren pivoxil)
 spiramycin
 Spirulina Pacifica
 Sporanox oral solution (itracona-
  zole)
 Sporicidin
 squalamine
 SSKI (saturated solution of
  potassium iodide)
 Staarvisc (sodium hyaluronate)
 Stadol, Stadol NS (butorphanol
  tartrate)
 Staphylococcus aureus immune
  globulin intravenous (human)
  (SA-IGIV)
 Starlix (nateglinide)
 stavudine (Zerit, d4T)
 Stemgen
 Sterecyt (prednimustine)
 sterile porfimer sodium (Photofrin)
 Stimate (desmopressin acetate)
  nasal spray
 Stoxil (idoxuridine)
 Streptase (streptokinase)
 streptogramin
 streptokinase (Kabikinase,
  Streptase)
 stroma-free hemoglobin (SFHb)
  solution
 Stromagen

medication *(cont.)*

Stromectol (ivermectin)
strontium chloride Sr 89
  (Metastron)
St. Thomas' solution
Suby's solution G (Suby G)
succimer (Chemet)
Sucraid (sacrosidase)
sucralfate (Carafate)
Sulamyd (sulfacetamide sodium)
Sular (nisoldipine)
sulfacetamide sodium (Sulamyd)
Sulfamylon (mafenide acetate)
sulindac (Clinoril)
sumatriptan succinate (Imitrex)
superabsorbent polymer (SAP)
superparamagnetic iron oxide
  (SPIO) contrast medium
SuperVent
Supprelin (histrelin acetate)
suramin
Surfaxin (lucinactant)
Surgicel Nu-Knit absorbable
  hemostatic agent
Surgidine
Surgi-Prep (povidone iodine;
  Betadine)
Surodex (dexamethasone)
Survanta (beractant)
Sustiva (efavirenz)
Sygen (ganglioside)
Symlin (pramlintide)
Symmetra I-125 brachytherapy
  seeds
Synagis (palivizumab)
Synarel (nafarelin acetate)
Synercid (quinupristin; delfopristin)
Syn-Rx (pseudoephredrine HCl/
  guaifenesin)
Synsorb Cd
Synsorb Pk
Synvisc
Syringe Avitene
TAC (triamcinolone cream)

medication *(cont.)*

Tace (chlorotrianisene)
tacrine (Cognex)
tacrolimus (Prograf)
Tagamet (cimetidine)
talc poudrage
talc slurry
Tamiflu (oseltamivir phosphate)
tamoxifen citrate (Nolvadex, TAM,
  TMX)
Tao (troleandomycin)
Targocid (teicoplanin)
Targretin (bexarotene) gel 1%
Tasmar (tolcapone)
TAT inhibitor
Taxol (paclitarel)
Taxotere (docetaxel)
tazarotene (Tazorac)
Tazidime (ceftazidime)
Tazocin (Zosyn)
Tazorac (tazarotene topical gel)
^{99m}Tc Abbokinase (urokinase)
  thrombolytic agent
^{99m}Tc glucarate "hot spot"
^{99m}Tc-GSA (Albunex)
TcHIDA
TCN-P (triciribine phosphate)
TCR (T-cell receptor) peptide
  vaccine
TDR (thymidine deoxyriboside,
  Zerit)
teboroxime (CardioTec or
  CardioTek)
TEC chemotherapy protocol
teceleukin (interleukin-2,
  recombinant)
Techneplex (^{99m}Tc penetate)
Technescan MAG3
technetium 99m albumin
technetium 99m albumin aggre-
  gated
technetium 99m albumin colloid
technetium 99m bicisate
technetium 99m colloid

medication *(cont.)*
technetium 99m diethylene contrast
   medium
technetium 99m diethylene-triamine
   pentaacetic acid-galactosyl-
   human serum-albumin
technetium 99m disofenin
technetium 99m etidronate
technetium 99m ferpentetate
technetium 99m furifosmin contrast
   medium
technetium 99m Glucarate hot spot
technetium 99m gluceptate
technetium 99m HIDA
technetium 99m iron-ascorbate-
   DTPA (Renotec)
technetium 99m lidofenin
technetium 99m macroaggregated
   albumin (^{99m}Tc MAA)
technetium 99m medronate
   (Macrotec)
technetium 99m mertiatide
   (Technescan MAG3)
technetium 99m oxidronate
technetium 99m penetate
   (Techneplex)
technetium 99m pertechnetate
technetium 99m PIPIDA
technetium 99m pyrophosphate
technetium 99m sestamibi
   (Cardiolite)
technetium 99m siboroxime
technetium 99m sodium
technetium 99m succimer
technetium 99m sulesomab
   (LeukoScan)
technetium 99m sulfur colloid
   (Tesuloid)
technetium 99m teboroxime
   (CardioTek or CardioTec)
technetium 99m tetrofosmin
technetium stannous pyrophosphate
   (TSPP)
tegaserod (Zelmac)

medication *(cont.)*
teicoplanin (Targocid)
teloxantrone HCl
temafloxacin (Omniflox)
Temodar (temozolomide)
TEMP chemotherapy protocol
10-EDAM (EDAM)
tenidap (Enable)
teniposide (VM-26, Vumon)
Tequin (gatifloxacin)
terazosin (Hytrin)
terbinafine (Lamisil)
terfenadine carboxylate (Allegra)
terlipressin (Glypressin)
teroxirone (alpha-TGI)
TeslaScan (mangafodipir trisodium)
Testoderm TTS (testosterone
   transdermal system)
Tesuloid
tetracycline
Teveten (eprosartan mesylate)
TGF-beta-2 (BetaKine)
thalidomide (Thalomid)
thallium 201 (Tl-201)
Thalomid (thalidomide)
Theochron (theophylline)
TheraCys (BCG live intravesical)
Theradigm-HBV
Theradigm-HPV
Therafectin (amiprilose HCl)
TheraSeed
Theratope-STn vaccine
Therex
Thermophore
thianamycin
Thioplex (thiotepa)
thiotepa (Thioplex)
13-cis-retinoic acid (13-CRA,
   isotretinoin)
3F8 monoclonal antibody
ThromboSol
Thunder God vine
thymalfasin (Zadaxin)
thymic humoral factor

medication *(cont.)*
thymidine deoxyriboside (TDR)
Thymoglobulin (antithymocyte
  globulin [rabbit])
thymopentin (Timunox)
thymostimuline (TP-1)
Thyrogyn (thyrotropin alfa)
tiagabine (Gabitril)
Tiazac (diltiazem HCl)
Tice (intravesical BCG)
Ticlid (ticlopidine)
ticlopidine (Ticlid)
TIL (tumor-infiltrating lympho-
  cytes)
Timoptic XE (timolol)
Timunox (thymopentin)
tioconazole (Vagistat)
tirofiban (Aggrastat)
tissue plasminogen activator (t-PA)
tissue-selective estrogens
TI-23 (CMV monoclonal antibody)
tizanidine (Zanaflex)
TLC G-65 (gentamicin liposome)
TMP-SMZ (trimethoprim-
  sulfamethoxazole)
TNF (tumor necrosis factor)
TNK-tPA
tNOX (quinol oxidase)
TNP-470
toborinone
TobraDex (tobramycin and
tolrestat (Alredase)
Tomudex
Topamax (topiramate)
Topiglan (alprostadil)
topotecan (Hycamptin)
Toprol XL (metoprolol succinate)
Toradol (ketorolac tromethamine)
torsemide (Demadex, Presaril)
Tostrex
Total toothpaste
t-PA (tissue plasminogen activator)
TPDCV chemotherapy protocol
TP-40

medication *(cont.)*
TpP (thrombus precursor protein)
TP10 complement inhibitor
TRA (all-trans retinoic acid,
  tretinoin)
tramadol HCl (Ultram)
transferrin
Trasylol (aprotinin)
Travasorb MCT
Treptase (urokinase)
tretinoin (Vesanoid)
tretinoin emollient cream (Renova)
trichosanthin (compound Q)
triciribine phosphate (TCN-P)
Tricomin
Tricor (micronized fenofibrate)
tricyclic antidepressant
Trileptal (oxcarbazepine)
trimethoprim-sulfamethoxazole
  (TMP-SMZ, Bactrim, Septra)
trimetrexate gluconate (TMQ,
  TMTX, NeuTrexin)
Tri-Nasal Spray (triamcinolone
  acetonide)
Triphasil (levonorgestrel, esthinyl
  estradiol)
triple antibiotics
Tritec (ranitidine bismuth citrate)
TroCam
trofermin (Fiblast)
troleandomycin (Tao)
Trovan (trovafloxacin)
Trovan/Zithromax Compliance Pak
Trovert
troxacitabine (formerly BCH-4556)
Tru-Scint AD imaging agent
Trusopt (dorzolamide HCl)
TSPP (technetium stannous
  pyrophosphate)
T-2 protocol
tumor-infiltrating lymphocytes
  (TIL)
tumor necrosis factor (TNF)
TUNEL stain

medication *(cont.)*
Tutoplast
Twinrix (hepatitis A inactivated and
  hepatitis B [recombinant]
  vaccine)
2A11 monoclonal antibody
2-CdA (2-chlorodeoxyadenosine)
Uendex (dextran sulfate)
Ultane (sevoflurane)
UltraJect morphine sulfate
UltraKlenz wound cleanser
Ultram (tramadol HCl)
ultrasmall superparamagnetic iron
  oxide (USPIO) imaging agent
UltraThon
Ultravate (halobetasol propionate)
Ultravist (iopromide)
Uniprost (prostacyclin)
Uniretic (moexipril/hydrochloro-
  thiazide)
Univasc (moexipril HCl)
University of Wisconsin solution
Uprima (apomorphine)
uracil mustard
uridine rescue
urofollitropin (Metrodin)
urokinase (Abbokinase, Treptase)
Urso (ursodiol)
ursodeoxycholic acid (ursodiol)
ursodiol (Actigall)
VAB-6 chemotherapy protocol
VAC chemotherapy protocol
VACA chemotherapy protocol
VACAD chemotherapy protocol
VACP chemotherapy protocol
VAD chemotherapy protocol
VAD/V chemotherapy protocol
Vagifem vaginal tablets (estradiol
  hemihydrate)
vaginal contraceptive film (VCF)
Vagistat tioconazole
VAI chemotherapy protocol
valacyclovir HCl (Valtrex)
valganciclovir
VALOP-B chemotherapy protocol

medication *(cont.)*
Valtrex (valacyclovir HCl)
VAM chemotherapy protocol
VAMP chemotherapy protocol
Vancenase Pockethaler
Vaniqa cream
Vanlev (omapatrilat)
Vantin (cefpodoxime proxetil)
VAPE (vincristine, Adriamycin,
  procarbazine, etoposide)
varicella vaccine (Varivax)
Varivax (varicella vaccine)
Vascor (bepridil)
Vascu-Guard
vascular targeting agent
Vasomax (phentolamine mesylate)
VAT chemotherapy protocol
Vaxid
VaxSyn HIV-1
VBC chemotherapy protocol
VBMCP chemotherapy protocol
VBMF chemotherapy protocol
VBP chemotherapy protocol
VeIP chemotherapy protocol
Velban (vinblastine)
Veldona interferon alfa lozenge
velnacrine maleate (Mentane)
Velosulin BR (buffered regular)
  insulin
venlafaxine (Effexor)
verapamil (Covera-HS)
Verdia (tasosartan)
Verluma (nofetumomab) diagnostic
  imaging agent
Versed syrup
Vesanoid (tretinoin)
vesnarinone
Vestra (reboxetine mesylate)
Vexol (rimexolone)
Viadur (leuprolide acetate implant)
Viagra (sildenafil citrate)
VIC chemotherapy protocol
Vicoprofen (hydrocodone bitartrate
  and ibuprofen)

medication *(cont.)*

vidarabine (adenine arabinoside, Ara-A, Vira-A)

Videx (didanosine, dideoxyinosine, ddI)

VIE chemotherapy protocol

vigabatrin (Sabril)

viloxazine (Catatrol)

VIMRxyn (synthetic hypericin)

Vincasar (vincristine)

vindesine sulfate (Eldisine, Navelbine, VOB)

vinorelbine tartrate (Navelbine)

Vioxx (rofecoxib)

Viozan

VIP chemotherapy protocol

VIP-B chemotherapy protocol

Viprinex (ancrod)

Viracept (nelfinavir mesylate)

Viramune (nevirapine)

Virazole (ribavirin)

Virend

Viruzilin

Viscoat (hyaluronate sodium; chondroitin sulfate sodium)

Visidex, Visidex II

Visipaque (iodixanol) contrast medium

Vistide (cidofovir)

Visudyne (verteporfin for injection)

Vitrase

Vitravene (fomivirsen)

Vitreon (perfluorophenanthrene)

Vivelle; Vivelle-Dot (estradiol transdermal system)

Vleminckx's solution

VMP chemotherapy protocol

Volmax (albuterol)

Voltaren delayed-release tablets (diclofenac sodium)

Voltaren eye drops (diclofenac sodium)

VPCA chemotherapy protocol

VPP chemotherapy protocol

medication *(cont.)*

Vumon (teniposide)

water-soluble contrast medium (WSCM)

Welchol (formerly Cholestagel)

Wellferon (interferon alfa-n1)

WinRho SD

Xalatan (latanoprost solution)

Xatral OD (alfuzosin)

Xcytrin (motexafin gadolinium) injection

Xeloda (capecitabine)

Xenical (orlistat)

xenon 133 (^{133}Xe)

Xerecept (corticotropin-releasing factor)

XomaZyme-H65

Xopenex (levalbuterol HCl) inhalation solution

xylazine

Xyrem (gamma hydroxybutyrate)

yohimbine

Zacutex (lexipafant)

Zadaxin (thymalfasin)

Zaditen (ketotifen)

Zaditor (ketotifen fumarate)

zafirlukast (Accolate)

Zagam (sparfloxacin)

zalcitabine (Hivid)

Zanaflex (tizanidine)

Zanfel

Zanosar (streptozocin)

Zantac Efferdose

Zaroxolyn (methyl metolazone)

ZDV (zidovudine)

Zebeta (bisoprolol)

Zefazone (cefmetazole)

Zelapar (selegiline HCl)

Zeldox (ziprasidone hydrochloride)

Zelmac (tegaserod)

Zenapax (dacliximab) monoclonal antibody

Zenker's fixative

Zerit (stavudine, d4T)

medication *(cont.)*
Zestoretic
Zestril (lisinopril) tablets
Zevalin (ibritumomab tiuxetan)
Ziac (bisoprolol fumarate-
hydrochlorothiazide)
Ziagen (abacavir)
Zicam
ziconotide
zidovudine (AZT, Aztec, Retrovir)
ZIG vaccine
Zinecard (dexrazoxane)
Zithromax (azithromycin, Z-Pak)
Zixoryn (flumecinol)
Zocor (simvastatin)
Zofran (ondansetron)
Zoladex (goserelin acetate implant)
Zoloft (sertraline hydrochloride)
zolpidem tartrate (Ambien)
Zomaril (iloperidone)
Zomax (zomepirac sodium)
zomepirac sodium (Zomax)
Zometa (zoledronic acid for
injection)
Zomig (zolmitriptan)
Zonalon (doxepin hydrochloride
cream)
Zonegran (zonisamide)
zopiclone
Zosyn (piperacillin sodium,
tazobactam sodium)
Zovirax (acyclovir)
Z-Pak (Zithromax)
Zyban (bupropion HCl)
Zydone (hydrocodone bitartrate/
acetaminophen) tablets
Zyflo (zileuton)
Zyprexa (olanzapine)
Zyrtec (cetirizine HCl)
Zyvox (linezolid)

medicinal botanicals—term used for therapeutic natural products ignored by medical providers for many years but perceived by many to be more cost-effective and gentle, with fewer side effects, than traditional prescription medications. Some botanicals and their purported uses include bilberry (strengthens vessels, improves night vision), *Echinacea* (enhances immune system, prevents colds), kava kava and valerian (relaxants), garlic (improves HDL/LDL ratios, lowers blood pressure), ginseng (increases endurance), *Gingko biloba* (increases blood flow to brain and extremities), feverfew (treats migraine headache), ginger (acts as an antinauseant), hawthorne (improves heart, blood, and oxygen flow), St. John's wort (reduces anxiety and depression). Most are now sold as dietary supplements.

Medicon instruments—for vascular and cardiac surgery.

Medifil—collagen hemostatic wound dressing.

Mediflex-Bookler—holding and positioning devices.

Mediflex-Gazayerli retractor—endoscopic retractor-dissector that can be introduced through a rigid straight port and then reshaped.

Medigraphics 2000 analyzer—used in testing exhaled gases in cardiopulmonary exercise study.

Medipore Dress-it—a precut surgical dressing of a porous material with a cloth backing.

Medi-Ject—needle-free insulin injection system.

Medi-Jector Choice—needle-free insulin injector.

MediPort—a totally implanted vascular access device for continuous or intermittent outpatient delivery of fluids and medications. May be used with externalized catheters.

Medisense Pen 2—self blood glucose monitor. See *SBGM*.

Medisorb drug delivery system—allows controlled, sustained release of injectable drugs.

Mediterranean lymphoma—small intestine malignant lymphoma. The disease is characterized by a diffuse, intense plasma cell infiltrate in the lamina propria of the small intestine that may give rise to a malignant lymphoma. See *IPSID*.

MedJet microkeratome—a cutting device for vision correction and corneal transplant procedures.

Medline—medical bibliographical computer database, through which a search of the current literature on almost any medical subject can be conducted.

Mednext bone dissecting system—a high-speed system used in neurosurgery, otolaryngologic surgery, and plastic-craniofacial surgery.

Medoff sliding fracture plate.

Medrad automated power injector—injects a set amount of iodinated contrast medium at the therapist's discretion.

Medrad Mrinnervu (also MRinnervu) endorectal colon probe.

medroxyprogesterone (Amen, Curretab, Cycrin, Depo-Provera, Premphase, Prempro)—a hormone given to postmenopausal women for symptoms of vaginal atrophy and hot flashes, as well as abnormal uterine bleeding.

meds—brief form for *medications*.

MEDS (microsurgical extraction of ductal sperm)—in infertility.

MedSpeak/Radiology—with Windows NT, a real-time continuous speech recognition system developed by IBM.

Medstone STS shock-wave generator—used to produce shock waves for dissolving kidney stones and gallstones. Also, *Medstone STS lithotripsy system*.

MED (microendoscopic diskectomy) **system**.

Medtronic Activa tremor control therapy—uses an implanted device to suppress essential tremor and tremor associated with Parkinson's disease. The implanted system delivers mild electrical stimulation to block brain signals that cause tremor.

Medtronic Gem automatic implantable defibrillator—protects survivors of cardiac arrest and others whose hearts beat dangerously fast.

Medtronic Hancock II—tissue valve, available in both aortic and mitral models.

Medtronic Hemopump—a cardiac assist device used in minimally invasive heart surgery. This system allows the surgeon to perform some procedures without stopping the heart completely. In addition, blood does not actually leave the body as it does in more conventional perfusion techniques.

Medtronic Inspire—a system of implantable devices that deliver electrical stimulation to the hypoglossal nerve for control of obstructive sleep apnea.

Medtronic Jewel AF—implantable arrhythmia management device.

Medtronic Micro Jewel II—very small implantable defibrillator, about the size of a small pager.

Medtronic Octopus—a tissue stabilizing system used in coronary artery bypass graft surgery. It stabilizes the beating heart in order to facilitate suture placement.

Medtronic Pulsor Intrasound—pain reliever using sound vibrations.

Medtronic Sprint lead for cardioverter-defibrillators.

Medtronic SynchroMed pump—implantable subcutaneous infusion pump used to deliver chemotherapy drugs.

Medtronic temporary pacemaker.

Medtronic tremor control therapy device—an implanted device, similar to a cardiac pacemaker, that delivers electrical stimulation to block or override brain signals that cause tremor.

medullaris—conus medullaris.

MedX physical therapy device.

Mees' lines—transverse lines on the fingernails, strongly suggestive of arsenic poisoning. Cf. *Beau's line*.

mefenamic acid (Ponstel)—a nonsteroidal anti-inflammatory drug. Used for arthritis and menstrual cramps.

mefloquine (Lariam)—believed to be effective against some resistant strains of malaria. It is considered the oral drug of choice for persons traveling in areas where resistant strains of malaria are endemic.

MEG (magnetoencephalogram).

Megace (megestrol acetate).

MegaDyne all-in-one hand control—used in laparoscopic surgery for aspiration, irrigation, and cauterization.

Megadyne/Fann E-Z clean laparoscopic electrodes—Teflon-coated electrodes that do not have to be removed from the operating port for cleaning after coagulation.

megahertz (mHz)—thousand cycles per second, used as measurement in audiograms. See *hertz*.

megakaryocyte growth and development factor (MGDF)—reduces the duration and severity of thrombocytopenia in cancer patients following chemotherapy.

Megalink biliary stent—for the treatment of malignant obstructions of the biliary duct.

megestrol acetate (Megace)—synthetic version of progesterone for breast and endometrial cancers in women. Also approved for treating weight loss and anorexia in AIDS patients, based on the side effect of weight gain frequently seen in female cancer patients who were treated with the drug. It was noted that the weight gain was due to increased appetite rather than water retention.

MEI (metastatic efficiency index).

meibomian cyst—see *chalazion*.

meibomian froth (Path).

meibomian gland—one of the sebaceous glands of the eyelid.

Meige's ("mezh'uhz") **disease** or **syndrome**—dystonia of facial and oromandibular muscles with blepharospasm, grimacing mouth movements, and protrusion of the tongue. Also called *Brueghel's syndrome*, illustrated in Brueghel's painting *De Gaper*. First described by Dr. Henry Meige in 1910. Primarily affects middle-aged and elderly adults, women more often than men. Do not confuse with *Meigs' syndrome*.

Meigs' ("megz") **syndrome**—ascites and hydrothorax, seen with pelvic tumors, including ovarian fibromas. Named for Dr. Joe Vincent Meigs, an American surgeon. Do not confuse with *Meige's syndrome*.

Melacine (melanoma cell lysate vaccine).

melanin—the dark brown to black pigment normally present, predominantly in the hair, skin, the choroid coat of the eye, and substantia nigra of the brain. Also in some tumors, e.g., melanoma. Cf. *melena*.

melanocytes—see *cultured autologous melanocytes*.

melanoma cell lysate vaccine—see *Melacine*.

melanonychia—see *longitudinal melanonychia*.

melanotic—referring to the presence of melanin. Often confused with *melenic*. *Melenic* stools, not *melanotic* stools. Cf. *melenic*.

MELAS (mitochondrial myopathy, encephalopathy, lactic acidosis, and stroke-like episodes).

melena—passage of dark, tarry stools, indicating bleeding in the lower gastrointestinal tract. Cf. *melanin*.

melenic—referring to or marked by melena, as in *melenic stools*. Cf. *melanotic*.

melolabial flap—a flap from the medial cheek, used as a transposition flap, to repair a defect on the side of the nose. It is used for deep nasal defects, providing thick sebaceous skin and subcutaneous fat for rebuilding tissue lost in surgery and, folded on itself, can recreate an alar rim. Erroneously referred to as *nasolabial flap*.

meloplasty—face-lift; plastic surgery of the cheek.

melorheostosis—an uncommon bone disorder characterized by cortical thickening of the bone with irregular dense hyperostosis along the cortex. It most often affects the lower limbs but can affect the hands. The cause is still unknown, although it was first described in 1922.

melphalan (Alkeran)—used to treat multiple myeloma and unresectable epithelial ovarian carcinoma; investigational for malignant melanoma.

memantine—neuroprotective agent.

memapsin 2—protein-cutting enzyme, or protease, believed to be directly responsible for Alzheimer's disease. Also known as *beta-secretase*.

membrane delamination wedge (Oph)—an instrument that allows the surgeon to separate proliferative membranes from the retina effectively and safely. Used to decrease the risk of iatrogenic retinal tears that may complicate procedures to treat proliferative vitreoretinal diseases.

membrane stripping (Obstetrics)—used to induce labor at term, thus avoiding oxytoxic drugs or amniotomy. It is done by digital separation of the membranes from the lower uterine segment.

membranous croup—the bacterial cause of serious airway obstruction in children. Also called *membranous laryngotracheobronchitis* or *bacterial tracheitis*.

Memorial Sloan-Kettering Cancer Center, New York. Also, MSK Cancer Center.

Memorial Sloan-Kettering protocol—a chemotherapy protocol.

MemoryLens—a foldable intraocular lens (IOL).

MemoryTrace AT—ambulatory cardiac monitor which automatically records an EKG when it senses an arrhythmia in the patient's heart. The EKG is stored electronically and can be transmitted over the telephone to a cardiologist.

Memotherm—a nitinol self-expanding stent used for peripheral artery procedures.

MEN (multiple endocrine neoplasia).
Mengert's index—in pelvimetry.
meningococcal supraglottitis—a recent clustering of cases caused by *Neisseria meningitidis* suggests this may be an emerging infectious syndrome.
meninx—the singular form of the membrane covering the brain and spinal cord; meninges (plural) consist of the dura, pia, and arachnoid.
meniscal (*not* menisceal) (adj.)—usually refers to one of the crescent-shaped structures of the knee joint.
"menisceal"—mispronunciation of *meniscal*. See *meniscal*.
Menke's steely hair syndrome.
MEN I (multiple endocrine neoplasia, type I) **syndrome**.
Menorest (transdermal 17-beta-estradiol)—hormone replacement patch for treatment of menopausal symptoms and prevention of postmenopausal osteoporosis.
menotropins (Humegon)—used to induce ovulation in anovulatory nonfertile patients whose cause of anovulation is functional and not due to primary ovarian failure.
mental status examination—see *test*.
Mentane (velnacrine).
Mentax (1% butenafine hydrochloride) cream—topical antifungal drug used for treatment of tinea pedis, tinea corporis, and tinea cruris.
mentis—see *non compos mentis*.
Mentor Alpha 1 inflatable penile prosthesis.
Mentor BVAT—computer screen chart used in testing visual acuity.
MEP (motor evoked potential)—used to monitor descending pathways in neurosurgery.
MEP (multimodality evoked potential)—a combination of visual, somato-sensory, and brain stem auditory evoked potential.
Mepitel contact-layer wound dressing.
Mepore absorptive dressing.
mEq (milliequivalent).
meralgia paresthetica—a neuropathy, usually due to compression of the lateral femoral cutaneous nerve, producing pain, paresthesias, and sensory disturbances. See *Roth-Bernhardt's disease*, which is synonymous.
M/E ratio (myeloid/erythroid).
mercaptopurine (Purinethol)—chemotherapy drug used to treat acute lymphatic leukemia.
Mercator atrial high-density array catheter—used in the right atrium for diagnosing and mapping complex arrhythmias that may be difficult to identify using conventional mapping systems alone.
Mercedes tip cannula—used for liposuction.
mercury artifact (Radiol)—mercury seen in unexpected places in the body, after the breaking of a Cantor tube that was weighted with mercury to stay in the stomach.
mercury-in-Silastic strain gauge (Vasc Surg)—used for determination of the blood flow.
Meridia (sibutramine HCl)—serotonin, dopamine, and norepinephrine reuptake inhibitor specifically used for treatment of obesity. Meridia apparently suppresses hunger but is said to cause less serotonin toxicity than Redux and Pondimin (both discontinued 1997) because Meridia does not increase the release of serotonin from nerve cells, thus reducing risk of heart problems seen reportedly with fen-phen products.

meridian therapy—acupuncture, identifying 14 main meridians running vertically up and down the surface of the body. Acupuncture points are specific locations where the meridians come to the surface of the skin and are easily accessible by "needling," moxibustion, and acupressure: Yuan-Source points, Xi-Cleft points, Back-Shu and Front-Mu points, Luo-Connecting points, Eight Influential points.

Merindino procedure—distal esophagectomy, 50% gastrectomy, jejunal interposition, with esophagojejunostomy, pyloroplasty and vagotomy, and jejunojejunostomy.

Merkel cell carcinoma (MCC)—rare and aggressive neuroendocrine tumor of dermal origin.

Merlin bendable blade (ENT).

Merocel sponge—a compressed, lint-free, nonfiber sponge that expands when in contact with nasal secretions, used in postoperative nasal packing. It may be used in other settings.

meropenem (Merrem)—an antibiotic that can be used as an alternative to Primaxin in treating intra-abdominal infections.

Merrem I.V. (meropenem)—a broad-spectrum intravenous antibiotic.

MERRF (myoclonus epilepsy associated with ragged-red fibers).

Merry Walker ambulation device—a device modeled on a baby walker and designed for adults with ambulation problems.

Mersilene (*not* Mersiline)—a braided nonabsorbable suture that becomes encapsulated in the body tissues. Used in cardiovascular, general, and plastic surgery as retention sutures. Colors: green and white.

Mersilk—a braided silk suture.

MESA (microepididymal sperm aspiration or microsurgical epididymal sperm aspiration)—used in infertility treatments.

mesalamine (5-ASA, Asacol, Rowasa, Pentasa)—anti-inflammatory drug for ulcerative colitis. Rowasa is prescribed as a rectal suspension. Oral Asacol is a time-release tablet which dissolves in the terminal ileum. Pentasa, also oral, may be taken four times daily for up to 8 weeks.

Mesalt dressing—crystalline sodium chloride-impregnated dressing used to cleanse infected wounds.

mesh—see *graft*.

mesh plug hernioplasty—a hernia repair procedure using a cone-shaped plug of Marlex mesh to close the hernia defect. See *PerFix*.

mesna (Mesnex)—used only for patients receiving ifosfamide. It prevents the side effect of hemorrhagic cystitis.

Messerklinger sinus endoscopy set.

met, mets—unit of measurement for treadmill scoring; 1 met = 3.5 ml O_2/kg/min. Cf. *mets, "Metz."*

metacarpal—refers to the bones of the metacarpus, that part of the hand between the wrist and the fingers. Cf. *metatarsal*. The above words are often confused, even by the dictators, so be aware of the anatomic area referred to.

metachronous seeding—metastases occurring from a secondary tumor rather than directly from the primary tumor.

Metadate ER (extended-release methylphenidate)—for treatment of attention-deficit/hyperactivity disorder.

Meta DDDR pacemaker.

metaiodobenzylguanidine (MIBG).

metallic stent placement—used to relieve acute colonic obstruction secondary to colorectal carcinoma.

metaphyseal lesion of the distal femur —a common site to indicate abuse in an infant.

metaphysis—the wide part at the end of the shaft of a long bone, adjacent to the cartilaginous disk of the epiphysis. In childhood, this is composed of spongy bone and contains the growth zone. In the adult, it is continuous with the epiphysis. Cf. *metastasis*.

metastasis—spread of cancer from one organ or part of the body to another not necessarily contiguous with it; it may spread through the lymphatic system or venous system, etc. See *metaphysis*. Cf. *met, mets*.

metastatic efficiency index (MEI)— "The MEI value for the eye is by far the highest, indicating a very favorable environment for the growth of cancer cells."

Metastron (strontium chloride Sm 89).

Metasul—metal-on-metal hip prosthesis.

metatarsal—refers to the bones of the metatarsus, that part of the foot between the ankle articulation and the toes. See *metacarpal*.

methazolamide tablets (Neptazane).

methemoglobin (metHb)—does not carry oxygen through the blood. A small amount of methemoglobin is normally present in the blood, but if hemoglobin is converted to excess methemoglobin through injury or exposure to toxic agents, cyanosis can result.

methicillin-resistant *Staphylococcus aureus* (MRSA, "mer'sa")—a strain of *S. aureus* that is resistant to methicillin, gentamicin, and ciprofloxacin. Now treated with vancomycin. This resistant gram-positive bacterium often inhabits the nares of healthy individuals. See *MARSA*.

methionine-enkephalin—drug used to treat immunodeficiency and AIDS. See *homocysteine*.

methisoprinol (inosine pranobex).

method (see also *operation*)
  bench
  Cherry-Crandall
  Crede's
  CSQI
  flow cytometry
  flush
  Holdrinet
  Ionescu
  Ko-Airan bleeding control
  Lown and Woolf
  Mauriceau-Smellie-Veit
  Oliver-Rosalki
  Pfeiffer-Comberg
  piggybacking
  Pulver-Taft weave
  Roche-Microwell Plate Hybridization
  Sigma CPK serum testing
  Smellie
  Sub-Q-Set
  Turner-Warwick
  Wheeless
  Wroblewski testing serum LDH

methotrexate (MTX, Mexate)—antineoplastic agent, usually used in combination with other chemotherapeutic agents in treatment of various types of cancer. Also used as an immunosuppressive agent.

methoxsalen (Oxsoralen)—for treatment of psoriasis; taken orally and then followed by blacklight lamp or sunlamp treatment; palliative for cutaneous T-cell lymphoma.

Methylin (methylphenidate)—drug used to treat attention-deficit disorder.

Methylin ER (methylphenidate HCl)—extended release form for treatment of ADHD.

methylmalonic acidemia—a nutritional deficiency thought to be responsible for certain skin diseases.

methylmethacrylate—a cement used in orthopedics and neurosurgery.

methylmethacrylate beads—a method of providing an antibiotic to prevent postfracture osteomyelitis. Impregnated with an antibiotic, the beads of methylmethacrylate are strung on a surgical wire, implanted in the area of an open fracture (following surgical debridement and irrigation with an antibiotic solution). The beads dissolve, releasing the antibiotic in situ at therapeutic levels over several weeks.

methylphenidate (Methylin; Ritalin)—drug used to treat attention-deficit disorder.

methyl tertiary butyl ether (MTBE).

metipranolol (OptiPranolol)—a topical drug which belongs to the class of beta-blocking agents used to treat chronic open-angle glaucoma. The drug acts to decrease intraocular pressure by decreasing the production of aqueous humor.

metoclopramide (Neu-Sensamide).

metoprolol succinate (Toprol XL)—a once-a-day treatment for hypertension and angina pectoris in a sustained release tablet. Cf. *metoprolol tartrate*.

metoprolol tartrate (Lopressor)—cardioselective beta blocker drug used for hypertension and angina; also for migraine headaches. Cf. *metoprolol succinate*.

Metrix atrial defibrillation system—an implantable device designed specifically for patients suffering from recurrent symptomatic episodes of atrial fibrillation.

metrizamide—a water soluble contrast medium used in myelograms and other studies.

Metrodin (urofollitropin).

mets (plural of met)—unit of measurement in treadmills. See *met*.

"mets"—slang for metastases. Cf. *meds, met, "Metz."*

metyrosine (Demser)—antihypertensive for pheochromocytoma.

"Metz"—slang for Metzenbaum scissors. Cf. *mets*.

Meuli arthroplasty.

Meurman classification of congenital aural atresia.

Mevacor (lovastatin).

Mexate (methotrexate).

Mexitil (mexiletine)—an antiarrhythmic agent.

Mezlin (mezlocillin sodium).

mezlocillin—a fourth-generation broad-spectrum penicillin. Cf. *Mezlin*.

MFG (magnetic field gradients).

MFG (manofluorography).

MFH (malignant fibrous histiocytoma).

MGBG—a polyamine synthesis inhibitor for treatment of brain tumors.

MGDF (megakaryocyte growth and development factor).

MG II total hip system.

MHA-TP (microhemagglutination test for *Treponema pallidum*, the organism that causes syphilis).

MHz (megahertz) (1 million hertz)—a term often used in radiology and audiology. A hertz equals 1 cycle per second.

MI (migration index).

Miacalcin (calcitonin)—a nasal spray used to treat osteoporosis in estrogen-averse women who are more than 5 years postmenopausal.

Miami Acute Care (MAC) **collar**—for cervical support.

Miami J collar—cervical immobilization for ICU patients restricted to the supine position.

MIBG (metaiodobenzylguanidine)—a synthetic antineoplastic drug, used in combination with others in beginning therapy of nonlymphatic leukemia. It has a cytocidal effect on both proliferating and nonproliferating human cells.

Micardis (telmisartan)—taken once-daily for the treatment of hypertension.

MIC disposable cytology brush.

MIC gastroenteric tube—a dual lumen catheter which allows access to the stomach and the jejunum, for use in patients who need both gastric decompression and jejunal feeding. (MIC, Medical Innovations Corp.)

Michaelis-Gutmann bodies—lamellar inclusion bodies found in the cytoplasm of Von Hansemann cells, consistent with diagnosis of malacoplakia of kidney.

Michel deformity—complete failure of development of the inner ear.

MIC-Key G and **MIC-Key J** (pronounced "Mickey")—gastrostomy tubes.

miconazole nitrate vaginal cream—a 7-day, over-the-counter treatment for vaginal yeast infections.

Micral chemstrip—urine test for microalbuminuria.

Micral urine dipstick test—detects low levels of albumin.

micro-, prefix meaning small or abnormally small. Cf. *macro-*.

Micro-Aire pulse lavage system—for debriding bone surfaces in hip and knee implantation procedures.

microbial keratitis—see *keratitis*.

microbipolar forceps—electronic forceps in straight and curved versions; used in microsurgery.

Microblator—small joint ArthroWand.

microbubble contrast agent for color Doppler ultrasound on breast masses—a minimally invasive technique that enables accurate differentiation of benign masses from carcinomas through the use of anatomic and dynamic features.

microcalcification—very small deposit of calcium in breast tissue, as seen in a mammogram. Clustered microcalcifications are highly suggestive of malignancy.

microchimerism—findings related to the presence of donor cells in a graft recipient that can mimic infection.

Micrococcus sedentarius—a coagulase-negative organism. Can be confused with *Staphylococcus epidermidis*, but *S. epidermidis* ferments glucose and micrococci do not.

Micro Diamond-Point microsurgery instruments.

"microdots"—panstromal occurrence of fine, highly reflective structures appearing in the eyes of chronic contact lens wearers.

Microdot technique for precision suture placement.

microendoscopic diskectomy (MED) **system**—used in herniated disk surgery. This microsurgical instrumentation is used to perform back surgery through a one-half-inch incision.

Microflo test strip—used with Precision QID glucose monitoring system.

Microfoam surgical tape (*not* Microform).

MicroGlide reciprocating osteotome—high-speed microreciprocating osteotome used in rhinoplasty.

micrognathia-glossoptosis syndrome. See *Pierre Robin syndrome*.

Micro-Imager—high-resolution digital camera.

Microjet-based cutting and debriding devices—used as alternatives to scalpel and laser surgery approaches for common ophthalmic procedures.

microkatals per liter—a katal is a unit of measure proposed to express enzymatic activity. The abbreviation for *katal* is *kat*.

MicroKlenz wound cleanser.

Microknit vascular graft prosthesis—a fine-knit, thin-walled Dacron prosthesis that comes as a straight tube or patch graft. It is said to handle much like normal arterial tissue. It has also been marketed under the names of *Weaveknit* and *Wesolowski* prostheses.

MicroLap and MicroLap Gold—a microlaparoscopy system used in diagnosis and treatment of pelvic pain, infertility, and tubal ligation.

Microlase transpupillary diode laser (Oph).

Microlight—see *Lasermedic Microlight*.

microlumbar diskectomy (MLD)—a rigid microsurgical operative technique which uses microscopic-aided dissection throughout rather than just at the point of disk dissection.

MicroMewi multiple sidehole infusion catheter—a microcatheter used to deliver drugs into the peripheral vasculature for therapeutic embolization. Named for Mark Mewissen, M.D., interventional radiologist.

Micro Minix pacemaker—a smaller version of the Minix pacemaker. The term *Micro* is part of the trade name.

Micronase (glyburide)—for type II diabetics (NIDDM) who do not respond to diet alone.

Micron bobbin ventilation tubes—made of titanium; used in surgery.

micronized fenofibrate (Tricor)—a formulation of fibric acid derivative fenofibrate, indicated for treatment of patients with type IIa, IIb, III, or IV dyslipidemia. This formulation has improved absorption characteristics compared to the standard preparation, allowing a lower daily dosage and once-daily administration.

Micron Res-Q—implantable cardioverter-defibrillator.

Microny SR+ single-chamber, rate-responsive pulse generator.

MicroPlaner soft tissue shaver—used to shave facial soft tissue. It is said to be less traumatic than conventional tissue aspiration techniques.

Microprobe laser (Oph)—an ophthalmic laser microendoscope that provides both laser function and illumination in one instrument. It is used to visualize and treat retinal or choroidal vascular disease, retinal tears or detachments and also treats the ciliary processes in intractable neovascular glaucoma.

Micro-Probe tip—used for microdissection.

Micropuncture Peel-Away introducer—used to introduce balloon, electrode, and other catheters. Knobs allow the sheath to be peeled away and removed.

microscope, microscopy
  atomic force (AFM)
  biomicroscope (slit lamp)
  confocal
  dark-field
  DIC (differential interference
    contrast)
  scanning acoustic (SAM)
  Wild operating
microSelectron-HDR (high dose rate)
  —an afterloader used in radiation
  therapy.
MicroSmooth probe—a vitreoretinal
  probe for attachment to an ocutome.
microsomal triglyceride transfer protein (MTP).
MicroSpan microhysteroscopy system—a 1.6 mm hysteroscope and
  MicroSpan sheath that allow atraumatic access to the uterus without
  cervical dilatation.
MigraSpray—an herbal remedy for
  migraine available in a saline solution
  containing the herb feverfew (*Tanacetum parthenium*). It is sprayed
  under the tongue or inside the cheek,
  allowing instant absorption of the
  herb and direct passage into the
  blood stream, bypassing the GI tract
  and eliminating the need to swallow
  bulky pills.
microsurgery—see *transanal endoscopic microsurgery*.
microsurgical denervation of the spermatic cord—an effective testicular-sparing surgical alternative for treatment of chronic orchialgia.
microsurgical DREZ-otomy—a procedure to treat spasticity and pain in
  lower limbs. (DREZ, dorsal root
  entry zone.)
microsurgical epididymovasostomy
  (MSEV)—for congenital and acquired vasoepididymal obstruction.

microsurgical extraction of sperm from epididymis (MASE)—an infertility procedure.
MicroTeq portable belt—device worn
  for home treatment as augmentation
  for TENS.
microtome—see *Stadie-Riggs microtome*.
microtubule-associated proteins
  (MAPs).
microvascular angiopathy (MVA).
microvascular free tissue transfer—a
  procedure used in near-total or total
  glossectomy following reconstruction
  with a latissimus dorsi flap modified
  to create a muscle sling attached to
  pterygoid and masseter stumps. The
  flap is then reinnervated by anastomosis of the hypoglossal nerve stump
  to the nerve of the latissimus dorsi.
Microvasive Glidewire—see *Glidewire*.
Microvasive Rigiflex TTS balloon—
  see *Rigiflex TTS balloon*.
Microvasive stiff piano wire guidewire.
Microvit cutter—used in vitreoretinal
  surgery in cutting the vitreous, in
  posterior segment surgery.
microwave cardiac ablation system—a
  minimally invasive system used to
  treat cardiac arrhythmias.
microwave nonsurgical treatment—for
  benign prostatic hypertrophy. Performed under local anesthesia.
  Ultrasound defines the size and
  shape of the prostate gland, and the
  physician uses a computer to guide
  the procedure. A catheter is inserted
  through the urethra to the prostate.
  Microwave energy from an antenna
  inside the catheter heats and destroys
  enlarged cells in the gland. The
  equipment has a cooling and flushing
  provision. Heated cells dissolve and

microwave *(cont.)*
are absorbed by the body, with resultant shrinkage of the prostate and
return of normal urinary function.

microwave thermoradiotherapy (Oph)
—used to treat uveal melanoma.

Micro-Z—wearable, high-volt-pulsed,
galvanic neuromuscular stimulator.

MIC Thermal Option—disposable biopsy forceps.

MIC-TJ—transgastric jejunal tube.

MID (multi-infarct dementia).

Midas Rex pneumatic instruments—
used in working on bone and articular cartilage; in cement removal and
in polyethylene and metal cutting.

MIDCAB (minimally invasive direct
coronary artery bypass) **procedure**.

middle cerebral artery (MCA).

midgut—distal duodenum, jejunum,
ileum, and right colon. See *foregut*
and *hindgut*.

midinfrared laser—alternative to excimer, which uses ultraviolet light.

midline shift—displacement of a structure that is normally seen at or near
the midline of the body, such as the
pineal gland or the trachea.

midodrine (ProAmatine)—drug used to
treat orthostatic hypotension.

midparental height—a term used in
discussion of patients with possible
growth hormone deficiency. One of
the factors which must be taken into
consideration is the height of the
patient's parents, as short stature
might simply be a familial characteristic. Therefore, the heights of both
parents are added together and divided by 2 (the midparental height),
and if this is low, it indicates that the
patient's short stature is normal for
that family and not necessarily a
growth hormone failure. Conversely,
if the midparental height is relatively
high, consideration might be given to
institution of supplemental growth
hormone therapy.

Miescher's cheilitis granulomatosa—
noncaseating granulomas of the lips,
a manifestation of Melkersson-Ro-
senthal syndrome.

Mifegyne (mifepristone)—an oral anti-
progesterone for therapeutic abortion, breast cancer, and Cushing syndrome.

Mifeprex (mifepristone, RU-486)—induces spontaneous abortion when
administered in early pregnancy
(before seven weeks) and followed
by administration of misoprostol approximately two days later.

migraine equivalent—symptom-com-
plex of migraine (aura, autonomic
instability, transient neurological
deficits, aphasia, or other features)
without the headache component.

Migra-Lieve—combination of herbal
and nutritional supplements used to
support cardiovascular tone and reduce platelet aggregation.

Migranal (dihydroergotamine mesylate)
nasal spray—treatment for migraine
headaches.

migration index (MI)—hip dysplasia
measurement in children with cerebral palsy.

Mijnhard electrical cycloergometer—
a device for measuring the heart rate
under stress; a type of exercise tolerance test.

MiKasome—liposomal formulation of
the antibiotic amikacin, reportedly
longer-acting than other formulations.

mil—unit of measurement equals 0.001
inch. Often used to express diameter
of wire sutures.

milestones—see *developmental milestones*.

miliaria—heat rash. Cf. *malaria*.

militate—to affect, to carry weight, used with the word "against": "His long smoking history would militate against a very good prognosis." Cf. *mitigate*.

milk leg disease—the edematous, uniformly swollen, white extremity seen in femoroiliac thrombophlebitis.

Millar MPC-500 catheter—a high-fidelity microtipped catheter used in transesophageal echocardiography.

Millenia balloon catheter—for use during percutaneous transluminal coronary angioplasty.

Millen technique retropubic prostatectomy—a transverse row of sutures, with the "smile" removed from upper margin of bladder neck.

Miller-Abbott tube—a double-lumen long gastrointestinal tube.

Miller Galante I condylar total knee system.

mill-house murmur—a loud, continuous churning sound heard over the precordium (sometimes even without the use of a stethoscope). May be diagnostic of a venous air embolism.

millicurie (mc, mCi) (1/1000th of a curie)—the unit of measurement of radioactivity.

milliequivalent (mEq)—the unit of measurement used in writing electrolyte values and dosage of potassium chloride.

Milligan-Morgan technique—for treatment of hemorrhoids.

millijoule (mJ) ("mil-e-jul") (1/1000th of a joule)—measurement used in YAG laser and argon laser applications.

milliliter (mL).

millimoles per liter (mmol/L).

milliner's needle—a straight needle with an eye, used primarily for suturing skin or readily accessible tissue.

milliosmole (mOsm).

Millon's reagent—a nitric acid/mercuric nitrate solution that reacts with tyrosine and other phenols, turning red or orange in the presence of proteins. Since tyrosine is present in most proteins, Millon's reagent is a good indicator of the presence of protein in urine.

milrinone lactate (Primacor)—a vasodilator used to treat congestive heart failure.

Milroy's disease—manifested by congenital lymphedema; the patient has an inborn error of development of the lymphatic channels.

Miltex surgical instruments.

Mima polymorpha—see *Acinetobacter lwoffi*.

MIMCOM (multimode imaging confocal optical microscope)—a class of optical microscopes providing novel imaging modalities, including biological imaging.

MindSet toe splint—a plastic toe splint for broken or injured toes that can be worn inside a regular shoe. Allows the patient to remain active and in less pain.

MINE (mesna [rescue], ifosfamide, Novantrone, etoposide)—a chemotherapy protocol for advanced lymphomas.

Minerva neurosurgical robot.

Minerva-type cast—used for odontoid fracture.

Minesse (gestodene, progestin, and ethinyl estradiol)—low-dose oral contraceptive pill with 24 active pills and four placebo pills in a 28-day pill pack.

Mini-Acutrak—a small-bone fixation system.

miniarousals (*not* many arousals)—a term used in sleep studies.

MINI Crown stent—specifically engineered for smaller vessels.

mini-FES (functional endoscopic sinus) **surgery** (ENT)—made possible by the use of microdebriders. Reportedly causes few complications in patients, especially children, undergoing sinus surgery.

mini Hoffmann external fixation system.

Mini-Hohmann podiatric retractor.

minilap—minilaparotomy staging pelvic lymphadenectomy

minilaparotomy pelvic lymph node dissection—found to be significantly cheaper but just as successful in surgically staging prostate cancer, as laparoscopic pelvic lymph node dissection.

minilaparotomy incision—used in vesicolithotomy, ureterolithotomy, suprapubic tube insertion, and bladder neck suspension.

minilaparotomy staging pelvic lymphadenectomy.

minimally invasive surgery—an all-inclusive term used for procedures including laparoscopy, thoracoscopy, or percutaneous diskectomy. Generally employs a number of tiny incisions through which trocars are placed. Retractors, dissecting instruments, scopes, graspers, and suturing devices are all inserted through strategically placed incisions, and any resected organs or tissue is removed via the same incisions. Minimally invasive surgery, properly performed, results in quicker recovery, fewer complications and side effects, shorter hospital stays, and more rapid return to normal activities.

Mini-Med continuous glucose sensor—implanted device that continuously records patient's glucose levels, then downloads data to an external computer for analysis.

Mini-Mental State Examination (MMSE)—a formal mental status test used to evaluate Alzheimer's disease. A score of 10-26 correlates with Alzheimer's of mild to moderate severity.

MiniSite laparoscope with 2 mm access site.

Minnesota antilymphoblast globulin—given to post-transplantation patients experiencing allograft rejection.

Minnesota Multiphasic Personality Inventory (MMPI)—mental status examination.

Minnesota Test for Differential Diagnosis of Aphasia (MTDDA)—a test to assess neurological deficit following such incidents as a subarachnoid hemorrhage. The test consists of seven subtests, including reading comprehension, reading rate, oral reading, describing a picture, writing letters dictated by the examiner, writing sentences dictated by the examiner, and arithmetic problems.

minor vestibular adenitis—see *vulvar vestibulitis syndrome.*

minoxidil—a cardiac drug also used for penile erectile dysfunction.

miotic—(1) an agent that causes the pupil to contract; (2) pertaining to, or causing, contraction of the pupil.

MIP (maximum intensity projection) — a term used in MRI and CT scans.

Miragel—hydrophilic sponge material used in the IMEX scleral implant.

Mirage nasal ventilation mask system
—used for treatment of obstructive
sleep apnea.

Miraluma—nuclear medicine test used
in breast imaging.

Mirapex (pramipexole dihydrochloride
tablets)—a dopamine agonist drug
used in the treatment of Parkinson's
disease.

Mirena—a levonorgestrel-releasing intrauterine contraceptive designed to
be long-acting (5 years) and provide
reversible contraception.

Mirizzi's syndrome—common hepatic
duct obstruction caused by extrinsic
compression from an impacted stone
in the cystic duct.

mirror image breast biopsy—a biopsy
of the same spot in the opposite
breast as the location of an earlier
lesion (the same, but opposite, as in
a mirror).

mirror-imaging—can affect a physician's sense of orientation within the
cavity being operated. It occurs in
laparoscopy due to the placement of
viewing port and instrumentation
port such that the instrument comes
toward the viewer, rather than both
pointing in the same direction.

mirroring—a phenomenon in which
one extremity cannot move without
the other moving in an identical
manner.

mirtazapine (Remeron)—antidepressant drug.

Miskimon retractor.

misoprostol—used to prevent the formation of gastric and duodenal
ulcers associated with the use of nonsteroidal anti-inflammatory drugs.

missed ostium sequence (MOS)—
caused by the inadequate surgical
removal of the most anterior portion
of the uncinate process during endoscopic sinus surgery. It is postulated
to be the cause of FES (functional
endoscopic sinus) surgical failure.

**Mississippi Scale for Combat-Related
Posttraumatic Stress Disorder**—a
psychiatric test for measuring post-
traumatic stress disorder.

Mississippi 3-class system—a scoring
system for HELLP syndrome that is
based on the mother's platelet count.
HELLP syndrome (hemolysis, elevated liver enzymes, low platelets) is
a severe form of preeclampsia/
eclampsia that can lead to pleural
effusion, ascites, and even liver necrosis and is thought to have a genetic origin.

Mitchell distal osteotomy—to correct
hallux valgus.

Mitchell technique—for epispadias repair.

Mitek anchor system—used in medial
canthoplasty for reattaching the
medial canthal tendon to the medial
orbital wall. The operation can be
performed through a small incision
as well and may not be as invasive
as other conventional procedures. It
also has the advantage of being an
easy technique with very accurate
placement of the anchor and, conse-
quently, reduced operating time.

Mithracin (plicamycin).

mitigate—to make milder, less severe,
as "We might attempt to mitigate his
symptoms with phototherapy." Cf.
militate.

mitolactol—chemotherapy drug.

mitomycin (mitomycin-C, Mutamycin)
—a chemotherapy drug used to treat
gastric, pancreatic, and bladder carcinoma. Cf. *mithramycin* (now *plicamycin*).

mitotic chromosomes.

mitoxantrone (Novantrone)—chemotherapy drug which, in combination with steroids, has been shown to help alleviate pain related to hormone-refractory prostate cancer.

Mitraflex wound dressing—sterile multilayer wound dressing which is very thin and can be used over the entire face or around the shoulder, for example.

mitral regurgitation artifact (cineangiography)—induced if the catheter is too close to the mitral valve in left ventricular angiography.

mitral valve homograft—mitral valves taken from cadavers, reducing chance of rejection that occurs with animal or mechanical valves. Valves are taken from young organ donors and can be preserved for up to 10 years, thus making use of hearts that are not suitable for whole-heart transplants. Transplant of human valves does not require lifelong use of blood thinners, and it is expected that these valves will last longer than animal valves.

mitral valve prolapse (MVP).

Mitrofanoff appendicovesicotomy—a technique for continent urinary diversion.

Mitrofanoff neourethra procedure—creates a neourethra for a continent abdominal stoma. A neourethra is developed by implanting a tubular segment into the bladder, which, when brought out through the skin, creates a continent, catheterizable neourethra.

Mitsui scale—"Anterior chamber pigment was measured on a modified Mitsui scale."

mittelschmerz—pain midway between the menstrual periods.

Mittendorf's dot—also known as *hyaloid corpuscle*. Represents the attachment of a hyaloid vessel to the posterior capsule.

Mivacron (mivacurium).

mivacurium (Mivacron)—a short-acting neuromuscular blocker, a muscle relaxant, and an adjunct to anesthesia.

MIVR (minimally invasive valve repair or replacement).

mixed angina—a widely used term with controversial definitions. The simplest definition seems to be "the coexistence of effort angina and rest angina, without any judgment as to the etiology." Also called *variable threshold angina*.

mixed connective tissue disease (MCTD).

mixed leukocyte culture (MLC).

Miya hook ligament carrier—used in sacrospinous ligament suspension.

Miyazaki-Bonney test—for stress incontinence. It duplicates the effects of the Burch bladder neck suspension procedure to determine if surgery will help the patient. See also *Bonney test*.

mJ (millijoule).

MKC-442—a non-nucleoside reverse transcriptase inhibitor for the treatment of HIV disease.

MKM AutoPilot stereotactic system—allows the operator to visualize navigation during surgery.

M-K (McCarey-Kaufman) **medium**.

mL (milliliter)—equivalent to a cubic centimeter (cc).

MLC (mixed leukocyte culture)—a trial in a test tube to determine in advance if donor and recipient tissues are compatible.

MLD (microlumbar diskectomy).

MLD (minimum lethal dose)—refers to ingestion of poisons or toxins.

MLH$_1$ gene—the second defective gene linked to colon cancer discovered by the team that discovered MSH$_2$. See *MSH$_2$*.

MLNS (mucocutaneous lymph node syndrome).

MLS (mini lag-screw)—see *Alphatec*.

MMCM (macromolecular contrast medium)—MRI term.

MMEF (maximum midexpiratory flow rate).

M-mode echocardiogram.

mmol/L (millimoles per liter)—an SI (International System) unit of measurement of serum values.

MMOPP (methotrexate, mechlorethamine, Oncovin, procarbazine, prednisone)—chemotherapy protocol for astrocytoma and neuroectodermal tumor.

MMSE (Mini-Mental State Examination).

MMS-10 tympanic displacement analyzer—a device to measure the perilymphatic pressure in patients with Meniere's disease.

MND (motor neuron disease).

MN rgp120—an AIDS vaccine that has shown encouraging results by inducing HIV-1 MN antibody production.

MNTI (melanotic neuroectodermal tumor of infancy)—rare neoplasm occurring most often in the first year of life.

MOAB, MoAb, MAb (monoclonal antibody).

Mobetron intraoperative radiation therapy (IORT) **treatment system** —a mobile, self-shielded electron linear accelerator that directly delivers IORT to patients as they are undergoing cancer surgery.

Mobic (meloxicam)—drug for treatment of osteoarthritis.

mobilize—move. Cf. *immobilize*.

Mobin-Uddin umbrella filter—for transvenous vena cava interruption in prevention of pulmonary emboli. See also *Kim-Ray Greenfield filter*, which is *not* synonymous.

MOBS (Montefiore Organic Brain Scale).

MOCB (medial olivocochlear bundle).

moccasin-type tinea pedis—characterized by scaling, hyperkeratosis, minimal inflammation, particularly refractory to topical therapy and usually requiring an oral antifungal agent.

MOCNI ("mock-ney") (method of collection not indicated) (Path).

modafinil (Provigil).

Modic's classification of disk abnormality—numbered 1, 2, 3, 4, 4A, 4B, and 4C; based on MRI findings.

modified Hughes procedure—reconstruction of large defects of the lower eyelid.

modified Isshiki type 4 thyroplasty—used in treatment of unilateral cricothyroid muscle paralysis.

modified Pereyra bladder neck suspension.

modified Rodnan total skin-thickness score technique—used to determine skin thickness in scleroderma.

MODS (multiple organ dysfunction syndrome)—thought to be a more accurate term than *MOF (multiple organ failure)*.

Modulap—reusable electrosurgical cutting and coagulation probe for use in general laparoscopic surgical procedures.

Modulith SL 20—a third-generation lithotriptor equipped with fluoro-

Modulith SL 20 *(cont.)*
scopic and ultrasound localization systems.

Modulock posterior spinal fixation.

MODY (maturity-onset diabetes of the young)—a distinct form of non-insulin-dependent diabetes mellitus.

Moe—instrumentation and wiring of the spinous processes for scoliosis.

Moebius' sign—in exophthalmos, one or both eyes fail to converge on attempting to look at an object close to midline.

moexipril hydrochloride (Univasc).

MOF (MeCCNU, Oncovin, fluorouracil)—chemotherapy protocol for rectal adenocarcinoma.

MOF (multiple organ failure)—see *multisystem organ failure*.

Mogadon (nitrazepam)—a sedative for treating myoclonic epilepsy.

Mohs' fresh tissue chemosurgery—used primarily in basal cell carcinoma. After fixation in vivo with zinc chloride paste, the tumor is then excised under microscopic control. Named for surgeon Dr. Frederick E. Mohs.

moiré artifact (Radiol)—a pattern, sometimes seen in expensive silks, caused by the superimposition of two grids with linear patterns running in almost the same direction; the slight variation causes the moiré phenomenon.

Moire topographic assessment—scoliosis screening test that is more expensive and time-consuming than the Adams test.

moisture vapor permeability (MVP).

molar pregnancy—refers to a hydatidiform mole, an abnormal pregnancy which results from an ovum which has been converted to a mole. (This has nothing to do with molar teeth.)

molars—see *mulberry molars*.

molding—the shaping of the fetal head by the birth canal. Also, *moulding*.

molecular coincidence detection (MCD) **imaging**—imaging technology that is able to detect lung cancer and show the location and extent of the disease.

molecular recognition unit (MRU)—pharmacologic technology based on monoclonal antibodies but physically much smaller. MRUs link with drugs or diagnostic radiology agents and allow them to reach more fully into body tissues. See *ThromboScan MRU*.

molgramostim (Leucomax)—a granulocyte/macrophage colony-stimulating factor derived from *E. coli*.

molluscum contagiosum virus (MCV)—a poxvirus that results in persistent skin infection, often manifesting itself in AIDS patients.

Molnar disk—plastic disk to anchor a nephrostomy tube in place.

Molteno filtering bleb (Oph).

Molteno implant drainage device (Oph).

Molteno seton—a tube which allows aqueous humor to flow from the anterior chamber to the subconjunctival space to decrease intraocular pressure.

Molt periosteal elevator.

molybdenum—see *SMo*, stainless steel with molybdenum.

MOM (milk of magnesia).

Monaghan 300 ventilator—a pressure-cycled ventilator that forces air into the lungs until an airway pressure (which has previously been determined) is obtained.

Monday crust—the phenomenon of patients being less open to analysis after a weekend.

Mondini's dysplasia.

Mondor's disease—superficial thrombophlebitis of the skin of the breast, usually occurring spontaneously in the upper outer quadrant. The condition often mimics the appearance of cancer.

mongoloid fissure—groove in the lateral canthus of the eyelid.

Monistat (*not* Monostat) (miconazole nitrate)—for local treatment of cutaneous or vulvovaginal candidiasis and other superficial fungal infections.

monkeypox—an orthopox virus with an appearance and behavior very similar to smallpox. One of its most interesting features is that it appears to have both human-to-human and animal-to-human transmission. Outbreaks of this disease, which was thought to have been eradicated many years ago, have occurred in the Republic of Congo (formerly Zaire) in what has been described as epidemic proportions.

monobactams—class of antibiotics for gram-negative bacteria. Example: azetreonam (Azactam).

monochromatization—filtering technique that permits the passage of only certain x-rays that fall within a narrow band of energy levels.

monoclonal antibody (MAb; MoAb; MOAB)—an antibody derived from a single cell ("clone") in the laboratory. Monoclonal antibodies to T-cells are called *OKT antibodies* and are used to study the T-cell populations (or T-cell subsets) in patients. See also *antibody*; *medication*.

monoclonal antibody-based enzyme immunoassay.

monoclonal antibody-specific immobilization of platelet antigens (MAIPA) **assay.**

Monocryl suture (polyglecaprone 25) —a pliable, synthetic, absorbable, monofilament suture.

Monodox (doxycycline, Vibramycin)— an antibiotic.

Monoflex lens—intraocular lens made of PMMA.

Monojector—see *fingerstick devices for blood glucose testing.*

Monoket (isosorbide mononitrate)—for prevention of angina pectoris.

monolaurin (Glylorin).

Monolyth oxygenator—extracorporeal membrane oxygenation system used during cardiac bypass procedures.

Monopril (fosinopril)—antihypertensive.

Monoscopy locking trocar with Woodford spike—a locking trocar which features an intra-abdominal locking mechanism. Used in laparoscopic procedures.

monosomy 7 syndrome.

Monospot test—a rapidly performed serum agglutination test for infectious mononucleosis. Note: *Monospot* is one word, *not* two.

Monostrut cardiac valve prosthesis.

Monro, foramen of—brain anatomy.

Monsel's solution—a hemostatic solution. "There was a small amount of oozing from the cervical biopsy site, and Monsel's solution was used to stop this bleeding."

monster rongeur.

Montefiore Organic Brain Scale (MOBS).

Monteggia fracture-dislocation—fracture of the ulna, with a radial head dislocation.

Montevideo units—measurement of the length and strength of uterine contractions.

Montgomery Safe-T-Tube—used in patients with acute tracheal injuries,

Montgomery *(cont.)*
to support the trachea post reconstruction, and also to support an
intrathoracic tracheal stenosis.

Monticelli-Spinelli system—a circular
external fixation system for fractures
of the leg and for leg lengthenings.

Monurol (fosfomycin tromethamine)—
a single-dose antibiotic used for
treating urinary tract infections.

Moolgaoker forceps—for spontaneous
vaginal delivery assist.

Moon Boot brace—used as an external
support to brace fracture of the distal tibia and fibula.

moon face (or *facies*)—a pronounced
rounding of the cheeks in Cushing's
syndrome or prolonged adrenocortical therapy.

MOP (mechlorethamine, Oncovin,
prednisone; mechlorethamine, Oncovin, procarbazine)—chemotherapy
protocols.

MOPP (mechlorethamine, Oncovin,
procarbazine, and prednisone)—chemotherapy protocol for adult Hodgkin's disease.

Moranyl (suramin)—antiparasitic.

Moraxella lwoffi—see *Acinetobacter
lwoffi*.

morcellation—see *morselize*.

Morgagni's ("mor-gah-nyee") **appendix**.

Morgagni's crypt.

Morganella morganii—newer name for
what was called *Proteus morganii*.

Morganstern continuous-flow operating cystoscope.

moribund—dying.

moricizine (Ethmozine)—sodium channel blocker used as an antiarrhythmic and indicated for the treatment
of life-threatening ventricular arrhythmias.

Moro reflex—seen normally in infants
up to 3 or 4 months of age. An infant is placed supine, and a sudden
noxious stimulus is made (usually a
loud noise by slapping the table
alongside). The child will respond
by extending and then flexing the
arms (in a protective or embracing
attitude) and flexing the hips and
knees. Also called *embrace* or *star-
tle reflex*.

Morscher titanium cervical plate—for
treatment of complex cervical spine
disorders.

morselize (verb)—to take small pieces
(morsels) of bone or cartilage in
nasal surgery or orthopedic surgery.
"The distal fibula was morselized
and the bone chips packed tightly
into the arthrodesis site laterally
after the fibrous tissue had been
curetted out." (English dictionaries
have *morsel, and* medical dictionaries have *morcellation* as main entries. The need for the verb form
frequently used in surgical dictation
is not recognized in nonmedical dictionaries.)

Morse taper stem—"The hip was then
redislocated and the trial head was
taken off and the final cobalt
chromium head was placed on the
Morse taper. It was pounded into
position using ten taps."

morsicatio buccarum—the nervous
habit of biting or chewing the buccal
mucosa.

mortise—a slot, or wedge-shaped cut
into bone (or timber) into which will
fit a tenon. This is also a carpenter's
or furniture-maker's word. Cf. *Webster's* definition of *tenon* (*not* tendon).
The ankle mortise is the normal
articulation between the talus and the
distal tibia and fibula.

MOS (missed ostium sequence).

mosaic perfusion (Radiol)—used in radiologic description of lung in bronchiolitis and other conditions.

mosaicplasty—technique to repair talar injuries resulting from osteochondritis dissecans, which generally strikes active children, young adults, and athletes. Mosaicplasty has also been used to repair knee joints.

Mosaic valve—a bioprosthetic heart valve designed to reduce valve calcification and maintain the natural shape and function of the valve, reducing mechanical stress on the tissue.

Moschcowitz procedure—obliteration of the cul-de-sac.

Mosley method—for anterior shoulder repair.

mOsm (milliosmole).

mosquito clamp.

Moss G-tube PEG kit—for PEG and laparoscopic procedures. Rigid introducer for simplified duodenal placement of "J" wire and G-tube. For simple gastric feeding without decompression.

Moss Miami load-sharing spinal implant system—provides anterior column support in balancing natural forces of spine.

Moss nasal tube, Mark IV—esophageal/duodenal decompression device for enteral hyperalimentation.

Moss Suction Buster tube—see *Suction Buster catheter*.

Moss T-anchor needle introducer gun —used to implant nylon T-anchors in the Moss percutaneous endoscopic gastrostomy regimen.

moth-eaten appearance—radiologic appearance reflecting increased density and rarefaction in the long bones of children with congenital syphilis.

mother and baby endoscope—same as *mother-daughter scope*; physicians may refer to each scope separately as *motherscope* and *babyscope*.

Mother2Be—line of natural skin and body care treatments designed to soothe, heal, and protect the skin of pregnant women.

Motilium (domperidone).

Motor Control Test (MCT)—used in conjunction with computerized dynamic posturography.

motorcyclist's knee—see *O'Donoghue's Unhappy Triad* (OUT).

motor evoked potential (MEP).

motor meal barium GI series—shows transit time, stomach to colon (normal transit time, 60 minutes).

Motrin Migraine Pain (ibuprofen)—over-the-counter ibuprofen product developed for migraines.

MOTT (*Mycobacterium* other than tuberculosis).

Mouchet's syndrome—paralysis of the cubital nerve following fracture of the external humeral condyle.

moulding—see *molding*, which seems to be the preferred spelling.

mouse units (MU)—used in an endocrinology test to measure levels of circulating pituitary hormones.

mouthwash—see *Peridex mouthwash*.

moving-bed infusion-tracking MRA —method for imaging the entire peripheral vascular tree with only one bolus of Magnevist over a scanning time of four minutes.

moxa—a Chinese herb used to boost the effects of acupuncture. Moxa works directly on the skin, wrapped around the tip of an acupuncture needle or in a stick form that's passed over a tender joint. See *moxibustion* and *sparrow-picking technique*.

moxibustion—treatment of disease by applying heat to acupuncture points. Used for ailments such as bronchial asthma, bronchitis, certain types of paralysis, and arthritic disorders.

moyamoya ("puff of smoke")—angiographic diagnosis of bilateral stenosis or occlusion of the internal carotid arteries above the clinoids.

MPC scissors—automated intravitreal scissors.

MPD (main pancreatic duct) **stent**.

MPGR (multiplanar gradient-recalled) **echo.**

MPHR (maximum predicted heart rate) —a term used in exercise tolerance tests. See *Bruce protocol, ETT.*

MPIF-1 (myeloid progenitor inhibitory factor-1).

MPM hydrogel dressing.

mPower PET scanner—by Positron.

MPR (multiplanar reformation).

MP-RAGE (magnetization prepared three-dimensional gradient-echo) **sequences**—MRI term.

M-protein, M-component—used in reference to chemotherapy response in patients with multiple myeloma (and perhaps other diseases).

MRA (magnetic resonance angiography)—gated inflow technique. See *3DCE MRA technique.*

MRC (magnetic resonance cholangiography).

MRCP (magnetic resonance cholangiopancreatography).

MRCP using HASTE with a phased array coil—noninvasive technique for revealing the pancreaticobiliary tract in young children. See *HASTE.*

MR hydrography—technique that displays static or slow-moving fluids as bright structures against the dark background of the rest of the body.

The images show fluid-containing structures, such as ducts, cysts, sacs, and spaces, as white on black; thus, calculi can be readily identified as filling defects.

MRI (magnetic resonance imaging) **terms** for quick reference:
acquisition time
adiabatic fast passage
A-FAIR
AMT-25-enhanced MR images
analog-to-digital converter
angular frequency
angular momentum
antenna
array processor
artifact
axial proton-density-weighted image
axial T2-weighted image
Bloch equation
Boltzmann distribution
bone marrow edema pattern
breath-hold fast spin-echo images
bright signal
Carr-Purcell-Meiboom-Gill sequence
Carr-Purcell sequence
chemical shift
chemical shift imaging (CSI)
cine study
coherence
coil
continuous wave
contrast enhancement
conventional spin-echo images
coronal SPIR image
coronal T1-weighted MR image (spin echo)
crossed coil
cryomagnet
cryostat
demodulator
detector
diamagnetic

MRI terms *(cont.)*
 diffusion
 digital-to-analog converter
 echo, echoes
 echo planar imaging
 echo time (TE)
 eddy currents; eddies
 edge detection (ED)
 endorectal coil
 endovaginal coil
 excitation
 Exorcist respiratory compensation
  technique
 Faraday shield
 fast-Fourier transform
 fast spin-echo acquisition, 2-D
  or 3-D
 fat- and water-suppressed
  T2-weighted images
 ferromagnetic
 field gradient
 field lock
 field of view (FOV)
 filling factor
 filtered-back projection
 FLAIR (fluid-attentuated inversion
  recovery)
 flip angle
 flow artifact
 flow-related enhancement
 flow-related phase shifts
 fMRI (functional MRI)
 FNH (focal nodular hyperplasia)
 Fourier transform
 free induction decay (FID)
 free induction signal
 frequency
 FSE-T2 (fast spin echo) with fat
  suppression
 functional
 gadolinium-enhanced T1-weighted
  images
 gauss
 Golay coil

MRI terms *(cont.)*
 gradient coil
 gradient-echo pulse sequence
 gradient magnetic field
 gyromagnetic ratio
 half-dose enhanced MRI with
  MT (magnetization transfer)
 half-fourier acquisition single-shot
  turbo spin-echo (HASTE)
 HASTE (half-fourier acquisition
  single-shot turbo spin-echo)
 Helmholtz coil
 hertz (Hz)
 homogeneity
 HRARE (hybrid rapid acquisition
  with relaxation enhancement)
 image acquisition time
 inductance
 inhomogeneity
 interface
 interpulse time
 intravascular signal intensity in MR
  angiography
 inversion
 inversion recovery
 inversion time (TI)
 kilohertz (kHz)
 Larmor equation
 Larmor frequency
 lattice
 line imaging
 line scanning
 line width
 LMR (localized magnetic
  resonance)
 long echo train fast spin-echo
  sequence
 longitudinal magnetization
 longitudinal relaxation
 Lorentzian line
 macroscopic magnetization moment
 macroscopic magnetization vector
 magnetic dipole
 magnetic field

MRI terms *(cont.)*
    magnetic gradient
    magnetic induction
    magnetic moment
    magnetic resonance
    magnetic resonance signal
    magnetic susceptibility
    magnetization
    magnetization transfer (MT)
      saturation
    MIP (maximum intensity projection)
    MMCM-enhanced MR imaging
    MP-RAGE (magnetization prepared
      3-D gradient-echo) sequences
    MRCP using HASTE with a phased
      array coil
    multiple line-scan imaging (MLSI)
    multiple plane imaging
    multiple sensitive point
    multishot spin-echo echo-planar
      imaging
    nidus patency
    nuclear magnetic resonance
    nuclear signal
    nuclear spin
    nuclear spin quantum number
    nucleon
    number of excitations
    nutation
    opposed loop-pair quadrature
      magnetic resonance coil
    orientation
      axial
      coronal
      sagittal
      transverse
    paramagnetic
    partial saturation
    PASTA (polarity-altered spectral
      selective acquisition) imaging
    PC (phase-contrast) technique
    percentage signal intensity loss
      (PSIL)
    permanent magnet

MRI terms *(cont.)*
    permeability
    phantom
    phase
    phase contrast
    phase imaging
    phase sensitive detector
    phase shift
    pixel (picture element)
    planar spin imaging
    point imaging
    point scanning
    precession
    precessional frequency
    proton density
    PSIL (percentage signal intensity
      loss)
    pulsed gradients
    pulse length
    pulse, radiofrequency
    pulse sequences
    pulse width
    rature detector
    rature surface coil system
    quality factor
    quenching
    radian
    rapid acquisition with relaxation
      enhancement (RARE)
    rapid imaging
    RARE (rapid acquisition with relax-
      ation enhancement) technique
    readout delay
    receiver
    receiver coil
    reconstruction
    reduced signal intensity
    relaxation rate
    relaxation time
    repeated FID (free induction decay)
    rephasing gradient
    resistive magnet
    resolution, spatial
    resonance

MRI terms *(cont.)*
  resonant frequency
  respiratory triggered fast SE
    technique
  respiratory triggering
  RF (radiofrequency) coil
  RF (radiofrequency) pulse
  ROC (receiver operating charac-
    teristic)
  ROPE (respiratory ordered phase
    encoding)
  rotating frame of reference
  saddle coil
  sagittal T1-weighted image
  saturation recovery
  saturation transfer
  selective excitation
  selective irradiation
  sensitive plane
  sensitive point
  sensitive volume
  sequence time
  sequential plane imaging
  sequential point imaging
  shaded surface display (SSD)
  shim coil
  shimming
  signal-to-noise ratio (SNR or S/N
    ratio)
  simultaneous volume imaging
  single shot fast spin echo (SSFSE)
  single slice fast dynamic in vivo
  skin depth
  solenoid coil
  spectrometer
  spectrum
  spin
  spin density
  spin echo
  spin-echo imaging
  spin-lattice relaxation time
  spin-spin relaxation time
  spin-warp imaging
  SPIR (selective partial inversion-
    recovery)

MRI terms *(cont.)*
  SPIR fat-suppression images
  SPIR-FLAIR images or sequences
  SSD (shaded surface display)
  standard-dose enhanced conven-
    tional T1-weighted images
  steady state free precession (SSFP)
  STEAM (stimulated echo acquisi-
    tion mode) sequence
  STIR (short inversion time
    inversion-recovery) sequence
  superconducting magnet
  surface coil
  TE (echo time)
  tesla (T)
  three-dimensional Fourier
  3-D TOF (time-of-flight) MR angio-
    graphic sequences
  TI (inversion time)
  time-of-flight (TOF) echoplanar
    imaging
  time-of-flight (TOF) method
  TOF (time of flight)
  T1 (spin-lattice or longitudinal
    relaxation time)
  TR (repetition time)
  transform imaging
  transverse magnetization
  TRIADS (time-resolved imaging by
    automatic data segmentation)
  T1-weighted fat-suppressed
    gadolinium-enhanced SE images
  T1-weighted gadolinium-enhanced
    SE images
  T2 (spin-spin or transverse
    relaxation time)
  T2-weighted fast SE images
  T2-weighted turbo SE images
  tuning
  tunnel
  2-D or 3-D fast spin-echo acquisi-
    tion
  3-D TurboFLAIR (fluid-attenuated
    inversion-recovery)
  transaxial fat-saturated 3-D images

MRI terms *(cont.)*
   triple-dose gadolinium-enhanced
      MR imaging without MT
      (magnetization transfer)
   turbo spin-echo sequences
   turbo STIR images
   two-dimensional Fourier
   vector
   velocity encoding
   venetian blind artifacts
   volume acquisition
   volume analysis
   volume imaging
   volume rendering
   volumetric
   voxel (volume element)
   zeugmatography, Fourier
      transformation
MRM (magnetic resonance mammography).
MRN (magnetic resonance neurography).
mRNA (messenger RNA).
MRP (magnetic resonance pancreatography).
MR peritoneography—a study in which the imaging agent is instilled into the peritoneal cavity, magnetic resonance scanning is performed with the peritoneal cavity filled, and after complete drainage of the contrast material, a scan is again performed. Images are reviewed for evidence of peritoneal leaks, hernias, loculated fluid collections, and adhesions. MR peritoneography is particularly useful in continuous ambulatory peritoneal dialysis.
MRS (magnetic resonance spectroscopy).
MRSA (methicillin-resistant *Staphylococcus aureus*).
MRU (magnetic resonance urography).
MRU (molecular recognition unit).

MSAFP (maternal serum alpha-fetoprotein).
MSBP or **MSP** (Munchausen syndrome by proxy).
MS Classique catheter—balloon dilatation catheter for angioplasty.
MSEV (microsurgical epididymovasostomy).
MSH₂ gene—the gene responsible for the most common forms of inherited colon cancer. Identification of this gene may lead to a broadly used genetic cancer screening. The MSH$_2$ gene normally "corrects" mistakes that occur when cells are damaged or divide. However, a flawed gene may allow mistakes to accumulate, thus triggering the growth of cancerous neoplasms.
MSI (magnetic source imaging).
"m-site"—see *Emcyt*.
MSL-109 monoclonal antibody—a drug used to treat patients with AIDS.
MSLT (multiple sleep latency test).
MSP, MSBP (Munchausen syndrome by proxy).
MSTS (Musculoskeletal Tumor Society) **staging system**—for soft-tissue sarcomas.
MSUD (maple-sugar urine) **disease**.
MTBE (methyl tertiary butyl ether)—a drug instilled under local anesthesia to dissolve large cholesterol stones in the gallbladder. Via transhepatic catheter, the bile is aspirated from the gallbladder, and 5 to 10 ml of MTBE is instilled in the gallbladder. As the stone dissolves, the MTBE containing dissolved cholesterol is removed, and more MTBE instilled. This process is continued until fluoroscopy reveals complete dissolving of the stones. Cf. *Actigall, Chenix*.

MTC (mitomycin).

MTD (maximum tolerated dose).

MTM (modified Thayer-Martin medium, a culture medium)—used in culturing *Neisseria gonorrhoeae*.

MTP (microsomal triglyceride transfer protein)—a protein linked to low levels of LDL and thus indicative of low risk for heart attack or stroke.

MTP-PE—see *muramyl-tripeptide*.

MT (magnetization transfer) **saturation** —MRI term.

MTSS (medial tibial stress syndrome).

MTX (methotrexate).

Much's ("mooks") **granules**—found in the sputa of patients with tuberculosis. They are visible on Gram's stain but not on stain for acid-fast bacilli or by other methods.

mucocutaneous lymph node syndrome (MLNS)—affects prepubertal children almost exclusively, mostly males, with a peak incidence during the first 18 months. See *Kawasaki's disease*.

mucolipidosis III (pseudo-Hurler deformity)—a rare congenital abnormality which includes clawhand, ground-glass corneas, aortic valvular disease, and other orthopedic and biochemical abnormalities. Onset is around age three.

mucormycosis—rare and often fatal mycotic infection caused by one of the sporophytic fungi of the order Mucorales. It is known to affect patients who are immunocompromised. The most common form is rhinocerebral, although primary infections of the skin, lungs, and GI tract have also been reported. Involvement of the GU tract is primarily limited to the kidneys. Mucormycosis (*not* mucomycosis)

may also be referred to as *phycomycosis* or *zygomycosis*.

mucosa (pl., mucosae)—the mucous membrane. See *mucous, honeycomb mucosa*.

mucosal ileal diaphragms—diaphragm-like mucosal strictures of GI tract, associated with use of nonsteroidal anti-inflammatory drug use.

mucous (adj.)—pertaining to mucus, or secreting mucus, as *mucous membrane*; the epithelium-covered membrane that lines certain organs, such as the eyes, nose, mouth, throat, and vagina. Cf. *mucus*.

MUCP (maximum urethral closure pressure) (Urol).

mucus (noun)—viscid secretion produced by mucous membranes. See *mucous*.

Mueller's (Müller) **muscle**—in the upper and lower eyelids; involved in correction of eyelid retraction in Graves' ophthalmopathy.

Muercke's lines—seen on the fingernails and toenails in patients with hypoalbuminemia. The lines run across the nail and are parallel to each other.

MUGA (multiple gated acquisition) **scan**—a blood pool radionuclide study of cardiac shape and dynamics in which a radionuclide is introduced into the circulation. Radioactive emissions from the heart are electronically monitored, stored, and analyzed, resulting in a composite scan consisting of a series of successive images all taken at the same point in the cardiac cycle.

mulberry molars—five-pointed molars are a sign of congenital syphilis. Also, *Hutchinson's teeth and hutchinsonian molars*.

Mulder sign—a click felt between the metatarsal heads when diagnosing Morton's neuroma in the web space of the toes.

Mullen prognostic nutritional index.

Mullins cardiac device.

Multibite biopsy forceps—biopsy forceps that allow the surgeon to obtain multiple samples with only one pass through the scope.

MultiBoot—an orthosis that provides pressure-free positioning of the ulcerated heel.

multicentric angiofollicular hyperplasia (MAFH)—a disease characterized by diffuse lymphadenopathy, splenomegaly, anemia, polyclonal hypergammaglobulinemia, and constitutional symptoms. It is the multicentric form of Castleman's disease, a localized form of mediastinal lymphoid hyperplasia. See *Castleman's disease.*

Multiclip—a disposable surgical ligating clip device.

Multidex wound-filling material.

multidrug-resistant tuberculosis (MDR-TB).

multi-echo images—a series of spin echo images obtained with various pulse sequences in MRI scans.

Multifire Endohernia clip applier—used in laparoscopic herniorrhaphy.

Multifire GIA, Multifire Endo GIA (30 or 60)—stapling device used in laparoscopic surgery.

multiflanged Portnoy catheter—for hydrocephalus shunts.

Multi-Flex stent—a hydrophilic-coated urologic stent with inner lumen hydrogel coating to ensure ease of placement over a guide wire.

multifocal chorioretinitis—small, multifocal retinal lesions with intra-ocular inflammatory cells. Usually classified as one of the white dot syndromes.

multigenic carcinogenesis—involvement of multiple genes in the origin of carcinomas and other malignant neoplasms.

multi-infarct dementia (MID).

Multikine (leukocyte; interleukin)—an immunotherapy drug used to treat patients with head and neck cancer and prostate cancer.

Multileaf Collimator (MLC)—a device used in radiation oncology that allows the radiation beam to automatically follow the shape of a tumor, irradiating only cancerous tissue and not adjacent healthy tissue.

Multilok hand operating table.

multimer assay.

multimode imaging confocal optical microscope (MIMCOM).

Multi-Operatory Dentalaser (MOD)—used for composite curing and teeth whitening.

MultiPad absorptive dressing.

multiplanar gradient-recalled (MPGR) **echo**—MRI term.

multiplanar mode; technique—MRI terms.

multiplanar reformation (MPR).

multiple endocrine adenopathies, or **abnormalities** (MEA).

multiple endocrine neoplasia (MEN), **type 2b**—a syndrome, often familial, characterized by medullary carcinoma of the thyroid, pheochromocytoma, mucosal neuromas, Marfan's body structure, and ophthalmologic manifestations.

multiple evanescent white dot syndrome—seen usually in young adults, mostly women. It is characterized by unilateral visual loss,

multiple evanescent *(cont.)* occasionally preceded by viral-like symptoms. It appears to be self-limiting, with recovery in approximately seven weeks. The syndrome takes its name from the widespread white dots seen at the posterior pole, deep in the retina or at the level of the retinal pigment epithelium.

multiple gated acquisition scan—see *MUGA*.

multiple organ dysfunction syndrome (MODS).

multiple organ failure (MOF).

multiple sleep latency test (MSLT)—used to diagnose the sleep apnea syndrome, narcolepsy, and other sleep disorders.

multiple sort flow cytometry—a flow cytometer used in detection and identification of cancer cells.

Multi Podus (boot) **system**—bracing device for the treatment of foot and ankle abnormalities including contractures, foot drop, pressure sores, spasticity, inversion and eversion, rotation, tendinitis, sprains, and stress fractures. It is also used postoperatively after ligament and tendon repairs.

Multipurpose-SM catheter.

multisystem organ failure (MSOF)—the most common cause of death in patients in the ICU. Multisystem organ failure, by definition, involves the simultaneous failure of two or more of these body systems: lungs, liver, kidneys, GI tract, circulatory system, or central nervous system.

MultiVac—suction ArthroWand.

multivitamin formula (M.V.I.-12).

MultiVysion PB assay—a genetic test that can be used to identify chromosomal abnormalities in genetic mate-rial released by the ovum prior to, and immediately following, fertilization.

Mumford-Gurd procedure—arthroplasty used in separation of the acromioclavicular joint.

Munchausen's syndrome—named for the fictional Baron Munchausen, who told greatly exaggerated tales. In this syndrome the patient gives exaggerated and dramatic symptoms of a disease he does not have. Because the book about the fictional baron was written in English and his name spelled with a single *h* and no umlaut, *Munchausen* is the spelling used today in a medical context.

Munchausen syndrome by proxy (MSP, MSBP)—a bizarre variation of Munchausen syndrome involving a mother (or other caregiver) and a child. The mother (often a healthcare professional) seems concerned and caring, while actually causing physical symptoms in the child or sometimes reporting the unconfirmed occurrence of such symptoms. The child may suffer through numerous medical and surgical interventions. This is a serious and potentially lethal form of child abuse which apparently has its psychological roots in the mother's need for a relationship with a physician due to her own profound sense of early abandonment as a child. This syndrome presents a confusing number of symptoms but may result in the child's death, if undiagnosed. See *Munchausen syndrome*.

mupirocin (Bactroban)—an antibiotic ointment applied to the nares and umbilical cord of premature infants to eliminate MRSA (methicillin-

mupirocin *(cont.)*
resistant *Staphylococcus aureus*), a common source of infection in high-risk infants.

muramyl-tripeptide (MTP-PE)—drug used to treat patients with Kaposi's sarcoma.

murmur grades—may use either roman or arabic numerals:
grade I or 1, barely audible, must strain to hear
grade II or 2, quiet, but clearly audible
grade III or 3, moderately loud
grade IV or 4, loud
grade V or 5, very loud; may be heard with the stethoscope partly off the chest
grade VI or 6, so loud that it can be heard with the stethoscope just off the chest wall

Muromonab–CD3—a murine monoclonal antibody to the T3 (CD3) antigen of human T cells which acts as an immunosuppressant. This drug reverses graft rejection of renal and other transplants by blocking T-cell functions.

Murphy skid (Ortho).

muscimol—one of the poisons from the deadly mushroom *Amanita muscaria*.

muscle-splitting incision.

MUSE (medicated urethral system for erection) **urethral suppository** (alprostadil)—noninvasive transurethral system for treatment of male impotence, composed of a prefilled plastic applicator for delivery of alprostadil in suppository form.

mushroom worker's disease (or **lung**)—pulmonary symptoms caused by exposure to *Thermoactinomyces* organisms in the compost in which mushrooms grow.

Mustang steerable guide wire—used to introduce and place catheters during angioplasty procedures.

mustard—see *L-phenylalanine mustard*.

Mustardé procedure—flap otoplasty. Cf. *Mustard procedure*.

Mustard procedure—for transposition of the great vessels. Cf. *Mustardé procedure*.

Mutamycin (injectable mitomycin)—used with other chemotherapeutic agents in combination for treatment of disseminated adenocarcinoma of the pancreas, stomach, breast, colon, head, neck, and lung.

MUSTPAC—a portable medical ultrasound 3-D communications system that can be carried as a backpack. It enables a technician in a remote location to scan patients and transmit 3-D images many miles away.

mute toe signs—equivocal Babinski reflexes.

mutton fat KPs (keratitic precipitates)—clusters of inflammatory cells and white cells that adhere to the corneal endothelium. Found in patients with uveitis.

MVA (microvascular angiopathy).

MVAC or **M-VAC** (methotrexate, vincristine, Adriamycin, cisplatin)—chemotherapy protocol for adenocarcinoma of the uterus and cervix, and transitional cell carcinoma of the breast.

M-Vax—therapeutic cancer vaccine for postsurgical stage III metastatic melanoma, made by modifying a patient's own tumor cells with a molecule called a "hapten."

M.V.C.9+4—an intravenous multivitamin complex, containing 9 water-soluble and 4 fat-soluble vitamins.

MVF (mitoxantrone, vincristine, fluorouracil)—chemotherapy protocol for breast carcinoma.

M.V.I.-12—intravenous multivitamin infusion.

MVP (mean platelet volume).

MVP (mitral valve prolapse).

MVP (moisture vapor permeability).

MVT (mitoxantrone, VP-16, thiotepa)—chemotherapy protocol for multiple myeloma and lymphomas.

MVV (maximal voluntary ventilation).

myalgic encephalomyelitis (ME)—the British term for what in the U.S. is called *chronic fatigue syndrome.* Also called *postviral fatigue syndrome* and *yuppie flu.*

Myambutol (ethambutol)—used to treat tuberculosis as well as MAC infection in AIDS patients.

mycelium—a mat of fungal growth consisting of hyphae.

MycoAKT latex bead agglutination test—used for the identification of *Mycobacterium* species, needed because of the increasing frequency of nontuberculous mycobacterial diseases associated with AIDS.

Mycobacterium abscessus—a rapidly growing, opportunistic organism, known to cause disease by inoculation after trauma. It is the suspected cause of refractory post-tympanostomy tube otorrhea.

Mycobacterium avium **complex**—see *MAC infection.*

Mycobacterium avium-intracellulare **infection**—see *MAI infection.*

Mycobacterium **cell wall complex** (MCC)—anticancer technology prepared from the nonpathogenic *Mycobacterium phlei (M. phlei).* It interacts synergistically with chemotherapeutic agents, thus significantly enhancing their ability to inhibit growth of malignant melanoma cells.

Mycobacterium gordonae—has been cultured from tap water, soil, sputum, and gastric lavage specimens.

Mycobutin (rifabutin)—used for treating MAC infection in AIDS patients.

mycophenolate mofetil (CellCept)—used investigationally against rejection of kidney transplants.

mycosis fungoides—lymphoma (white blood cell malignancy) which occurs in the skin.

mycosis fungoides palmaris et plantaris—an infection that manifests primarily on the palms and soles and clinically may mimic various inflammatory palmoplantar dermatoses.

MycroMesh biomaterial—inert, expanded polytetrafluoroethylene material used in repair of hernias.

myelodysplastic syndrome (MDS)—hematopoietic stem cell disorders characterized by bone marrow dysplasia and various combinations of anemia, leukopenia, and thrombocytopenia.

myeloid/erythroid (M/E) **ratio**.

myeloid progenitor inhibitory factor-1 (MPIF-1)—a human protein in development that may allow cancer patients to be treated with more potent chemotherapy.

myelomere—spinal cord segment.

Myers-Briggs Personality Inventory.

Myers Solution—includes a patented instrument and technique designed to close the groin wound that is created when introducing a cardiac catheter. It debrides the surrounding adventitia and delivers a form of human glue to the puncture site. The solution can be activated by laser light, reducing the risk of hemor-

Myers *(cont.)*
rhage at the puncture site and speeding recovery time.

Myhre syndrome—rare inherited disorder characterized by mental retardation, short stature, unusual facial features, and skeletal abnormalities. Other findings may include hearing impairment, muscular hypertrophy, and/or joint stiffness. The syndrome is thought to be inherited as an autosomal dominant genetic trait.

Mylotarg (gemtuzumab ozogamicin; CMA-676)—antibody-targeted chemotherapeutic agent for the treatment of CD33-positive relapsed acute myeloid leukemia. Mylotarg is the combination of a monoclonal antibody directed at CD33, a protein expressed only by myeloid leukemic cells, and calicheamicin, a cytotoxic antibiotic. This antibody-drug conjugate delivers treatment directly to the leukemia cells while sparing normal cells.

Myobock artificial hand—the Utah artificial arm, a myoelectric prosthesis for amputations above the elbow. Available with either a hook or an artificial Myobock hand.

myocardial adrenergic signaling—the normal physiological stimulation of heart function. It is generated when chemical transmitters known as catecholamines bind with certain receptors on the surfaces of heart cells, triggering a series of events which results in increased heart rate and force of contraction of the heart. In congestive heart failure, the heart is often unable to respond adequately to catecholamines.

myocardial remodeling—a feature in the progression of myocardial failure involving changes in the structure and function of the myocardium.

myoclonus epilepsy associated with ragged-red fibers (MERRF).

myocutaneous graft.

myofascial release—a physical therapy method of light-touch techniques designed to release tight fascial restrictions throughout the body. It is often used in conjunction with other therapies such as NDT (neurodevelopmental techniques) and SI (sensory integration).

Myoscint (imciromab pentetate)—the monoclonal antibody Fab to myosin, labeled with indium 111. Used to detect myocarditis and signs of rejection in patients after heart transplant.

myositis ossificans (MO)—benign muscle tumor, mostly of young men. This is difficult for radiologists, orthopedic surgeons, and pathologists to differentiate from much more serious conditions. Plain films are the most reliable method of making the diagnosis, as MRI scans, radionuclide scans, and smears from biopsies can offer misleading information. This condition has a string sign. See *string sign*.

MYOterm XP—cardioplegia delivery system.

MyoTrac and **MyoTrac 2 EMG monitoring**—a biofeedback medical device used to help prevent repetitive strain injury. EMG electrodes are placed on the back and shoulders to measure muscle tension and relaxation. The device can be worn all day to maintain healthy working and resting positions.

Myotrophin (mecasermin, previously known as recombinant human insulin-like growth factor-1, rhIGF-1)—

483 Myotrophin • M-Zole

Myotrophin *(cont.)*
used to treat amyotrophic lateral sclerosis. May be used to treat various peripheral neuropathies, including chemotherapy-induced peripheral neuropathy, post-polio syndrome, and diabetic neuropathy as well as acute kidney failure.

Myoview—an imaging drug used in scintigraphic imaging of the heart during resting and exercise to delineate cardiac ischemia.

myxoma—a tumor of mucoid (mucous) material.

M-Zole 3 Combination Pack—antifungal vaginal suppositories and cream

M-Zole 7 Dual Pack—antifungal vaginal suppositories and cream. Also called *M-Zole 7 Combination Pack.*

N, n

Nabi-HB (hepatitis B immune globulin [human])—for treatment of acute exposure to blood containing HB_sAg (hepatitis B surface antigen), perinatal exposure of infants born to HB_sAg-positive mothers, sexual exposure to HB_sAg-positive persons, and household exposure to persons with acute hepatitis B virus (HBV) infection. Administration by intramuscular injection.

Nabi-NicVAX—nicotine vaccine for the prevention and treatment of nicotine addiction.

nabumetone (Relafen)—a nonsteroidal anti-inflammatory drug for rheumatoid arthritis and osteoarthritis. It belongs to a class of NSAIDs known as naphthylalkalones and is thought to have fewer GI side effects than other NSAIDs.

NAC (N-acetyl-L-cysteine)—an investigational drug used for AIDS treatment. See *anti-TNF drugs*.

NAD (no appreciable disease).

Nadbath akinesia—facial nerve block given behind the ear in preparation for cataract surgery.

nadir—the lowest point; in hematology-oncology, the lowest point reached by the white cell count after chemotherapy has been administered. When the WBC count falls below 1000, the chemotherapeutic agent may be discontinued until the white cell count rises. Pronounced like (Ralph) Nader.

NAET (Nambudripad's Allergy Elimination Technique).

nafamostat mesylate—useful agent for stabilizing the coagulant and fibrinolytic systems in hepatic resection. A serine protease inhibitor and potent antifibrinolytic agent. Prevents coagulation and fibrinolysis leading to massive blood loss during hepatic resection.

nafarelin (Synarel)—synthetic version of gonadotropin-releasing hormone used to treat endometriosis. The formation of painful endometrial implants within the pelvic area is facilitated by the hormone estrogen. Rising estrogen during the first half of the menstrual cycle causes proliferation of the endometrium and also

nafarelin *(cont.)*
causes endometrial implants in the pelvic area to swell. Later these implants bleed, slough off, and produce inflammation and scarring within the pelvis and abdomen. Nafarelin suppresses the release of estrogen from the ovaries and stops the menstrual cycle while the patient is on the drug, thereby treating the endometriosis. It is administered intranasally because it cannot be absorbed in the GI tract following oral administration.

Nagahara phaco chopper and phaco chop technique—nucleus emulsification device and technique developed by Dr. Kunihiro B. Nagahara for removal of cataracts.

Naganol (suramin)—antiparasitic.

nail—see *device.*

nail bed *(not* nailbed)—the skin surface just under the nail.

Nakao snare I and **II**—a snare that combines the actions of polyp transection and retrieval into one. It snares and transects a polyp while the polyp is in the capture pouch.

nalmefene HCl (Revex).

naltrexone hydrochloride—a narcotic in dosage form for the treatment of opiate addiction.

Nambudripad's Allergy Elimination Technique (NAET)—acupuncture technique that eliminates allergies by use of muscle testing. The patient holds a vial of allergen; the practitioner then applies pressure to see if the muscles weaken. If they do, the patient is allergic, and acupuncture is then done to eliminate the allergic reaction.

NANB hepatitis *(not* NA&B)—non-A, non-B hepatitis (now called hepatitis C), an acute viral hepatitis that does not have antibodies or antigens of either hepatitis A or B.

nanogram (millimicrogram)—used in plasma testosterone measurement, growth hormone assay results; given in nanograms per cubic centimeter (ng/cc).

nanowalker—three-legged device with a probe that can measure and image a surface with nanometer precision over a large area.

naphthylalkalones—a class of nonsteroidal anti-inflammatory drugs for treating rheumatoid arthritis and osteoarthritis. Thought to have fewer GI side effects than other kinds of NSAIDS. See *nabumetone.*

Naphuride (suramin)—antiparasitic.

Naprelan (naproxen sodium)—a once-a-day formulation of Naprosyn, an NSAID used to treat osteoarthritis and rheumatoid arthritis.

naproxen (Aleve, Anaprox, Napron X, Naprosyn, Naprelan)—nonsteroidal anti-inflammatory drug.

Nardi test (morphine-prostigmine)—for ampullary stenosis of pancreaticobiliary sphincters.

Naropin (ropivacaine hydrochloride)—local anesthetic to control pain postoperatively and during labor and delivery, and for major surgical procedures such as cesarean sections, orthopedic, abdominal, and major nerve blocks.

narrowband UV-B (NBUVB)—therapeutic light exposure of narrowband ultraviolet B light in the treatment of psoriasis. Narrowband has been found to facilitate faster clearing and more complete disease resolution than broadband UV-B.

narrowed pulse pressure—the difference between the systolic and diastolic pressures.

Nasacort AQ (triamcinolone acetonide) —used for treatment of seasonal and perennial allergic rhinitis for patients age six and older. It is a well-tolerated, odorless, taste-free, once-daily medication, reportedly providing rapid relief of symptoms.

nasal flaring—involuntary outward movement of nasal alae in newborns with respiratory distress and in patients with some types of heart disease. Also called *alar flaring*.

nasal T-cell/natural killer cell lymphoma—a locally destructive disease typically presenting with obliteration of the nasal passages and maxillary sinuses. Involvement of the adjacent alveolar bone, hard palate, orbits, and nasopharynx is found in more than 50% of cases and is associated with extensive soft-tissue masses. Presence of bone erosion on x-ray is suggestive but not diagnostic of the disease.

Nasarel (flunisolide)—aqueous-based, fragrance-free reformulation of Nasalide.

Nascobal gel (cyanocobalamin)—vitamin B_{12} intranasal gel developed for once-weekly self-administration as alternative to once-monthly vitamin B_{12} injections. Gel is absorbed through the nasal mucous membranes for treatment of vitamin B_{12} deficiency and pernicious anemia.

Nashold TC electrode—for making dorsal root entry zone (DREZ) lesions in the spinal cord.

nasogastric (NG) **feeding tube.**

nasojejunal (NJ) **feeding tube.**

Nasonex (mometasone furoate monohydrate) **aqueous nasal spray**—once-daily nasal corticosteroid for the treatment of seasonal allergic and perennial rhinitis.

NAT (nucleic acid testing)—can detect HIV and hepatitis C in donated blood.

natatory ligament—a term used in surgery of the hand, particularly in the context of Dupuytren's contracture.

nateglinide—monotherapy drug for type 2 diabetes, or combination therapy when administered with metformin.

National Institute for Allergy and Infectious Diseases (NIAID).

National Notifiable Disease Surveillance System (NNDSS)—an arm of the Centers for Disease Control and Prevention. States submit annual reports on incidence of certain diseases in order to assess effectiveness of vaccination programs and need for additional preventive measures.

National Organizations Responding to AIDS (NORA).

native tissue harmonic imaging (NTHI)—used in echocardiography on difficult-to-image patients. It allows for deep penetration while maintaining high resolution images of the body's native tissue.

Natrecor (nesiritide)—for treatment of congestive heart failure. It is a genetically engineered form of the naturally occurring cardiac human b-type natriuretic peptide, which is produced primarily in the ventricle of the heart. It is the body's natural response to a failing heart.

natriuresis—excretion of abnormal amounts of sodium in the urine.

Natural-Hip prosthesis.

Natural-Knee system—implants used to surgically manage the arthritic knee.

Naughton cardiac exercise treadmill test—used for patients who cannot stand for prolonged periods as required in traditional treadmill tests.

Navarre—devices for interventional radiology.

Navelbine (vinorelbine tartrate)—chemotherapeutic agent for treatment of non-small cell lung carcinoma.

Navigator flexible endoscope.

Naviport deflectable tip guiding catheter—has open lumen or tube designed for delivery of diagnostic or therapeutic microcatheters into the chambers and/or the coronary vasculature of the heart.

Navratil retractor (Ob-Gyn). Also, *Breisky-Navratil retractor*.

NBIH cardiac device.

N-butyl-deoxynojirimycin (DNJ)—antiviral AIDS treatment.

NCP (NeuroCybernetic Prosthesis) **system**—vagal nerve stimulation device for treatment of epilepsy that has proven refractory to antiseizure medication and surgical therapy.

NCV (nerve conduction velocity).

NDT (neurodevelopmental techniques) —a physical therapy method to facilitate active, functional movement of patients suffering from lack of muscle tone, sensory loss, and diminished range of motion.

Nd:YAG (neodymium:yttrium-aluminum-garnet) **laser**. See *neodymium*.

Nd:YAG CTLC (contact transscleral laser cytophotocoagulation)—used in treatment of glaucoma.

Nd:YLF (neodymium:yttrium-lithium fluoride) **laser**.

near-infrared spectroscopy (NIRS).

near-miss—adjective describing near-fatal occurrence, e.g., *near-miss SIDS, near-miss drowning*.

nebacumab (Ha-1A monoclonal antibody)—used to treat gram-negative shock.

NebuPent (aerosolized pentamidine)— for prevention of *Pneumocystis carinii* pneumonia in AIDS patients.

NEC ("neck") (necrotizing enterocolitis)—develops in premature infants unable to tolerate formula.

necrotizing enterocolitis (NEC).

necrotizing fasciitis—a fulminating group A streptococcal infection beginning with severe or extensive cellulitis that spreads to involve the superficial and deep fascia, producing thrombosis of the subcutaneous vessels and gangrene of the underlying tissues. A cutaneous lesion usually serves as a portal of entry for the infection, but sometimes no such lesion is found. Also called "flesh-eating bacteria." See *streptococcus A infection*.

NED (no evidence of disease).

nedocromil sodium (Tilade)—inhaled to treat bronchial asthma or reversible obstructive airway disease. It has an anti-inflammatory action but is not a steroid or bronchodilator.

needle
Accucore II biopsy
Atraloc surgical
B-D spinal
Bierman
Biopty cut
Boynton needle holder
Brockenbrough
butterfly
Cardiopoint
Charles flute
Chiba

needle *(cont.)*
   Cibis ski
   CIF-4
   coaxial sheath cut-biopsy
   Cobb-Ragde
   Colapinto curved
   Colorado microdissection
   Control-Release pop-off
   Cook endoscopic curved
   Core aspiration/injection
   Core CO_2 insufflation
   C-type acupuncture
   cut-biopsy
   Dieckmann intraosseous
   docking
   Dos Santos
   D-TACH removable
   Echo-Coat ultrasound biopsy
   Endopath Ultra Veress
   Ethalloy TruTaper cardiovascular
   Franseen stereotactic
   French-eye
   GraNee (Riza-Ribe grasper)
   Gripper
   Hawkeye suture
   Hawkins breast localization
   Howell biopsy aspiration
   Huber
   J
   Keith
   Klatskin
   Koch nucleus hydrolysis
   Lewis Pair-Pak
   Madayag biopsy
   milliner's
   Nottingham colposuspension
   PC-7
   P.D. Access
   Pencan spinal
   PercuCut cut-biopsy
   Pereyra
   Plum-Blossom
   Protect Point
   Punctur-Guard

needle *(cont.)*
   Quincke spinal
   Riza-Ribe
   Rosen
   Rosenthal
   Sabreloc spatula
   SafeTap tapered spinal
   Safety AV fistula
   Sahli
   SC-1
   Seldinger gastrostomy
   self-aspirating cut-biopsy
   Sensi-Touch anesthesia
   side-cutting spatulated
   Skinny
   SmallPort
   SmartNeedle
   Solitaire
   spatulated half-circle
   Stamey
   steel-winged butterfly
   Steis
   stereotactic biopsy
   Stifcore aspiration
   Teflon-coated hollow-bore
   Terry-Mayo
   THI
   Thomas
   Tru-Cut
   Tuohy
   Unimar J
   Veress
   Visi-Black surgical
   Voorhees
   Waterfield
   Westerman-Jensen
   Whitacre spinal
   Wright
Neer classification of shoulder fractures—I, II, III.
Neer hemiarthroplasty.
nefazodone (Serzone)—an antidepressant. Symptoms of depression can be caused by decreased levels of the

nefazodone *(cont.)*
neurotransmitters norepinephrine and serotonin in the brain. Nefazodone corrects the serotonin deficiency by inhibiting its reuptake by nerve terminals, thus allowing an increase in its relative concentration.

negative stroke margin—On fine-needle biopsy, the breast is compressed before the needle is inserted. However, breast compression to 3.5 cm or less may pass the needle through the back wall of the breast. This danger is termed "negative stroke margin."

negative symptoms of schizophrenia—apathy, depression, emotional unresponsiveness, social withdrawal. Cf. *positive symptoms of schizophrenia.*

Negri body (inclusion body found in rabies).

Neiguan point—acupressure point P6, which is located approximately three fingerwidths up from the wrist crease, between the flexor tendons on the medial aspect of the forearm.

Neisseria—now split between the genus *Branhamella* and the genus *Neisseria.*

Neisseria meningitidis—the cause of meningococcal meningitis.

Nélaton dislocation of the ankle.

Nélaton rubber tube drain.

nelfinavir (Viracept)—nonpeptide HIV protease inhibitor.

Nellcor Symphony—blood pressure monitoring system.

NEMD (nonspecific esophageal motility disorder) (Radiol, GI).

neoadjuvant hormonal therapy (NHT)—drug therapy in conjunction with radiation therapy, which is reported to offer significantly improved clinical outcomes.

Neocate One+ (*not* Neocare)—hypoallergenic formula for children allergic to cow's milk, soy, casein, and whey (multiple food protein intolerance).

neochoana—artificially created choana.

Neocontrol—magnet technology embedded in the seat of a chair. The patient who is treated for urinary incontinence sits in the chair with clothes on for 20 minutes, twice a week for 8 weeks. As the magnetic field pulsates at a controlled rate, muscles contract in the pelvic floor, improving muscle strength and bladder control.

neodymium:yttrium-aluminum-garnet laser (Nd:YAG laser)—used in glaucoma procedure combining a nonpenetrating trabeculectomy with a Nd:YAG trabeculectomy. It forms through-and-through filtration under a scleral flap without actually entering the anterior chamber. See *laser.*

Neoflex bendable knife—electrocautery with a flexible pencil-like device that provides the surgeon access to difficult-to-reach areas.

NeoKnife electrosurgical instrument—for cutting, fulguration, and desiccation.

neonatal acne—nonfollicular pustulosis of the newborn; recent findings indicate it is caused by *Malassezia furfur* yeasts. Cf. *Malassezia furfur pustulosis.*

NeoNaze—nasal function restoration device for laryngectomy patients.

neon particle protocol—focal radiation therapy.

Neoprobe 1000 detector—handheld gamma-detection probe, used for lymphatic mapping in patients with breast cancer.

Neoprobe 1500 portable radioisotope detector—handheld device that detects gamma rays and can be used externally and intraoperatively to track an injected radiopharmaceutical within the body.

Neoral (cyclosporine for microemulsion)—for treatment of severe rheumatoid arthritis. In the form of capsules and oral solution, it is used for the prophylaxis of organ rejection in kidney, liver, and heart allogenic transplants.

neoscrotum—constructed, using skin flaps or a split-thickness graft fashioned into a neopouch, after blunt trauma has damaged the scrotum.

Neo-Sert umbilical vessel catheter insertion set—used in neonates.

Ne-Osteo bone morphogenic protein (BMP)—a combination of bone factors within a collagen matrix, used as an alternative to autograft and the necessity for bone harvesting. Ne-Osteo is used with the BAK interbody-fusion system. Additionally, Ne-Osteo BMP may be used in dental applications, e.g., the treatment of bone loss due to periodontal disease.

NeoTect (depreotide)—second in a class of new disease-specific diagnostic imaging agents designed to help physicians identify and localize the specific disease they are seeing by imaging techniques.

Neotrend system—provides multiparameter blood gas monitoring in premature infants without drawing blood.

Neotrofin (AIT-082, leteprinim potassium)—used for nerve repair and regeneration, including the treatment of Alzheimer's disease.

Neovastat—for the treatment of solid tumor cancers.

NephrAmine—essential amino acid injection formulated for patients with renal disease.

nephritogenic—causing or relating to causing nephritis.

nephrostomy-type catheter.

nephrotic syndrome—defined as serum albumin greater than 3.0 gm/dl and proteinuria of 3.5 gm or more in 24 hours.

nephroureterectomy—a procedure consisting of en bloc removal of a cuff of bladder around the ipsilateral ureteral orifice. Traditional management of transitional cell carcinoma of the renal pelvis. Now replaced by local surgical resection alone or in combination with other local therapies.

Nepro—diet supplement formulated to meet electrolyte needs in renal patients with fluid restrictions.

nerve block infusion kit—provides continuous infusion of local anesthetic near a nerve for regional pain management during orthopedic and general surgery.

nerve conduction velocity (NCV)—a diagnostic test which may be performed along with an EMG. It tests the integrity of peripheral nerves by measuring the time it takes for an impulse generated by an electric stimulator, placed over a nerve, to travel over a segment of it.

nerve growth factor (NGF)—a substance produced in the brain. Levels of nerve growth factor may be decreased in patients with Alzheimer's disease. Without NGF, neurons die; future therapy for Alzheimer's disease may involve supplementation with NGF.

nerve of Latarjet ("Lat´ar-zhay")—continuation of the vagus nerve along the stomach. In a proximal gastric

nerve of Latarjet *(cont.)*
vagotomy procedure, tiny branches of this nerve to the stomach are divided, which decreases the acid output of the stomach and protects against ulcer disease.

nerve of Wrisberg—there are two nerves with the same name: the medial cutaneous nerve of the arm and the intermediate nerve. Named for an 18th century German anatomist.

NervePace—noninvasive nerve conduction testing machine that measures sensorimotor latencies to assess compression neuropathies, as in carpal tunnel syndrome.

network—see *artificial neural networks (ANNs)*.

Neumega (oprelvekin) (recombinant human interleukin-11)—platelet growth factor that helps prevent recurrent severe chemotherapy-induced thrombocytopenia.

Neupogen (filgrastim)—a recombinant G-CSF used to support peripheral blood progenitor cell transplantation. Neupogen-mobilized PBPC transplantation for cancer patients is said to be rapidly replacing bone marrow transplant procedures.

Neuprex—used for treatment of fungal infections.

neural tube defects (NTD)—birth defects such as spina bifida. Some research indicates that obese women are twice as likely to have children with neural tube defects.

neurapraxia (*not* neuropraxia)—a conduction block (either partial or total) of a segment of nerve fiber, causing a temporary paralysis, as in "The patient has a right ulnar nerve neurapraxia."

neurilemmoma (schwannoma)—proliferation of cells forming a nerve sheath; a common peripheral nerve tumor.

neuroacanthocytosis—a frontosubcortical type of dementia.

neuro-Behçet's disease.

Neurobehavioral Cognitive Status Examination—neurological test.

NeuroCell-HD—a porcine neural cell product for transplantation into people with advanced Huntington's disease. It integrates into the patient's brain tissue and restores damaged neural circuitry. See also *NeuroCell-PD*.

NeuroCell-PD—a porcine neural cell product for transplantation into people with advanced Parkinson's disease. See also *NeuroCell-HD*.

NeuroCybernetic prosthesis system—a seizure-control device that works by stimulating the vagus nerve. It consists of a generator implanted under the collar bone and connected by wire to the vagus nerve in the neck, where it delivers electrical signals to the brain to control seizures.

neuroendovascular interventional procedures (Rad).

neurofibrillary tangles—snarled neurofilaments of cortical neurons, seen on biopsy, diagnostic of Alzheimer's disease.

neurogastroenterology—medical field that deals with the enteric nervous system, which refers to a "second brain" in the human body, located in the gut. The central nervous system brain and the gut's brain function independently but also react to each other. Many gastrointestinal problems, such as colitis and irritable bowel syndrome, can be attributed to

neurogastroenterology *(cont.)* the gut's brain. Also, many links exist between the two brains, as seen in certain food allergies as well as autoimmune diseases like Crohn's disease and ulcerative colitis.

neurogram—see *pudendal neurogram.*

neuroimmune dysfunction—increased density of nerve fibers reactive to immune system neuropeptides associated with production of pain linked to inflammation. Investigators think that this triggers the pain associated with appendicitis, without the usual inflammation, leading to a normal-appearing appendix at the time of operation.

NeuroLink II—an EEG data acquisition system that converts analog brain wave data into digital signals.

Neurolite—a radiologic imaging agent, technetium 99m bicisate, used in a CT scan to pinpoint regions in the brain with altered blood flow after the patient has had a stroke.

neurological signs—see *localizing* or *focal neurological signs, soft neurological signs.*

NeuroMate—robotic technology for use in stereotactic brain surgery. NeuroMate consists of a robotic arm assembly and a PC-based positioning system.

Neuromed Octrode implantable device for chronic pain management.

Neuromeet nerve approximator—single-use clamp used in reattachment of damaged nerve endings. Once aligned, entire nerves may be sutured concentrically by rotating the approximator.

neuronal apoptosis inhibitory protein (NAIP)—naturally occurring protein that has been found to prevent brain cell death and holds promise in human clinical trials.

neuron specific enolase (NSE)—a tumor marker.

Neurontin (gabapentin)—adjunctive therapy in the treatment of partial seizures in adults with epilepsy. It is also used to treat manic-depressive disorder.

Neuroperfusion pump—used to treat stroke victims. Oxygenated blood is pumped from an artery in the groin to the brain through a catheter or hollow tube to a vein in the neck to the damaged region of the brain.

neuroprobe—a pain management system said to be able to modulate pain at every known level of the nervous system. It uses five modes of stimulation and is laser compatible.

NeuroSector—trade name for an ultrasound system. See *real-time ultrasonography.*

neurotmesis—complete transection of a nerve, which results in cell death.

Neuro-Trace—an instrument that provides pulsating low current stimulation for location of nerves during operative procedures.

Neurotrend—system designed for continuous monitoring of blood gases for determination of cerebral ischemia and/or hypoxia in patients suffering from closed-head trauma and during surgical intervention.

Neutralase—used for heparin reversal.

NeuTrexin (trimetrexate glucuronate)—used to treat *Pneumocystis carinii* pneumonia in immunocompromised patients. May also be used to treat colorectal cancer.

neutrophil attachment level.

neutrophil elastase-releasing capacity.

NEV (noninvasive extrathoracic ventilator)—similar to the old "iron lung."

Neville-Barnes forceps—for spontaneous vaginal delivery assist.

Neville tracheal and **tracheobronchial prostheses**—for tracheal reconstruction in patients with benign tumor, primary or secondary carcinoma, or stenosis caused by intubation or other trauma.

nevirapine (BI-RG-587)—an antiviral drug used for treatment of HIV. (BI, Boehringer Ingelheim is the manufacturer.)

Nevyas drape retractor—a disposable stick-on arched frame, which is placed over the patient's forehead, and the sterile surgical drape is placed over it, thus permitting the patient to breathe more easily.

New England Baptist acetabular cup —used for total hip arthroplasty.

New Mind Set toe splint—for ambulation during healing process.

Newport MC hip orthosis—a brace consisting of pelvic and femoral braces linked by a metal rod. It is used to keep the leg in abduction following total hip arthroplasty, while permitting ambulation. *MC* stands for *maximum control.*

new variant Creutzfeldt-Jakob disease (nvCJD)—name given to the type of bovine spongiform encephalopathy that is transmitted to humans. It is a subject of debate whether nvCJD is truly any different from standard CJD.

Newvicon vacuum chamber pickup tube—for video camera used in arthroscopy. Also, *Circon video camera, Saticon vacuum chamber pickup tube, Vidicon.*

Nexacryl—a medical cohesive product used to treat corneal lacerations and perforations.

NexGen complete knee replacement —femoral components for total knee arthroplasty.

Nexium (esomeprazole magnesium)—a proton pump inhibitor derived from Prilosec (omeprazole). It is used in the treatment of certain gastrointestinal acid-related disorders.

NexStent carotid stent—a nitinol-based continuous-mesh carotid stent.

Nextep—a line of walkers and braces used to treat foot, ankle, and lower limb injuries. Functional knee brace with a bipivotal hinge.

Nexus implant—a cemented chrome cobalt femoral implant.

Nexus 2 linear ablation catheter— used in treatment of atrial arrhythmias.

Nezelof's syndrome—see *DiGeorge syndrome.*

Nezhat-Dorsey Trumpet Valve hydrodissector—includes SmokEvac electrosurgical probe for hydrodissection of tissue, aspiration of fluids, lavage, blunt dissection, smoke evacuation, and the delivery of laser and electrical energy. For precise fingertip control of suction and irrigation in laser surgery.

NF-ATc—proteins that have been found to play a key regulatory role in the immune response and in cardiac hypertrophy; also referred to as "NFAT-3."

NG (nasogastric) **feeding tube.**

NGD 95-1—an antiobesity compound.

N-geneous HDL cholesterol test— measures how much high-density lipoprotein cholesterol is present in a patient's serum.

NGF (nerve growth factor).

N High Sensitivity CRP (C-reactive protein) **assay**—offers physicians

N High Sensitivity *(cont.)*
the ability to assess risk of cardiovascular and peripheral vascular disease many years before its occurrence by detecting low levels of C-reactive protein in the blood, allowing the opportunity for implementing preventive health measures.

NHL (non-Hodgkin's lymphoma) **tumors.**

NHT (neoadjuvant hormonal therapy).

NIAID (National Institute for Allergy and Infectious Diseases).

Niaspan (niacin)—once-nightly administration to increase HDL cholesterol in patients with dyslipidemia. Previously approved as an adjunct to diet for reduction of elevated total cholesterol and LDL cholesterol and reduction of triglyceride levels.

Nibbler—a device for dissection, morcellation, suction, and irrigation.

Nibblit—laparoscopic device that provides for aquadissection, sharp and blunt dissection for lysis of adhesions, biopsy, and specimen retrieval in one instrument.

nicardipine hydrochloride (Cardene)—used for treatment of angina and hypertension.

NicCheck-I—a test that measures the level of nicotine and its metabolites in the urine, classifying nicotine usage as high or low.

NicCheck-II—a more sensitive version of NicCheck-I, this test is able to detect passive exposure to smoke.

NicErase-SL—a sublingual tablet used as a therapeutic aid to stop smoking.

Nichol procedure—a vaginal suspension procedure for urinary stress incontinence.

nicked free beta subunit of human chorionic gonadotropin—a potential marker for Down syndrome screening.

Nicoderm—a transdermal patch containing nicotine, available by prescription only, for use by smokers to avoid nicotine withdrawal symptoms when they try to quit smoking. Also, *Habitrol, ProStep.*

Nicolet Nerve Integrity Monitor-2 (NIM-2)—used in surgery to locate and identify the facial and other cranial nerves quickly. It also helps to map the course of each nerve and to ascertain whether it is functioning.

Nicorette (nicotine polacrilex)—chewing gum used as an aid by smokers who want to stop.

Nicorette inhaler—delivers pure nicotine in amounts lower than smoking but adequate to relieve the physical craving for nicotine.

Nicotrol inhaler—an inhaled version of nicotine replacement therapy that not only helps to control the physical craving for cigarettes but also provides the hand-to-mouth behavioral component of smoking.

NicVAX—a nicotine conjugate vaccine to help patients quit smoking.

Nidek EC-5000 excimer laser system—used in LASIK procedures.

Nidek MK-2000 keratome system—ophthalmic keratome system for the creation of a lamellar flap on the cornea during keratoplasty and other refractive procedures.

nidus ("nest")—the point of origin or focus of a morbid process.

Niebauer prosthesis—Silastic metacarpophalangeal joint.

Niemann-Pick disease—a rare form of familial lipidosis, resulting in mental retardation, growth retardation, and progressive blindness.

NightBird nasal CPAP (continuous positive airway pressure)—for treatment of obstructive sleep apnea. (No space in NightBird.)

night nurse's paralysis—a variant of the narcolepsy/cataplexy syndrome, also called *cataplexy of awakening*. A temporary paralysis which quickly disappears.

NightOwl pocket polygraph—a small recording device used to diagnose sleep disorders.

Nilandron (nilutamide)—a once-a-day, nonsteroidal antiandrogen drug for the treatment of advanced prostate cancer.

nil disease—synonym for lipoid nephrosis, so-called because so little evidence of disease is seen on light microscopy of a renal biopsy in a case of lipoid nephrosis.

nilutamide (Anandron; Nilandron).

Nimbex (cisatracurium)—neuromuscular blocking agent used with general anesthesia during tracheal intubation or for skeletal muscular relaxation during surgery or mechanical ventilation.

nimodipine (Nimotop)—calcium channel blocker also used to treat manic-depressive disorder. Its therapeutic action is based on the fact that calcium ions, which it blocks, must enter a nerve cell before a neurotransmitter can be released. Also, treatment for subarachnoid hemorrhage.

NIM-2 (Nicolet Nerve Integrity Monitor-2).

ninety-ninety (90/90) **intraosseous wiring**—used to obtain rigid fixation for digital replantation or for transverse fractures. Two intraosseous wires are placed perpendicular to each other (hence, 90° angle or 90/90).

Nipah virus—human pathogen identified in recent outbreaks of disease and death in Malaysia.

Nipent (pentostatin) **injection**—an antineoplastic agent for use in the treatment of adult patients with hairy cell leukemia refractory to alpha-interferon treatment. It may also be used for the treatment of cutaneous T-cell lymphoma and chronic lymphocytic leukemia.

NIR Primo Monorail stent system—coronary stent system used in PTCA procedures for the treatment of coronary artery disease.

NIRS (near-infrared spectroscopy)—a device which uses light to assess and quantify various characteristics of human blood and tissue.

NIR with SOX—over-the-wire coronary stent system for treatment of coronary artery disease. The SOX system stent sleeves protect the proximal and distal ends of the stent for a smooth interface between the stent system and arterial wall.

nisoldipine (Sular)—oral extended-release calcium channel blocker.

Nissen fundoplication—procedure to control gastroesophageal reflux.

Nissen laparoscopic fundoplication—surgical procedure for the treatment of reflux esophagitis and gastroesophageal reflux disease.

Nissl's granules—cytoplasmic bodies in nerve cell bodies. (Franz Nissl, German neuropathologist.)

Nissl's stain (Path).

nitazoxanide (NTZ; Cryptaz)—used for the treatment of cryptosporidiosis in HIV positive and AIDS patients.

nitinol mesh-covered frame—used for laparoscopic herniorrhaphy.

nitinol mesh stent.

nitrazepam (Mogadon)—sedative; also used to treat myoclonic epilepsy.

nitrendipine (Baypress)—vasodilator and calcium channel blocker for hypertension.

nitrogen-13 ammonia—a radioactive tracer used to perform a PET scan to evaluate heart function at rest and during stress. Nitrogen-13 ammonia has a longer half-life than rubidium-82. Therefore, the stress portion of the test may be done with an exercise bike or treadmill.

nitroglycerin (Cardio)—a vasodilator administered as sublingual tablets or spray, by injection, or topically (as an ointment) to treat angina pectoris. See *"nitro paste."*

Nitrol ointment—a brand of nitroglycerin ointment. See *"nitro paste."*

"nitro paste" (Cardio)—careless jargon widely used by physicians for nitroglycerin ointment. The dosage of this coronary vasodilator is measured in inches of ointment (or fractions thereof) as it comes from the tube. The patient is supplied with disposable ruled applicators, with which the ointment is measured out and smeared over the skin in much the same way as one spreads mucilage or wallpaper paste—hence, probably, the popular misnomer "paste." When "nitro paste" is dicated, "nitro" should be expanded to "nitroglycerin," and "paste" should be translated "ointment"—unless departmental rules forbid using the right words when the dictator uses the wrong ones. Note that the name of one brand of nitroglycerin, Nitrol, is easily mistaken for "nitro" in dictation.

NitroQuick (nitroglycerin) **sublingual tablets**—indicated for the acute relief of an attack or prophylaxis of angina pectoris due to coronary artery disease. Equivalent to Nitrostat.

Nizoral (ketoconazole)—antifungal agent used, in conjunction with cyclosporine (also cyclosporin), in treatment of heart transplant patients. The cyclosporine (an immunosuppressant) keeps the body from rejecting the transplant. The ketoconazole slows down the metabolizing of the cyclosporine, thus prolonging its effect and reducing the amount of cyclosporine needed. Infection and organ rejection were less frequent than in those receiving only cyclosporine.

NJ (nasojejunal) **feeding.**

NK (natural killer) **cell**—evaluated in specific and nonspecific immunotherapy and in cytotoxicity assays.

NLP (no light perception).

NMES (neuromuscular electrical stimulation) **protocol**—see *ReAct device.*

N-methyl-D-aspartate (NMDA) **receptor antagonists**—drugs that are said to protect the brain from toxic neurotransmitters released after stroke or head injury.

NMP (nuclear matrix protein).

NMP22 test—for the early detection of transitional cell carcinoma of the bladder.

NMR (nuclear magnetic resonance) **scan**—early term for what is now called MRI (magnetic resonance imaging) scan. The name is said to have been changed because of patients' resistance to the word *nuclear.*

NNDSS (National Notifiable Disease Surveillance System).

Nocardia—the fungus causing nocardiasis, more devastating than usual in the AIDS patient.

nocturnal polysomnography.

node
Aschoff-Tawara
Bouchard's
Flack's
jugulodigastric
Koch's
Osler's
Rouviere
SA or S-A (sinoatrial)
sentinel
shotty
signal
singer's (of a vocal cord)
Sister Mary Joseph
Troisier's
Virchow's

node of Rouviere—situated in retropharyngeal space.

nodules—see *siderotic nodules of the spleen.*

Noiles posterior stabilized knee prosthesis.

Noiles rotating hinge total knee prosthesis.

Nolvadex (tamoxifen citrate) **tablets**—used to reduce the incidence of breast cancer in women at high risk for developing the disease, and to reduce the occurrence of contralateral breast cancer in patients receiving adjuvant Nolvadex therapy for breast cancer. May be used as adjuvant treatment of ductal carcinoma in situ in women following breast surgery and radiation.

no man's land in the hand—the area between the distal palmar crease and the proximal interphalangeal joints (the web space between the thumb and index finger). Until modern microsurgical techniques were developed, tendon repair in the palm was usually unsuccessful, as the swelling of the newly sutured tendon in this tight part of the hand led to ischemia. Hand microsurgeons are now able to do primary tendon repair in no man's land in the hand.

Nomos—pin-free attachment stereotactic system.

nonballoon therapies—used for treatment of ischemic heart disease in suitable coronary anatomy. They include *stents* (Palmaz-Schatz and Gianturco-Roubin), *atherectomy* (directional, rotational, and extraction), and *excimer laser angioplasty.*

noncholecystokinin—a substance that is thought to be important in regulating gallbladder contraction and emptying.

noncomitant—see *comitant, concomitant.*

noncompliant—said of patients who do not follow their physician's directions and advice regarding diet or medicinal treatment.

non compos mentis—a psychiatric and legal term for a patient not of sound mind and in need of guardianship.

noninvasive extrathoracic ventilation (NEV).

nonionic contrast media (Radiol)—more expensive but safer than low-osmolar media (ionic media). Nonionic contrast media are almost universally used in the U.S., and radiologists invariably indicate thus in their dictation for medicolegal reasons. The words "nonionic contrast medium" begin more sentences, by a large margin, in reports involving contrast than the name of the pharmaceutical itself or the dose.

nonionic *(cont.)*
See *ionic contrast media, low-osmolar contrast media.*

non-nasal CD56⁺T/NK (natural killer) **cell lymphoma**—uncommon tumors that show predominantly extranodal presentation, high-stage disease, a highly aggressive course, and strong association with Epstein-Barr virus.

nonoxynol 9—over-the-counter spermatocide, a component in most contraceptive creams, gels, and foams, which reliably kills the AIDS virus and STDs on contact.

non-Q-wave myocardial infarction (NQWMI).

nonrapid eye movement (NREM).

nonrheumatic valvular aortic stenosis.

nonseminomatous germ cell tumor (NSGCT).

non-small cell lung carcinoma (or **cancer**) (NSCLC)—all types of lung cancer other than small cell lung carcinoma (SCLC). This group of cancers includes adenocarcinoma, squamous cell carcinoma, and large cell carcinoma. See *Navelbine.*

NonSpil drug delivery system—a spill-resistant liquid that can be used with a wide variety of both over-the-counter and prescription drugs.

nonsyncytium-inducing (NSI) **variant of the AIDS virus**—not as virulent as the SI (syncytium-inducing) strain. This quickly changing virus can mutate into a more aggressive strain. See *SI* and *HlV phenotype test.*

nonspecific esophageal motility disorder (NEMD).

nonspecific urethritis (NSU).

nonweightbearing—see *weightbearing.*

NoProfile balloon catheter (Cardio).

norastemizole—third-generation non-sedating antihistamine, a fast-acting,
once-daily treatment for perennial and seasonal allergic rhinitis.

Norco ulnar deviation support—hand therapy product.

Nordan-Ruiz trapezoidal marker—used in refractive eye surgery.

NordiPen—a pen system used to deliver Norditropin SimpleXx.

Norditropin (somatropin)—indicated for long-term treatment in children with growth failure due to inadequate production of growth hormone by the pituitary gland.

Norditropin SimpleXx (somatropin [rDNA origin] for injection)—a liquid formulation of human growth hormone delivered in a pen system, NordiPen, designed to make daily injections more convenient.

no-reflow phenomenon—failure of a significant proportion of capillaries within the tissue to re-perfuse upon restoration of blood flow in the arteries supplying the tissue, such as might occur in reconstructive surgery. Oxygen free radicals such as human manganese superoxide dismutase that scavenge or inhibit formation of reactive O_2 metabolites are being investigated as possible treatment.

Norelin—used for the treatment of prostate cancer. It is a therapeutic vaccine that stimulates antibodies to gonadotropin-releasing hormone that reduces levels of sex hormones, including testosterone.

norfloxacin (Chibroxin, Noroxin)—a fluoroquinolone antibiotic. Chibroxin is used to treat conjunctivitis. Oral Noroxin is used to treat urinary tract infections.

Norian SRS (skeletal repair system)—an injectable bone substitute paste or

Norian *(cont.)*
cement used in fracture treatment procedures.

Noritate (metronidazole) **cream**—for topical treatment of inflammatory lesions and erythema associated with rosacea.

Norland bone densitometry.

normal pressure hydrocephalus (NPH).

normal spontaneous vaginal delivery (NSVD).

Normiflo (ardeparin sodium injection)—low molecular weight heparin used for prevention of deep vein thrombosis in patients undergoing knee replacement therapy.

Normigel hydrogel dressing.

Noroxin (norfloxacin)—fluoroquinolone antibiotic used to treat urinary tract infection.

Norplant (levonorgestrel)—a synthetic progestin, now used for contraception. Tiny silicone tubes filled with levonorgestrel are implanted under the skin of a woman's upper arm and, over about a five-year period, the hormone is gradually released. This is a reversible method, as the tubes can be removed if fertility is again desired.

Norrie syndrome—inherited neurodevelopmental disorder characterized by blindness in both eyes at birth. Some children with this disorder may experience varying degrees of mental retardation. Other symptoms may include mild to profound hearing loss, growth delays, and/or diabetes. Cataracts may develop during early infancy, and the eyeball may shrink. The gene responsible for Norrie syndrome is inherited as an X-linked recessive genetic trait.

Norvasc (amlodipine).

Norvir (ritonavir) **capsules and oral solution**—protease inhibitor now approved for treatment of children ages 2-12 with HIV/AIDS, having previously been approved only for adults. A soft-gelatin capsule (100 mg), to replace the previously marketed semisolid capsule, has been approved for marketing.

Norwood operation—performed for hypoplastic left-sided heart syndrome. See *Fontan; Gill/Jonas; Sade.*

nosocomial disease—disease originating in a hospital.

No Sting barrier film—provides sting-free, alcohol-free protection for wound care.

notochord *(not* notocord) (chorda dorsalis)—seen in the embryo; in adults the nuclei pulposi are the vestigial notochord.

Nottingham colposuspension needle—for bladder neck elevation. Malleable tipped, colposuspension needle that is adjustable to any angle for use in Stamey bladder neck suspension procedures.

Nottingham introducer—used to place a tube as a palliative procedure in patients with esophageal cancer. See *Atkinson tube stent.*

NovaCath multi-lumen infusion catheter.

Novacor left ventricular assist system (LVAS)—an implantable pump that keeps blood circulating in patients with end-stage heart disease. It is designed as both a "bridge" to heart transplant and a long-term alternative to transplant.

NovaGold breast implant—water-based (PVP-hydrogel-based) breast implant that contains radiolucent biocompatible polymer filling.

NovaLine Litho-S DUV excimer laser—provides high spectral purity.

Novantrone (mitoxantrone for injection concentrate)—used to slow the progress of neurologic disability and reduce the relapse rate in patients with clinically worsening forms of relapsing-remitting and secondary progressive multiple sclerosis. Also used as a chemotherapy agent, in combination with steroids, to treat patients with pain related to hormone-refractory prostate cancer and treatment of acute myelogenous leukemia.

Novapren—a drug used to treat HIV-positive patients.

NovaPulse CO$_2$ laser—for cosmetic skin resurfacing facial cosmetic surgery to remove blemishes, scars, and birthmarks.

NovaSaline inflatable saline breast implant—for breast augmentation and breast reconstruction surgery. Also, *NovaSaline pre-filled breast implant.*

Novasome (nonoxynol-9)—spermicidal contraceptive.

Novastan (argatroban)—direct thrombin inhibitor used as an injectable anticoagulant.

Novel erythropoiesis stimulating protein (NESP)—a recombinant protein that stimulates red blood cell production. It is used to treat anemia in patients with chronic renal failure.

NovolinPen device—holds cartridges of insulin. A patient can select and inject correct dose without need for syringes or insulin vials.

NovoNorm (repaglinide)—member of a new class of oral antidiabetic agents for treating type 2 diabetes.

NovoSeven (factor VIIa, recombinant)—treatment for hemophilia patients who have developed antibodies against coagulation factors VIII or IX.

Novus Verdi diode-pumped green photocoagulator—for treatment of retinal diseases and glaucoma.

NOX (number of excitations)—MRI term. The initialism *NOX* is often dictated.

NOX-100—drug designed to block excess production of nitric oxide in the blood, a key event that can lead in a "chain reaction" to sepsis.

N.P. or **NP**—nurse practitioner.

NPH (normal pressure hydrocephalus).

NREM sleep—non-rapid eye movement in which the heart rate is slowed and regular, the blood pressure is low, the brain waves are slow and of high voltage, and sleep is dreamless, interspersed with occasional periods of REM sleep. See *REM sleep.*

NRSI (nonrapid sequence induction)—orotracheal intubation.

NSAIDs (nonsteroidal anti-inflammatory drugs)—a category of drugs commonly used for treatment of rheumatoid arthritis and osteoarthritis are acetylsalicylic acid (aspirin) and ibuprofen (Motrin). Pronounced "en´sayds" or "en´seds." Not to be confused with the trade name *Ansaid,* an NSAID.

NSA (neck-shaft angle) **of femur**—hip dysplasia measurement in children with cerebral palsy.

NSCLC (non-small cell lung carcinoma, or cancer).

NSE (neuron specific enolase).

NSI (nonsyncytium-inducing) **variant of HIV.**

NSO (non-nutritive sucking opportunities)—used to stimulate premature

NSO *(cont.)*
babies suffering from lack of stimulation. They were given pacifiers four times a day and did better than other high-risk infants.

NSR (normal sinus rhythm).

NSU (nonspecific urethritis).

NSVD (normal spontaneous vaginal delivery).

NTD (neural tube defects).

N-Terface—contact-layer wound dressing.

NTG (normal-tension glaucoma).

NTHI (native tissue harmonic imaging).

NTM (nontuberculous mycobacterium).

NTx Assay—see *Osteomark test.*

NTZ (nitazoxanide).

nuchal cord—umbilical cord wrapped around the neck of the fetus can result in hypoxia or even death.

nuchal translucency—ultrasound appearance of fluid accumulation in neck of a fetus that may indicate Down syndrome.

nuclear contour index (NCI) **on blood lymphocytes**—used as the criterion for differential diagnosis of erythrodermic actinic reticuloid vs. Sezary syndrome.

nuclear magnetic resonance imaging (NMR)—see *magnetic resonance imaging.*

nuclear matrix protein (NMP)—used to enable detection and monitoring of prostate, cervical, colorectal, breast, and bladder cancers using urine, serum, and cell-based NMP.

nuclear signal; spin; spin quantum number—MRI terms.

nuclear-tagged red blood cell bleeding study (Radiol).

nuclectomy—excision of nucleus pulposus.

nucleic acid sequence-based amplification—a rapid research-targeted method for isolating DNA or RNA sequence in a specimen that has excellent specificity. Cf. *polymerase chain reaction.*

nucleic acid testing (NAT).

nucleolar pattern of ANA (antinuclear antibodies)—associated with scleroderma.

nucleolus (pl., nucleoli)—a part of the nucleus which is spherical and more hyperchromatic than the nucleus.

nucleoside analogue—one of a class of synthetic compounds, like AZT, ddI, and ddC, that inhibit replication of the HIV virus.

Nucleotome Endoflex—an instrument used to cut away herniated disk during an endoscopic microdiskectomy. This instrument includes a light source, the visual imaging of a steerable, flexible endoscope, and the cutting ability of a Nucleotome.

Nucleotome Flex II—a flexible cutting probe for removing herniated nucleus pulposus material during spinal surgery. Its flexible probe can rotate from 0 to 90° within the disk space. Used in percutaneous diskectomy.

Nuclepore prep (Path).

Nucletron—radiotherapy products for the treatment of cancer.

nucleus (pl., nuclei)—central cellular core containing DNA. See *Westphal-Edinger nucleus.*

nucleus lateralis of Le Gros Clark—dorsal portion of the lateral mamillary nucleus of Rose.

nucleus of Darkschewitsch—located in the rostral part of the midbrain. See *Darkschewitsch.*

nucleus of Gudden—dorsal tegmental nucleus.

nucleus of Luys—see *body of Luys*.

nucleus of Perlia—central nucleus of the oculomotor nerve.

nucleus of Rose—also *lateral mamillary nucleus of Rose*. See *nucleus lateralis of Le Gros Clark*.

nucleus pulposus *(not* pulposis*)*—the semifluid inner portion of the intervertebral disk.

NuDerm—hydrocolloid dressing material.

NUG (necrotizing ulcerative gingivitis).

Nu Gauze dressing (marketed by Johnson & Johnson). *Not* Nu-gauze.

Nu-Gel—clear hydrogel wound dressing for wounds with light to medium exudate, burns, and skin reactions to oncological procedures.

Nu-Knit—see *Surgical Nu-Knit*.

null cell lymphoblastic leukemia.

null-type non-Hodgkin's lymphoma.

NuLytely bowel prep—for use in GI endoscopy.

number of excitations (NOX)—MRI term. *NOX* is often dictated.

Numby Stuff—needle-free method for delivering local anesthesia in children. It uses lidocaine HCl 2% with epinephrine 1:100,000, and drug delivery electrodes that penetrate the skin 10 mm deep within 7 to 10 minutes.

Nuport PEG tube—a percutaneous endoscopic gastrostomy tube.

Nurolon suture—a braided nylon suture with extremely low tissue reaction (made by Ethicon).

Nuromax (doxacurium chloride).

nutcracker esophagus (Radiol).

Nu-Tip disposable scissor tip—with reusable handle and shaft.

nutmeg appearance of liver (Radiol).

nutratherapy—vitamin and/or mineral supplementation.

Nutricath—silicone elastomer catheter.

Nu-Trim—dietary fat substitute said to be good for the heart. It contains a high concentration of beta-glucans, the soluble fibers found in oats and barley and known to lower LDL cholesterol and total cholesterol; they may also play a role in lowering blood sugar levels.

NutriMan TNT (*Tribulus terrestris* extract)—a natural sexual stimulant said to have the libido-enhancing properties of Viagra without the dangerous side effects. It works by helping to regulate secretion of hormones, increases muscle tone and sexual endurance, and is a natural testosterone precursor.

Nutropin (somatropin)—for the treatment of growth failure associated with Turner syndrome.

Nutropin AQ—liquid recombinant human growth hormone.

Nutropin Depot—sustained-release injection.

Nuvance (interleukin-4 receptor)—asthma drug which reportedly increases forced expiratory volume and decreases wheezing, shortness of breath, coughing, chest tightness, and nocturnal asthma.

Nuvolase 660—medical laser system used in the treatment of benign cutaneous vascular and pigmented lesions.

nvCJD (new variant Creutzfeldt-Jakob disease).

NVE (native valve endocarditis).

NWB (nonweightbearing).

Nycore cardiac device.

nyctalopia—night blindness.

NYHA (New York Heart Association) classification of congestive heart failure:
class I, asymptomatic
class II, slightly symptomatic
class III, congestive heart failure symptoms
class IV, severe congestive heart failure

Nyhus/Nelson tube—gastric decompression and jejunal feeding tube which permits gastric decompression and enteral feeding simultaneously.

Nylen-Bárány maneuver (Neuro).

Nylok self-locking nail (Ortho).

Nymox urinary test—used (in addition to brain and spinal fluid studies) to diagnose Alzheimer's disease.

Nyotran (nystatin)—liposomal formulation for treatment of systemic fungal infections.

Nyquist limit (Cardio).

nystagmus—a rhythmic horizontal or vertical oscillation of (usually both) eyeballs, generally more pronounced when looking in certain directions. See *periodic alternating nystagmus* and *optokinetic nystagmus*.

Nystatin LF (liposomal formulation)—an antifungal drug.

O, o

OA (osteoarthritis).

O&P test (ova and parasites)—examination of stool, urine, or other material for parasites or their ova (eggs). "Stools for O&P x 2 [times two] were obtained and were negative."

Oasis thrombectomy system—catheter-based system which removes blood clots that develop in access grafts of dialysis patients. Uses a low-pressure water jet to break up the clot and remove fragments from the occluded graft.

Oasis wound dressing—for management of full-thickness skin injuries.

Obecalp (*placebo* spelled backwards)—given as a medication.

Ober-Barr brachioradialis transfer—for weakness of the triceps muscle.

Obetrol—see *Adderall*.

obliterative bronchiolitis—not the same as bronchiolitis obliterans. The pathologic hallmark of this disease is the presence of submucosal and peribronchiolar fibrosis. It is less common than bronchiolitis obliterans with organizing pneumonia (BOOP).

OBS (organic brain syndrome).

obsessive-compulsive disorder (OCD)—a psychiatric disorder characterized by persisting or recurring thoughts or impulses (obsessions) and repetitive, ritualized, stereotyped acts (compulsions), such as hand washing, touching all the posts of a fence, or carrying out a series of actions in a certain order. Sometimes these symptoms overlap with the tics (with the absence of intention), twitching of the face, blinking, throat-clearing, hyperactivity, tearing hair, gnashing teeth, etc., of Tourette's disease.

Obsessive Compulsive Drinking Scale (OCDS)—a 14-item quick and reliable self-rating instrument that provides a total and two subscale scores that measure some cognitive aspects of alcohol "craving." It is used as an alcoholism severity-and-treatment outcome instrument.

obstructive sleep apnea (OSA).

obturator—a rod or wire placed inside a catheter, trocar, endoscope, or other tubular instrument to close the opening in its tip during insertion. In an arthroscopic temporomandibular

obturator *(cont.)*
joint procedure: "A sheath with a sharp obturator was inserted into the superior joint space. After the space was entered, the sharp obturator was replaced with a dull one to further direct the sheath into the joint."

obturator hernia—hernia through the obturator foramen, a cause of small bowel obstruction.

obturator sign—may be positive in appendicitis or when there is fluid or blood in the pelvis. The flexed thigh is rotated both internally and externally, and hypogastric pain is elicited when there is an inflammatory process in contact with the obturator externus muscle.

obtuse marginal (OM) coronary artery.

Obwegeser-Dalpont internal screw fixation—used in sagittal split ramus osteotomy.

Obwegeser sagittal mandibular osteotomy technique—Salyer and Bardach modifications.

O-Cal f.a.—prescription oral multivitamin with calcium and folic acid.

occipitofrontal circumference (Peds) —a term used in measurement of the head.

occult—in medicine, something that is present in such a tiny quantity that it is effectively hidden. Usage: "We still must rule out the possibility of occult neoplasm." See also *fecal occult blood test* and *occult blood*.

occult blood—blood present in stool, urine, or other material in too small an amount to be detected by naked-eye observation, but detectable by chemical testing or microscopic examination. See *fecal occult blood test*.

occupational contact dermatitis.

occur, occurred (past tense); **occurring**. Frequently misspelled.

OCD (obsessive compulsive disorder).

OCD (osteochondral defect).

OCG (oral cholecystogram).

OCT (optical coherence tomography).

OCT (optimal cutting temperature).

OCT (oxytocin challenge test).

octopus test—measures peripheral vision. The patient is seated before a large screen, holding a counter. Each time the patient sees a light reflected at any angle on the screen, he presses the hand counter, which is monitored in another room by a technician.

OctreoScan (indium 111 pentetreotide) **radiologic imaging agent**—used to detect metastatic neuroendocrine tumors that contain somatostatin receptors. Cf. *octreotide*.

octreotide (Sandostatin)—for control of severe diarrhea in patients with vipomas and AIDS. Also for tumors with somatostatin receptors. Cf. *OctreoScan*.

Ocufen (flurbiprofen sodium)—used for inhibition of intraoperative miosis.

Ocuflox (ofloxacin)—ophthalmic solution for treatment of bacterial infections.

OcuHist (formerly AK-Con-A)—an antihistamine eye drop, now available over the counter.

ocular rosacea—involvement of the eye secondary to acne rosacea, which affects facial skin and the eye. It may result in mild blepharoconjunctivitis or in blindness.

OcuLight SL (Oph)—diode laser.

oculogyric crisis—occurs when the eyeballs become fixed in one position for a considerable period of time,

oculogyric *(cont.)*
minutes to hours. Seen in encephalitis or postencephalitic parkinsonism. "She is having an acute extrapyramidal reaction. She is drooling, unable to speak coherently; no evidence of oculogyric crisis."

oculoplethysmography/carotid phonoangiography (OPG/CPA)—examination used in evaluating suspected intracranial cerebrovascular disease. A noninvasive test, serial angiography of the internal carotid artery, using the OPG-Gee instrument, to determine the degree of occlusion of the internal carotid. The ophthalmic systolic pressure is correlated with the brachial systolic pressure (as determined by arm cuff and auscultation) which is measured immediately after the OPG study.

Ocupress (carteolol HCl) **ophthalmic solution**—used to lower intraocular pressure and may be used in patients with chronic open-angle glaucoma and intraocular hypertension.

Ocutech Vision Enhancing System—autofocusing glasses that allow distance vision for patients whose eye conditions cannot be corrected with regular glasses.

ocutome—a device to remove vitreous; e.g., O'Malley ocutome.

O.D. *(oculus dexter*, right eye).

o.d. *(omni die)*—every day (also *q.d.*).

OD (overdose).

OD'd—slang for overdosed.

O_2 (oxygen) **debt**—when available oxygen is less than oxygen requirements, in reference to resuscitation of newborns and in exercise physiology.

O'Donoghue's Unhappy Triad (OUT)—a triple injury of damage, with joint cartilage and both outside and inside knee ligaments being torn. Also called *motorcyclist's knee.*

odontoid view of cervical spine (Radiol)—x-ray view of the odontoid process of the second cervical vertebra, also called the *dens.*

OD (ocular or optical density) **values**—antibody titer determination on amniotic fluid for erythroblastosis fetalis.

Odyssey phacoemulsification system (Oph).

off-pump coronary artery bypass (OPCAB).

ofloxacin (Floxin, Ocuflox)—a broad-spectrum antibiotic given intravenously or orally to treat respiratory and urinary infections as well as sexually transmitted diseases. Ocuflox eye drops are given for bacterial conjunctivitis.

Ogden anchor—used to anchor soft tissue to bone.

Ogilvie's syndrome—pseudo-obstruction or adynamic ileus of colon.

Ogura tissue and cartilage forceps.

Ohashiatsu—a form of shiatsu massage developed by the Ohashi Institute of New York City, consisting of techniques to alleviate symptoms common to pregnancy (fatigue, aching, general discomfort) and the delivery process through the use of pressure to specific body areas.

OHSS (ovarian hyperstimulation syndrome).

oil drop change—a localized brown color, a sign of psoriasis in the nail bed.

"oil droplet" reflex—seen on retinoscopy.

oil red O stain (Oph)—a dye used in histologic demonstration of neutral fats. "Oil red O stain for intracytoplasmic fat was present."

Oklahoma ankle joint—orthosis for ambulation in children with cerebral palsy and myelomeningocele. Made of polypropylene vacuformed in plastic.

OKN (optokinetic nystagmus) (Neuro).

OKT3—see *Orthoclone OKT3*.

OKT4—monoclonal antibody to human T-4 cells. Also, *antihuman T-4 cell*, *antihuman inducer/helper T-cell*.

OKT8—the monoclonal antibody to human T-8 cells. Also called *antihuman T-8 cell*, and *antihuman suppressor/cytotoxic T-cell*.

olanzapine (Zyprex)—antipsychotic drug for schizophrenia.

Olean (olestra)—a fat-based substitute for conventional fats, used in certain snack foods. It adds no fat or calories to food, but it may cause abdominal cramping and diarrhea in some people and inhibits the absorption of certain vitamins and nutrients.

Olerud and Molander fracture classification.

olestra—see *Olean*.

oligoclonal bands.

oligodendroglioma—derived from cells forming and maintaining the myelin sheaths in the central nervous system.

oligoteratoasthenozoospermia syndrome—spermatozoa reduced in number with poor motility and an increased number of abnormal shapes.

oligozymes—catalytically interactive oligomers used to treat diseases and to aid in pharmaceutical or genomic research.

Oliver-Rosalki method of testing serum CPK—see also *Sigma*.

olive wire; ring—used in Ilizarov limb lengthening procedure.

Ollier's disease—enchondromatosis.

OLM (ophthalmic laser microendoscope)—see *Microprobe*.

olsalazine (Dipentum)—for ulcerative colitis, particularly in patients who cannot tolerate the standard treatment because they are allergic to sulfa drugs (olsalazine is not a sulfa drug). After being given orally, it is converted in the colon to 5-ASA, a topical anti-inflammatory, which is the active ingredient.

Olsen cholangiogram clamp.

OLT (orthotopic liver transplantation).

Olympia VACPAC—a support device used in back surgery that is able to be molded under the patient during inspiration and hardened by suction while an inflated urologic irrigation bladder is under the abdomen. After hardening, the irrigation bladder is deflated and a vacant space is left under the abdomen that decreases extradural venous pressure. Lumbar respiratory movements are also minimized by the technique. Cf. *Andrews spinal frame/table, Hastings frame*.

Olympus CF-1T100L—forward-viewing video colonoscope.

Olympus CF-200Z colonoscope—provides high-power magnified observation of the surface of colorectal neoplasms.

Olympus CYF-3 OES cystofiberscope—used in urinary endoscopy.

Olympus ENF-P2 scope—flexible laryngoscope.

Olympus EVIS 140—endoscope reprocessing system.

Olympus EVIS Q-200V—video endoscope.

Olympus FBK 13 forceps—endoscopic biopsy forceps.

Olympus GF-UM3 and **CF-UM20 ultrasonic endoscope**—designed to allow a limited visual exam of upper GI tract and endoscopic ultrasonography of organs adjacent to esophagus, stomach, and duodenum.

Olympus GIF-EUM2 echoendoscope—side-viewing gastroscope or duodenoscope with ultrasound probe.

Olympus GIF-1T10 and **GIF20 echoendoscope**—forward-viewing gastroscope with ultrasound probe.

Olympus JF1T10 fiberoptic duodenoscope.

Olympus JF-UM20 echoendoscope—endoscopic ultrasonography instrument for ERCP and pancreatic-biliary ultrasonography.

Olympus One-Step Button—short gastrostomy tube (the thickness of the stomach wall) with an internal button to hold it in place and an external opening with an attached plastic plug. Inserted endoscopically and used for tube feedings.

Olympus OSF scope—flexible sigmoidoscope.

Olympus SIF10 enteroscope.

Olympus TJF-100 endoscope—with reusable biopsy channel caps.

Olympus UM-1W endoscopic probe—transendoscopic ultrasound probe to be used with regular endoscopes, rather than with specially made ultrasonograph endoscopes.

Olympus URF-P2 translaparoscopic choledochofiberscope—used in the management of biliary tract disease including removal of cystic and common bile duct stones.

Olympus VU-M2 and **XIF-UM3 echoendoscope**—a side-viewing gastroscope with ultrasound probe.

Olympus XQ230 gastroscope.

OMB (obtuse marginal branch)—one of the coronary arteries.

Omed bulldog vascular clamp—for atraumatic occlusion of vessels.

Omega splinting material—used in hand therapy.

omeprazole (Prilosec)—used to treat gastroesophageal reflux.

omeprazole plus amoxicillin—in some studies found to be most effective combination treatment for *H. pylori*. See *Helicobacter pylori*.

Omiderm—transparent adhesive film dressing.

OmniCath atherectomy catheter.

Omnicef (cefdinir)—broad-spectrum cephalosporin antibiotic.

omni die (o.d.)—every day.

OmniFilter—mounted on a guide wire, it prevents blood clots from reaching various organs of the body.

Omnifit HA hip stem—prosthesis of hydroxyapatite.

Omnifit Plus—enhanced offset cemented hip system.

Omni-Flexor—a handheld physical therapy device that allows for all six ranges of wrist movement. Because it is small, the patient can use it at home after proper instruction.

Omniflox (temafloxacin).

Omniloc dental system—used in tooth restorations.

Omnipaque (iohexol)—a nonionic imaging agent used like iopamidol or metrizamide in various radiological special procedures.

OmniPulse-MAX holmium laser—a pulsed laser system for use in lithotripsy procedures.

Omni retractor.

Omniscan (gadodiamide) **contrast medium**—second-generation nonionic contrast agent used in MRI scans.

Omniscience—single leaflet cardiac valve prosthesis.

OmniStent—a stent used in angioplasty and atherectomy procedures. Used to reduce restenosis in blood vessels.

Omni-Tract—adjustable wishbone retractor.

omphalodiverticular band.

OMS Concentrate—oral morphine sulfate in solution.

Oncaspar (pegaspargase).

oncogene—a tumor gene that can, in normal cells, somehow be turned on by viruses, certain chemicals, and other substances, to cause cancer. See *gene*.

Oncolym—radiolabeled monoclonal antibody for single-dose treatment of non-Hodgkin's B-cell lymphoma.

On-Command catheters (male and female)—used to treat urinary incontinence and retention.

Onconase—a cytotoxic ribonuclease used to treat solid tumors resistant to other cancer therapies.

Oncophage—cancer vaccine.

OncoScint CR103 (colorectal) and **OV103** (ovarian)—monoclonal antibody B72.3 labeled with indium 111, used as a radioactive imaging agent to detect colorectal or ovarian carcinomas.

OncoScint CR/OV (satumomab pendetide) **contrast medium**—indium 111 in satumomab pendetide, a radionuclide agent that targets the cell-surface antigen, TAG-72, common to both pelvic and extrahepatic abdominal carcinomas.

ondansetron (Zofran)—an intravenous antiemetic drug given for postoperative nausea and vomiting, and for chemotherapy patients.

Ondine's curse—periodic breathing. Chronic alveolar hypoventilation together with unresponsiveness of the carotid body to hypoxemia.

One-Shot anastomotic instrument—allows the surgeon to complete a vascular anastomosis, as in coronary artery bypass grafting, in two minutes with one squeeze of the handle (compared to 20 to 25 minutes for hand sewing). It is based on the VCS vascular clip technology, which allows the surgeon to join two vessels by individually placing a series of titanium clips to complete the anastomosis. The One-Shot automates this process by simultaneously placing 12 clips.

One Touch blood glucose meter—for self-testing by diabetics.

onlay graft—a bone graft, not to be confused with inlay graft. Both are used in craniofacial surgery. Cf. *inlay graft*.

OnLineABG monitoring system—attached to the patient to deliver arterial blood gas values within 60 seconds.

"ONP"—see *O&P* (ova and parasites).

Ontak (denileukin diftitox)—a "fusion protein" produced by genetically fusing protein from the diphtheria toxin to interleukin-2, a naturally occurring immune system protein, in order to treat certain patients with advanced or recurring cutaneous T-cell lymphoma.

onychopachydermoperiostitis—see *psoriatic onychopachydermoperiostitis*.

Onyx—a liquid embolic system for the treatment of aneurysms and arteriovenous malformations.

Onyx finger pulse oximeter.

opacification—increase in the density of a tissue or region, with increased resistance to x-rays.

opacities—see *snowball opacities* (Oph).

Opal Photoactivator—used with Visudyne (verteporfin for injection) therapy for treatment of the wet form of age-related macular degeneration.

OPART—open MRI with access to all four sides.

OPCAB (off-pump coronary artery bypass)—surgery performed while the heart is still beating. Uses a stabilizer arm attached to the device that holds the chest open during surgery. The arm touches the heart and temporarily stops movement in one spot, allowing the surgeon to attach grafts to the arteries without stopping the entire heart.

opening snap—an important finding on physical examination because an audible opening snap in mitral or tricuspid stenosis implies a flexible valve.

open mesh-plug hernioplasty—used for preperitoneal hernioplasty and femoral hernia repair. Mesh is inserted through the trocar; the plug has a fluted outside layer combined with an inside arrangement of mesh "petals" that expand or contract to fit the hernia defect.

open-mouth odontoid view—a view of the odontoid process of the second cervical vertebra for which the x-ray beam is aimed through the patient's open mouth.

open reduction and internal fixation (ORIF)—an orthopedic procedure to correct a severely fractured bone.

"open sky" MRI—see *FONAR-360 MRI scanner*.

open-sky vitrectomy—operative procedure to remove vitreous from the eye by first removing a button of cornea. The vitreous is then removed through the pupil, after the lens has been extracted.

OPERA (outpatient endometrial resection/ablation)—minimally invasive alternative procedure to hysterectomy for patients suffering from abnormal uterine bleeding (AUB).

OPERA STAR SL—a hysteroscope used in OPERA (outpatient endometrial resection/ablation) procedures. STAR is an acronym for specialized tissue aspirating resectoscope.

Operating Arm system—mechanical arm used as a pointer in image-guided and intraoperative navigation for neurosurgery (i.e., during surgical procedure).

operation or **procedure**—a quick-reference list of diagnostic procedures and studies (invasive and non-invasive) and surgical procedures, approaches, maneuvers, methods, techniques, therapies, and treatments of all kinds. See individual entries in alpha order throughout the book for descriptions.

Abbe repair
Abbe-McIndoe vaginal construction
abdominal-sacral colpoperineopexy
ab-externo laser sclerotomy
ab-interno laser sclerotomy
ablative therapy with bone marrow
    rescue
ACAT (automated computerized
    axial tomography)
acetabuloplasty
active specific immunotherapy (ASI)
acupressure without needles
Acuson computed sonography
adaptive cellular therapy
    (RIGS/ACT)

operation *(cont.)*
adenosine echocardiography
advanced cardiac mapping
affinity chromatography
agarose gel electrophoresis (AGE)
air contrast barium enema
alcohol ablation
Alliston GE reflux repair
ALT (argon laser trabeculoplasty)
Altemeier's perineal rectosigmoidectomy
ALT-RCC (autolymphocyte-based
treatment for renal cell
carcinoma)
amnioinfusion
Ancure endovascular repair
antecolic anastomosis
antecolic gastrojejunostomy
antegrade scrotal sclerotherapy
anthropometry
anti-aliasing technique on x-ray
antifibrin antibody imaging
antiperistaltic technique
aortobifemoral reconstruction
apheresis
APLD (automated percutaneous
lumbar diskectomy)
appendicovesicotomy
applanation tonometry
argon laser trabeculoplasty (ALT)
Aries-Pitanguy correction of
mammary ptosis
arterial switch
A-scan ultrasound
aspiration biopsy cytology (ABC)
astigmatic keratotomy
Auchincloss modified radical
mastectomy
Aufranc-Turner arthroplasty
auricular acupuncture
autoaugmentation
autologous transfusion
automated percutaneous lumbar
diskectomy (APLD)

operation *(cont.)*
auxiliary transplant
aversion therapy
axillofemoral bypass
Bacon-Babcock rectovaginal fistula
Baffe's anastomosis
BAK interbody fusion surgical
procedure
Baldy-Webster correction of uterine
retrodisplacement
balloon catheterization
Ball treatment of pruritus ani
band-snare technique
Bankart shoulder dislocation repair
Barcat modified technique
Bardenheuer's modified bifurcation
procedure
barrel-stave osteotomy
Bassini inguinal hernia repair
Batchelor modified procedure to
correct hindfoot valgus deformity
Batista left ventriculectomy
BEAM (brain electrical activity
mapping)
Belsey Mark IV fundoplication
Bennett's quadriceps plastic procedure
Billroth gastroenterostomy
biosurgery
Bishop-Koop ileostomy
Blalock-Hanlon cardiac surgery
Blalock-Taussig cardiac surgery
blind esophageal brushing (BEG)
Blumgart hepaticojejunostomy
Blythe uvulopalatoplasty
Boerema hernia repair
Bohlman triple-wire technique
bone density measurement
Booth wire osteotomy
Bosker transmandibular recon-
structive surgery
Brackin ureterointestinal anastomosis
brachytherapy
Brandt-Daroff exercises
breast-conserving therapy (BCT)

operation *(cont.)*

breast reduction technique
breath-hold MR cholangiography
Bricker ureteroileostomy
Bristow repair of shoulder dislocation
bronchial artery embolization
bronchial sleeve procedure
Brooke ileostomy
Brostrom ankle repair
Brown two-portal endoscopic carpal
    tunnel release
Bruhat laser surgery neosalpingos-
    tomy
bubble ventriculography
Buerhenne stone basket
bundle-nailing treatment of bone
    shaft fractures
bunionectomy
Bunnell tendon transfer
Burch colposuspension for stress
    incontinence
Burch iliopectineal ligament
Burch laparoscopic procedure
butterfly flap technique
buttonpexy fixation of stomal
    prolapse
callus distraction technique
Camey ileocystoplasty
Camitz palmaris longus abductor-
    plasty
canalith repositioning maneuver
    (CRP)
capillary electrophoresis (CE)
capnography
capsulorrhexis
cardiac hybrid revascularization
cardiac shock wave therapy
    (CSWT)
cardiokymography
Cardiolite scan
cardiomyoplasty
CardioTec scan
cardiotocography
carotid angioplasty with stenting

operation *(cont.)*

carotid endarterectomy (CEA)
catheter balloon valvuloplasty
catheter-directed thrombolysis and
    endovascular stent placement
Cavitron ultrasonic surgical
    aspiration of tumor
CECT (contrast enhancement of
    computed tomographic) head
    and body imaging
celiacography
cervicectomy
cervicography or cervigram
cheilectomy
chelation therapy
chemoprevention
chevron osteotomy
Chiari medial displacement pelvic
    osteotomy
cholescintography
Chonstruct chondral repair
chorionic villi biopsy
Chow technique
Chrisman and Snook correction of
    ankle instability
chromohydrotubation
chymonucleolysis
cine CT (computed tomography)
circulator boot therapy
circumduction-adduction shoulder
    maneuver
cisternography
Clagett-Barrett esophagogastrostomy
Clark perineorrhaphy
classic abdominal Semm hysterec-
    tomy (CASH)
claviculectomy
clitoridectomy
closed intramedullary pinning
    (CIMP)
closing base wedge osteotomy
    (CBWO)
coagulum pyelolithotomy
Coblation

operation *(cont.)*
 Coblation Channeling
 Cody tack operation
 Coffey ureterointestinal anastomosis
 cold cup biopsy
 Collin-Beard resection of levator
  muscle
 Collis-Nissen fundoplication
 Collis-Nissen gastroplasty
 colocolponeopoiesis
 color Doppler sonography
 colpocystourethropexy (CCUP)
 computed dental radiography (CDR)
 computed tomographic angiography
  (CTA)
 computed tomography angiographic
  portography (CTAP)
 computed tomography laser
  mammography (CTLM)
 computer-assisted minimally
  invasive surgery
 computerized dynamic posturography (CDP)
 computerized phonoenterography
 conjunctivodacryocystorhinostomy
  (CDCR)
 contact transscleral laser cytophotocoagulation (CTLC)
 continent supravesical bowel urinary
  diversion
 continuous arteriovenous hemofiltration (CAVH)
 continuous circular capsulorrhexis
  technique
 continuous curvilinear capsulorrhexis (CCC)
 continuous wave Doppler examination
 contoured tilting compression
  mammography
 contrast echocardiography
 contrast material enhanced scan
 Copalis (coupled particle light
  scattering)

operation *(cont.)*
 corner mouth lift
 coronary artery bypass graft
  (CABG)
 coronary artery scan (CAS)
 coronary atherectomy
 coronary radiation therapy (CRT)
 coronary remodeling
 corpus cavernosum penile
  electromyography
 corset platysmaplasty
 corticomedullary junction (CMJ)
  phase imaging on CT scan
 Cosgrove-Edwards annuloplasty
 Costello's laser ablation of prostate
 Cotton cartilage graft to cricolaryngeal area
 cough CPR
 counterflow centrifugal elutriation
 coupled suturing
 craniosacral therapy (CST)
 Crawford-Adams arthroplasty
 Crawford's graft inclusion
  reattachment
 cribogram
 Crikelair otoplasty
 Cröhnlein
 crossed-swords technique
 crossfire radiation therapy
 crowncork tympanoplasty
 crural steal procedure
 cryoablation for prostate cancer
 cryosurgery
 cryosurgical ablation of hepatic
  tumor
 CT (computed tomography)
 CTHA (CT during hepatic arteriography)
 CTLM (computed tomography laser
  mammography)
 CT/SPECT fusion
 CT with slip-ring technology
 cupping (acupuncture)
 Cushieri maneuver

operation *(cont.)*

Cutler-Beard eyelid operation
Cyclops reconstruction to cover defect
Cyriax physiotherapy
cystocolpoproctography
cytoablative therapy
cytoreductive surgery
dacryocystorhinostomy (DCR)
Damus-Kaye-Stansel congenital heart defect repair
Darrach ulnar tenodesis
Davydov vagina construction
Dennis-Varco pancreaticoduodenostomy
Dennyson-Fulford extra-articular subtalar arthrodesis
DentaScan
dermabrasion
De Vega tricuspid annuloplasty
DEXA radiographic technique
DEXA (dual energy x-ray absorptiometry) scan
diaphanography
Dibbell unilateral cleft lip nasal reconstruction
diffraction-enhanced imaging (DEI)
diffusion-weighted ultrafast MRI imaging
digital radiography
digital subtraction angiography (DSA)
digital subtraction macrodacryocystography
DioPexy probe
dipyridamole echocardiography
directional coronary angioplasty (DCA)
directional coronary atherectomy (DCA)
direct myocardial revascularization (DMR)
direct vision internal urethrotomy (DVIU)

operation *(cont.)*

distortion product otoacoustic emission (DPOAE)
dobutamine stress echocardiography (DSE)
Döderlein (or Doederlein) laparoscopic hysterectomy
donor island harvesting
donor-specific transfusion
Doppler echocardiography
Doppler tissue imaging (DTI)
Dotter-Judkins PTA
double contrast arthrography
double contrast barium enema
double-orifice repair
DREZ-otomy
DS (duplex sonography)
dual photon densitometry
Duecollement hemicolectomy
Duhamel pull-through anastomosis, laparoscopic
duodenal seromyectomy
duodenal switch
duplex ultrasound
DuVal pancreaticojejunostomy
DuVries hammer toe repair
DVIU (direct vision internal urethrotomy)
Dwyer correction of scoliosis
Dwyer osteotomy
dynamic computerized tomography
dynamic conformal therapy
dynamic graciloplasty
dynamic spiral CT lung densitometry
echocardiography
Eckhout vertical gastroplasty
ECMO (extracorporeal membrane oxygenation)
EDAS (encephaloduroarteriosynangiosis)
Egan's mammography
ELCA (excimer laser coronary angioplasty)

operation *(cont.)*
elective lymph node dissection
    (ELND)
electrocardiographic gating with
    electron-beam CT technology
electrochemotherapy
electrocochleography
electrocorticography
electroejaculation
electrohydraulic lithotripsy (EHL)
electron beam angiography of
    coronary arteries
electron beam computed
    tomography
electron beam intraoperative radio-
    therapy (EBIORT)
electron beam tomography (EBT)
electro-oculogram
electroporation therapy
electroretinogram
Elmslie triple arthrodesis
embryoscopy
Emmet-Studdiford perineorrhaphy
en bloc transplantation of small
    pediatric kidneys into adult
    recipients
en bloc vein resection
embolotherapy
encephaloduroarteriosynangiosis
    (EDAS)
Endocare renal cryoablation
endometrial ablation
endometrial resection and ablation
    (ERA)
endopyelotomy
endoscopic aspiration mucosectomy
endoscopic band ligation (EBL)
endoscopic biliary endoprosthesis
endoscopic brow lift
endoscopic division of incompetent
    perforating veins
endoscopic injection therapy (EIT)
endoscopic laser cholecystectomy
endoscopic laser dacryocysto-
    rhinotomy

operation *(cont.)*
endoscopic ligation
endoscopic mucosal resection
    (EMR)
endoscopic mucosectomy
endoscopic papillectomy (EP)
endoscopic retrograde cholangi-
    ography (ERC)
endoscopic retrograde cholangio-
    pancreatography (ERCP)
endoscopic sphincterotomy (ES)
endoscopic strip craniectomy
endoscopic transpapillary catheteri-
    zation of the gallbladder (ETCG)
endoscopic ultrasonography
endoscopic ultrasound-assisted band
    ligation
endoscopic ultrasound-guided fine
    needle aspiration (EUS-FNA)
endoscopic variceal ligation (EVL)
endoscopic variceal sclerotherapy
    (EVS)
endosonography
end-stage coxarthrosis
enhanced external counterpulsation
    (EECP)
EnSite cardiac mapping procedure
enteroenterostomy
Entero-Test
enucleation
epididymovasostomy
episcleral plaque brachytherapy
ErecAid treatment of erectile
    impotence
esophageal sling procedure
ethoxysclerol procedure
EVac CAT procedure
EVAL embolization
Evans tenodesis
Eve transfer operation
evisceration
exenterative surgery for pelvic
    cancer
excimer laser coronary angioplasty
    (ELCA)

operation *(cont.)*

Exogen SAFHS (sonic accelerated fracture healing system)

Exorcist respiratory compensation

extended right hepatectomy

external beam radiation therapy (EBRT)

external cephalic version (ECV)

extracorporeal photoimmune therapy

extracorporeal shock-wave lithotripsy

extracranial-intracranial (EC-IC) bypass

extraperitoneal excision of lower one-third of ureter with bladder cuff without an initial vesicotomy

ex vivo liver-directed gene therapy

facilitated angioplasty

Faden retropexy

falloposcopy

fascia lata suburethral sling

fast spin-echo acquisition technique

FDG (18-fluorodeoxyglucose) positron emission tomography

female genital mutilation (FMG)

fetal neuron allotransplantation

fetal pig cell transplantation

fetal ventral mesencephalic tissue transplantation

fiberoptic bronchoscopy

fibroid embolization

Fick sacculotomy

flap tracheostomy

flicker electroretinogram (ERG)

fluorescein angiography

fluoroscopic cystocolpoproctography

flush aortogram

Flutter chest percussion therapy

FOAM (fluorescence overlay antigen mapping)

Fobi pouch procedure

focused heat technology

operation *(cont.)*

Fontan anastomosis

Fontan-Kreutzer repair

four-flap Z-plasty

Fourier transform infrared spectroscopy

Fourier transform Raman spectroscopy

Fowler-Stephens orchiopexy (orchidopexy)

fractionated stereotaxic radiation therapy

Frank nonsurgical perineal autodilation for vaginal construction

free toe transfer

full-bladder ultrasound

full-column barium enema

functional endoscopic sinus surgery (FESS)

functional MRI technique

Furniss ureterointestinal anastomosis

gadolinium-enhanced subtracted MR angiography, 3-D

galactography

Galileo intravascular radiotherapy

gallium scan

galvanic vestibular stimulation (GVR)

gamete intrafallopian transfer (GIFT)

gamma-ribbon radiation therapy

gas chromatography

gastric neobladder procedure

gating

generalized nephrographic (GNG) phase imaging

GenESA System pharmacological stress test

gene therapy

Giampapa suturing technique

Giannestras step-down modified osteotomy

Gillies elevation

Girdlestone-Taylor

operation *(cont.)*
Gittes urethral suspension
Glenn anastomosis
GliaSite radiation therapy
Goldman procedure
Goulian mammoplasty
granulocyte transfusion
great toe arthroplasty implant
(GAIT)
Grice-Green correction of hindfoot
valgus deformity
gum sculpting
Gustilo-Kyle arthroplasty
HAART (highly active antiretroviral
therapy)
Halban culdoplasty
HALS (hand-assisted laparoscopic
surgery)
Halsted inguinal herniorrhaphy
hammer toe repair
hand-assisted laparoscopic surgery
(HALS)
hang-back technique
harvesting
Hauser transplantation of patellar
tendon insertion
heater probe thermocoagulation
heavy ion irradiation
Heineke-Mikulicz pyloroplasty
Heller-Belsey correction of
achalasia of esophagus
Heller-Dor laparoscopic procedure
Heller-Nissen correction of
achalasia of esophagus
helmet-molding therapy
hematopoietic stem cell (HSC)
transplant procedure
hemicallotasis
hemicolectomy
hemi-Fontan
hemofiltration
Henning arthroscopic meniscal
repair
hepatic resection

operation *(cont.)*
hepatic segmentectomy
hepatobiliary scintigraphy
hepatopancreatoduodenectomy
hexagonal keratotomy
HHH or triple-H (hypertensive
hypervolemic hemodilution)
therapy
HIDA scan
Higgins ureterointestinal
anastomosis
high-resolution storage phosphor
managing
high-speed rotational atherectomy
(RA)
high-voltage pulsed galvanic
stimulation
Hill cluster harvest micrograft
Hill esophageal antireflux repair
Hill gastropexy fundoplication
Hoffa's tendon shortening
Hoffman and Mohr repair of
unicoronal cranial synostosis
Hoffman-Clayton podiatric
treatment of rheumatoid arthritis
Hofmeister gastroenterostomy
Hofmeister-Shoemaker gastro–
jejunostomy
home ambulatory inotropic therapy
Ho:YAG LTK (noncontact
holmium:YAG laser thermal
keratoplasty)
HRARE (hybrid rapid acquisition
with relaxation enhancement)
HS-tk gene therapy
Hunter open cord tendon implant
Hunter tendon rod insertion
Hunt-Lawrence pouch
hyperbaric oxygen therapy
hyperoxia
hypertension optimal treatment
(HOT)
hyperthermia, whole body
hysterosalpingosonography (HSSG)

operation *(cont.)*
hysterosonography
ICG (iodocyanine green)
   fluorescein angiography
ICSI (intracytoplasmic sperm
   injection)
ileal pouch-anal anastomosis (IPAA)
Ilizarov limb lengthening
image-guided surgery
immunoscintigraphy
impedance plethysmography (IPG)
IMRT (intensity modulated radiation
   therapy)
incentive spirometry
indium 111 scintigraphy scan
indocyanin green angiography
infibulation
injection technique
inotropic therapy
Integris 3-D RA (rotational
   angiography)
intensity-modulated radiation
   therapy (IMRT)
Intensive Narcotic Detoxification
intentional transoperative
   hemodilution
intermittent exotropia
interpleural analgesia
in-the-bag IOL lens implantation
intra-aortic endovascular
   sonography
intracardiac amobarbital sodium
   procedure
intracaval endovascular ultrasonography
intracoronary artery radiation
intracoronary ultrasonography
intracytoplasmic sperm injection
   (ICSI)
intradiscal electrothermal (IDET)
   annuloplasty
intrahepatic cholangioenterostomy
intralesional laser therapy
intraluminal brachytherapy

operation *(cont.)*
intraoperative cholangiography
   (IOC)
intraoperative high dose rate
   (IOHDR) brachytherapy
intraoperative hippocampal cooling
intraoperative lymphatic mapping
intraoperative radiation therapy
   (IORT)
intraoperative radiolymphoscintigraphy
intraoperative radiotherapy (IORT)
intraoperative transmyocardial
   revascularization (ITMR)
intraoperative ultrasonography
   (IOUS)
intraperitoneal hyperthermic
   chemotherapy (IPHC)
intraperitoneal onlay mesh hernia
   repair (IPOM)
intraportal endovascular ultrasonography (IPEUS)
intravascular MRI technique
intravascular red light therapy
   (IRLT)
intravascular ultrasound (IVUS)
intravenous fluorescein angiography
   (IVFA)
intravenous pyelogram (IVP)
invasive procedure
inversion-ligation appendectomy
inverted U-pouch ileal reservoir
in vitro fertilization (IVF)
in vivo optical spectroscopy
   (INVOS)
iodocyanine green (ICG)
   fluorescein angiography
iontophoresis
iridectomy
iridencleisis
isolated heat perfusion of an
   extremity
isotopic cisternography
Isshiki thyroplasty type I

operation *(cont.)*

IVOX artificial lung procedure
Jatene arterial switch procedure (correction of transposed great arteries in neonate)
Jenckel cholecystoduodenostomy
Jones first-toe repair
Joplin bunionectomy
Judd ventral hernia repair
Judkins coronary arteriography
Kalamchi osteotomy
Kapandji-Sauve technique for distal radial-ulnar joint repair
karate chop phaco technique
Karydakis procedure
Kasai peritoneal venous shunt
Kech and Kelly osteotomy
keel excision
Kelikian modified Z osteotomy
Keller arthroplasty
Keller bunionectomy
Kestenbach-Anderson eye surgery
Kestenbaum repair of nystagmic torticollis
keyhole resection
Kiricuta reconstructive breast procedure
Kirsch laser welding technique
Klagsbrun harvest of chondrocytes
Kocher-Langenbeck ilioinguinal approach to fracture repair
Koch lens insertion
Kock modified pouch
Koenig arthroplasty
Kono patch enlargement of aorta
Kreuscher bunionectomy
Kropp bladder neck reconstruction
Krupin valve with disc
krypton (red) laser photocoagulation
Kun colocolpopoiesis
LABA (laser-assisted balloon angioplasty)
lacrimal scintigraphy
Ladd correction of malrotation of bowel

operation *(cont.)*

Lange tendon lengthening
laparoscopic-assisted colorectal resection
laparoscopic bladder neck suture suspension procedure
laparoscopic cholecystectomy
laparoscopic Heller myotomy
laparoscopic intracorporeal ultrasound
laparoscopic laser-assisted auto-augmentation of bladder
laparoscopic laser cholecystectomy
laparoscopic Nissen and Toupet fundoplication
laparoscopic pneumodissection
laparoscopic radical prostatectomy
laparoscopic transcystic duct exploration
laparoscopic transcystic papillotomy
laparoscopic ultrasound (LUS)
laparoscopic urinary diversion procedure
laparoscopic uterine nerve ablation (LUNA)
laparoscopic videolaseroscopy
laparoscopy under local anesthesia (LULA)
Lap-Band adjustable gastric banding (LAGB)
lap Nissen (laparoscopic Nissen fundoplication)
LAR/CAA (low anterior resection in combination with coloanal anastomosis)
large loop excision of the transformation zone (LLETZ)
large particle biopsy
large-skull implant surgery
LARS (laparoscopic antireflux surgery)
laryngeal framework surgery (LFS)
laryngoplastic phonosurgery
laser angioplasty

operation *(cont.)*
  laser-assisted balloon angioplasty
    (LABA)
  laser-assisted microanastomosis
  laser-assisted tissue welding
  laser-assisted uvulopalatoplasty
    (LAUP)
  laser biomicroscopy of vitreoretinal
    structures
  laser correlational spectroscopy
    (LCS)
  laser image custom arthroplasty
    (LICA)
  laser in situ keratomileusis (LASIK)
  laser myringotomy
  laser nucleotomy
  laser uterosacral nerve ablation
    (LUNA)
  laser photoablation
  laser sclerostomy
  laser stapedotomy
  laser thermal keratoplasty (LTK)
  laser trabeculodissection (LTD)
  Lasertrolysis
  laser welding
  Lash hysterectomy
  lateral acetabular shelf osteotomy
  lateral crural steal (LCS) for nasal
    tip reconstruction
  Latzko vesicovaginal fistula
  Lazarus-Nelson peritoneal lavage
  Leadbetter-Politano ureterovesico-
    plasty
  LeDuc-Camey ileocystoplasty
  LeDuc ureteral anastomosis
  LEEP (loop electrosurgical excision
    procedure)
  LeFort I apertognathia repair
  LeFort II and III fracture repairs
  LeFort uterine prolapse repair
  Lejour-type breast reduction,
    modified
  lens-sparing external beam radiation
    therapy (LSRT)

operation *(cont.)*
  Lester Martin modification of
    Duhamel procedure
  Lewis-Tanner esophagectomy
  LICA (laser image custom
    arthroplasty)
  Lich-Gregoire repair
  Lichtenstein hernia repair
  Lich ureteral implantation
    for neobladder construction
  ligamentum teres cardiopexy
    fundoplication
  light reflection rheography
  Lindseth's kyphectomy with
    posterior crisscross wires
  Lindseth's osteotomy
  lip lift
  liquid crystal thermography
  LITT (laser-induced thermotherapy)
  liver-directed ex vivo gene therapy
  LLETZ (large loop excision of the
    transformation zone)
  loop electrosurgical excision
    procedure (LEEP)
  loopogram (ileostogram)
  Lortat-Jacob hepatic resection
  Lovaas autism treatment program
  low-dose screen-film technique
  LUNA (laser uterosacral nerve
    ablation)
  LVRS (lung volume reduction
    surgery)
  lymphapheresis
  lymphoscintigraphy
  MAA lung scan
  Madden incisional hernia repair
  Madigan prostatectomy
  Magerl screw placement
  Magnuson-Stack shoulder
    arthrotomy
  magnetic resonance angiography
    (MRA)
  magnetic resonance cholangi-
    ography (MRC)

operation *(cont.)*

magnetic resonance elastography (MRE)

magnetic resonance mammography

magnetic resonance neurography (MRN)

magnetic resonance spectroscopy (MRS)

magnetic resonance urography

magnetic stimulation of fracture

magnetoencephalogram (MEG)

MAGPI (meatal advancement, glanduloplasty, penoscrotal junction meatotomy)

Ma-Griffith anastomosis

Malbran transscleral fixation of intraocular lens

mammary ptosis

mammoplasty

Mammotest breast biopsy

Maquet elevation of tibial crest

Marshall-Marchetti-Krantz vesico-urethral suspension

Marx osteoradionecrosis (ORN)

Masimo SET (signal extraction technology)

Masket lens insertion

masking technology

Mason abdominotranssphincteric resection

Mason vertical-banded gastroplasty

maternal blood clot patch therapy

matricectomy

Matsner median episiotomy

Mau osteotomy, modified

Mayday distal first metatarsal osteotomy for hallux valgus

Mayo culdoplasty, modified

maze procedure (ablation of refractory atrial fibrillation)

McCall posterior culdoplasty

McCraw gracilis myocutaneous flap for vaginal construction

McDonald cervical cerclage

operation *(cont.)*

McIndoe vaginal construction

McKee-Farrar total hip arthroplasty

McRoberts maneuver

McVay hernia repair

meatal advancement, glanduloplasty, penoscrotal junction meatotomy (MAGPI)

median sternotomy

mediastinotomy

medical holography

meloplasty

membrane stripping

meridian therapy

Merindino GI procedure

MESA (microepididymal sperm aspiration)

mesh plug hernioplasty

metrizamide CT cisternogram

Meuli arthroplasty

Microdot technique

microendoscopic diskectomy (MED)

microlumbar diskectomy

microsurgical denervation of the spermatic cord

microsurgical epidymovasostomy (MSEV)

microvascular arterial bypass surgery for impotence

microvascular free tissue transfer for glossectomy

microwave nonsurgical treatment for benign prostatic hypertrophy

microwave thermoradiotherapy

MIDCAB (minimally invasive direct coronary artery bypass)

Millen retropubic prostatectomy

Milligan-Morgan hemorrhoidectomy

mini-FES (functional endoscopic sinus) surgery

minilaparotomy pelvic lymph node dissection

minilaparotomy staging pelvic lymphadenectomy

operation *(cont.)*

Mitchell distal osteotomy
Mitchell epispadias repair technique
Mitek anchor system
Mitrofanoff appendicovesicotomy
Mitrofanoff neourethra procedure
MIVR (minimally invasive valve repair or replacement)
M-mode echocardiogram
modified Hughes eyelid procedure
modified Isshiki type 4 thyroplasty
modified Pereyra bladder neck suspension
Moe scoliosis
Mohs' chemosurgery
monochromatization filtering technique
mosaicplasty
Moskowitz obliteration of cul-de-sac
Mosley anterior shoulder repair
moxibustion
microsurgical epidymovasostomy (MSEV)
moving-bed infusion-tracking MRA
MRCP (magnetic resonance cholangiopancreatography)
MRCP using HASTE with a phased-array coil
MR hydrography
MRP (magnetic resonance pancreatography)
MR peritoneography
MT (magnetization transfer) saturation
MUGA (multiple gated acquisition) scan
Mumford-Gurd arthroplasty
Mustardé flap otoplasty
Mustard transposition of great vessels
myofascial release
Nagahara phaco chopper and phaco chop technique

operation *(cont.)*

Nambudripad's Allergy Elimination Technique (NAET)
native tissue harmonic imaging
NDT (neuro-developmental techniques)
Nd:YAG CTLC (contact trans-scleral laser cytophotocoagulation)
near-infrared spectroscopy (NIRS)
Neer hemiarthroplasty
neoadjuvant hormonal therapy (NHT)
nephroureterectomy with en bloc removal of cuff of bladder
neuroendovascular interventional procedures
New England Baptist arthroplasty
Nichol vaginal suspension
ninety-ninety intraosseous wiring
Nissen laparoscopic fundoplication
Nissen total fundoplication
non-breath-hold MR cholangiography
Norland bone densitometry
Norwood (Fontan modification)
Norwood (Gill/Jonas modification)
Norwood (Sade modification)
nuclectomy
Numby Stuff needle-free method
Ober-Barr brachioradialis transfer
Obwegeser's sagittal mandibular osteotomy
oculoplethysmography-carotid phonoangiography (OPG/CPA)
off-pump coronary artery bypass (OPCAB)
OPART
open mesh-plug hernioplasty
open reduction and internal fixation (ORIF)
open-sky vitrectomy
OPERA (outpatient endometrial resection/ablation) procedures

operation *(cont.)*
optical coherence tomography
(OCT)
Oriental flap technique
Orr-Loygue transabdominal
proctopexy
Orr rectal prolapse repair
orthotopic transplantation
osteomanipulative therapy (chiropractic)
osteoradionecrosis (ORN)
out-in-out technique
oxygen cisternography
palladium 103 brachytherapy
pallidal brain stimulation procedure
pallidotomy guided by microelectrode recording
pancreatic enzyme therapy
pancreaticoduodenectomy
pancreatoduodenectomy
PANDO (primary acquired nasolacrimal duct obstruction).
panretinal photocoagulation (PRP)
and focal laser therapy
pants-over-vest repair
Pap Plus speculoscopy
PARK (photoastigmatic refractive
keratectomy)
Parker-Kerr closed end-to-end
enteroenterostomy
partial encircling endocardial
ventriculotomy
partial liquid ventilation
Partipilo gastrostomy
PC-IOL (posterior chamber intraocular lens) implantation
Pearce trabeculectomy
PEARL (physiologic endometrial
ablation/resection loop)
pelvic floor electrical stimulation
(PFS)
Pember circumacetabular osteotomy
Pemberton's acetabuloplasty
PEMF (pulsed electromagnetic
field)

operation *(cont.)*
penile vein ligation
percutaneous aortic balloon
valvuloplasty
percutaneous automated diskectomy
percutaneous balloon mitral
valvuloplasty
percutaneous bladder neck stabilization (PBNS)
percutaneous cholecystolithotomy
(PCCL)
percutaneous choledochoscopy
percutaneous coronary rotational
atherectomy (PCRA)
percutaneous dilational tracheostomy (PDT)
percutaneous endoscopic
gastrostomy (PEG)
percutaneous endoscopic
jejunostomy (PEJ)
percutaneous epididymal sperm
aspiration
percutaneous gastroenterostomy
(PEG)
percutaneous gastrostomy (PG)
percutaneous intracoronary
angioscopy
percutaneous mitral balloon
valvotomy (PMBV)
percutaneous nephrostolithotomy
(PCNL)
percutaneous pinning of fractures
percutaneous radiofrequency
catheter ablation
percutaneous resection of
transitional cell carcinoma
percutaneous transatrial mitral
commissurotomy
percutaneous transhepatic
cholangiography (PTHC)
percutaneous transhepatic cholecystolithotomy (PCTCL)
percutaneous transhepatic liver
biopsy with tract embolization
(PBTE)

operation *(cont.)*

percutaneous transluminal angioplasty (PTA)

percutaneous transluminal myocardial (or transmyocardial) revascularization (PTMR)

percutaneous transluminal renal
angioplasty (PTRA)

percutaneous transluminal septal
myocardial ablation

percutaneous transperineal seed
implantation

percutaneous transvenous mitral
commissurotomy (PTMC)

Perfix hernioplasty

perfusion-weighted MRI imaging

perineal surgical apron technique

PerioChip

periosteal stripping

peripheral excimer laser angioplasty
(PELA)

peripheral laser angioplasty (PLA)

peripheral scatter photocoagulation

peritomy

peritoneography MR

periurethral collagen injection

permanent brachytherapy

petaling the cast procedure

PET (positron emission
tomography) scan

PET with 3D SSP (positron
emission tomography with 3-D
stereotaxic surface projection)

pharaonic circumcision

phonocardiography

photoangioplasty

photoastigmatic refractive
keratectomy (PARK)

photocoagulation

photodynamic therapy (PDT)

photo epilation

photon correlation spectroscopy

photorefractive keratectomy (PRK)

phototherapeutic keratectomy (PTK)

operation *(cont.)*

photothermal sclerosis

phytotherapy

PIPIDA scan

plasmapheresis

platform posturography

pleural tent construction

plicectomy

plugged liver biopsy

P-MRS (phosphorus nuclear magnetic resonance spectroscopy)

pneumatic retinopexy

polydioxanone plating procedure

Ponka herniorrhaphy

Port-Access minimally invasive
cardiac surgery

portoportal anastomosis

posterior capsulorrhexis with optic
capture

posterior chamber intraocular lens
(PC-IOL) implantation

posterior lumbar interbody
fusion (PLIF)

posteromedial release of clubfoot
(PMR)

power Doppler sonography

Prentiss orchiopexy

pressure support ventilation

Pringle maneuver

Profore four-layer bandaging

profundaplasty

proliferative retinopathy photocoagulation

prolotherapy

ProstaSeed ^{125}I radiation treatment

ProstRcision

proton magnetic resonance
spectroscopy

proximal row carpectomy (PRC)

psoralen inactivation technique

PTFE (polytetrafluoroethylene)

pubovaginal sling procedure

Puestow pancreaticojejunostomy

pulsed dose therapy

operation *(cont.)*

pulsed dye laser therapy
pulsed electromagnetic field
(PEMF) therapy
push enteroscope/enteroscopy
Putti-Platt arthroplasty
pylorus-preserving pancreatoduodenectomy (PPPD)
pylorus-preserving Whipple (PPW)
modification
PYP (pyrophosphate) scan
quantitative computed tomography
(QCT)
quantitative coronary arteriography
(QCA)
QUART (quadrantectomy, axillary
dissection, and radiotherapy)
radial keratotomy
radial thermokeratoplasty
radical prostatectomy (RP)
radiocolloid mapping
radiofrequency (RF) ablation
radiofrequency catheter ablation
(RFA)
radiofrequency percutaneous myocardial revascularization
(RF-PMR)
radioimmunoluminography (RILG)
radioimmunoscintimetry
radiolymphoscintigraphy
radionuclide cholescintography
radionuclide scan
Raman spectroscopy
Rashkind balloon atrial septotomy
Rastelli cardiac procedure
Raz sling for urinary incontinence
real-time ultrasonography
recombinant enzyme replacement
therapy
rectal endoscopic ultrasonography
(REU)
rectilinear biphasic waveform
for external defibrillation
REDS (remote endoscopic digital
spectroscopy)

operation *(cont.)*

reduced liver transplant (RLT)
reduction columelloplasty
reflectance-guided laser selection
remote afterloading brachytherapy
(RAB)
remote brachytherapy
remote endoscopic digital
spectroscopy (REDS)
retrograde cerebral perfusion (RCP)
retroperitoneoscopy
retropubic prostatectomy
Reverdin-Green osteotomy
Revo rotator cuff repair
RHCT (renal helical CT) imaging
rheography, light reflection
rhinolaryngostroboscopy (RLS)
rhizotomy, functional posterior
RICE (rest, ice, compression,
elevation) treatment
RIGS/ACT (adaptive cellular
therapy)
Ripstein rectal prolapse repair
Rocabado technique for manipulative (physical) therapy
rollerball endometrial ablation
Rosomoff cordotomy
Ross aortic valve replacement
procedure
rotational atherectomy (RA)
rotational scarf osteotomy
ruptured abdominal aortic
aneurysm (RAAA)
rush immunotherapy
Rutkow sutureless plug and patch
sacral nerve stimulation (SNS)
therapy
sacrospinous colpopexy
SAFHS (sonic-accelerated fracture
healing system) therapy
sagittal split ramus osteotomy
(SSRO)
saline-enhanced MR arthrography
of shoulder

operation *(cont.)*
saloon door approach in MIDCAB procedures
Salter osteotomy
same-day microsurgical arthroscopic lateral-approach laser-assisted (SMALL) fluoroscopic diskectomy
Sand process
sandwich treatment
SASMA (skin-adipose superficial musculoaponeurotic) facelift
Sauve-Kapandji distal radioulnar joint reconstruction
Scanning-Beam Digital X-ray (SBDX)
scaphotrapeziotrapezoid (STT) arthrodesis
scarf osteotomy bunionectomy
Schepens-Okamura-Brockhurst retinal detachment repair
Schiotz tonometry
Schlein elbow arthroplasty
Schuknecht cochleosacculotomy
scintirenography
scleral buckling procedure
sclerouvectomy, partial lamellar
second-look laparotomy
sector scan echocardiography
SeedNet cryotherapy
seminal vesiculography (SVG)
Semont maneuver
serial scans
sestamibi Tc-99m SPECT with dipyridamole stress test
Sever-L'Episcopo shoulder repair
SharpShooter tissue repair
Sharrard kyphectomy
Shepherd lens insertion
Shirodkar cervical cerclage
shoelace technique for delayed fasciotomy closure
Shouldice hernia repair
SI (sensory integration)

operation *(cont.)*
single-field hyperthermia combined with radiation therapy
Silastic bead embolization
single photon planar scintigraphy (SPPS)
Sinu-Clear procedure
skeletal targeted radiotherapy (STR)
Skoog release of Dupuytren's contracture
sleeve pneumonectomy
small-bowel enteroscopy (SBE)
SMALL (same-day microsurgical arthroscopic lateral approach laser-assisted) fluoroscopic diskectomy
SMART (surgical myomectomy as reproductive therapy)
SmartBeam radiotherapy
smasectomy rhytidectomy technique
Smead-Jones closure
snare resection (band and snare)
Soave abdominal pull-through procedure
soft tissue shaving cannula liposhaver
somato-emotional release (SER)
Sones coronary arteriography
sonic-accelerated fracture healing system (SAFHS) therapy
sonohysterography
sonopuncture
Southwick osteotomy
sparrow-picking technique
SPECT (single photon emission computed tomography) scan
spectral Doppler
speculoscopy
sperm aspiration technique
spinal myeloscopy
spiral x-ray computed tomography (SXCT)
split anterior tibial tendon transfer (SPLATT)

operation *(cont.)*
stacked scans
STAE (subsegmental transcatheter arterial embolization)
STA-MCA (superficial temporal artery–middle cerebral artery) bypass
Stamey bladder suspension
Stamm gastrostomy
Stanmore shoulder arthroplasty
stapled lung reduction
Steel osteotomy
step-oblique mammography
stereotactic pallidotomy
stereotactic radiosurgery (SRS)
stereotactic tractotomy
stereotaxically guided interstitial laser therapy
stereotaxic core needle biopsy (SCNB)
stereotaxy
STING (subureteric Teflon injection)
Stoppa laparoscopic hernia repair
stress cystogram
stress-injected sestamibi-gated SPECT with echocardiography
stress perfusion and rest function by sestamibi-gated SPECT
stress perfusion scintigraphy
strip-biopsy
Strother acrochordonectomy
subclavian flap aortoplasty (SFA)
subfascial endoscopic perforator surgery (SEPS)
submucosal saline injection technique
subperiosteal corticotomy
subplatysmal face-lift technique
suburethral sling procedure
suction-assisted lipectomy (SAL)
suction-assisted lipoplasty (SAL)
Sugiura paraesophagogastric devascularization

operation *(cont.)*
Sunna circumcision
supraglottoplasty
surface electromyography (sEMG)
Swanson PIP joint arthroplasty
Swenson's abdominal pull-through
Swiss ball therapy
Syed-Neblett brachytherapy method
Syme's amputation of foot
Syme's external urethrotomy
TACE (transcatheter arterial chemoembolization)
TAPET (tumor amplified protein expression therapy)
Targis microwave catheter-based system
TcHIDA scan
TCP (total cavopulmonary connection)
tease procedure
teboroxime scan
TECAB (totally endoscopic coronary artery bypass)
TechneScan MAG3
technetium scan
Teflon paste injection for incontinence
tendon Z-lengthening around the knee and ankle
Tennison-Randall cleft lip repair
TEP (totally extraperitoneal) hernia repair
terminal sedation (TS)
Tesla imaging system
T-graft configuration technique
Thal esophageal stricture repair
thallium stress test
Thera Cool cold therapy
ThermaChoice uterine balloon therapy
thermal quenching
thermistor-plethysmography
Thermoflex water-induced thermotherapy (WIT)

operation *(cont.)*
  Thiersch-Duplay urethroplasty
  thin-layer chromatography
  Thom flap laryngeal reconstruction
  thoracoabdominal aortic aneurysm
    (TAAA) surgery
  thoracophrenolaparotomy
  thorascopic apical pleurectomy
  thorascopic talc pleurodesis
  3DCE (three-dimensional contrast-
    enhanced) MR angiography
    technique
  3DFT magnetic resonance
    angiography
  thromboelastograph (TEG)
  ThromboScan MRU
  thyroplasty type I
  thyroxine radioisotope assay
    (T_4RIA)
  Tikhoff-Linberg shoulder resection
  time-resolved imaging by automatic
    data segmentation (TRIADS)
  TIPSS (transjugular intrahepatic
    portosystemic shunt)
  tissue engineering
  TKA (total knee arthroplasty)
  TMR (transmyocardial revascular-
    ization)
  tomodensitometic examination,
    abdominal
  tonsillar Coblation
  topodermatography
  Torkildsen shunt ventriculo-
    cisternostomy
  total cavopulmonary connection
  total hip replacement (THR)
  total lymphoid irradiation (TLI)
  total mesorectal excision (TME)
  Toupet hemifundoplication
  Toupet partial posterior
    fundoplication
  T-PRK (tracker-assisted photo-
    refractive keratectomy)
  trachelotomy

operation *(cont.)*
  tracheoesophageal puncture (TEP)
  tracheotomy
  Trager therapy
  transabdominal preperitoneal
    (TAPP) hernia repair
  transanal endoscopic microsurgery
    (TEM)
  transbronchial biopsy (TBB)
  transcarotid balloon valvuloplasty
  transcatheter arterial embolization
    (TAE)
  transcervical balloon tuboplasty
    (TBT)
  transconjunctival removal of
    cavernous hemangioma
  transcoronary ablation of septal
    hypertrophy (TASH)
  transcranial color-coded sonography
  transcutaneous neuromuscular
    electrical stimulation (TNMES)
  transesophageal echocardiogram
    (TEE)
  transfemoral liver biopsy
  transferred immune response
  transhepatic embolization (THE)
  transient evoked otoacoustic
    emission (TEOAE)
  transjugular intrahepatic porto-
    systemic shunt (TIPSS)
  transjugular liver biopsy
  translabyrinthine removal of large
    acoustic neuromas
  transluminal endovascular graft
    placement
  transmyocardial revascularization
    (TMR)
  transnasal endoluminal ultra-
    sonography
  transpapillary endoscopic chole-
    cystotomy
  transplanted stamp graft
  transpupillary thermotherapy
  transrectal ultrasound (TRUS)

operation *(cont.)*
transthoracic echocardiogram
transthoracic needle aspiration biopsy
transumbilical breast augmentation
(TUBA)
transurethral balloon Laserthermia
prostatectomy
transurethral incision of the prostate
(TUIP)
transurethral microwave thermotherapy (TUMT)
transurethral needle ablation
(TUNA)
transurethral ultrasound-guided
laser-induced prostatectomy
(TULIP)
transvaginal sacrospinous culpopexy
transvaginal ultrasound-guided
urethral reconstruction
transvenous liver biopsy
Traverso-Longmire technique
triangular vaginal patch sling
triple-H therapy (hypertensive
hypervolemic hemodilution)
TSPP (technetium stannous pyrophosphate) rectilinear bone scan
tumescent liposuction technique
Turco's posteromedial release of
clubfoot
Turner-Warwick urethroplasty
"turn-up" plasty
TVT (tension-free vaginal tape)
continent procedure
2-D echocardiography
2-D IVUS (two-dimensional
intravascular ultrasound)
two-layer latex and Marlex
closure technique
two-stage capsulorrhexis
ultrafast CT electron beam
tomography
ultrasonic aspiration
ultrasound biomicroscopy (UBM)
ultrasound-guided anterior subcostal
liver biopsy

operation *(cont.)*
ultrasound-guided pseudoaneurysm
compression
ultrasound-guided transcervical
tuboplasty
umbilical artery velocimetry
unenhanced scan
UPLIFT (uterine positioning via
ligament investment fixation and
truncation) procedure
ureterorenoscopy
ureteroscopy
urethrovesical suspension
urinary undiversion procedure
urocytogram
Urowave thermotherapy
uterine balloon therapy
uvulopalatopharyngoplasty (UPPP)
vaginal flap reconstruction of
urethra and vesical neck
vaginal interruption of pregnancy,
with dilatation and curettage
(VIP-DAC)
vaginal wall sling surgery
vagus nerve stimulation (VNS)
valvuloplasty
vascular brachytherapy
vascular targeting agent technology
VAX-D (vertebral axial decompression) therapy
VCAB (ventriculocoronary artery
bypass)
vectorcardiography
velolaryngeal endoscopy
vertical-banded gastroplasty (VBG)
ventricular endoaneurysmorrhaphy
vertical tripod fixation (VTF)
vesicoureterogram (VCUG)
vesicourethral suspension
vibroacoustic stimulation
video-assisted thoracic surgery
video densitometry (VD)
videoendoscopic swallowing study
(VESS)

operation *(cont.)*
  videolaseroscopy
  Vineberg cardiac revascularization
  vitrectomy
  voiding cystourethrogram (VCUG)
  Voxgram
  V/Q (ventilation/perfusion) scan
  Waldhausen subclavian flap repair
  Wardill palatoplasty
  Warthin-Starry technique
  water-induced thermotherapy
    (WIT)
  Watson-Jones tenodesis
  Weir nasal alar excision
  Wheeless construction of J rectal
    pouch
  whiplash technique
  Whipple pancreaticoduodenectomy
  Williams vulvovaginoplasty
  Wirsung dilatation procedure
  Witzel duodenostomy
  Womack splenectomy
  Woods screw maneuver
  Wu bunionectomy
  Wyse reduction mammoplasty
  xenotransplantation
  Young-Dees-Leadbetter bladder-
    neck reconstruction
  Y stenting angioplasty
  Zancolli clawhand deformity repair
  Zavanelli maneuver
  zonulolysis
  Z-plasty, four-flap
  zygote intrafallopian transfer (ZIFT)
OPG/CPA—see *oculoplethysmography/
  carotid phonoangiography.*
ophthalmic pneumocystis—see *AIDS-
  associated ophthalmic pneumocystis.*
ophthalmodynamometry—measures
  the relative central retinal artery pressures and indirectly assesses carotid
  artery flow on each side. See *Bail-
  liart's ophthalmodynamometer.*

ophthalmoscopy—allows examination
  of the interior of the eye after dilation.
Opmilas CO_2 multipurpose laser.
Opmilas 144 Plus laser system—used
  for soft tissue applications in arthroscopic and general surgery. Uses
  Nd:YAG laser for gynecologic, urologic, and general surgery.
OPPA (Oncovin, procarbazine, prednisone, Adriamycin)—chemotherapy
  protocol for Hodgkin's lymphoma.
opportunistic infection or **organism**—
  a microorganism that does not ordi-
  narily cause disease but becomes
  pathogenic under certain circumstances (e.g., impaired immune response, or predisposing factors such
  as neoplasm or trauma). AIDS patients or patients who are immunocompromised are giving a new
  meaning to this term and to our
  understanding of the immune system.
  Opportunistic infections are responsible for approximately 90% of
  AIDS-related deaths.
**opposed loop-pair quadrature mag-
  netic resonance coil**—MRI term.
opposition—the act of being opposite,
  or the state of being set in opposite
  manner, as "The thumb and index
  finger could be placed in opposition." Cf. *apposition.*
Opsis DistalCam video system—used
  in laparoscopic surgery.
OpSite—watertight polyurethane dressing that adheres to the skin around
  the wound, but not the wound itself.
OpSite Flexigrid transparent adhesive
  film dressing.
opsonizing antibodies—antibodies that
  make bacteria susceptible to phago-
  cytes.

optical coherence tomography (OCT) —a noninvasive, noncontact imaging technology capable of producing cross-sectional images of the retina in vivo with high resolution to obtain multiple cross-sectional images of the fovea, peripapillary retina, and macula.

optical pachometer—used in determining the depth of corneal pathology in an eye.

Optical Tracking System—LED wand used by neurosurgeons for image-guided intraoperative navigation (i.e., during surgical procedure).

optical trapping—see *LaserTweezers.*

optic neuritis—inflammation of that portion of the optic nerve that is not ophthalmoscopically visible.

Opti-Gard patient eye protector.

OptiHaler—a drug delivery system for use with metered dose inhalers.

optimal cutting temperature (OCT)— a synthetic water-soluble glycol and resin mounting medium; used to embed and mount tissue for cutting frozen sections.

Optimed glaucoma pressure regulator—a tiny implant.

Optipore wound-cleaning sponge.

OptiPranolol (metipranolol).

Optiray (ioversol)—a nonionic contrast medium.

Optisol—"The donor corneoscleral button with a 3 mm rim was preserved in Optisol."

Optison—ultrasound contrast agent.

Optistat—a power injector by Mallinckrodt that introduces contrast media into the body in a controlled manner.

optokinetic nystagmus (OKN).

Optrin (motexafin lutetium; Lu-Tex)— used for photodynamic therapy of patients with age-related macular degeneration.

Optro (recombinant human hemoglobin, formerly known as rHb 1.1)— used to restore blood volume and oxygen delivery for the treatment of acute intraoperative blood loss.

Opus cardiac troponin I assay—a test used to diagnose acute myocardial infarction within 22 minutes after receipt of a blood sample by the lab. A heart attack disrupts blood flow as well as delivery of oxygen to heart muscle. The result is destruction of cells and the release of cardiac troponin I into healthy tissue and the bloodstream. Measurement of cardiac troponin I and other cardiac markers permits the quick finding of heart attack. Cardiac troponin I is present in the blood from 4 to 6 hours after acute onset of myocardial infarction following heart muscle damage and remains elevated as long as 7 days.

OR, O.R. (operating room).

Oracle Focus—a line of combined ultrasound imaging and PTCA catheters.

Oracle Megasonics catheters (interventional radiology)—a line of high-pressure PTCA catheters.

Oracle Micro catheter.

Oracle Micro Plus—PTCA and ultrasound imaging catheter.

oral—pertaining to the mouth, as in oral intake, oral surgery. Cf. *aural.*

Oralease—a proprietary oral gel formulation of diclofenac (nonsteroidal anti-inflammatory drug) that relieves pain from oral ulcers.

Oralet lollipop (fentanyl citrate).

Oralex—ultrasound imaging agent.

Oralgen—oral insulin administered using a metered dosage aerosol applicator, for treatment of type 1 and type 2 diabetes.

OralScreen 3-panel oral fluids test—for illicit drugs, including marijuana, cocaine, and opiates. Results are available within 10 minutes.

Oramorph SR—sustained release tablets of oral morphine sulfate.

orascope—microfiberoptic endoscope that allows a dentist or endodontist to see inside a tooth.

OraSure—an oral specimen collection device used to screen for the presence of antibodies to HIV.

OraTest—used for detection of oral cancer.

Orbasone system—noninvasive therapeutic device used to treat joints, muscles, and ligaments.

Orbis-Sigma cerebrospinal fluid shunt valve—has three pressure/flow stages, and reportedly a much lower failure rate than standard valves.

orbital rim stepoff (Oph)—an indication of fracture (and slight displacement). "Examination for fracture revealed no orbital rim stepoff."

Oreopoulos-Zellerman catheter—used for peritoneal dialysis.

Orfizip cast—a wrist cast that goes from the palm to the elbow. It closes over the forearm by means of a zipper, hence the name.

organic brain syndrome (OBS).

organ of Corti (in the cochlea)—contains hair cells, transmitting stimuli to the cochlear branch of cranial nerve VIII (acoustic, or vestibulocochlear, nerve).

organoaxial gastric volvulus—occurs when the stomach rotates along a longitudinal axis. It is rarely mesenteroaxial or vertical.

orgotein—used to treat familial amyotrophic lateral sclerosis.

Oriental flap technique—creation of a V-Y flap.

oriented times four (oriented x 4)—oriented to person, time, place, and future plans.

oriented times three (oriented x 3)—oriented to person, time, and place.

ORIF (open reduction and internal fixation).

Origin balloon, tacker, trocar—instruments for laparoscopic surgery.

origin of a vessel (Radiol)—the commencement of a vessel as it branches off from a larger vessel.

Orion anterior cervical plate—internal fixation system made of a titanium alloy, a locked screw-to-plate system used to stabilize the cervical spine after trauma, or multilevel diskectomy.

ORLAU (Orthotic Research and Locomotor Assessment Unit) **swivel walker**—orthosis for ambulation in children with cerebral palsy and myelomeningocele.

orlistat (Xenical)—a drug treatment for obesity that blocks the body's absorption of dietary fat.

Ormond's disease—idiopathic retroperitoneal fibrosis.

ORN (osteoradionecrosis).

Ornidyl (eflornithine).

OR1—incorporates all components of the surgical suite into a single electronic system. Developed by Karl Storz Endoscopy-America, Inc., the system includes control of endoscopic devices with options for activation by touch screen and remote control, all using PC-based architecture.

orotracheal intubation, NRSI (non-rapid sequence induction).

orphan drug—a drug used to treat a rare disease for which the manufacturer could not expect to recoup drug development and production

orphan drug *(cont.)*
costs due to the small number of patients who would use the drug. The Orphan Drug Act supports the development of orphan drugs by allowing tax credits to the pharmaceutical company and shortened FDA approval time.

Orr-Loygue transabdominal proctopexy—for complete rectal prolapse.

Orr rectal prolapse repair.

ortho—when an ophthalmologist uses the word *ortho*, it usually refers to *orthophoric* or *orthophoria*.

Ortho-Cept (progesterone desogestrel, ethinyl estradiol)—oral contraceptive.

Orthoclone OKT3—anti-CD3 monoclonal antibody for acute graft rejection in kidney transplant patients.

Ortho Dx—an electromedical stimulator for postsurgical knee rehabilitation.

OrthoDyn—bone substitute material used to fill voids in bone as well as in multiple applications for fracture repair.

Ortho-Est (estropipate).

Ortho-evac—a postoperative autotransfusion system designed especially for orthopedic use, including knee, hip, and spinal surgery.

Orthofix Cervical-Stim—noninvasive cervical bone growth stimulator.

Orthofix external fixator.

Orthofix intramedullary nail.

OrthoGen/OsteoGen—an implantable stimulator for nonunion of fractures.

Ortho HCV 2.0 ELISA test system—a blood screening test for hepatitis C. Detects antibodies to three HCV antigens.

Ortho-Ice Multipaks—a complete system for cryotherapy (cold) or heat therapy. Special holders allow application at any joint.

Ortholav—equipment for pulsed irrigation and suction. Used with Ritter double- or single-orifice tip or Yankauer multi- or single-orifice tip.

Ortholinum (botulinum toxin, type F)—used to treat torticollis. See *Clostridium botulinum toxin, type A*.

Ortholoc Advantim knee revision system.

Ortho-mune—the brand name used by Ortho Diagnostic Systems, Inc., for its line of monoclonal antibodies, which includes OKT4 and OKT8, and many others.

OrthoNail—an intramedullary fixation device.

OrthoPak II bone growth stimulator—a bone growth stimulator with electrodes. The battery-powered OrthoPak II weighs only 4 ounces and can be mounted directly on a cast or carried from a belt clip or in a pocket.

orthopedic hardware—wires, pins, screws, plates, and other devices of metal or other material implanted in or attached to bone in the course of a surgical procedure.

orthophoria—parallelism of the visual axes; the normal muscle balance.

orthoplast jacket—a specially molded jacket used for correction of scoliosis. It is worn for 23 hours a day until skeletal maturity has taken place or until the spine has straightened and correction can be maintained out of the jacket.

orthopnea, three-pillow; two-pillow—difficulty breathing unless positioned in a semisitting position. Often measured roughly by how many pillows the patient needs in order to breathe comfortably while sleeping upright in a semi-sitting position.

Ortho-Prefest (17[beta]-estradiol/nor-gestimate)—drug to treat vasomotor symptoms associated with menopause, treatment of vulvar and vaginal atrophy, and prevention of osteoporosis.

Orthoset cement—radiopaque bone cement.

orthosis—an orthopedic appliance or apparatus applied externally to correct deformities, to support or improve the function of a joint. See also *prosthesis.*
Caligamed ankle
Gillette joint
GunSlinger shoulder
LSU (Louisiana State University) reciprocation-gait
Malleoloc anatomic ankle
MultiBoot
Newport MC hip
Oklahoma ankle joint
ORLAU swivel walker
Rebel knee
Rochester HKAFO
Select joint
SportsFit thumb
Thera-Soft hand/wrist
TLSO (thoracolumbosacral orthosis)
Toronto parapodium
UCBL (University of California Berkeley Laboratory)
Viscoheel K, Viscoheel N
Viscoheel SofSpot

Orthosorb absorbable pin—absorbable fixation device used to fix fractures of the phalanges or metacarpals. The pin is absorbed within six months.

orthotopic transplantation—transplantation of an organ and placing it in the recipient in its normal anatomic position. Examples: heart and liver transplantation.

Orthovisc—naturally derived hyaluronic acid used in intra-articular injection to reduce joint pain and other symptoms related to osteoarthritis.

Ortolani's sign—a click at the hip joint, in congenital dislocated hip.

Orudis KT (ketoprofen)—a nonprescription-strength version of the prescription pain killer Orudis, now sold over-the-counter.

Oruvail (ketoprofen)—a once-a-day form of the nonsteroidal anti-inflammatory drug ketoprofen.

O.S. (*oculus sinister*, left eye).

OSA (obstructive sleep apnea).

OSCAR—an ultrasonic bone cement removal system used in hip revision procedures.

Osciflator balloon inflation syringe—used in angioplasty procedures.

oscillating saw (Ortho).

OSCM (oil-soluble contrast medium).

OS-5/Plus, OS-5/Plus 2 brace—noncustom multifunctional knee brace for postoperative and rehabilitation applications. Made by Omni Scientific (OS).

OSI arthroscopy tools, including the well-leg holder, the arthroscopic leg holder, and the extremity elevator.

Osler's nodes—small tender nodules (2 to 5 mm in diameter) seen about the tips of the fingers or toes; may be found in patients with bacterial endocarditis, acute and subacute.

OsmoCyte pillow—a highly absorptive wound dressing that cushions the wound and absorbs excess moisture/exudate over a longer period of time than a standard dressing.

osmolality—a test of concentration of a solution. It is used to determine the concentration of urine or serum, and results are expressed in milliosmoles

osmolality *(cont.)*
  per kilogram (mOsm/kg). Cf. *osmolarity.*
osmolarity—concentration of an osmotic solution, e.g., urine or blood serum; expressed in osmoles per liter (Osm/l). Cf. *osmolality.*
osseous—bony.
ossification of the posterior longitudinal ligament (OPLL)—one of the well-known causes of cervical radiculomyelopathy.
Ossoff-Karlen laryngoscope (ENT).
Ostase biochemical marker of bone turnover—a blood test that aids in management of postmenopausal osteoporosis. See *Access Ostase.*
osteal—bony (osseous). Cf. *ostial.*
osteoarthritis radiographic grading
  grade I, small osteophytes
  grade II, osteophytes without joint
    space impairment
  grade III, osteophytes with moderate
    loss of normal joint space
  grade IV, osteophytes with significant loss of joint space and
    sclerosis of subchondral bone
  grade V, grade IV with subluxation
osteochondral defect (OCD) **of the glenoid fossa**—occurs most often as a result of acute trauma and has a high association with instability, labral tear, and intra-articular bodies.
osteochondritis dissecans *(not* dessicans)—see *König disease.*
Osteo-Clage cable system—used in orthopedic cerclage fixation.
OsteoGen HA (hydroxyapatite)—dental implant material.
Osteogenics BoneSource—a synthetic bone replacement material.
Osteo-Gram—a bone density test for osteoporosis used in conjunction with the OsteoView desktop hand x-ray device.

osteomanipulative therapy (chiropractic).
Osteomark—an enzyme-linked monoclonal antibody-based agent for monitoring the breakdown of bone mass, used to track developing osteoporosis and response to treatment.
Osteomark test (NTx Assay)—a simple urine test that measures the rate of bone resorption or loss.
osteomesopyknosis—a rare, benign osteosclerotic bone disorder limited to the axial skeleton and diagnosed from radiographs of the area. It is distinguished from superficially similar sclerosing bone conditions such as osteopetrosis, pyknodysostosis, renal osteodystrophy, and atypical axial osteomalacia.
Osteonics-HA coated implant (Ortho).
Osteonics Omnifit-HA hip stem.
Osteopatch—a transdermal patch used in the diagnosis and management of osteoporosis. It collects sweat and checks for biochemical markers of bone loss.
osteophytes—bony excrescence or osseous outgrowth. See *bridging osteophytes.*
Osteosal—rapid office test to detect increased bone breakdown indicating the risk of osteoporosis and to monitor the adequacy of therapy.
Osteoset—bone graft substitute.
OsteoStim—implantable bone growth stimulator.
osteotomy
  Chiari medial displacement pelvic
  Kalamchi
  lateral acetabular shelf
  Mayday
  Pember circumacetabular
  Salter
  Steel

OsteoView—a self-contained desktop device for taking hand x-rays. It is used in conjunction with OsteoGram bone density test in the diagnosis of osteoporosis.

OsteoView 2000—digital imaging system used to diagnose osteoporosis and arthritis.

ostial—pertaining to an ostium (an opening). Cf. *osteal*.

ostiomeatal—denoting the opening of the auditory, nasal, or urinary meatus. The word does not have anything to do with osteo (bone).

ostiomeatal stent (ENT)—a temporary tube placed following functional endoscopic sinus surgery for the purpose of preventing adhesions and maintaining patency of a middle meatal antrostomy. In children, the stent allows postoperative suctioning, usually necessary after about three weeks, without general anesthesia.

ostium—opening into a tubular organ.

os trigonum—a separate ossicle of the lateral tubercle of the posterior aspect of the talus of the ankle. A true os trigonum forms as a secondary ossification center which does not fuse with the talus after skeletal maturation.

os trigonum syndrome (also known as *talar compression syndrome*)—produces significant pain due to inflammation of the ankle joint capsule, a fracture of the os trigonum, or pathology of the Steida process of the talus.

OTA (oligoteratoasthenozoospermia).

OTC (over-the-counter) **drug**—generally considered safe for consumers to use (as determined by the FDA) if the label directions and warnings are properly followed. Available without a prescription.

OTFC (oral transmucosal fentanyl citrate, Oralet)—fentanyl available in a candy-like oral tablet (to be sucked), to relieve severe pain in pediatric patients.

otoacoustic emission (OAE) **testing**—a hearing test for patients who cannot (because of disability or because they are too young) give adequate feedback required in the standard hearing test.

OtoLam—laser technology for treatment of middle ear infections in children, said to sharply reduce antibiotic utilization and help to avoid need for insertion of ventilation tubes in the operating room.

otospongiosis/otosclerosis syndrome—a type of genetic deafness. Treatment with sodium fluoride in very low doses is a promising therapy where there is early detection of this syndrome.

Ototemp 3000—measures core body temperature by reading the temperature of the tympanic membrane, without actually touching the membrane, giving an accurate reading in five seconds.

ototoxic—anything harmful to the structures or process of hearing, such as some drugs causing tinnitus, or extremely loud noises (or music). Aminoglycoside antibiotics are well known for their ototoxic side effects. "She denied the use of ototoxic drugs and has no history of ear trauma or recurrent infections."

Ottawa Ankle Rules (OARs)—a decision-making process used by orthopedists to decide if an x-ray is necessary to evaluate an acute ankle

Ottawa Ankle Rules *(cont.)*
injury. Currently, this assessment is validated for adult use only, but it is being tested for pediatric use. Adult statistics indicate that this simple assessment could safely decrease the use of x-rays by 25%.

OTW (over the wire).

O.U., OU *(oculus uterque,* each eye).

Ouchterlony double diffusion technique—"Circulating immune complexes, C3, hemolytic complement, and precipitating antibodies by Ouchterlony are pending."

OutBound—a disposable syringe infusion system used in the administration of chemotherapy.

outcomes management—use of monitored data in a way that allows individuals and healthcare systems and providers to learn from experience and make changes in the way services are provided and administered. Also called *outcomes measurement* and *outcomes monitoring.*

Outerbridge ridge (named for R. E. Outerbridge, M.D., British Columbia, Canada)—a ridge of varying height, crossing the medial femoral condyle at its osteochondral junction, described by Outerbridge in 1961. He suggested that at least one cause of patellar chondromalacia might be friction against the medial patellar facet cartilage as the patella rides this ridge in normal movement of the knee. See *Outerbridge scale.*

Outerbridge scale—for assessing joint damage or articular surface damage in chondromalacia patellae:
grade 1, softening and swelling of the cartilage.
grade 2, fragmentation and fissuring in an area half an inch or less in diameter.

grade 3, same as grade 2, but involves an area more than half an inch.
grade 4, erosion of cartilage down to bone.

out-in-out technique—for suturing in an intraocular lens (posterior chamber) for aphakia.

outlet view (Radiol)—an x-ray showing a tangential view of the coracoacromial arch in the sagittal plane of the scapula.

outpatient endometrial resection/ablation (OPERA).

outpatient endometrial resection/ablation (OPERA) **specialized tissue aspirating resectoscope** (STAR).

outrigger splint—used following metacarpophalangeal joint arthroplasty.

oval window—see *vestibular window.*

OvaRex MAb—immunotherapy for treatment of advanced ovarian cancer.

ovarian hyperstimulation syndrome (OHSS)—a complication of hormonal therapy for in vitro fertilization. This syndrome includes massive ovarian enlargement, ascites, pleural effusions, and electrolyte and coagulation imbalances.

ovarian remnant syndrome—a condition in which remnants of ovarian cortex left behind after surgical removal of the ovaries become functional and cystic. It most often occurs in patients who have experienced a difficult oophorectomy.

O-Vax—a therapeutic vaccine for advanced ovarian cancer.

OVD (ophthalmic viscosurgical device) —see *Cellugel OVD.*

overshooting—failure to stop a voluntary movement when its goal or purpose has been achieved.

over-the-counter (OTC) **drug.**

Oves cervical cap—for use in artificial insemination procedures.

Oves fertility cap—used by couples having difficulty conceiving as a result of low sperm counts, reduced sperm motility, or a chronically hostile vaginal environment (such as one caused by a yeast infection).

OV-1 surgical keratometer (OV, Ophthalmic Ventures).

OvuStick—a urinary dipstick used to detect luteinizing hormone surge in infertility patients.

oxandrolone (Oxandrin)—an anabolic steroid for growth disorders in boys; also for muscle wasting and weakness in AIDS patients.

ox cell hemolysin test.

Oxifirst—fetal oxygen monitoring system.

Oxilan (ioxilan)—a low-osmolar, triiodinated radiographic contrast agent for intra-arterial and intravenous administration.

oximeter—a photoelectric device that measures the oxygen saturation of the blood. "Oxygen saturation was monitored by ear or finger oximeter." Used in assessing sleep disorders by polysomnogram. There is no "air" oximeter.

oxothiazolidine carboxylate (Procysteine).

Oxsoralen (methoxsalen).

oxyazolidinones—a new class of antibiotics that disrupts the initiation of bacterial protein synthesis at an earlier stage of the cycle than other antibiotics. The bacteria are then unable to manufacture proteins and are unable to reproduce. An example is the antiobiotic Zyvox (linezolid).

oxycodone and acetaminophen capsules—a Duramed product that has bioequivalency and therapeutic interchangeability with Tylox.

oxycodone HCl (Roxicodone)—analgesic with habit-forming properties similar to morphine. Used for moderate to moderately severe pain, particularly in an oncology setting.

Oxycontin (oxycodone HCl)—used for providing prolonged relief of moderate to severe pain.

oxygen cisternography—technique for the diagnosis of acoustic tumors. In some cases where air will not enter the internal auditory canal, Pantopaque may be introduced into the posterior fossa for cisternography.

oxygen saturation—see SaO_2 (arterial oxygen saturation).

Oxygent (perflubron emulsion)—temporary blood substitute used in surgery, reducing the need for donor blood.

Oxylator EM-100 emergency resuscitation device.

oxymetholone (Anadrol-50)—for anemia resulting from treatment with chemotherapy drugs.

Oxymizer—oxygen-conserving device used to provide adequate oxygen saturation at lower flow rates. It permits a portable oxygen source to last longer, thus allowing patients to be away from their primary oxygen source for longer periods.

oxyphenbutazone—a nonsteroidal anti-inflammatory drug.

oxyphil cell.

oxytocin challenge test (OCT).

Oxytrak pulse oximeter and Dinamap blood pressure monitor—measures oxygen saturation.

P, p

p—If you can't find a word anywhere, try looking in the *p's* in a dictionary. Often an initial *p* is silent, as in *phthisis, pneumonia, psoas, psoriasis, psyllium, pterygium, pterygoid,* and *ptosis.*

Pa (pascal).

PAB-Esc-C (Platinol, Adriamycin, bleomycin, escalating doses of Cytoxan)—chemotherapy protocol.

PAC (papular acrodermatitis of childhood). Cf. *Gianotti-Crosti syndrome.*

PACE (Platinol, Adriamycin, cyclophosphamide, etoposide)—chemotherapy protocol.

Pace bipolar pacing catheter.

pacemaker (cardiac)
  Activitrax
  Addvent atrioventricular
  Autima II dual chamber
  Dash
  DDD
  Diamond II DDR
  dual chamber Medtronic.Kappa 400
  Elite dual chamber rate-responsive
  Enterra
  Entity
  Ergos O_2

pacemaker *(cont.)*
  escape
  Integrity AFx AutoCapture
  Jade II SSI
  Kairos
  Kappa 400 Series
  Medtronic temporary
  Micro Minix
  Pacesetter Synchrony
  Relay cardiac
  Ruby II DDD
  SAVVI synchronous
  Topaz II SSIR
  Trilogy DC+
  Trilogy SR+
  Triumph VR
  Unity-C
  Ventak AICD
  Vitatron Diamond II

pacemaker adaptive rate—the rate that the pacemaker adapts automatically to increases or decreases in the natural (intrinsic) heart rate. Also, *rate-adaptive, rate-responsive, or rate-modulated.*

pacemaker code system—a three-letter code often used to describe various types of pacemakers. The first letter

pacemaker code *(cont.)*
represents the chamber of the heart which is stimulated to contract (i.e., paced) by an attached electrode. The second letter represents the chamber(s) in which the pacemaker can sense ongoing normal electrical activity. The third letter indicates the type of response (i.e., mode) of which the pacemaker is capable (inhibited from competing with normal heart contractions, triggered by abnormal heart activity). Example: A DDD pacemaker serves the electrical activity of both the atrium and ventricle, paces (stimulates) both the atrium and ventricle to beat, may cause (trigger) the atrium to contract while sending no signal (inhibited) to the ventricle depending on what natural electrical activity is occurring in the heart at that time.

Pacesetter APS—a portable, pocket-size pacemaker programmer.

Pacesetter Synchrony pacemaker—a permanent rate-responsive dual chamber pacemaker.

Pacesetter Trilogy DR+ pulse generator.

pachometer—instrument that measures the thickness of the cornea.

Pach-Pen—a device that measures corneal thickness in thousandths of a millimeter.

Pacifico post-suture inflation technique—reduces postoperatively induced astigmatism using CU-8 bicurve needle.

Pacis BCG—immunotherapy against bladder cancer.

pack-year smoking history—as "The patient has a 50-pack-year smoking history." The patient has smoked a pack a day for 50 years, or two packs a day for 25 years, or five packs a day for ten years (or ten packs a day for five years!). It is the packs per day multiplied by the number of years of smoking; the cumulative result is the important factor.

paclitaxel (Taxol).

PACS (Picture Archiving and Communications Systems).

PACU (postanesthesia care unit)—a newer name for the recovery room.

PAD (public access defibrillation)—a program that seeks to distribute external defibrillators at specific sites where sudden cardiac arrest may frequently occur, e.g., public places (such as airports and casinos) where large numbers of older people may be under stress.

Padgett baseline pinch gauge—records thumb-finger grasp.

Padgett hydraulic hand dynamometer—measures hand strength.

pad test—test for urinary incontinence, confirmed by one gram or more of urinary leakage in 60 minutes.

Paecilomyces variotiia—a fungus that is an infrequent human pathogen. It has caused complications associated with prosthetic cardiac valves, synthetic lens implants, and cerebrospinal fluid shunts.

PAFD (percutaneous abscess and fluid drainage).

PAG (periaqueductal gray) **matter**. Stimulation of the PAG matter with deep brain electrodes inhibits pain. See *PVG matter*.

Pagoclone—used for treatment of anxiety and panic attacks.

PAH acid (para-aminohippuric)—used in kidney function test. See *Stamey test*.

PAI (plasminogen activator inhibitor-1).

PAIgG (platelet-associated IgG).

PainBuster disposable infusion pain management kit—based on I-Flow's elastomeric infusion technology, it provides continuous infusion of a non-narcotic local anesthetic (bupivacaine HCl) directly into the intraoperative site for postoperative pain management for a 24- to 48-hour period.

pain management techniques
(electrically generated)
CES (cranial electrical stimulation)
DCS (dorsal column stimulator)
galvanic stimulation
HVS (high-voltage stimulation)
interferential current therapy
iontophoresis
Liss CES
LV-MS (low-voltage microampere stimulation)
PEMT (pulsed electromagnetic therapy)
PENS (percutaneous electrical nerve stimulation)
TENS (transcutaneous electrical nerve stimulation)

painter's encephalopathy—chronic organic brain syndrome secondary to exposure to fumes from some types of paints.

PAI-1 (plasminogen activator inhibitor)—substance that inhibits the activity of tissue plasminogen activator (t-PA) and thus is felt to be associated with increased cardiovascular risk.

PAI (Preadmission Acuity Inquiry) **tool**—designed to assess functional levels of independence and acuity of applicants to long-term care facilities.

PAK (percutaneous access kit)—see *Denver PAK*.

palisading (Path)—a lining up of cells such that their long axis is perpendicular to some other structure. Usage: peripheral palisading.

palladium 103 (^{103}Pd) **implantation**—ultrasound-guided transperineal implantation as brachytherapy for prostate cancer.

pallidal brain stimulation—treatment for Parkinson's disease. A thin wire electrode implanted in the globus pallidus of the brain is connected to a pulse generator implanted in the chest. The pulse generator sends an electric current to the brain, jamming nerve signals from the globus pallidus.

pallidotomy guided by microelectrode recording—may be more successful in treating Parkinson's disease than the traditional electrical stimulation pallidotomy.

palmar beak ligament (Ortho)—"It has been suggested that instability resulting from incompetence of the palmar beak ligament is responsible for initiating the progression of degenerative joint disease."

palmar erythema (erythema palmare)—redness of the palms that persists; it may be seen in patients with liver disease, rheumatoid arthritis, and a number of other diverse medical problems.

Palmaz balloon-expandable stent—for use in patients with narrowed or blocked iliac arteries after unsuccessful balloon angioplasty.

Palmaz Corinthian—transhepatic biliary stent and delivery system.

Palmaz-Schatz stent (PSS)—a balloon-expandable articulated, slotted tube stent comprised of rigid segments attached by a central articulation.

Palmaz-Schatz stent *(cont.)*
The biliary stent is used to treat biliary duct stenosis. The coronary stent is used to teat focal saphenous vein graft.

Palmaz vascular stent—a cylinder of stainless steel mesh. The stent is placed over a balloon catheter and inserted into an occluded artery after angioplasty is performed. The balloon is inflated once the catheter is positioned at the site of the occlusion. The balloon is then deflated, but the stent retains its expanded shape and remains permanently at the site of the occlusion, holding the vessel walls apart and facilitating blood flow. Also, *Palmaz-Schatz stent.*

Palmer classification of cartilage tear.

palmomental—refers to the palm of the hand and the mentalis muscle. See *palmomental reflex.*

palmomental reflex—contraction of the ipsilateral mentalis and orbicularis oris muscles, with slight elevation and retraction of the angle of the mouth in response to scratching the thenar area of the hand; seen occasionally in an exaggerated form in patients with corticospinal tract lesions. Also called *palmomental reflex of Marinesco-Radovici.*

palpation—the act of feeling with the fingers in examination of the body. Inspection, palpation, and auscultation are the three methods of examination used most. Cf. *palpitation, papillation.*

palpitation—the subjective feeling of an irregular or abnormally rapid heart beat. Cf. *palpation, papillation.*

palsy—see *tardy palsy.*

Palumbo knee brace—custom-fitted knee brace used with chondromalacia patellae.

PAM (potential acuity meter)—used in testing vision.

pamidronate disodium (Aredia)—used to decrease the hypercalcemia associated with malignancy. Also known as *disodium pamidronate.*

PAN (periodic alternating nystagmus).

Panacryl absorbable suture—used for soft tissue approximation and/or ligation during general and orthopedic (tendon and ligament repair) procedures. It is used for extended wound support up to six months.

Panafil enzymatic debriding agent.

Panafil White ointment—for wound debridement.

pancreatic enzyme therapy—used in treatment of pain in chronic pancreatitis.

pancreaticoduodenectomy—surgical resection of the primary tumor in peripancreatic cancer.

pancreatic polypeptide (PP).

pancreatic sepsis in acute pancreatitis—treated with therapeutic concentrations of antibiotics in the pancreatic tissue in pancreatitis.

pancreatoduodenectomy, pylorus preserving (PPPD).

Pancrecarb MS-8 (pancrelipase)—used for pancreatic enzyme insufficiency.

pancrelipase—used for cystic fibrosis therapy.

pan-cultured—as in "The urine was pan-cultured." The specimen is cultured to determine which organisms are present and to determine which antibiotics are specific for that organism. The prefix *pan* means *all, every.*

PANDO (primary acquired nasolacrimal duct obstruction).

P&K (Polaroids and Kodachromes)—photographs of specimens. "P&K were taken," or "Polaroids and Kodachromes were taken."

panic disorder patients—function assessed by two types of medical outcomes study: (1) the 20-item short-form survey that covers physical functioning, role functioning, social functioning, mental health, current health perception, and bodily pain; and (2) the 36-item short-form survey which covers all of the areas in the 20-item survey and also includes energy/fatigue and general health perceptions.

Panje ("pan-gee") **voice button**—a laryngeal prosthesis to improve esophageal speech in patients who have had laryngectomies. See also *Blom-Singer valve,* a similar prosthetic device.

Pannaz (phenylephrine and phenylpropanolamine)—decongestant.

panniculus, hanging. See *apron.*

PanoGauze hydrogel-impregnated gauze.

PanoPlex hydrogel dressing.

Panoramic 200 nonmydriatic ophthalmoscope—combines advances in laser and optical imaging technology to digitally capture over 80% of the retina in less than 1/2 second without use of dilating drops or contact with the eye. The system is patient-activated and uses very low levels of light.

panretinal photocoagulation (PRP).

Panretin (alitretinoin) **topical gel**—treatment for AIDS-related Kaposi's sarcoma cutaneous lesions.

pan-sensitive—sensitive to everything.

PANTA (polymyxin B, amphotericin B, nalidixic acid, trimethoprim, and azlocillin).

pantaloon embolus—see *saddle embolus.*

pantaloon hernia—results when direct and indirect hernias occur simultaneously. Also called *combined hernia.*

pantoprazole (Pantozol)—a drug for the treatment of erosive esophagitis.

Pantozol (pantoprazole).

pants-over-vest repair (Surg).

PAP (peroxidase-antiperoxidase)—see *immunoperoxidase stain.*

papaverine topical gel—used to treat sexual dysfunction in spinal cord injury patients.

Papercuff—a disposable blood pressure cuff with an outer paper layer that doesn't stretch, thus transferring all of the inflation pressure to the underlying artery. The inner plastic layer does stretch, conforming closely to the patient's arm, resulting in a significantly higher pressure pulse amplitude being transmitted to cuff signal detecting devices.

papilla, optic—point at which the optic nerve fibers leave the eyeball. Also called *optic disk.*

papillation—the presence of small projections or elevations (as the papillae on the tongue). Cf. *palpation, palpitation.*

papilledema—swelling of the nerve head from increased intracranial pressure or interference with the venous return from the eye.

papilloma, inverted schneiderian—see *schneiderian papilloma.*

papillotomy—incision of a papilla, as of the duodenal papilla. See *laparoscopic transcystic papillotomy.*

PapNet—increases sensitivity of standard Pap tests by combining automated microscopy and computerized analysis to reduce screening errors.

papova—an acronym for a group of DNA viruses thought to cause warts in humans. (See *HPV.*) Comes from the first two letters of the names of the viruses:

pa   papilloma virus
po   polyoma virus
va   vacuolative virus

PAPP A (pregnancy-associated plasma protein A).

Pap Plus speculoscopy—a visual cervical screening exam, using a small disposable blue-white light source called Speculite, as an adjunct to the traditional Pap smear.

papular acrodermatitis of childhood (PAC).

PAPVR (partial anomalous pulmonary venous return).

para—the number of times a woman has given birth. This word is frequently followed by four numbers separated by hyphens (for example, para 3-1-0-3). The first numeral refers to the number of full-term deliveries, in this case three; the second indicates the number of premature births (one); the third numeral is the number of abortions or miscarriages (none); the fourth numeral indicates the number of living children (three). See also *gravida*; *GPMAL.*

para–aminohippuric (PAH).

paraconal fascia—relatively unknown fascia that is located between the lateral aspect of the perirenal fascia and the posterior parietal peritoneum. Important because it protects delicate retroperitoneal organs (duodenum, pancreas, celiac axis, and superior mesenteric artery). Locating this condensed fascia is an important step in the dissection of the high retroperitoneum in advanced videoendoscopy.

paradoxus—see *pulsus paradoxus.*

paraesophageal hernia, type II—occurs when the distal esophagus is located in its normal position, anchored by the phrenoesophageal ligament, and a defect in the diaphragm allows the stomach and hernia sac to travel into the chest. Because this condition is usually asymptomatic, it may reach tremendous size with complex herniation before diagnosis is made. Surgical correction is universally advised due to the risk of sudden catastrophic gastric volvulus and death.

parafascicular thalamotomy (PFT).

paraffin block or **section**—tissue embedded in paraffin for sectioning and subsequent staining for microscopy. See *permanent section.*

Paragon coronary stent.

parallel squat exercise—a rehabilitation exercise used for patients without an anterior cruciate ligament. The patient squats until the knee is at 90° and the femur is parallel to the floor.

paramagnetic artifact (MRI)—can be seen in the soft tissues after surgery.

Paramax cruciate guide system—simplifies endoscopic cruciate reconstruction, using soft tissue and bony component grafts.

parameter—one of a number of ways to test, describe, or evaluate a person or an object. Cf. *perimeter.*

Paraplatin (carboplatin)—chemotherapy drug.

Parasmillie—double-bladed knife for patellar tendon graft harvesting.

parathormone (parathyroid hormone, PTH).

Paratrend 7 and 7+—a tiny sensor placed in the brain for monitoring blood gases of brain-injured patients.

paravariceally—beside a varix.

parecoxib—an injectable COX-2 inhibitor for hospital-based management of acute pain.

parenteral—a route of drug administration not involving the gastrointestinal tract (intravenous, intramuscular). Cf. *enteral*.

Parham bands—used to hold the fracture fragments of long bones securely in place.

Parietex—composite mesh for hernia surgery. It contains a resorbable collagen layer to prevent development of intra-abdominal adhesions, and the product can be used in either open or laparoscopic incisional and ventral hernias.

Parinaud's oculoglandular syndrome—granulomatous conjunctivitis with swelling in preauricular lymph nodes. It is caused by *Bartonella henselae* infection.

Paritene—mesh graft for hernia surgery. The material has a larger weave designed to provide greater elasticity, less density, and less rigidity.

parity—a woman's reproductive history.

PARK (photoastigmatic refractive keratectomy)—a laser surgery procedure for correction of astigmatism. The cornea is reshaped using a cold-beam laser that removes corneal tissue without damaging surrounding tissue. The reshaped cornea allows light to focus directly on the retina for clearer distance vision.

Park blade septostomy (Cardio).

Parker-Kerr closed method—of end-to-end enteroenterostomy.

Parker-Kerr intestinal clamps.

Parkland formula—used to guide initial fluid resuscitation during the first 24 hours after burn trauma. The formula calls for 4 mL over the first 24 hours. Half of the fluid is administered over the first 8 hours post burn, and the remaining half is administered over the next 16 hours. The volume of fluid given is based on the time elapsed since the burn.

Parona's space—the tissue plane over the pronator quadratus in the distal forearm that is deep to the ulnar and radial bursae.

parosteal osteosarcoma—a low-grade, well-differentiated, malignant tumor arising from the surface of the bone. Although similar in meaning, parosteal is used as the disease entity modifier, not periosteal.

paroxetine (Paxil)—a 5HT (serotonin) receptor blocker which inhibits the reuptake of serotonin and increases levels of it. Used to treat depression which is caused by low levels of serotonin.

paroxysmal atrial tachycardia (PAT).

paroxysmal nocturnal dyspnea (PND).

paroxysmal nocturnal hemoglobinuria (PNH).

paroxysmal supraventricular tachycardia (PSVT).

PARP (poly ADP-ribose polymerase)—naturally occurring enzyme, overproduction of which is believed responsible for brain cell death in stroke victims. Research is ongoing to develop a PARP inhibitor.

Parrot's sign—dilation of the pupils when the skin of the neck is pinched, as in meningitis.

Parsol 1789—an ingredient commonly used in European, Canadian, and Australian sunscreens, now approved for wider use in suncare products distributed in the U.S.

partial agonist—a compound that possesses both agonist and antagonist properties.

partial anomalous pulmonary venous return (PAPVR).

partial encircling endocardial ventriculotomy—see *ventriculotomy.*

partial liquid ventilation—a technique that involves introducing the chemical perflubron into a premature infant's malfunctioning lungs and then pumping oxygen into the liquid. Because it is so efficient at absorbing oxygen, perflubron allows lower ventilator pressure settings. Standard ventilator therapy with surfactants at high force can cause permanent lung injury and lead to bronchopulmonary dysplasia. See *perflubron.*

partial saturation technique—a magnetic resonance technique in which single excitation pulses are delivered to tissue at intervals equal to or shorter than T1.

party wall—a wall between two contiguous structures.

parvovirus—see *human parvovirus B19.*

PAS (periodic acid-Schiff) **stain**—a test for collagen disease and also for the presence of Whipple's disease. See *Whipple's disease.*

PAS (physician-assisted suicide).

PAS (pulsatile antiembolic system).

PASA (proximal articular set angle) (Ortho).

PASAT (paced auditory serial addition task)—a test in which the patient is asked to mentally add a series of numbers from 1 to 10, stating the sum as each new number is presented. Used to assess closed head trauma.

pascal (Pa)—unit of measurement of pressure in the SI system. You will be hearing about this in relation to blood gases. Blood pressures will most probably continue to be given in millimeters of mercury (mmHg). See *SI, International System.*

Paser (aminosalicylic acid)—used in treatment of tuberculosis, in combination with other agents.

P.A.S. (peripheral access system) **Port catheter**—implanted in the antecubital fossa for administration of chemotherapy drugs, for long-term TPN, or for administration of intravenous antibiotics. Also made with double lumens. *P.A.S. Port* is a trademark.

P.A.S. Port Fluoro-Free—implantable peripheral access system that incorporates the Cath-Finder system that tracks the catheter tip during placement without the use of fluoroscopy. Implanted in the antecubital fossa for administration of chemotherapy drugs, for long-term TPN, or for administration of intravenous antibiotics. Also made with double lumens.

Passage catheter—balloon catheter used to dilate biliary strictures. Passage is a trade name.

Passager introducing sheath.

Passy-Muir tracheostomy speaking valve—an attachment that allows ventilator-dependent patients to speak more easily.

PASTA (polarity-altered spectral selective acquisition) **imaging** (MRI).

Past Feelings and Acts of Violence (PFAV) **Scale**—assesses such indicators of violence as past history of arrests, violence against family mem-

Past Feelings *(cont.)*

bers, violence against strangers, use of weapons.

past-pointing *(not* passed pointing)—a test used to determine the presence of incoordination in voluntary movements. When the patient is asked to touch the examiner's finger or nose, or his own nose, he goes past it. A variant of this test is used in otolaryngology to test for vestibular problems.

PASYS ("paces") and **PASYS ST**—a single chamber cardiac pacing system.

PAT (paroxysmal atrial tachycardia).

Patanol (olopatadine hydrochloride ophthalmic solution)—for treatment of allergic conjunctivitis.

patches, Peyer's—see *Peyer's patches.*

patella alta—a "high-riding" patella, associated with some knee problems.

patella baja—caused by abnormal shortness of the patellar tendon, a low-riding patella. See *patella alta.*

Patella's disease—pyloric stenosis occurring in tuberculous patients after fibrous stenosis. Named for an Italian physician, V. Patella.

patellaplasty *(not* patelloplasty).

patellar apprehension test (Ortho).

pathergy—refers to the phenomenon of trivial trauma evoking new lesions or exacerbating old ones, similar to the clinical course of some keloids.

Pathfinder—a microcatheter system, manufactured by Cardima, used in the treatment of atrial fibrillation.

Pathfinder DFA (direct fluorescent antigen) **test**—detects genital *Chlamydia trachomatis.*

pathogen (including bacteria, fungi, parasites, and viruses)—a quick-reference list. See individual entries.

pathogen *(cont.)*

Acanthamoeba keratitis
Achromobacter lwoffi
Acinetobacter lwoffi
Actinobacillus actinomycetem comitans
adenovirus
aeroallergen
Aeromonas sobria
Afipia felis
Alcaligenes bookeri
Alternaria
Alteromonas putrefaciens
Andes virus
Aquaspirillum itersonii
arbovirus (arthropod-borne virus)
Arcanobacterium haemolyticum
ARV (AIDS-related virus)
Aspergillus
avian influenza A (H5N1) virus
bacillus Calmette-Guérin (BCG)
Bacillus circulans
Bacillus coagulans
Bacteroides corrodens
baculovirus (genetically engineered)
Bartonella bacilliformis
Bartonella elizabethae
Bartonella henselae
Bartonella quintana
Basidiomycetes
Bayou (BAY) virus
Bdellovibrio
Bio-Tract
Black Creek Canal virus
Bordetella
Borrelia burgdorferi
Branhamella catarrhalis
Brevibacterium linens
Calmette-Guérin, bacillus (BCG)
Campylobacter fetus
Campylobacter jejuni
Candida albicans
Candida glabrata
Cardiobacterium hominis

pathogen *(cont.)*
Chaetomium
Chlamydia pneumoniae
Chlamydia trachomatis
CobactinE
Coxiella burnetii
Cryptococcus neoformans
Cryptosporidium
Curvularia
Dermatophagoides farinae
Dermatophagoides pteronyssinus
Döderlein's bacillus
Ducrey's bacillus
Eaton agent *(Mycoplasma pneumoniae)*
E. coli H157:H7
Eikenella corrodens
Entamoeba histolytica
Enterobacter liquefaciens
Enterobacter sakazakii
Epstein-Barr virus (EBV)
Francisella tularensis
Friedländer's bacillus
Fusarium (a slime mold)
gamma-herpesvirus
Gardnerella vaginalis
GAS (group A streptococcus)
Giardia lamblia
gram-negative organism
Haemophilus aphrophilus
Haemophilus ducreyi
Haemophilus vaginalis
Hafnia alvei
Helicobacter hepaticus
Helicobacter pylori
Helminthosporium
Herellea vaginicola
herpes simplex virus (HSV)
herpes zoster virus (HZV)
H5N1 virus
HHV-8 (human herpesvirus-8)
Hib or HIB (haemophilus influenza type B)
Histoplasma capsulatum

pathogen *(cont.)*
HIV (human immunodeficiency virus)
HIV-1E virus
Hormodendrum
HTLV-I retrovirus (human T-cell leukemia/lymphoma virus)
HTLV-III (human T-cell lymphotropic virus)
human immunodeficiency virus (HIV)
human herpesvirus 6 (HHV-6)
human mammary tumor virus (HMTV)
human papillomavirus (HPV)
human parvovirus B19 (HPV B19)
Iodamoeba buetschlii
Isospora parasite
Ixodes dammini
Ixodes pacificus
Juquitiba virus
Kingella kingae
Klebsiella oxytoca
Klebsiella pneumoniae
KSHV (Kaposi sarcoma-associated virus)
Laguna Negra virus
Legionella pneumophila
Leishmania donovani
lentivirus
leukovirus
lymphocytic choriomeningitis virus (LCMV)
MARSA (methicillin-aminoglyco side-resistant *Staphylococcus aureus)*
McKrae strain herpes simplex virus
MCV (molluscum contagiosum virus)
methicillin-resistant *Staphylococcus aureus* (MRSA)
Micrococcus sedentarius
Mima polymorpha
molluscum contagiosum virus (MCV)

pathogen *(cont.)*
monkeypox
Moraxella lwoffi
Morganella morganii
MRSA (methicillin-resistant
 Staphylococcus aureus)
Mycobacterium avium
Mycobacterium avium-intracellulare
 complex
Mycobacterium gordonae
Mycobacterium tuberculosis
Mycoplasma pneumoniae (Eaton
 agent)
Neisseria
Neisseria meningitidis
Nipah virus
Nocardia
nonsyncytium-inducing (NSI)
 variant of the AIDS virus
oncogenic retrovirus
opportunistic infection or organism
Paecilomyces variotiia
Penicillium
Penicillium marneffei
Phoma (a slime mold)
picornavirus
Pneumocystis carinii
porcine endogenous retrovirus
 (PERV)
Propionibacterium
Pseudallescheria boydii
Pseudomonas exotoxin
Pseudomonas maltophilia
Pseudomonas stutzeri
Psorospermium haeckelii
Pullularia (a slime mold)
respiratory syncytial virus (RSV)
retrovirus
Rhizopus nigricans
Rhodococcus equi
Rhodotorula
RNA virus
Rochalimaea henselae (changed to
 Bartonella henselae)

pathogen *(cont.)*
rotavirus
Rous sarcoma virus
Saccharomyces
Serratia liquefaciens
Serratia marcescens
Sin Nombre virus (SNV)
Spondylocladium
Staphylococcus aureus
Staphylococcus epidermidis
Stemphyllium
Stenotrophomonas (formerly
 Xanthomonas) *maltophilia*
Streptococcus milleri
Streptococcus mitis
togavirus
Torula histolytica
Toxoplasma gondii
Trichosporon beigelii
Ureaplasma urealyticum
vancomycin-resistant enterococci
 (VRE)
vancomycin-resistant *Enterococcus
 faecium* (VREF)
varicella zoster virus (VZV)
virus
virus-like infectious agent (VLIA)
West Nile virus
xenotropic donor organisms
Yersinia pestis
zoonotic retroviruses
pathognomonic—characteristic or diagnostic of a particular disease.
PATI (Penetrating Abdominal Trauma
Index).
patient-controlled analgesia (PCA)
system.
patient motion artifact (Radiol)—blurring on plain films; multiple bands
or ghosts, mostly in the phase-
encoding direction, on MRI scans.
Patient Outcomes Research Team
(PORT).

Patil stereotaxic system—for biopsy, hematoma evacuation, angiographic targeting, epilepsy implants, stereotaxic craniotomy.

patty or **pattie, cottonoid**—see *cottonoid patty (pattie), Cellolite.*

paucity—deficiency, shortage. "There is a paucity of objective findings, so we will have to undertake further laboratory tests before we can make a diagnosis in this patient."

Paufique knife (Oph).

Pauwel's classification of femoral neck fractures—based on the location of the fracture line. Uses roman numerals. See *Garden's classification.*

PAVe (procarbazine, melphalan, and vinblastine)—chemotherapy protocol for adult Hodgkin's disease.

paving stone degeneration—atrophic condition in which sharply outlined, rounded lesions appear in the peripheral retina. Also, *cobblestone degeneration.*

Pavlik harness—used to correct congenital hip dysplasia in infants under six months of age. Also, *Kicker Pavlik harness.*

PAWP (pulmonary artery wedge pressure).

Paxene (paclitaxel)—Canadian version of Taxol; used for treatment of Kaposi's sarcoma in patients who have failed prior liposomal anthracycline therapy.

Paxil (paroxetine HCl)—for treatment of social anxiety disorder, or social phobia; also used for the treatment of depression, panic disorder, and obsessive compulsive disorder.

PBC (primary biliary cirrhosis).

PBLs (peripheral blood lymphocytes).

PBNS (percutaneous bladder neck stabilization).

PBPC (peripheral blood progenitor cell)—used in bone marrow transplants.

PBPI (penile brachial pressure index).

PBSC (peripheral blood stem cell collections)—for allogeneic bone marrow transplantation.

PBTE (percutaneous transhepatic liver biopsy with tract embolization).

PBV (percutaneous balloon valvuloplasty).

PCA (porous-coated anatomic) **knee prosthesis**—a cementless implant that permits biologic union between the implant and the bone which infiltrates into the textured surface of the prosthesis.

PCA (patient-controlled analgesia) **system**—to administer analgesics as needed. Several manufacturers are marketing a portable computerized pump with a chamber that holds a prefilled syringe. The physician programs the pump and determines the total amount of the drug that the patient can receive over a given period of time and the amount of each dose. When the patient is in pain, he can push a button on a cord attached to the pump; the pump then dispenses a small dose of the medication into the patient's I.V. line. The patient is quite likely to need less medication this way because he feels in control and therefore less anxious and less tense than when waiting for someone to dispense the medication.

PCBS (percutaneous cardiopulmonary bypass support).

PCCL (percutaneous cholecystolithotomy).

PC (phase-contrast) **technique** (MRI).

PCD (programmable cardioverter-defibrillator)—for detection and reversal of ventricular tachycardia.

PCD Transvene implantable cardioverter-defibrillator system.

PCE (Platinol, cyclophosphamide, etoposide)—chemotherapy protocol for small cell carcinoma of the lung.

PCHA (proliferating cell nuclear antigen) (ENT, Neuro)—a technique to assess the growth rate of vestibular schwannomas.

PC-IOL (posterior chamber intraocular lens) **implantation**—performed bilaterally to correct pediatric aphakia.

PCL (posterior cruciate ligament).

PCNL (percutaneous nephrostolithotomy)—uses ultrasound waves to disintegrate kidney stones.

PCO (polycystic ovary).

PCO (posterior capsular opacification).

PCP (phencyclidine)—a street drug.

PCP (*Pneumocystis carinii* pneumonia).

PC Polygraf HR—a device that evaluates lower esophageal sphincter and esophageal motility disorders.

PCR (polymerase chain reaction).

PCRA (percutaneous coronary rotational atherectomy).

PC-7 needle—a curved needle used in intraocular lens procedures.

PC-SPES—a combination of eight Chinese herbs said to offer new hope for men with advanced prostate cancer.

PCTCL (percutaneous transhepatic cholecystolithotomy).

PCV (procarbazine, CCNU, vincristine)—chemotherapy protocol for anaplastic astrocytoma.

PCW (pulmonary capillary wedge).

PD (peritoneal dialysis).

PDA (patent ductus arteriosus).

P.D. Access with Peel-Away needle introducer—used to place central venous lines in infants and adults for long-term intravenous delivery of antibiotics, chemotherapy agents, and nutritionals.

PDB (preperitoneal distention balloon)—permits easy separation of the preperitoneal layers in laparoscopic extraperitoneal herniorrhaphy, and the transparent balloon allows for constant visualization.

PDC (peritoneal dialysis catheter).

PDS (pancreatic duct sphincter).

PDS (pigment dispersion syndrome).

PDS (polydioxanone suture) **II Endoloop suture.**

PDT (percutaneous dilational tracheostomy).

PDT (photodynamic therapy)—a colloquial term for *laser surgery*. See *Levulan*.

PEA (pulseless electrical activity)—formerly called EMD (electromechanical dissociation). PEA covers EMD, pseudo-EMD, and idioventricular rhythms.

peak-and-trough levels—maximum and minimum blood levels of a therapeutic agent, determined by drawing blood at strategic intervals after administration. This method provides more precise information than doing random blood levels and is particularly useful with drugs having a narrow margin between effective and toxic levels. "The following studies were considered: BUN, creatinine clearance, two urinalyses, and three drug assays one peak-and-trough level each, initially, and a repeat trough level at the end of seven days."

peak flow—see *Wright peak flow.*

peak latencies of pattern electroretinogram (PERG).

peakometer—used in testing the peak flow of the urinary bladder.

peanut—operating room slang for a small sponge.

Pearce nucleus hydrodissector—used during cataract surgery.

Pearce trabeculectomy—a type of glaucoma surgery in which trabecular meshwork is excised.

Pearce Tripod—implant cataract lens.

PEARL (physiologic endometrial ablation/resection loop).

pearl chains—chains of cells or vesicles brought into alignment during electro-cell fusion, prior to electroporation. See *electroporation*.

Pearl Omega—an anti-AIDS drug.

peau d'orange ("po-do-rahnj"') (Fr., orange peel)—dimpled appearance of the skin due to interstitial edema and particularly seen in breast cancer.

PEB (Platinol, etoposide, bleomycin)—chemotherapy protocol used to treat malignant germ cell tumor.

pectus excavatum—depression of the sternum. *(Not* pectus recurvatum.)

Pedi PEG tube—a percutaneous endoscopic gastrostomy tube.

PEEP ("peep")—positive end-expiratory pressure.

PEFR (peak expiratory flow rate)—a pulmonary function test.

PEG–ADA (pegademase bovine).

pegademase bovine (PEG-ADA, Adagen)—used to treat a rare congenital genetic disorder known as *severe combined immunodeficiency disease* (SCID) or *bubble boy disease*, in which the patient is missing the enzyme adenosine deaminase. Bone marrow transplantation is an alternative treatment that is not always successful. Pegademase replaces the missing ADA enzyme and allows the immune system to produce antibodies in patients who are not candidates for a bone marrow transplant. The term *bovine* refers to the source of the drug—cows. The drug is specially treated to reduce the risk of allergic reactions to this heterologous product.

pegaspargase (Oncaspar)—an alternative form of the chemotherapy drug L-asparaginase (Elspar). Oncospar is manufactured in a water-soluble base of PEG (polyethylene glycol). It is prescribed for patients with acute lymphoblastic leukemia who are hypersensitive to L-asparaginase, which is derived from the bacterium *E. coli*.

Pegasus Nd:YAG—surgical laser.

Pegasys (PEG-interferon alfa-2a)—a long-acting form of interferon for once weekly administration in the treatment of chronic hepatitis C.

PEG (polyethylene glycol)**-hemoglobin** —see *polyethylene glycol (PEG)-hemoglobin*.

PEG interleukin-2 (PEG IL-2)—drug used to treat AIDS patients.

PEG-Intron—used for treatment of hepatitis C.

PEG-Intron A (interferon alfa-2b conjugated polyethylene glycol)—used for treatment of patients with chronic myelogenous leukemia.

PEG-LES—polyethylene glycol electrolyte lavage solution for colonoscopy preparation.

PEG (percutaneous endoscopic gastrostomy) **tube**—the preferred method for patients who need long-term enteral feedings. Also, *PEG-24 system.*

"pegylated"—referring to drug formulations containing polyethylene glycols (PEG). "This HIV-positive patient was given PEG interleukin-2."

pegylated-liposomal doxorubicin—used in treatment of AIDS-associated Kaposi's sarcoma.

PEH (papillary endothelial hyperplasia).

PEI (percutaneous ethanol injection).

PEJ (percutaneous endoscopic jejunostomy).

Pelger-Huët cells—seen in acute myelogenous leukemia.

pelgeroid—refers to Pelger-Huët nuclear anomaly of neutrophils and eosinophils.

peliosis hepatis—hemorrhagic cysts in the liver. (Note: *hepatis*, not *hepatitis*.)

Pelizaeus-Merzbacher disease—familial disease of the myelin sheath.

pellet artifact (Radiol)—shotgun pellets found in the GI tract of patients who have eaten wild game.

Pelorus stereotactic system.

pelvic floor electrical stimulation (PFS, *not* PFES)—to reduce urinary incontinence in women with stress urinary incontinence. May be effective in men and women with mixed and urge urinary incontinence.

Pemberton's acetabuloplasty—procedure to correct congenital dislocation or subluxation of the hip.

PEMF (pulsed electromagnetic field) **therapy**. See *PEMT, AMT*.

Pemoline C-IV—stimulant drug used in treatment of attention-deficit/hyperactivity disorder.

PEMT (pulsed electromagnetic therapy) —used in treatment of nonunion of bone secondary to trauma.

Pencan spinal needle—reportedly allows a faster flow rate than other needles.

penciclovir (Denavir)—a topical prescription treatment for cold sores, in 1% strength.

Penderluft syndrome—a disturbance in air exchange in which the diaphragm is out of synchronization with inhalation and expiration.

Penetrating Abdominal Trauma Index (PATI)—a system of scoring abdominal trauma which takes into account the number of abdominal organs injured. A low PATI correlates with less severe injuries. Patients with a PATI of less than 25 could be surgically managed by primary closure of their abdominal wounds without the need for a colostomy. Although primary closure always carries the risk of intraabdominal infection and possible leaks from the suture lines, a colostomy involves known psychological complications, additional surgical complications, and additional financial considerations. The PATI is used to determine which surgical course to pursue.

Penetrex (enoxacin).

Penfield retractor—"A Penfield retractor could be placed behind the T11 vertebral body, as well as inferiorly along the L1 vertebra."

Penicillium—one of the molds most prevalent in damp interior areas. See also *Aspergillus*.

Penicillium marneffei—AIDS-related illness from Southeast Asia.

penicilloyl polylysine (PPL, Pre-Pan).

penile brachial pressure index (PBPI) —Doppler study of blood flow in the penile arteries to assess cardiovascular disease. A value of 0.65 or less indicates possibility of impending myocardial infarction or stroke.

penile gangrene and penile necrosis—often occur in patients with diabetes mellitus and end-stage renal disease.

penile prosthesis—see *prosthesis*.

penile vein ligation—for impotence from venous leakage.

Penlac nail lacquer (ciclopirox)—broad-spectrum antifungal topical therapy approved for treatment of toe- and fingernail fungus.

Pennig dynamic wrist fixator—used to treat distal radius fractures while allowing for use of the hand.

Pennig minifixator—fracture fragment fixator for use in minimally invasive surgery of the hands and feet.

Penn pouch—for continent urinary diversion. Uses terminal ileum or cecum to form pouch.

Pennsaid topical lotion (diclofenac HCl)—for relief of osteoarthritis pain.

PENS (percutaneous *electrical* nerve stimulation)—not the same as percutaneous *epidural* neurostimulator. See *percutaneous electrical nerve stimulation*.

PENS (percutaneous *epidural* neurostimulator)—not the same as percutaneous *electrical* nerve stimulation.

Pentacarinat (pentamidine isethionate).

pentagastrin stimulated analysis.

pentamidine isethionate (Pentam 300)—an antiprotozoal agent used against *Pneumocystis carinii* pneumonia.

pentamidine isethionate, aerosolized (NebuPent, Pentacarinat, Pneumopent)—inhaled to prevent *Pneumocystis carinii* pneumonia in AIDS patients.

Pentam 300 (pentamidine isethionate).

Pentasa (mesalamine).

Pentax EUP-EC124 ultrasound gastroscope—a forward-viewing fiberoptic gastroscope.

Pentax FG-36UX—linear scanning echoendoscope.

Pentax-Hitachi FG32UA—endosonographic system.

People-Finder—a handheld device that uses infrared to enable the deaf-blind to locate people, stoves, animals, and light sources.

PEP (progestogen-associated endometrial protein).

PepGen P-15 (peptide-enhanced bone graft)—bioengineered bone replacement graft material for the treatment of osseous defects resulting from moderate to severe periodontitis.

peppermint oil—may be used as a contrast agent with barium enema.

Peptamen—a liquid, complete isotonic elemental diet that can be used full strength from the initial feeding.

Perative—a nutritionally complete formula for metabolically stressed patients.

Perceptin—selective histamine H3 receptor antagonist for treatment of patients with central nervous system diseases involving attention, learning, and/or sleep disorders. It may also be used to treat attention-deficit/hyperactivity disorder, dementia associated with Alzheimer's disease, and narcolepsy.

Perclose closure device—from developers of the Techstar, Prostar, and Prostar Plus closure devices. In dictation, you may hear physicians use the developer's name to refer to the device rather than the brand name.

PercuCut cut-biopsy needles—used in soft tissue biopsies.

Percuflex Plus stent—flexible ureteral stent.

PercuGuide—used in diagnostic radiology for precise localization of non-palpable lesions.

PercuPump disposable syringe and injector.

percussion—rhythmic clapping with cupped hands on the patient's chest and back to loosen pulmonary secretions so they can be coughed up or suctioned out. Also called *frappage, chest PT.*

percutaneous abscess and fluid drainage (PAFD).

percutaneous access kit (PAK).

percutaneous aortic balloon valvuloplasty—performed in patients with cardiogenic shock and critical aortic stenosis.

percutaneous automated diskectomy—a procedure which uses a 2 mm suction cutting probe into the disk under fluoroscopy; performed under local anesthesia.

percutaneous balloon mitral valvuloplasty—see *percutaneous transvenous mitral commissurotomy.*

percutaneous balloon valvuloplasty.

percutaneous bladder neck stabilization (PBNS)—procedure for treatment of women with stress urinary incontinence, using bone-anchor suspension technique.

percutaneous cardiopulmonary bypass support (PCBS)—used to support patients following cardiac arrest, or used prophylactically for high-risk patients having cardiac catheterization or PTCA.

percutaneous choledochoscopy—a nonsurgical method for diagnosing and treating biliary tree problems. Percutaneous access is via T-tubes and transhepatic drains.

percutaneous coronary rotational atherectomy (PCRA)—procedure using a high-speed rotary device to grind obstructing atheroma into fine particles.

percutaneous dilational tracheostomy (PDT)—procedure that may be performed at bedside to relieve airway obstruction and remove tracheopulmonary secretions.

percutaneous diskoscope—device to visualize material removed in percutaneous lumbar diskectomy.

percutaneous electrical nerve stimulation (PENS)—only electrical impulses are administered via needles inserted through the skin into target areas for pain relief. Cf. *TENS.*

percutaneous endoscopic gastrostomy (PEG).

percutaneous endoscopic jejunostomy (PEJ).

percutaneous epididymal sperm aspiration—a nonsurgical method of obtaining sperm for in vitro fertilization that involves inserting a 21-gauge butterfly needle directly into the head of the epididymis. The procedure is significantly less costly than microsurgical aspiration, but it can cause scarring.

percutaneous ethanol injection (PEI)—a promising treatment modality for small liver cancers.

percutaneous gastroenterostomy (PGE)—insertion of a tube into the small bowel, rather than just into the stomach. PG and PGE are used to permit feeding into the stomach, duodenum, or jejunum, and for decompression of a gastric outlet obstruction, or for chronic obstruction of the small bowel. PG and PGE are also used in feeding patients with strokes, with malignancies of the esophagus, and in management of patients with burns or severe trauma.

percutaneous interosseous nerve (PIN).

percutaneous intracoronary angioscopy.

percutaneous mitral balloon valvotomy (PMBV).

percutaneous nephrostolithotomy (PCNL)—uses ultrasound waves to disintegrate kidney stones.

percutaneous patent ductus arteriosus closure—the insertion of occluding spring coils into the patent ductus employing cardiac catheterization techniques. Multiple techniques for patent ductus arteriosus closure exist, but this is one of the latest.

percutaneous pinning of proximal humerus fractures—circumvents extensive soft-tissue stripping. It is performed to maintain fracture alignment without ORIF (open reduction and internal fixation).

percutaneous radiofrequency catheter ablation—a potential cure for idiopathic ventricular tachycardia.

percutaneous resection of transitional cell carcinoma of the renal pelvis.

Percutaneous Stoller Afferent Nerve Stimulation System (PerQ SANS) —used for treatment of urge incontinence and urinary urgency and frequency. Employs low-frequency electrical stimulation delivered through a very fine gauge needle.

percutaneous transatrial mitral commissurotomy—nonsurgical technique for patients with rheumatic mitral stenosis.

percutaneous transhepatic cholangiography (PTC).

percutaneous transhepatic liver biopsy with tract embolization (PBTE).

percutaneous transluminal angioplasty (PTA).

percutaneous transluminal myocardial (or transmyocardial) revascularization (PTMR)—procedure using a laser to create pathways for oxygenated blood to feed ischemic (oxygen-starved) heart muscle.

percutaneous transluminal renal angioplasty (PTRA).

percutaneous transluminal septal myocardial ablation—used for patients with hypertrophic cardiomyopathy. It is a a primary, sometimes familial, and genetically determined form of myocardial hypertrophy with a dynamic left ventricular outflow tract obstruction.

percutaneous transperineal seed implantation—a procedure to radiate prostatic cancer locally. Small seeds of iodine 15 or palladium 103 radioactive material are inserted into prostatic tissue. The procedure is said to be cost-effective and avoid systemic radiation effects.

percutaneous transvenous mitral commissurotomy (PTMC)—an alternative to open heart surgical mitral commissurotomy that uses catheterization techniques and uses a balloon catheter to dilate the mitral valve. Bifoil and trefoil balloons used for this procedure contain two or three balloons on a single shaft, requiring one transseptal puncture and one guide wire in the left ventricle rather than the two required for a usual two-balloon method. Single balloons are not usually adequate to dilate the mitral valve sufficiently. The shaft and tip of the bifoil and trefoil balloon catheters, however, are stiffer and make the procedure somewhat more difficult, with the greater risk of left ventricular perforation.

percutaneous umbilical cord blood sampling (PUBS).

PerDUCER pericardial access device—used for delivery of therapeutic agents inside the pericardium.

Pereyra needle—a single-prong ligature carrier for use in bladder neck suspension.

Perfecta hip prosthesis—provides anatomic proximal fit with wedge-shaped cross-section in sagittal, coronal, and transverse planes.

PerFixation screws—used in tendon graft repairs

PerFix Marlex mesh plug—a preformed Marlex mesh hernia plug consisting of a fluted outside layer combined with an inside arrangement of eight mesh petals that allow it to maintain an open conelike shape.

perflubron—a colorless, odorless liquid that easily absorbs oxygen and breaks the surface tension of air sacs in the lungs, allowing them to open up and help the patient breathe more easily. Perflubron is inert and does not transfer across cell membranes; thus patients do not drown in their own fluids. See *partial liquid ventilation*.

perfluoropropane (C_3F_8) **gas**.

perfosfamide (Pergamid).

perfusion—pouring a fluid over an organ or tissue, or through vessels of an organ; used in kidney and heart perfusion surgery, and organ transplantation. Cf. *profusion*.

perfusion-weighted imaging—ultrafast MRI technique that shows which parts of the brain are still alive after a stroke but are still vulnerable because they are being starved of blood. Results of these scans may determine whether neuroprotective drugs will be effective.

PERG (peak latencies of pattern electroretinogram).

Pergamid (perfosfamide)—used to treat bone marrow in vitro before reinfusing it into patients treated for acute myelogenous leukemia.

periaqueductal gray electrode—not a proper name; it refers to the gray matter of the brain.

periarticular heterotopic ossification (PHO)—a complication of total hip arthroplasty in which ectopic bone growth occurs in the joint, causing decreased range of motion and pain. In severe cases, the head of the femur may actually become fused to the acetabulum. The cause is unknown. The Brooker system is used to classify PHO.

peribronchial cuffing—thickening of bronchial walls by fibrosis, as seen in asthma, emphysema, and other chronic respiratory disorders.

pericardial baffle.

pericardium—the fibrous sac surrounding the heart and roots of the great vessels. Cf. *precordium*.

Peridex mouthwash—used to reduce oral mucositis in patients receiving chemotherapy.

Periflow peripheral balloon catheters —used for angioplasty and the infusion of solutions to the peripheral vasculature.

perilunate fracture dislocation (PLFD).

perilymphatic fistula (PLF).

perimeter—circumference, edge. Cf. *parameter*.

Perimount RSR pericardial bioprosthesis—see *Carpentier-Edwards Perimount*.

perineal—refers to the perineum, the area between the scrotum and the anus in the male, and between the

perineal *(cont.)*
vulva and the anus in the female. Cf. *peritoneal, peroneal.*

perineal artery fasciocutaneous flaps—used in reconstructive surgery for stenotic vagina. Cf. *peroneal artery.*

perineal surgical apron—technique used in obstetrics and surgery.

perineurium—area surrounding nerves; fibrous connective tissue.

PerioChip—indicated as an adjunct to scaling and root-planing procedures in patients with adult periodontitis.

periodic acid-Schiff test (PAS stain)—a test for collagen or for presence of Whipple's disease.

periodic lateralized epileptiform discharges (PLEDS)—found in electroencephalograms.

periorbital infantile myofibromatosis—a lesion of the eyelid and medial canthus in an infant, treated with subtotal excision.

Periostat—investigational drug said to reduce or even reverse the progression of periodontal disease in adults.

periosteal stripping—a procedure performed in children with limb-length discrepancy to increase the length of long bones.

peripheral access system (PAS) **port**—an implantable port positioned subcutaneously in the antecubital area of the arm. See *P.A.S. Port catheter.*

Peripheral AngioJet system—used to retrieve clots.

peripheral blood lymphocytes (PBLs).

peripheral blood stem cell (PBSC) **collections.**

peripheral excimer laser angioplasty (PELA).

peripheral laser angioplasty (PLA).

peripherally inserted catheter (PIC)—intravenous catheter for long-term venous access in patients cared for at home or in nursing homes.

peripherally inserted central catheter (PICC).

peripheral scatter photocoagulation—for treatment of neovascularization of the vitreous base.

peripheral vestibular deficits (PVD).

peristaltic wave—a wave of muscular contractions passing along a tubular organ (such as the esophagus or intestines), by which its contents are advanced.

Peri-Strips Dry—thin strips of bovine pericardium sutured to a backing material and used to overlap staple lines. Used in lung resection procedures and other soft tissue repairs.

peritomy—an incision of the conjunctiva and the subconjunctival tissues, going around the entire corneal circumference. Used in cataract extractions, retinal detachment procedures, and enucleation. *Not* peridimy or peridomy.

peritoneal—refers to the peritoneum, the serous membrane lining the abdominal and pelvic cavities. Cf. *perineal, peroneal.*

peritoneal dialysis (PD).

peritonealize—to cover with peritoneum. Also, see *peritonize.*

peritoneal mouse (Radiol)—a free body sometimes seen on x-ray in the peritoneal cavity.

peritoneography—magnetic resonance imaging of the peritoneal cavity. Imaging agent is instilled into the peritoneal cavity, magnetic resonance scanning is performed with the peritoneal cavity filled, and after complete drainage of the contrast material, scan is again performed. Images are reviewed for evidence of

peritoneography *(cont.)*
peritoneal leaks, hernias, loculated fluid collections, and adhesions. MR peritoneography is particularly useful in patients using continuous ambulatory peritoneal dialysis.

peritoneum—serous membrane lining the abdomen.

peritonize—to cover with peritoneum. See *peritonealize.*

periurethral collagen injection—for the control of urinary incontinence in patients not responding to conservative therapy and who refuse surgery.

perivitelline space—the area around the yolk of an oocyte. Via a microinjection technique, sperm may be injected into the perivitelline space for in vitro fertilization.

Perkins Brailler—a braille embosser.

Perkins tonometer—measures intraocular pressure.

PERK (prospective evaluation of radial keratotomy) **protocol**—for correction of myopia.

perlèche—another term for cheilitis, or dryness and cracking around the mouth, from repeated licking or from a Candida infection.

Perlon suture (size 10-0)—a very fine (narrow) suture used in eye surgery.

PERM (Piattaforma Elettropneumatica per Riabilitazione Motoria)—developed in Italy. The English translation would be the Electropneumatic Platform for Motor Rehabilitation, but the PERM abbreviation will no doubt be used. It is a device that can be used in the treatment of the lower limbs to provide the patient with controlled and quantifiable mechanical stimuli, thus enabling the therapist to adopt a more rigorous approach to treatment even in the very early stages of rehabilitation. Alternatively, the system can be used in a different operating mode as a normal biofeedback system capable of displaying on-screen the extent to which voluntary load has been transferred to the lower limb.

Perma-Flow coronary bypass graft — synthetic blood vessel designed to be used in place of harvesting the patient's own blood vessels for bypass grafting. This graft can be implanted and the bypass procedure completed without having to stop the beating heart and place the patient on full coronary bypass.

Perma-Hand braided silk suture.

PermaMesh—a sheet of hydroxyapatite particles woven on absorbable suture material. This material can be molded and is used to hold graft material in place prior to wound closure.

permanent brachytherapy—Encapsulated radioactive "seeds" are inserted directly into a tumor, through needles, during the operative procedure. The radioactive material will deliver radiation over a few months, but will not be removed; it will gradually decay until it becomes basically inert. Low-energy radionuclides such as iodine 125 (^{125}I) and palladium 135 (^{135}Pd) are used.

permanent section (*paraffin section*; *paraffin block*)—technique in which tissue removed in an operation is embedded in paraffin for microscopic examination of the pathology present. This takes more time than frozen section but has certain advantages in that the specimen is permanent and not deteriorating, as in frozen section. Cf. *frozen section.*

Perma-Seal dialysis access graft.

PermCath—double-lumen ventricular access catheter.

Perneczky aneurysm clip—has an inverted spring mechanism to facilitate visual control during clip application.

peroneal—refers to the fibula or to the outer side of the leg and the muscles, nerves, and vessels thereof, the peroneus longus and the peroneus brevis. Cf. *perineal, peritoneal.*

peroxidase-antiperoxidase (PAP).

per primam (*not* primum)—first intention; primary union; healing directly, without granulation; the incision closes in minimal time, with no complications and with little resulting scar tissue.

Per-Q-Cath—peripherally inserted central catheter.

PerQ SANS (Percutaneous Stoller Afferent Nerve Stimulation System).

Persantine (dipyridamole) **thallium stress test**—a chemical equivalent of the treadmill stress test. It measures EKG reading, blood pressure, and heart rate in response to exertion on people who are not able to undergo a treadmill test. A small amount of radioactive thallium is injected IV (about as much radioactivity as you would get from a chest x-ray). The thallium will be carried to the heart, at which point a scanning device will demonstrate which areas of the heart are not getting sufficient blood.

persistent hyperplastic primary vitreous (PHPV).

persistent vegetative state (PVS).

Persona monitoring kit—a combination ovulation-prediction monitoring kit and birth control system. By testing hormones excreted in a woman's urine, the monitoring kit indicates a green light when pregnancy risk is low and a red light on the days she is at risk of becoming pregnant. It reportedly has a 95% accuracy rate, about the same as condoms.

person with AIDS (PWA)—term preferred over "AIDS victim" in AIDS self-help and awareness groups.

pertechnetate sodium (technetium solution) used as a diagnostic aid. See *technetium.*

PERV (porcine endogenous retrovirus).

pes anserine bursitis—occurs in elderly women with osteoarthritis. It can be treated with anti-inflammatory medication and drainage if necessary. It may be associated with anserine bursitis syndrome.

petal-fugal flow—"Angiography (for esophageal varices) was performed and showed petal-fugal flow." Also, mixed petal-fugal flow. See *hepatopetal* and *hepatofugal flow.*

petaling the cast—taping the edge of a rough or crumbling cast with short strips of tape or moleskin in overlapping fashion so that it looks like a series of petals.

petechia (pl., petechiae)—tiny, pinpoint round red spot caused by intradermal or submucous hemorrhage.

petit pas ("petty-pah") (Fr., small step) **gait**, as in "His gait was petit pas, but was otherwise normal."

PET (positron emission tomography) **scan**—uses deoxyglucose to distinguish tumor from necrosis.

PET with 3D SSP—helpful in accurate assessment of Alzheimer's disease.

Peutz-Jeghers syndrome—familial gastrointestinal polyposis, particularly in the small bowel, with mucocutaneous pigmentation.

Peyer's (rhymes with *flyers*) **patches**—elevated areas of closely packed lymphoid nodules on the mucosa of the small intestine.

Peyman intraocular forceps—with the functional capabilities of forceps, pick, and scissors.

Peyman vitrector—used in cataract extraction.

PFC Sigma—total knee system.

PFC (press-fit component) **total hip system**—has a porous-coated stem.

Pfeiffer-Comberg method—used radiographically to locate a foreign body in the eye.

p53 gene—mutation of which is responsible for many types of malignant tumors.

p55-IgG—p55 tumor necrosis factor receptor fusion protein.

PF (parafascicular) **nucleus** (Neuro).

PFS (pelvic floor electrical stimulation).

PFT (parafascicular thalamotomy).

PFTE (polyfluorotetraethylene)—plastic graft material; shunt.

PG (percutaneous gastrostomy)—radiologic alternative to surgical and endoscopic gastrostomy. See *PGE*.

PGE (percutaneous gastroenterostomy).

PGH (placental growth hormone).

PGK (Panos G. Koutrouvelis, M.D) **stereotactic device**—floor-mounted stereotactic device that allows accurate insertion of the Nucleotome aspiration probe at the L5-S1 level for percutaneous lumbar diskectomy.

P-glycoprotein (also known as *P-170 glycoprotein*)—a substance present in some types of cancer cells. When present, it enables those cells to expel chemotherapy drugs and resist their cytotoxic effects. Cancer patients with P-glycoprotein positive cells (leukemia, multiple myeloma, non-Hodgkin's lymphoma, and renal cell carcinoma) respond poorly to chemotherapy regimens. The P-glycoprotein efflux mechanism has been found to be inactivated by certain calcium channel blocking drugs that allow the chemotherapy agent to enter the cancer cell and be more effectively cytotoxic. See *calcium channel blockers*.

PgR (progesterone receptor).

pH—the measure of the relative balance between the acids and bases in a system. It has to do with the hydrogen ions in solutions, such as urine or serum. The normal pH of arterial blood is between 7.35 and 7.45. A pH below 7.0 or greater than 7.8 is not compatible with life. See *intracellular pH* (pHi).

PHA (phytohemagglutinin antigen)—a skin test for cellular-based immunity (not antibodies).

PHA (progressive hemifacial atrophy).

PHACE syndrome—neurocutaneous syndrome consisting of:

posterior fossa brain malformations, **h**emangiomas

arterial anomalies

coarctation of the aorta and cardiac defects

eye abnormalities

Phaco-Emulsifier—aspirator used in cataract extractions.

PhacoFlex II SI-30NB—foldable intraocular lens implant. See also *Single-Stitch PhacoFlex lens*.

Phadiatop test—a system for testing the blood to more quickly diagnose the cause of cold or allergy symptoms. Results of the yes/no test are available within a few hours.

phage typing of organisms.

phagocyte ("eating cell")—a cell which consumes other cells or foreign material.

Phalen's maneuver—to determine presence of carpal tunnel syndrome. See *Phalen's sign.*

Phalen's sign (*not* Phelan)—in carpal tunnel syndrome. Phalen's sign is present when paresthesias are produced or are exaggerated when the wrist is held in complete flexion for 30 seconds, which presses the median nerve against the upper edge of the transverse carpal ligament.

Phantom cardiac guide wire.

phantom limb pain—pain felt by the patient in an already-amputated limb, as though the limb were still there.

Phantom nasal mask—CPAP mask with built-in exhalation port. The mask conforms to the patient's face and minimizes leaks caused by facial hair and/or body movement.

Phantom V Plus catheter—dilating catheter used in common bile duct dilation and stone extraction.

pharaonic circumcision—a form of female genital mutilation. See *infibulation.*

pharmacogenomics—the study of variability of patient responses to drugs due to patients' inherent genetic differences.

pharmacokinetic parameters.

PharmaSeed palladium-103 seeds—radioactive ^{103}Pd seeds/implants used in brachytherapy for the treatment of prostate cancer.

PharmChek—sweat patch drug detection system.

phased-array study—inaccurate term for *phase image*, which is a form of gated blood pool study especially processed so that a little more infor-

mation is obtained from it. See *gated blood (pool) cardiac.*

phase image—MRI term. See *phased array study.*

phase sensitive detector—MRI term.

phen-fen—see *fen-phen diet.*

phenotype—see *Cellano phenotype, McLeod phenotype.*

phentolamine (Vasomax)—oral medication for erectile dysfunction.

pherogram—electrophoretic pattern.

pheromones—sexual odors which play an important part in insect, mammalian, and perhaps human reproductive behavior.

PHG (portal hypertensive gastropathy).

pHi (intracellular pH).

Philadelphia (Ph1) **chromosome**—a translocation from chromosome number 22 to chromosome number 9. The Philadelphia chromosome is found in the adult form of chronic myeloid leukemia. "A bone biopsy will be done, with Philadelphia chromosome cytogenic analysis."

Philips Tomoscan SR 6000 CT scanner.

Philips ultrasound machines—endovaginal and endorectal transducers.

phlyctenule ("flick-ten'-yule")—small nodular lesion found at the edge of the cornea; thought to be a cause of neovascularization.

PHNO (4-propyl-9-hydroxynaphthoxazine)—for Parkinson's disease.

PHO (periarticular heterotopic ossification).

Phocas syndrome (also, Tillaux-Phocas)—see *fibrocystic breast syndrome.*

PH-1 (primary hyperoxaluria, type 1).

phonocardiography—noninvasive cardiac diagnostic procedure which tests the occurrence, timing, and duration

phonocardiography *(cont.)*
of the various sounds in the cardiac cycle, determines the frequency (cycles per second) and intensity (amplitude), and demonstrates murmurs in low frequencies that can be missed by the ear.

Phoropter (*not* Foreopter)—American Optical Company's refractor.

phosphatidylglycerol levels—present with pulmonary maturity in a premature infant; levels decrease with lung maturity.

photic stimulation—flashing light stimulation, used in EEG testing.

photoablative refractive keratectomy (PRK)—alternative to radial keratotomy. Also, *phototherapeutic keratectomy.*

photoaged—premature aging process induced by overexposure to the sun, i.e., photoaged skin.

photoangioplasty—a treatment for atherosclerotic arteries that uses laser light to activate a photosensitive plaque-dissolving agent.

photoastigmatic refractive keratectomy (PARK).

photocatalytic air filtration system—uses light that reacts with a chemical catalyst to kill microbes, dust mites, and mold.

PhotoDerm—a computer-based machine that uses bright light similar to a camera's flashbulb to destroy spider veins by delivering controlled doses of light through a special handpiece. *PhotoDerm PL* is used to treat benign pigmented lesions (age spots, liver spots, freckles, birthmarks, melasma, hyperpigmentation, and tattoos), and *PhotoDerm VL* is used to treat noninvasive treatment of leg veins and other benign vascular lesions.

photodynamic therapy (PDT)—cancer treatment modality that utilizes light-activated drugs in combination with laser light sources to create highly reactive forms of oxygen that cause destruction of cancerous cells. Also called *light-activated therapy.* It is also used to treat age-related macular degeneration. See also *DHE, HPD, Photofrin.*

photo epilation—use of light energy through the surface of the skin to destroy follicles (or roots) of unwanted hair.

Photofrin (porfimer sodium)—a photosensitizing drug that selectively kills tumor cells while leaving normal tissue relatively unaffected. It is used as palliative treatment in esophageal cancer patients with obstruction who have failed on YAG laser therapy. It is also used for treatment of microinvasive endobronchial non-small cell lung carcinoma in patients not indicated for surgery and radiotherapy.

photometer—see *HemoCue photometer.*

photomotogram—timed Achilles tendon reflex.

Photon cataract removal system—uses ultrasonic phacoemulsification.

photon correlation spectroscopy—see *SpectRx.*

Photon Radiosurgery System (PRS)—x-ray delivery system for tumor therapy. Formerly approved only for treatment to the brain, the system is now FDA-approved for radiation therapy treatments anywhere in the body.

photopenic area—a coined word for the light area on a film or scan.

photophobia—unusual intolerance of light.

photophoresis—treatment used for cutaneous T-cell lymphoma, a rare immune system cancer. The patient is given doses of psoralen (a light-activated drug) orally. The patient is attached to a device that takes blood from one arm, separates the white cells from the red, and then exposes the white cells to a kind of ultraviolet light. The light-activated psoralen damages the cancerous white cells, which are then reinfused into the patient's other arm. After a few days, the cancerous white cells die. The treatment is repeated at intervals, and over a period of time the patient's immune system will be able to overcome the remaining infected white blood cells. See *psoralen.*

Photopic Imaging—ultrasound system that enhances visual acuity and helps clinicians more easily see signs of cancer or stroke.

PhotoPoint—laser therapy for exudative age-related macular degeneration. It seals leaking blood vessels in the macula without creating scar tissue that interferes with central vision.

photopsia—subjective sensation of sparks or flashes of light in retinal or optic diseases.

photorefractive keratectomy (PRK)—a procedure using computer-guided excimer laser ablation to reprofile the anterior corneal curvature in order to correct myopia. It is believed capable of correcting low and moderate myopic errors with a relatively high degree of accuracy and safety. See also *LASIK* and *T-PRK.*

photostimulable luminescence intensity—the higher the intensity, the better the radiographic image.

phototherapeutic keratectomy (PTK)—removal of anterior corneal pathology with the excimer laser.

photothermal sclerosis—method of treating varicose veins that are resistant to standard medical techniques, using a laser-like photothermal device.

PHPV (persistent hyperplastic primary vitreous).

PHRT (procarbazine, hydroxyurea, radiotherapy) **protocol.**

PHT (portal hypertension).

phthalocyanine ("thay-lo-cy-a-neen")—photosensitizing agent used in laser surgery.

phthisis ("ty-sis")—a wasting of part of the body. See *ptosis.*

phthisis bulbi—shrinkage and wasting of the eyeball.

phycobiliproteins—fluorescent pigments used in immunological diagnostic products.

phycomycosis—see *mucormycosis.*

Phylax AV—dual chamber implantable cardioverter-defibrillator.

physician-assisted suicide (PAS).

Physios CTM 01—noninvasive cardiac transplant monitoring system. It monitors the electrophysiologic performance of a transplanted heart to assist in the detection of acute allograft rejection.

Physio-Stim Lite—a bone growth stimulator used to promote healing of non-united fractures.

physostigmine—for treatment of glaucoma and mild or moderate Alzheimer's disease. It has improved memory and enhanced cognitive functioning in Alzheimer's patients.

phytochemicals—natural substances found in certain foods (wild blueberries, cruciferous vegetables) that are

phytochemicals *(cont.)*
believed to have cancer-fighting and anti-aging properties.

phytohemagglutinin antigen (PHA)—a plant product used for testing human T-cell response. An absent PHA response indicates an abnormally functioning T-cell system.

phytosterolemia—condition in patients on total parenteral nutrition (TPN), thought possibly to be a factor in the development of cholestatic liver disease, which often occurs in patients on TPN.

phytotherapy—treatment using plants.

PIA (Platinol, ifosfamide, Adriamycin)—chemotherapy protocol.

PIC (peripherally inserted catheter).

PIC (plasmin inhibitor complex).

pica—eating of materials not usually considered edible or nourishing (e.g., starch, dirt, clay, paint), usually by pregnant women or malnourished children. Cf. *PICA.*

PICA (posterior inferior communicating artery). Cf. *pica.*

Picasso phone—an innovative medical teleconferencing device. Physicians can send high-quality still images of patients and their medical conditions over standard analog phone lines, while simultaneously talking to the doctors on the other end of the connection. The phone on the sending end connects to a standard camcorder and to either a TV or PC screen. Using a computer mouse, the doctor can point out areas of interest.

PICC (peripherally inserted central catheter)—inserted into the cephalic or basilic vein in the arm and threaded into the superior vena cava. Made of silicone rubber (which is soft, flexible, durable, and reduces the risk of thrombosis). Use PIC catheter, *not* PICC catheter.

Picker Magnascanner—scintigraphy equipment to detect skeletal metastases.

Picket Fence leg positioner.

Pick inclusion body—found in Pick's disease.

picornavirus—extremely small, ether-resistant RNA virus, one of the group comprising the enteroviruses and the rhinoviruses.

Pico-ST II—low-profile balloon catheter used in percutaneous transluminal coronary angioplasty (PTCA) procedures.

Picture Archiving and Communications Systems (PACS)—an integrated information system that facilitates the practice of radiology and teleradiology. It includes, but is not limited to, picture archiving and voice reporting.

picture element (pixel)—MRI term.

PID (primary immune deficiency).

Pierre Robin ("pe-air ro-ban") **syndrome**—consisting of brachygnathia and cleft palate, giving a rather bird-like appearance. May also include displacement of the larynx backward and upward, and may produce feeding problems because sucking and swallowing are difficult. Often associated with glossoptosis. Cf. *Robin's syndrome, micrognathia-glossoptosis syndrome.*

Pierse tip forceps.

PIE (pulmonary infiltrates with eosinophilia) **syndrome**—adverse drug reaction to nonsteroidal anti-inflammatory drug. Suspected upper respiratory infections with fever, malaise, and pulmonary infiltrates may actually be PIE syndrome.

piezo electrical stimulator—used to stimulate acupuncture sites with small electrical shock.

Piezolith-EPL (extracorporeal piezoelectric lithotriptor).

Pigg-O-Stat (Radiol)—proprietary device resembling a clear plastic high chair that enables chest x-rays to be taken of very young children. It has two clear plastic doors; the child is placed inside and the arms raised so the doors will close and the arms will be out of the field of view of the chest. Without this device, the child's parent may be exposed to radiation when trying to keep the child's arms out of the field.

piggyback, piggybacking—a method by which more than one solution, and medication, can be infused simultaneously by introducing additional intravenous lines to the main solution line. Also, *piggyback probe.*

pigment dispersion syndrome (PDS) —a common cause of glaucoma in young adults; it is most often seen in myopic Caucasian males.

pigskin graft—see *porcine xenograft.*

pigtail catheter.

PIH (pregnancy-induced hypertension).

PilaSite—sustained-release pilocarpine for glaucoma.

Pilates ("puh-LAH-tees") **method of exercise**—a method of physical therapy, developed originally for bedridden patients in WWI prison camps. The method restores muscular balance in the bedridden, improves posture, eliminates muscular and soft tissue pain, and builds strength and flexibility. Dancers, athletes, actors, and singers have used it to refine strength, balance, and coordination.

Pillet hand prosthesis.

Pilling Weck Y-stent forceps—used for bronchoscopic inset of tracheobronchial stents.

pillion fracture—a T-shaped fracture involving the distal femur, and posterior displacement of the condyles, caused by a severe blow to the knee. "The patient is now status post grade II open fracture of the left tibia, with an ipsilateral minimally displaced left pillion fracture which was treated immediately following his injury."

pill-rolling tremor—involuntary rhythmic opposing movements, or circular rolling motion, of the thumb and index finger, characteristic of Parkinson's disease.

pilocarpine iontophoresis method—to measure sweat chloride levels. An elevated level of chloride in perspiration is a sign of cystic fibrosis.

pilomatrix carcinoma—a rare, low-grade malignant lesion arising from hair cortex cells, with a tendency to recur. It usually occurs as a solitary lesion on the head, neck, extremities, or trunk (in decreasing order).

pilosebaceous unit—the combination of a hair follicle with its oil gland, considered as an anatomic unit.

Pilostat eye drops (pilocarpine HCl)— topical antiglaucoma agent; direct-acting miotic.

Pilot audiometer—used for screening of hearing disorders in preschool children.

Pilot suturing guide—used to aid in closure of laparoscopic incisions.

pimagedine (Action-II)—a compound developed to inhibit or block abnormal glucose/protein complexes that lead to diabetic complications such as kidney disease.

PIMS (programmable implantable medication system).

pin—see *nail.*

PIN (percutaneous interosseous nerve) (Hand Surg).

pinacidil (Pindac)—a vasodilator used to treat hypertension.

Pinard's sign—in pregnancy, pain on pressure over the uterine fundus, after the sixth month. An indication of possible breech presentation.

PINC—polymer system for the delivery of gene-based products to muscle.

pinchcock mechanism—at the esophagogastric junction.

Pindac (pinacidil).

ping-pong fracture—an actual fracture or simply a concavity and depression in the skull, resembling the indentation that results from pressure by the fingers on a ping-pong ball.

ping-ponging—repeatedly reinfecting each other, when sexual partners are not treated simultaneously for a sexually transmitted infection.

pinguecula—a degenerative lesion of the conjunctiva appearing as a yellowish nodule near the limbus.

pin headrest (Neuro).

pinked up (verb) (Cardio).

pinkeye—any condition causing hyperemia of one or both eyes; usually, bacterial or viral conjunctivitis.

pink puffer—a patient with early respiratory failure, showing dyspnea but no cyanosis. Cf. *blue bloater.*

pink tetralogy of Fallot—tetralogy of Fallot with only mild cyanosis, mild pulmonary stenosis, and left-to-right shunt, and with the pulmonary pressure higher than normal. See *tetralogy of Fallot.* Cf. *Fallot's trilogy, Fallot's pentalogy.*

Pinky—see *Super Pinky.*

Pinn.ACL guide system—used to simplify and refine the posterior-entry ACL reconstruction.

Pinpoint stereotactic arm—used to deliver radioactive seed implants for CT-guided brachytherapy.

Pins' sign—disappearance of pleuritic pain when the patient assumes a knee-chest position.

pipecuronium (Arduan)—neuromuscular blocking agent used in anesthesia to relax skeletal muscles. Does not induce tachycardia, thus offering increased safety for cardiac patients undergoing surgery.

Pipelle endometrial suction catheter—used for endometrial dating, cancer screening, and monitoring the effects of hormone treatment.

pipestem sheathing—the appearance created by lipid deposition along retinal arterioles.

PIPIDA scan—a technetium ^{99m}Tc-PIPIDA hepatobiliary scan used in acute cholecystitis.

pirenzepine HCl (Gastrozepine)—tricyclic benzodiazepine agent for gastric and duodenal ulcers. It works by selective suppression of gastric acid secretion.

piritrexim isethionate—used to treat *Pneumocystis carinii*, *Toxoplasma*, and *Mycobacterium avium-intra-cellulare* in AIDS patients.

piroxicam (Feldene)—nonsteroidal anti-inflammatory drug used for osteoarthritis, rheumatoid arthritis, and some other inflammatory conditions.

Pisces spinal cord stimulation system—electrical stimulation of nerve structures, delivered by percutaneously implanted epidural electrodes.

pisotriquetral joint—in the area of the flexor carpi ulnaris.

piston stapes prosthesis—placed in the middle of the stapedectomy opening and crimped onto the long process of the incus, with the other end in an opening in the posterior-central portion of the footplate. This technique is said to bring back the normal vibratory performance of the ossicular chain.

Pitié-Salpetrière saphenous vein hook—used to retract the saphenous vein while clipping and ligating branches and to provide tension during dissection.

pitting edema—on firm finger pressure, a depression lasts for several minutes; due to fluid retention.

Pittman IMA retractor system—for use in coronary artery bypass surgery.

Pitt talking tracheostomy tube—used in patients with ventilator-dependent quadriplegia with severe phrenic nerve damage.

pituitary (hypophyseal) **stalk distortion** (PSD)—seen on MRI scan.

PIV (primary immune deficiency).

pivot-shift sign; **test** (Ortho).

Pixie minilaparoscope—a small laparoscope that is said to adapt to any video camera system.

Pixsys Flashpoint—a 3-D digitizer used in image-guided surgery.

"pizza" lung—a finding on pathologic examination of a lung that has sustained damage to the point where it resembles pizza.

PJC (premature junctional contraction) (Cardio).

PLA (peripheral laser angioplasty).

placebo ("plah-see'bo")—see *Obecalp*, which is *placebo* spelled backwards. *Placebo* is Latin for "I will please."

placental alkaline phosphatase test (PLAP)—elevated in patients with seminomas and nonseminomatous malignant germ cell tumors. PLAP may be useful as a serum marker in patients undergoing treatment for one of these tumors to determine progression or regression of the tumor. PLAP is elevated in smokers, so that must be taken into consideration in determining the usefulness of this test in those patients.

placental growth hormone (PGH)—a hormone that appears to have important implications for physiologic adjustment to gestation and in control of maternal insulin-like growth factor 1 levels. PGH is not detectable in fetal circulation.

plafond—the undersurface of a plateau, as in tibial plafond.

plain—simple, open, clear; used often in *plain film*, a radiographic study performed without contrast medium, as differentiated from contrast studies and tomograms. Cf. *plane*.

planar spin imaging—MRI term.

Plan B (levonorgestrel)—postcoital or "emergency" contraceptive.

plane—a specified level, as the plane of anesthesia; also, an anatomical area between two tissue layers where an incision may be placed. Cf. *plain*.

PLA-I—a platelet antigen. This protein is sometimes lacking on the surface of platelets in patients who have received red cell transfusions from donors who are PLA-I positive, causing severe bleeding, and may also cause post-transfusion purpura.

plasma cell mastitis—see *duct ectasia*.

plasma expander—see *artificial blood*.

plasma F—another term for *cortisol*.

Plasma-Lyte A pH 7.4; Plasma-Lyte R; Plasma-Lyte 56; Plasma-Lyte 148—intravenous nutritional/electrolyte therapy.

plasmapheresis—removal of plasma from blood taken from the patient, with retransfusion of the solid elements (red cells, platelets) into the patient. May be used for therapeutic purposes or for laboratory studies. Note the different root words in plasma**pheresis** and electro**phoresis**. Cf. *electrophoresis*.

Plasma Scalpel—a cutting tool used in uvulopalatophayrngoplasty (UPPP) and tonsillectomy. It operates at temperatures between 40-70°C, minimizing the thermal effect on surrounding tissue.

plasma thromboplastin component (PTC) in bleeding diseases.

plasmids—pieces of double-stranded circular DNA outside chromosomes, thought to be responsible for bacterial resistance.

Plastibell—used in circumcising infants.

Plasti-Pore—porous, high-density polyethylene material employed for the fabrication of ossicular replacement prostheses in otolaryngology, and for other grafts. It is used in the same way as Proplast. Cf. *Proplast*.

Plastiport TORP (total ossicular replacement prosthesis) (ENT).

Plastizote collar (Ortho).

Plast-O-Fit thermoplastic bandage system.

plate bender (Ortho)—used to bend dynamic compression plates. See *DCP*.

platelet antigen—see *PLA-I*.

platelet-derived growth factor—may be applied topically to aid healing in chronic, nonhealing wounds.

platelet membrane fluidity, increased—a biological risk factor for Alzheimer's disease.

platform posturography—used with other vestibular tests for patients with peripheral vestibular deficits, Ménière's disease, benign paroxysmal positional vertigo, and central nervous system vestibular impairment. Note: *Posturography* is a word related to *posture*, not urography, which is radiography of the urinary tract.

platinum coil (Radiol)—used in interventional neuroradiology in a nonsurgical repair of aneurysms in inoperable areas of the brain.

platyrrhine nose—a broad or flat nose (*platy-* meaning broad, flat). This term is somewhat redundant, as *rhine* means *nose*; nevertheless, it is dictated.

platysmaplasty—see *corset platysmaplasty*.

Plavix (clopidogrel bisulfate)—cardiovascular drug used to treat ischemia.

PLD (perilunate dislocations) (Ortho).

PLE (protein-losing enteropathy).

Pleatman sac—a rigid plastic sac used in laparoscopic procedures to isolate stones, bile, suspicious or infected tissue to prevent contamination. Prevents loss of specimen and avoids contamination of abdominal wall.

pleconaril—antiviral drug that inhibits the activity of enteroviruses and rhinoviruses. It is designed for the treatment of viral meningitis, viral respiratory infection, myocarditis, pericarditis, encephalitis, chronic meningoencephalitis, herpangina, otitis media, neonatal enteroviral disease, acute viral exacerbations in asthma, and colds.

pledgets—usually cotton. Cottonballs (sponges), rolled so that they have somewhat pointed ends; used to absorb blood or fluids at the operative site. In some parts of the country they are called "pollywogs."

PLEDs (periodic lateralized epileptiform discharges)—in electroencephalogram.

PlegiaGuard—safety device to prevent dangerous overpressure by inadvertent occlusion of cardioplegia line.

Plendil (felodipine)—a once-a-day calcium channel blocker for mild to moderate hypertension.

plesiotherapy—the same as brachytherapy. See *brachytherapy*.

Pletal (cilostazol)—drug approved for use in the reduction of symptoms of intermittent claudication, as indicated by an increase in walking distance.

pleural—refers to the pleura, the serous membrane lining each half of the thorax: pleural cavity, pleural effusion. Cf. *plural*.

pleural effusion—an abnormal accumulation of fluid in the pleural cavity, as seen on chest x-ray.

pleural tent—constructed apically by incising the thickened parietal pleura, bluntly dissecting it from the chest wall, and allowing it to drop down to the upper surface of the remaining tissue. Used where there are diffuse air leaks or where a significant residual pleural space is present following lung surgery.

PlexiPulse—postsurgical device that reduces incidence of deep vein thrombosis and postoperative edema, thereby promoting wound healing.

plexus of Santorini.

PLF (perilymphatic fistula).

PLFD (perilunate fracture dislocation).

plica (pl., plicae)—ridge, fold, band, or shelf of synovial tissue, as in the transverse suprapatellar, medial suprapatellar, mediopatellar, and infrapatellar plicae. These usually cause few problems, but occasionally are large enough to become symptomatic and may require surgical intervention. See *plicectomy*.

plicamycin (Mithracin)—chemotherapy drug for testicular carcinoma, when surgery or radiation is not an option.

plicectomy ("ply-kek´to-me")—excision of a plica. See *plica*.

PLIF (posterior lumbar interbody fusion).

PLL (posterior longitudinal ligament)—of the spine and spinal cord.

plombage ("plom-bahzh")—as in bone or chest plombage, the surgical filling of an empty space in the body with an inert material such as methylmethacrylate.

plop, tumor—heard with cardiac tumors on auscultation.

plugged liver biopsy—used in patients with impaired coagulation.

Plum-Blossom needle—used for acupuncture.

Plummer-Vinson syndrome—characterized by dysphagia, iron-deficiency anemia, and esophageal webs. Associated with an increased incidence of postcricoid carcinoma.

plural—more than one. Cf. *pleural*.

plus disease (Oph)—dilated, tortuous vessels exiting the optic disk, seen in retinopathy of prematurity, suggesting serious disease elsewhere in the eye.

PMBV (percutaneous mitral balloon valvotomy).

PMC (pseudomembranous colitis).

PM-81 monoclonal antibody—used to treat patients with acute myelogenous leukemia prior to bone marrow transplant.

PML (progressive multifocal leukoencephalopathy).

PMMA (polymethylmethacrylate) hard **contact lens** or **intraocular lens**.

PMPA—antiviral drug used in treatment of HIV patients.

PMR (posteromedial release).

P-MRS (phosphorus nuclear magnetic resonance spectroscopy)—measures energy metabolism in patients with migraine. Energy metabolism appears to be defective in migraine patients.

PMT AccuSpan tissue expander.

PMT halo system—head and neck brace, for immobilization of spine in cervical fractures.

PMT (pyridoxyl-5-methyl tryptophan) imaging agent.

P-MVAC (Platinol, methotrexate, vinblastine, Adriamycin, carboplatin) — chemotherapy protocol.

PMX-F (polymyxin B fibers)—investigational treatment for septic shock. PMX alone is toxic to the central nervous system and the kidney and thus cannot be used intravenously to treat endotoxemia; however, PMX-F makes it possible for use in the extracorporeal elimination of endotoxin. PMX-F is polymyxin B fixed to polystyrene fibers, making it nontoxic when used to detoxify endotoxin.

PND (paroxysmal nocturnal dyspnea).

pneumatic retinopexy—the fixation of the retina in its proper position with the injection of a bubble of gas into the interior of the eye in the vitreous cavity. With proper postoperative positioning, the retina can be pushed back into proper position and then the gas will spontaneously disappear in a few weeks. Gases used in this procedure may be either per fluoropropane (C_3F_8) or sulfur hexafluoride (SF_6).

pneumococcal conjugate vaccine—prophylaxis against pneumococcal diseases, e.g., otitis media, pneumonia, and meningitis.

Pneumocystis carinii **pneumonia** (PCP) —once a rare pneumonia, caused by a protozoan parasite, seen only in immunosuppressed patients, such as transplant patients or patients on chemotherapy. Now one of the leading causes of death in AIDS. See *AIDS, HIV, Kaposi's syndrome.*

pneumocystis choroidopathy—common in AIDS patients.

Pneumo-Needle—reusable instrument.

Pneumopent (aerosolized pentamidine isethionate)—for *Pneumocystis carinii* infection in AIDS patients.

pneumoparotitis—a rare cause of enlargement of the parotid gland. Swelling results from air forced through Stensen's duct; a transient or recurrent phenomenon. Recurrent parotid insufflation may predispose to sialectasias, recurrent parotitis, and even subcutaneous emphysema.

pneumophila, Legionella—the organism causing legionnaires' disease.

pneumoscrotum—occasionally occurs after blunt trauma and can serve as an early sign of pneumothorax.

Pneumo Sleeve—acts as an airlock during hand-assisted laparoscopic surgery (see *HALS*). It contains the CO_2 used to inflate the abdomen and provides working space.

PNH (paroxysmal nocturnal hemoglobinuria).

PNI (prognostic nutritional index).

PNK—see *P&K* ("P and K").

POAG (primary open angle glaucoma).

POAH (posterior occipitoatlantal hypermobility).

POC (point of care).

POCC (procarbazine, Oncovin, cyclophosphamide, CCNU)—chemotherapy protocol.

PocketDop—handheld Doppler monitor for vascular and obstetrical monitoring.

podagra—gout. "She comes to the emergency department complaining of acute podagra to the right big toe for the past two days."

Podiatrx-AF and **Podiatrx-TFM**—used in conjunction for treatment of fungal infections of the foot.

podophyllum—caustic agent used for removal of papillomas.

POEMS syndrome
P polyneuropathy
O organomegaly
E endocrinopathy
M monoclonal (M-) protein
S skin changes
This is a combination of sclerotic myeloma, polyneuropathy, and endocrinological disorder. Hepatomegaly may also be seen in these patients.

POH (presumed ocular histoplasmosis syndrome).

poikilocyte—an atypical red blood cell.

point-search instruments—identifies acupuncture points by means of electricity. Both light-band and digital instruments are available.

Polaris cage—an adjustable spinal cage implant that provides a supporting framework for bone in-growth in patients with spinal trauma, tumors, or degenerative diseases.

Polaris 1.32 Nd:YAG laser—for tissue melding.

polarity-altered spectral selective acquisition (PASTA) **imaging** (MRI).

polarity on an EEG—When "zero two zero negative polarity" is dictated, it should be written 0-2/0 negative.

Polar-Mate bipolar microcoagulator.

Polaroids and Kodachromes (P&K)—photographs of specimens. "Polaroids and Kodachromes were taken," or "P&K were taken."

Polarus proximal humeral fixation system.

Polar Vantage XL heart rate monitor—used by sports medicine and rehabilitation physicians to monitor patients from a distance, either at home or while in physical therapy.

Polatest vision tester—tests binocular vision.

pole of kidney—the upper or lower extremity of a kidney.

pollybeak nasal deformity—results from inadequate tissue resection from the anterior septal angle or postoperative edema and scar following rhinoplasty. The term is descriptive (like a parrot's beak), not indicative of a number (*poly*, many). It describes a bony deformity in which the nose is thin or narrowed at the top with tip projecting down over the lips, sometimes as much as at a 90° angle. May be further designated as *cartilaginous pollybeak* or *soft tissue pollybeak*.

pollywogs—see *pledgets*.

polycystic ovary (PCO).

Polydek—coated polyester suture used in plastic surgery.

Polyderm foam wound dressing.

Poly-Dial insert (Ortho)—hemispherical polyethylene cap that fits under the acetabular cup and over the metal ball of the femoral stem of S-ROM hip prosthesis to prevent excessive wear.

polydioxanone plating—a method of extraluminal laryngotracheal fixation used in the treatment of grade 2 or 3 subglottic stenosis.

polydioxanone suture (PDS).

polyethylene glycol electrolyte lavage solution (PEG-LES).

polyethylene glycol (PEG)-hemoglobin —a combination of PEG and specially treated blood from cows, used as a blood substitute. Because this blood has been made with a special chemical modification, the immune system does not recognize it as "foreign" and does not reject it. This is still investigational, but you could be hearing about it in the future. It should have a number of advantages, including no blood typing or cross-matching, and eliminating risk of blood-borne diseases.

polyfluorotetraethylene (PTFE)—plastic graft material.

PolyGIA stapler—a stapling device which fires absorbable staples instead of the usual metal staples.

polyglactin—a suture material.

polyglecaprone 25 (Monocryl)—pliable synthetic absorbable monofilament suture material.

PolyHeme—a chemically modified human hemoglobin-based oxygen-carrying blood substitute for treating acute blood loss. It is believed to be universally compatible with all blood types, is free of blood-borne disease including HIV and hepatitis, and has a shelf life of up to a year compared with 30 days for blood.

polylactide absorbable screw—alternative to stainless steel or titanium nonabsorbable implants for fixation of ankle fractures. Use of absorbable hardware has been found to create adequate syndesmosis and eliminates the necessity for a second operative procedure to remove metallic hardware.

PolyMem—foam wound dressing.

polymerase chain reaction (PCR)—a procedure used in many areas including prenatal diagnosis, human leukocyte antigen typing, paternity testing, infectious disease detection and confirmation, hematologic diagnosis, genetic disease markers, gene mapping, forensics, and screening blood supply for infectious disease. PCR uses an in vitro method of DNA replication specific for the DNA or RNA sequence targeted for amplification. That is, the targeted nucleic marker for a specific disease, virus, or other abnormal condition is identified and multiplied many times (amplification). Only a small sample (blood, tissue, bone) is required, and that sample need contain only a single intact RNA or DNA strand with the sequence of interest (e.g. only a single cell or hair is needed). Fresh samples are not needed (making it a valuable detection technique in forensics and archaeology), and the procedure is extremely sensitive. A disadvantage is that of contamination in view of the small sample size needed to conduct the test. See also *ligase chain reaction, repair chain reaction.*

polymorphous light eruption—intense reaction to sunlight.

polyribonucleotide (Ampligen).

Polyrox—Fractal active fixation lead used in cardiovascular devices.

Polyskin II—transparent, semipermeable dressing that helps prevent scab formation and dermal dryness.

polysomnogram—performed for evaluation of sleep apnea syndrome and sleep efficiency. Sleep stages are determined by EEG, EMG, and EOG recordings. Oxygen saturation is

polysomnogram *(cont.)*
monitored by ear or finger oximeter, and EKG is used to monitor cardiac rhythm. REM and NREM sleep, slow wave sleep, number of arousals, microarousals, awakenings, respiratory events (hypoxic and apneic) are recorded. Respiratory parameters are monitored by nasal and oral thermistors.

Polysorb suture—synthetic absorbable suture made from a proprietary braiding process, which gives it strength but allows it to glide through tissue effortlessly like a monofilament material.

Polystan—perfusion cannula and venous return catheter.

polytef soft-tissue patch (ENT)—used to reconstruct postparotidectomy defects and prevent Frey's syndrome.

polytene chromosomes.

Polytrim solution (trimethoprim sulfate, polymyxin B sulfate)—a broad-spectrum ophthalmic anti-infective.

polyurethane foam embolus—used in treatment of fistula of the carotid cavernous sinus. Under local anesthesia, a small compressed piece of polyurethane foam is attached to a suture, and the common carotid artery is entered and the foam embolus placed in the artery. Blood flow carries the embolus to the fistula site, and after a few minutes the foam expands and occludes the fistula site. Then the suture is attached to the arterial wall. Blood flow through the carotid artery continues unimpeded; only the fistula site is occluded.

polyvinyl alcohol splinting material—said to be easily molded, hypoallergenic, lighter than plaster of Paris, and transparent to x-rays.

PolyWic wound filling material.

POMP (prednisone, Oncovin, methotrexate, mercaptopurine)—a chemotherapy protocol for promyelocytic leukemia.

Pompe's glycogen storage disease, type II—an inherited form of infantile cardiomyopathy that may be treated therapeutically with secretion-reuptake of protein.

pomum adami (Adam's apple)—the prominence in the neck that is the thyroid cartilage.

Ponka technique—for local anesthesia in herniorrhaphy.

Pontén-type tubed pedicle (Plas Surg)—a fasciocutaneous flap.

Pontiac fever—nonpulmonary flu-like form of legionellosis. See *legionnaires' disease.*

pooling of blood in extremities.

POP (plaster of Paris)—POP ("pop") bandages.

pop-off needle—used in hard-to-get-at places, such as deep in the abdomen. A pre-attached needle is used to take one stitch only; the needle is then twisted slightly, and the suture "pops" off, leaving a long suture for later tying. A series of sutures can then be tied sequentially. It is faster to use than having needles threaded by a nurse. Trade names: D-Tach and Control-Release.

Poppen Ridge Sensitometer—used for edge/depth/gap perception test.

porcine endogenous retrovirus (PERV)—a zoonotic retrovirus that can be transmitted to humans through xenotransplantation.

porcine fetal lateral ganglionic eminence (LGE) **cells**—a xenotransplantation product under study for the treatment of chronic striatal and cortical strokes.

porcine xenograft—any graft of porcine, or pig, origin, including heart valves and skin grafts. When autograft material is not available in a severely burned patient, split-thickness grafts of pigskin are used to cover the burned areas. This is a temporary graft that reduces the pain, permits the wound to heal more rapidly, and helps prevent the loss of fluids through evaporation. It also helps to protect the wound from infection.

pore—small, mostly transient opening in a cell wall caused by application of a brief high electric field pulse.

pores of Kohn—communications between alveoli.

Porites coral—see *madreporic coral.*

Porocoat—a porous coating used in the interfacing surfaces of DePuy's interlocking (Tri-Lock Cup) acetabular cups. See *Proplast* and *Plasti-Pore* for other porous prosthetic materials.

porous-coated anatomic (PCA) knee prosthesis.

porous prosthetic materials—see *Plasti-Pore, Porocoat, Proplast.*

PORP (partial ossicular replacement prosthesis).

porphyrins—biochemical compounds in hemoglobin.

port—a small rubber stopper on the side of intravenous tubing used to administer drugs by I.V. push or to insert a needle to piggyback another smaller I.V. solution. See also *I.V. push; piggyback.*

PORT—a patented electrode design for delivery of radiofrequency (RF) energy.

PORT (Patient Outcomes Research Team)—used in psychiatric care settings to address use of antipsychotic drugs, methods of therapy, psychological and family interventions, vocational rehabilitation, etc.

portable blood irradiator—a device about the size of a pencil that uses the radioactive element thulium-170 to kill white blood cells in patients being treated for such cancers as leukemia and lymphoma and for immune diseases such as AIDS and the early rejection of bone-marrow transplants.

portable film—an x-ray picture taken with movable equipment at the bedside or in the emergency department or operating room, when it is not feasible to move the patient to the radiology department.

portable volume ventilator—designed to dispense oxygen from any source in institutions, ambulances, mobile military hospitals, or the home.

Port-A-Cath—an implantable port of plastic or stainless steel with a rubber-covered entry site for inserting drugs. The port is connected to a central venous catheter which is positioned in the subclavian vein. Both the port and the catheter are implanted subcutaneously. Drugs are injected by inserting the needle through the skin and subcutaneous tissue and into the rubber-covered entry site on the port.

portacaval H graft—a decompressive side-to-side shunt used in hepatic surgery.

Port-Access minimally invasive cardiac surgery—used in single- and multi-vessel bypass surgery and mitral valve repair and replacement. It allows the surgeon to operate on a stopped heart through a small inci-

Port-Access *(cont.)*
sion between the ribs, thus avoiding a sternotomy.

Portagen diet—medium chain triglyceride diet.

portal azygous collaterals—in hepatic surgery.

portal embolization (PE)—uses embolization material consisting of Gelfoam powder, thrombin, Urografin, and gentamicin. Embolization is followed by extensive resection, such as extended right hepatic lobectomy combined with pancreatoduodenectomy after portal embolization.

portal hypertension—a serious complication of chronic liver disease. Techniques for assessment of portal pressure include WHVP (wedged hepatic vein pressure) measurement, umbilical vein catheterization, direct transhepatic measurement using a thin needle, and hepatic parenchymal pressure measurement.

portal hypertensive gastropathy (PHG).

Porta-Lung noninvasive extrathoracic ventilator (NEV)—often used for ventilating children.

portal venous-dominant phase (PVP) **images** (CT scan).

Porta Pulse 3—portable defibrillator.

port of Wilmington—a portal located 1 cm lateral and anterior to the posterior lateral tip of the acromion for arthroscopic SLAP repair.

portogram—radiographic study of portal flow through transfemoral vein and shunt cannulation.

portoportal anastomosis—an anastomosis connecting a donor portal artery to a recipient portal artery, such as might be used in transplant surgery. When dictated, it may sound like the physician is stuttering.

POSICAM system—medical imaging device using PET (positron emission topography) technology.

Posicor (mibefradil)—used in treatment of hypertension and chronic angina.

positive acetowhite test—acetic acid applied to affected area (such as warts or a dysplastic area of the cervix), causing the area to become whitish and more conspicuous.

positive end-expiratory pressure (PEEP).

positive symptoms of schizophrenia—hearing voices, hallucinations, delusions of grandeur, and paranoia. Cf. *negative symptoms of schizophrenia.*

Positrol cardiac device.

positron emission tomography (PET) —a scanning technique in radiology using computers and radioactive isotopes to aid imaging and diagnosis. PET scanning depicts blood flow and measures metabolism.

POST (peritoneal oocyte and sperm transfer).

postage-stamp-type skin graft.

post balloon angioplasty restenosis—a condition following angioplasty that is more likely to occur in patients with white plaque than those with yellow plaque. Restenosis is also more likely in patients with higher levels of lipoprotein-A (Lp[a]). Knowing this, physicians may be able to predict outcomes better by noting the color of the plaque or the levels of Lp(a).

posterior blue (Oph).

posterior capsular opacification (PCO).

posterior capsulorrhexis with optic capture (Oph).

posterior chamber intraocular lens (PC-IOL) **implantation**—bilateral procedure performed to correct pediatric aphakia.

posterior occipitoatlantal hypermobility (POAH)—in Down syndrome.

posterior polymorphous dystrophy (PPMD) **of the cornea**—bilateral autosomal dominant condition, usually nonprogressive, affecting the deepest layers of the cornea. Associated with this may be secondary alterations in Descemet's membrane.

posterior subcapsular cataract (PSC).

posterior sulcus—the groove formed by the intersection of the diaphragm and the posterior thoracic wall, as seen in a lateral chest x-ray.

posteromedial pivot shift test—demonstrates posterior cruciate ligament rupture. In order for posteromedial pivot shift to occur, the posterior collateral ligament, the medial collateral ligament, and the posterior oblique ligament all must be interrupted. If even one of these ligaments is intact, the subluxation will not occur.

posteromedial release (PMR)—a one-stage correction for talipes equinovarus (clubfoot).

postoperative flexor tendon traction brace.

postoperative regimen for oral early feeding (PROEF)—a slushy mixture consisting of crushed ice and flavored grenadine syrup, with added electrolytes, vitamins, amino acids, trace elements, and simple sugars. It is used to prevent distention and nausea and vomiting after abdominal surgery, since it is absorbed entirely in the upper GI tract.

post-poliomyelitis muscular atrophy (PPMA)—found in 15% of people who have had polio in the past. It appears about 30 years later and manifests itself by extreme fatigue, often severe muscle pain, and with a muscular weakness that may be slowly progressive over a long period of time.

post-transplantation lymphoproliferative disorder (PTLD)—found in pediatric thoracic organ transplant recipients.

post-transplant diabetes mellitus (PTDM).

post-tussive (also, *posttussive*)—after coughing. Applied to rales and rhonchi that do not disappear after the patient tries to clear his trachea and bronchi by coughing.

postural drainage—positioning the body in various ways to loosen pulmonary secretions.

Posture S'port—a posture corrector worn to help patients sit up straight and eliminate back and shoulder pain.

posturing, decorticate and decerebrate—rigid involuntary positioning of unconscious patient giving evidence of brain damage.

posturography—see *platform posturography*.

postviral fatigue syndrome—see *myalgic encephalomyelitis, chronic fatigue syndrome, yuppie flu*.

potassium—see *KCl*; *SSKI*.

potassium hydroxide (KOH)—destroys human cells and thus facilitates identification of fungus or yeast in the specimen, when added to a specimen of skin, other tissue, or vaginal secretions before microscopic examination.

potential acuity meter (PAM)—used in testing vision.

Pott's puffy tumor—posttraumatic osteomyelitis of the skull, with resultant edema, but without laceration of

Pott's puffy tumor *(cont.)*
the overlying scalp. Also, subperiosteal abscess of frontal sinus origin. (Named for P. Pott.)

Potts scissors.

pouce flottant—French term for *floating thumb or great toe.* The condition is associated with a number of congenital defects and anomalies repaired by microvascular and plastic surgeons. Associated with club hand deformity, this condition is also known as *radial ray defect* or *intercalary defect of the pollical ray.* A modified Bardenheuer's bifurcation procedure is often used for correction of this problem.

pouch—see *device.*

pouchogram—coined word for contrast-enhanced, radiographic examination of continent urinary diversion pouch (reservoir).

poudrage ("poo-drahj")—application of a powder to a surface, as done to promote fusion of serous membranes (e.g., two layers of pericardium or pleura).

Pourcelot resistance index (Neuro).

powder—see *Karaya powder.*

"powder burn" spots—vesicular and hemorrhagic burnt-out lesions, resulting from untreated endometriosis, as seen at laparoscopy.

power Doppler sonography—noninvasive technique to differentiate small hepatocellular carcinoma from adenomatous hyperplasia in patients with cirrhosis of the liver. Cf. *color Doppler sonography.*

Powerheart—automatic external cardioverter-defibrillator device.

PowerSculpt cosmetic surgery system—includes powered reciprocating cannulas for precise sculpting and contouring of surgical sites. It is used in multiple facial and body applications.

PP (pancreatic polypeptide)—"PP is associated with bronchogenic carcinoma and is also associated with diarrhea, possibly mediated by prostaglandins."

PPD (purified protein derivative) **test**—a skin test for tuberculosis.

PPK (palmoplantar keratoderma)—see *Voerner's disease.*

PPL (penicilloyl polylysine, Pre-Pen)—used in skin testing along with penicillin G and penicilloic acid, for detecting IgE antipenicillin antibodies, and for identifying patients who are at risk for penicillin allergy.

PPMA (post-poliomyelitis muscular atrophy).

PPMD (posterior polymorphous dystrophy) **of the cornea.**

PPPD (pylorus-preserving pancreatoduodenectomy).

PPROM (preterm premature rupture of membranes) **in pregnancy.**

P pulmonale—an electrocardiographic syndrome of tall, narrow, peaked P-waves seen in leads II, III, and aVF, with a prominent initial positive P-wave component in V1 and V2.

Ppv (portal venous pressure).

pramipexole—antiparkinsonism drug thought to slow the progress of the disease if used in the early stages.

pramlintide (Symlin)—used by diabetic patients to improve glucose control.

Prandase (acarbose)—used to treat type 2 diabetes. It acts in the small intestine to slow down the breakdown of carbohydrates following a meal. It delays sugar absorption and results in a smoothing and lowering of the high glucose levels experienced after meals.

Prandin (repaglinide)—used for oral treatment of type 2 diabetes. It was developed to help manage meal-related (prandial) glucosc loads.

PRA test (plasma renin activity).

Pravachol (pravastatin).

pravastatin (Pravachol)—a drug used to lower the levels of LDL in patients with hypercholesterolemia that has not responded to dietary measures.

PRBCs (packed red blood cells).

PRC (proximal row carpectomy)—for SLAC (scapholunate arthritic collapse) deformity. See *SLAC*.

PRDPC (pooled random donor platelet concentrates).

Preadmission Acuity Inquiry (PAI) **tool**.

PreCare Conceive—a nutritional supplement to be used by both men and women before conception of a child.

precedence effect—used in hearing studies to determine the major stimulus events that affect ability to process sounds in reverberant spaces. It helps determine how the auditory system "ignores" echoes in reverberant environments so that the listener can distinguish the original sound as the source.

preceding (*not* preceeding)—occurring before. Cf. *proceeding*.

precessional frequency—MRI term.

Precision Osteolock—femoral component design system using LPPS (low-pressure plasma spray) hydroxyapatite for a stable cementless fixation.

Precision QID—compact handheld glucose monitoring system.

Preclude pericardial membrane—a Gore-Tex product.

precordial honk—an abnormal heart sound.

precordium—the area over the heart and the lower part of the thorax. See *pericardium*.

Precose (acarbose)—used for treating non-insulin-dependent diabetes mellitus. It slows down the digestion of carbohydrates without causing low blood sugar levels or weight gain. It is used in combination with diet therapy.

prednicarbate (Dermatop)—a medium-strength topical corticosteroid, a prednisolone derivative with no preservatives, propylene glycol, or hallogens, which makes it a more gentle corticosteroid for use on chronic dermatoses.

prednimustine (Sterecyt)—an antineoplastic for treatment of malignant non-Hodgkin's lymphoma.

preimplantation genetic diagnosis—the diagnosis of genetic abnormalities before embryo implantation. Embryos obtained through in vitro fertilization are sampled at the eight-cell blastomere stage, and DNA probes are used to identify the presence of a defective gene sequence for diseases such as sickle cell anemia, Tay-Sachs disease, X-linked disorders, and cystic fibrosis. Only genetically healthy embryos are selected for uterine implantation.

preinvasive urothelial neoplasia—described as generalized thickening of the urothelium, or hyperplasia; disordered arrangements of cells with nuclear atypia or dysplasia; fully developed carcinoma in situ.

Premarin, Prempro, Premphase—hormones used in clinical trials for treatment of Alzheimer's disease.

premature rupture of (amniotic) **membranes** (PROM).

PremesisRx—prescription prenatal vitamin and mineral tablet designed to reduce pregnancy-related nausea.

Premier Type-Specific HSV-1 and **Premier Type-Specific HSV-2 IgG ELISA tests**—used to distinguish herpes simplex virus (HSV) type 1 (oral herpes) from type 2 (genital herpes) by serological test methods.

Premium CEEA circular stapler—with a detachable anvil and stem, used in end-to-end anastomosis, as in the rectum.

Premium Plus CEEA disposable stapler—used in laparoscopic Nissen fundoplication with esophageal lengthening.

Premphase (conjugated estrogens and medroxyprogesterone acetate)—hormone replacement therapy.

Prempro (conjugated estrogen and medroxyprogesterone acetate)—hormone replacement therapy for prevention and management of osteoporosis and treatment of moderate to severe vasomotor symptoms in women with intact uterus.

Prentice position—an optometric term used to describe the position in which a light source is calibrated perpendicular to the face of a glass prism.

Prentiss maneuver—used to lengthen the spermatic cord by taking down the floor of the canal along with the epigastric vessels in a staged laparoscopic orchiopexy. See *Fowler-Stephens orchiopexy.*

preperitoneal distention balloon (PDB).

Prepidil Gel (dinoprostone cervical gel) —medication indicated for ripening an unfavorable cervix in pregnant women at or near term, with need (medical or obstetric) to induce labor.

Prepodyne solution—used as an operating room skin preparation.

prepped—a brief form for *prepared.* "The patient was prepped and draped in the usual sterile manner."

PREP System—thin-layer slide preparation technology for Pap smears.

PREs (progressive resistive exercises).

Presaril (torsemide)—now known as *Demadex.* See *torsemide.*

"presbyalgos"—a coined term meaning loss of pain sensibility with age.

presbyesophagus—esophageal motility disorder due to aging.

presbyopia—defect of vision in advancing age, involving loss of accommodation, or recession of near point. Onset usually occurs between 40 and 45 years of age. Synonym: farsightedness. See *SRP* (surgical reversal of presbyopia).

present (verb)—to present oneself to a physician, clinic, or hospital for treatment.

presentation—the initial overt features of an illness; also, the part of a fetus that enters the birth canal first is the presenting part.

pressured speech—a rapid, tense manner of speaking that betrays the anxiety of the speaker.

pressure-relieving cushions (as spelled by manufacturer)
AirLITE
Enhance
Isch-Dish
Quadtro
ROHO Dry Floatation
SlimLine
StimuLITE
Varilyte Solo
WAFFLE

PressureSense Monitor—checks for compartment syndrome.

pressure sore—an alternative term for *decubitus ulcer*. The term *pressure sore* seems to be used more frequently.

pressure support ventilation (PSV) (Resp Ther)—characterized by a unique combination of simultaneous spontaneous and mechanical breathing, so that the ventilatory and flow rates and tidal volume depend on the patient's breathing pattern and the set level of pressure support. It can be used as a stand-alone ventilatory support mode and alternative to volume-controlled ventilation, and it can be used in weaning patients from mechanical ventilation.

Pressure Ulcer Scale for Healing (PUSH) **tool**.

Presto cardiac device.

Preston pinch gauge—used to quantify pinch strength of the fingers.

presumed ocular histoplasmosis (POH) **syndrome**.

Prevacid (lansoprazole)—proton pump inhibitor used to heal erosive esophagitis. Not for long-term therapy.

Preven emergency contraceptive kit.

Prevnar—vaccine for prevention of invasive pneumococcal disease in young children.

PreVue—test for Lyme disease that searches for antigens made by the *Borrelia burgdorferi* bacteria responsible for the infection. The test can be done in the physician's office and should make it easier to diagnose the infection, which sometimes goes undetected until it has caused long-lasting damage.

PREZ (posterior root entry zone)—see *DREZ*.

Price and Brew staging scheme—for AIDS dementia complex.

prickle-cell layer of epidermis.

Priftin (rifapentine)—treatment of pulmonary tuberculosis.

Prilosec (omeprazole)—antisecretory drug in a sustained release capsule used to treat duodenal ulcers, gastroesophageal reflux disease, erosive esophagitis, and Barrett's esophagus. *Prilosec* is the trade name replacing *Losec* because of reports of confusion between Losec and Lasix in drug orders.

Primacor (milrinone lactate)—for congestive heart failure.

Primaderm—a semipermeable foam dressing.

Prima laser guide wire—used in angioplasty procedures. It can pass through totally occluded coronary arteries by dissolving tissue through photoablation.

Primapore absorptive wound dressing.

primaquine phosphate—antimalarial drug combined with the antibiotic clindamycin to treat *Pneumocystis carinii* pneumonia in AIDS patients.

primary biliary cirrhosis (PBC).

primary hyperoxaluria, type 1 (PH-1) —presents in childhood with recurrent urolithiasis. Also the cause of idiopathic renal failure in adults.

primary immune deficiency (PID)— found in children and adolescents in whom part of the immune system is missing or not functioning properly.

primary open angle glaucoma (POAG) (Oph)—the most common form of glaucoma, occurring when pressure in the eye gradually damages the optic nerve.

primary pure teratoma—a complex tumor with a histologically benign

primary pure teratoma *(cont.)* appearance, but an unpredictable course, and believed to have metastatic potential.

primary sclerosing cholangitis (PSC) —a chronic, progressive disease that damages the biliary tract. Associated with an increased risk of colorectal cancer.

Primbs-Circon indirect video ophthalmoscope system—can be used with either AO (American Optical) or Keeler indirect ophthalmoscope. It uses a beam splitter; a portion of the light goes to the eyepiece used by the surgeon, and the rest of the light goes to a video camera which televises (in color) the image seen through the ophthalmoscope (the televised image of intraocular, retinal, and vitreal pathology) to members of the surgical team.

PRIME (Primary Care Evaluation of Mental Disorders).

Prime ECG (electrocardiographic) **mapping system**.

PRIME-MD (computerized version of Primary Care Evaluation of Mental Disorders)—test for dependence, hypochondriasis, conversion disorder, and eating disorders. The computer-administered version was found to diagnose double the rate of substance abuse when compared with physician interview.

Primer—compression dressing or wrap.

Primsol solution (trimethoprim HCl oral solution)—for treatment of acute otitis media caused by susceptible organisms in children ages 6 months to 12 years.

Pringle maneuver—a technique for clamping the hepatic pedicle prior to hepatectomy.

Prinzide (hydrochlorothiazide, lisinopril)—combined diuretic and ACE inhibitor for hypertension.

Prinzmetal's angina—an angina pectoris variant in which the patient has attacks while resting, and exercise tolerance is not significantly decreased.

Prisma digital hearing aid—uses digital signal processing (DSP) and an advanced directional microphone.

PRK (photorefractive keratectomy). Also, *T-PRK.*

PRL (prolactin).

Pro-Air (procaterol).

ProAmatine (midodrine)—for treatment of neurogenic orthostatic hypotension.

proarrhythmia—the appearance of a new arrhythmia or worsening of arrhythmia in the context of antiarrhythmic drug therapy in comparison with drug-free condition. Certain antiarrhythmic drugs may actually worsen a minor cardiac arrhythmia, and such drugs are given only for life-threatening arrhythmias. See *propafenone.*

proband—a person, affected with what is probably a familial disease, diagnosed independently of his family in a genetic study. "A proband of this family was a seven-year-old girl with hyperextensible joints. Note: The family has several members with Ehlers-Danlos syndrome."

Pro-Banthine (propantheline promide) —peptic ulcer treatment adjunct; antispasmodic; antisecretory.

Probe cardiac device.

Procardia XL (nifedipine)—extended release for 24-hour control of hypertension and angina.

procaterol (Pro-Air)—a bronchodilator similar to Proventil in its action and the fact that it can be given either orally or by inhalation.

procedure—see *operation* for list of procedures, including diagnostic, radiographic, nonsurgical, surgical, and therapeutic procedures and studies.

Proceed—hemostatic surgical sealant composed of collagen-derived granules, thrombin, and patient fibrinogen. It provides both chemical and physical effects to speed clotting and thus seal bleeding tissue.

proceeding—progressing. Cf. *preceding*.

Pro-Clude—transparent film wound dressing.

procrastination (delayed action)—as in "His basic suggestions were that treatment remain conservative, and that procrastination be the procedure of choice for the time being." See also *tincture of time*.

Procrit (epoetin alfa)—used for anemic cancer patients with nonmyeloid malignancies on chemotherapy.

ProCross Rely over-the-wire balloon catheter.

Proctozone P (1% pramoxine HCl) and **Proctozone H** (1% hydrocortisone)—treatment for anorectal ailments, including pruritus ani and hemorrhoids.

Procuren—platelet-derived growth factor.

Procysteine (oxothiazolidine carboxylate)—a drug used to treat AIDS.

ProCyte—transparent adhesive film dressing.

Prodigy bone densitometer—includes DualFemur, Lateral Vertebral Assessment (LVA), and fast Total Body scanning, using standard DEXA technology.

Prodigy lens inserter—an intraocular lens inserter that requires little manipulation of the eye.

PROEF (postoperative regimen for oral early feeding).

profile—see *PULSES profile*.

Profile total hip system—has porous coating (Porocoat). Also, DePuy.

Profix component—used in joint replacements.

Pro-Flo XT catheter (Cardio).

Profore four-layer bandaging system —controls the underlying venous hypertension responsible for venous ulcers by providing effective levels of pressure and maintaining the pressure for a full week.

ProForma—double lumen papillotome.

profundaplasty, profundoplasty—surgical reconstruction of the profunda femoris, a procedure used in treatment of femoropopliteal occlusive disease.

profusion—abundance. "There was normal hair distribution and profusion." Cf. *perfusion*.

progesterone receptor (PgR).

prognostic nutritional index—one of the better known indices to provide a quantitative estimate of surgical risk and selection criteria for preoperative nutrition support. A highly significant increase in the incidence of postoperative complications, major sepsis, and death may be observed as the PNI increases.

Prograf (tacrolimus capsules and injection)—used for the prophylaxis of organ rejection in kidney transplant recipients.

progressive multifocal leukoencephalopathy (PML)—catastrophic HIV-

progressive multifocal *(cont.)* related encephalopathy for which there is, at present, no treatment.

progressive osseous heteroplasia—developmental disorder of heterotopic ossification that appears to affect only females.

progressive parenchymal restriction —see *bronchiolitis obliterans.*

progressive resistive exercises (PREs).

progressive systemic sclerosis (PSS).

ProHance (gadoteridol)—nonionic gadolinium MRI contrast medium.

Project Gargle—a data collection and analysis study on flu viruses. U.S. Air Force bases in various locations worldwide conduct active surveillance for flu viruses and submit throat swab specimens for virus isolation and characterization. The results of these laboratory analyses help determine the composition of the following year's influenza vaccine.

Prokop intraocular lens (implant).

prolactin levels (PRL)—elevated in patients with nonsecreting adenomas or other intrasellar and parasellar diseases (pseudoprolactinomas).

ProLease encapsulated sustained-release growth hormone—a sustained release version of human growth hormone, designed to reduce the need for daily injections.

Prolene (*not* Proline)—suture material.

Proleukin (aldesleukin)—used for treatment of metastatic melanoma.

proliferative retinopathy photocoagulation (PRP).

proliferative vitreoretinopathy (PVR).

PROloop—electrosurgical device for cutting, coagulation, and vaporization of tissues.

prolotherapy—injection of saline solution into a ligament or tendon at its attachment to bone. This causes localized inflammation, which then increases blood supply and flow of nutrients to the area and stimulates tissue to repair itself. Used in treatment of chronic pain.

PROM (premature rupture of membranes, amniotic) (Ob-Gyn).

ProMACE-CytaBOM (prednisone, methotrexate, Adriamycin, cyclophosphamide, etoposide, cytarabine, bleomycin, Oncovin, mitoxantrone) —chemotherapy protocol to treat Hodgkin's lymphoma.

ProMem (metrifonate)—for treatment of mild to moderate Alzheimer's disease.

Promensil—natural isoflavone-based dietary supplement derived from red clover. It is used to help women maintain estrogen levels and cardiovascular health during menopause.

Prometrium (progesterone, micronized)—oral form of progesterone used for estrogen replacement therapy in patients who have not undergone hysterectomy. It contains a progesterone synthesized from yams.

Promycin (porfiromycin)—a therapeutic agent that targets hypoxic cancer cells, which are known to be less susceptible to radiation therapy than other tumor cells

Pronova nonabsorbable suture—synthetic nonabsorbable monofilament suture. It is used for approximation and/or ligation of soft tissues during general surgical procedures.

ProOsteon implant 500—a bone-void filler fabricated to resemble cancellous bone. It is made of natural coralline hydroxyapatite. Provides a

ProOsteon implant *(cont.)*
matrix for bony ingrowth to improve stabilization. Replaces or augments autologous bone grafts.

propafenone (Rythmol)—an oral antiarrhythmic drug that decreases electrical conduction across the atria and ventricles. It is indicated for life-threatening arrhythmias only, as it may actually make minor arrhythmias more severe.

propantheline bromide (Pro-Banthine)—an antispasmodic for treating urinary urge incontinence; peptic ulcer adjunct.

Propaq Encore vital signs monitor—used to monitor neonatal and impedance respiration functions.

Propecia (finasteride)—an oral treatment for men with male pattern hair loss (androgenetic alopecia).

Propel cannulated interference screws—used in knee arthroscopy.

Pro/Pel coating (Cardio).

proper lamina; **ligament**; **membrane** (L., propria)—anglicized form of *lamina propria*, the form usually dictated.

Propionibacterium—an anaerobic organism, one of a group of normal skin flora.

Proplast—composite of Teflon polymer and elemental carbon. It resembles a black felt sponge and is 70 to 90% porous. It is used as graft material in fashioning prostheses. The host tissue, in effect, invades the pores of this material and transforms it into a similar tissue; it is biocompatible with many tissues, such as bone, soft tissue, and dura. Used in repair of dural defects and CSF leaks. See also *Plasti-Pore*.

ProPoint—point-search instrument used to localize acupuncture points.

proprietary medicine—the name given to trademarked, brand name medications, both prescription and over-the-counter drugs.

proprioception—relates to the sensory system mechanism that has to do with movement of the body, its posture, balance, and coordination.

proptosis—a forward displacement of the eyeball in exophthalmic goiter or in an inflammatory condition of the orbit. Cf. *ptosis*.

Propulsid (cisapride)—treatment for nocturnal heartburn due to gastroesophageal reflux disease. Discontinued July 2000 due to side effects of heart rhythm abnormalities and cardiac-related deaths.

Proscar (finasteride).

Prosed/DS—methenamine/benzoic acid analysis.

ProSol (amino acid injection)—adjunct in off-setting of nitrogen loss or in treatment of negative nitrogen balance. Also used to reduce fluid intake in patients who require both fluid restriction and total parenteral nutrition.

ProSom (estazolam)—a benzodiazepine type of sedative drug.

Prosorba column—an apheresis device that works much like dialysis to treat severe joint swelling and pain in rheumatoid arthritis patients who have not been helped by other therapies. The patient's blood is removed, the plasma separated and treated by the Prosorba machine, and the blood then remixed and transfused back into the body. The machine is a column filled with silica and "protein A" from the cell wall of a bacterium that clings to human antibodies. As plasma runs through the column, the "protein A" separates out a small

Prosorba *(cont.)*
amount of antibodies before the plasma is retransfused.

PROST (pronuclear-stage embryo transfer).

ProstaCoil—self-expanding stent used in treatment of urethral obstruction caused by enlargement of the prostate gland.

prostaglandin E1 (alprostadil) (Urol) —a special topical gel for the treatment of erectile dysfunction.

Prostalase laser system—an investigational Nd:YAG laser system used for TURP. See *transurethral balloon Laserthermia prostatectomy.*

Prostar, Prostar Plus, and **Prostar XL** percutaneous closure devices. See *Perclose closure device.*

ProstaScint (CYT-356 radiolabeled with 111 indium chloride)—a monoclonal antibody imaging agent for use in prostate cancer patients with suspected metastatic disease.

ProstaSeed ¹²⁵**I**—radiation treatment for prostate cancer.

prostate—the prostate gland, which surrounds the beginning of the urethra in the male. Cf. *prostrate.*

prostate-specific antigen (PSA)—a protease produced by prostatic epithelium, found elevated in primary and metastatic adenocarcinoma of the prostate as well as in some cases of prostatitis and benign prostatic hyperplasia.

prostate-specific antigen bound to alpha-1-antichymotrypsin—see *PSA-ACT.*

prostate-specific antigen (PSA) **free/ total index**—see *free/total PSA index.*

prostate-specific membrane antigen (PSMA)—a substance often ex-

pressed in the most aggressive clones of prostate cancer cells. Using a prostate cancer monoclonal antibody conjugate, a team of researchers targeted PSMA in an effort to detect circulating prostate cancer cells. With this test, much higher rates were found than with using prostate-specific antigen alone. Researchers believe this test may provide physicians with a method of identifying patients at high risk of advanced disease at the time of initial diagnosis or following therapy.

Prostatron—a mobile device that uses microwave energy to provide long-term relief from symptomatic benign prostatic hypertrophy. The procedure takes approximately one hour and can be done on an outpatient basis with local anesthesia. See *TUMT.*

ProStep (nicotine)—transdermal patch.

prosthesis—an artificial substitute or internal device to replace a body part, such as a hip, knee, joint, or cardiac valve; joint replacement material; and breast and penile implants. Also, an external device such as an arm, hand, leg, or foot, or an orthopedic appliance or device. May also be called *appliance, fixation device, implant, orthosis,* or *valve.*
Prostheses in this book include:
Acticon neosphincter
AcuMatch A Series acetabular
Airprene hinged knee
alumina-alumina total hip replacement
AMS (American Medical Systems) 700 CX inflatable penile
Angelchik antireflux
Apollo hip
Apollo knee
Atkinson endoprosthesis

prosthesis *(cont.)*
Austin Moore hip
Bateman UPF II bipolar endo-
prosthesis
Becker tissue expander/breast
Bio-Chromatic hand
bladder neck support continent
Blom-Singer indwelling low
pressure voice
Buechel-Pappas total ankle
Caffinière
Calnan-Nicolle synthetic joint
CardioFix Pericardium patch
Carpentier-Edwards Perimount
RSR pericardial bioprosthesis
CPHV OptiForm mitral valve
crutched-stick type endoprosthesis
DANA (designed after natural
anatomy) shoulder
Deon hip
Dilamezinsert penile
DoubleStent biliary endoprosthesis
Duraphase
Dynaflex penile
endoprosthesis
Finney Flexi-Rod penile
Finn hinged knee replacement
Flatt finger/thumb
Flowers mandibular glove
Freestyle aortic root bioprosthesis
GFS Mark II inflatable penile
Gianturco expandable (self-expand-
ing) metallic biliary stent
Groningen voice
Guepar II hinged knee
Hancock M.O. bioprosthesis
Hanger ComfortFlex knee
HD II (or 2) total hip
Inter-Op acetabular
IntraStent DoubleStrut biliary
endoprosthesis
Introl bladder neck support
J-FX bipolar head
Judet hip

prosthesis *(cont.)*
Kaster mitral valve
Kinematic rotating hinge
Leeds-Keio ligament
Link cementless reconstruction hip
Link Endo-Model rotational knee
Lord total hip
lunate
madreporic hip
McCutchen SLT hip
McNaught keel laryngeal
Mentor Alpha 1 inflatable penile
Metasul metal-on-metal hip
Microknit vascular graft
Monostrut cardiac valve
Natural-Hip
NCP (NeuroCybernetic Prosthesis)
NeuroCybernetic Prosthesis (NCP)
Neville tracheal and tracheo-
bronchial
Niebauer
Noiles posterior stabilized knee
Noiles rotating hinge total knee
Omnifit HA hip stem
Omniscience single leaflet cardiac
valve
Panje voice button laryngeal
Passy-Muir tracheostomy speaking
valve
PCA (porous-coated anatomic)
knee
Perfecta hip
Perimount RSR pericardial biopros-
thesis
Pillet hand
piston stapes
Pitt talking tracheostomy tube
porous-coated anatomic (PCA)
knee
Provox speaking valve
Richards hydroxyapatite PORP
and TORP
Ring hip
Sense-of-Feel

prosthesis *(cont.)*
Singer-Blom speech valve
Sivash
Small-Carrion penile
St. George total elbow
TARA (total articular replacement arthroplasty)
TMJ fossa-eminence
TORP (total ossicular replacement)
Townley TARA
UroLume endoprosthesis
Utah artificial arm
Vibrant D and Vibrant P soundbridge
Vitallium alloy cobalt-chrome
Wallstent iliac endoprosthesis
Wayfarer
Weaveknit vascular
Wehrs incus
Zweymuller

Prosthetic Disc Nucleus (PDN)—a device surgically implanted to treat patients with incapacitating, chronic low back pain resulting from degenerative disk disease.

prostrate—lying prone. Cf. *prostate.*

ProstRcision—an outpatient procedure that treats prostate cancer with a combination of seed implants followed by conformal beam irradiation.

protean—said of a disease having various symptoms in different patients.

protease inhibitor—a drug used to treat patients with AIDS.

ProtectaCap—a shock-absorbent foam whole-head protective cap which fastens under the chin. Designed for children under age 6, it has a colorful vinyl cover and none of the bulk or weight of commonly used helmets. Used to protect the skull following cranial surgery.

Protectaid contraceptive sponge.

Protect-a-Pass suture passer—used in percutaneous bladder neck stabiliza-tion for women with stress urinary incontinence. The passer utilizes a thumb lever that opens the suture channel and releases the suture, preventing entrapment of vaginal tissue in the open slot, and places a Z-stitch.

Protector suturing system—used in arthroscopic surgery for meniscal repair.

Protect Point needle—tapered tip reduces risk of glove puncture.

protein
ALZ-50
anti-Tamm-Horsfall
A68
autocrine motility factor (AMF)
bone morphogenic
BPI (bactericidal/permeability-increasing
C
CHUK (conserved helix-loop-helix ubiquitous kinase)
COUP-TF thyroid hormone receptor auxiliary
C-reactive (CRP)
CREB (cAMP response element binding)
cytokeratin
Endostatin
ESAT-6
estramustine binding (EMBP)
glial fibrillary acidic
GLQ223 (compound Q)
glycated
human Complement Factor H-related
ICAM-1 marker
IL-4R immune system
lactoferrin
Lp(a)
microtubule-associated
M-protein
neuronal apoptosis inhibitory (NAIP)

protein *(cont.)*
  Novel erythropoiesis stimulating (NESP)
  nuclear matrix (NMP)
  P-glycoprotein
  p24 antigen
  p55-IgG tumor necrosis factor receptor fusion
  phycobiliproteins
  Raf-1 human
  rhBMP-2 (recombinant human bone morphogenetic)
  ribonuclear (RNP)
  S
  SCA (single-chain antigen-binding)
  single-chain antigen-binding (SCA)
  solder
  Sonic Hedgehog (Shh)
  TGF-B (transforming growth factor-beta)
  TpP (thrombus precursor)

protein C—a naturally occurring anticoagulant protein that inhibits the coagulating activity of blood factors V and VIII. The protein C levels are of concern in patients with renal disease. See *protein S.*

protein-losing enteropathy (PLE).

protein S—a naturally occurring anticoagulant that is necessary for the activity of protein C in treating patients with renal disease. See *protein C.*

protein solder—human albumin preparation used for tissue welding, e.g., in urologic surgery, used in place of staples or sutures or clips, which have an inherent lithogenic reaction. It decreases operative time, promotes healing, and provides immediate intraoperative watertight seal in such procedures as arterial anastomoses, nerve coaptation, bowel anastomoses, and ureteral reconstruction. Also, *tissue solder, tissue glue.*

Protek joint implant.

Proteque SPS—steroid-sparing topical treatment for eczema and dermatitis.

Prothiaden (dothiepin HCl)—an antidepressant drug.

pro time—brief form used in dictation for *prothrombin time* (PT), a test for defects in blood clotting. (*Pro time* should be written as two words.)

protocol—see *medication* for chemotherapy protocols.

Protocult—stool sampling device that reduces the chance of contamination.

proton density images—MRI term.

Protonix (pantoprazole)—oral and I.V. formulations to treat esophageal diseases, such as erosive esophagitis, *H. pylori* infection, Zollinger-Ellison syndrome.

proton magnetic resonance spectroscopy—performed on the fetus via MRI. May serve as a noninvasive approach to monitoring the fetus.

proto-oncogene
  c-fms (growth factor receptor gene)
  c-myc/myb/fos (nuclear proteins)
  c-sis (growth factor gene)
  c-src (cytoplasmic protein tyrosine kinase)

Protouch—synthetic orthopedic padding.

Pro-Trac—cruciate reconstruction measurement device.

Protractor—a combination retractor and wound protector indicated for use during both laparoscopic and open surgical procedures.

Protropin and **Protropin II**—human growth hormone, genetically engineered. See *Genentech biosynthetic human growth hormone.*

protruding atheromas—cause embolic disease. Can be seen on transesophageal echocardiography.

PRO 2000 Gel—drug used for the prevention of HIV-1 infection and other sexually transmitted diseases.

proverbs, Benjamin (Psych).

Providencia rettgeri—newer name for the former *Proteus rettgeri;* commonly found in stool.

Provigil (modafinil)—used in the treatment of narcolepsy.

Provir—an oral drug used in treatment of diarrhea.

provocative maneuvers—on physical exam, diagnostic manipulations that reproduce the patient's symptoms in certain conditions, e.g., thoracic outlet syndrome.

Provox speaking valve—a type of laryngeal prosthesis implanted following laryngectomy. Air exhaled from the lungs is redirected through a surgical fistula in which the prosthetic speaking valve has been implanted. Advantages include more natural speech which is synchronized with breathing rather than speech using regurgitated air or the use of an external vibrator applied to the neck (which creates a mechanical, monotone-like speech). The name of the implant comes from the Latin *pro* 'for' and *vox* 'voice.'

proximal articular set angle (PASA).

Proximate flexible linear stapler.

Proximate linear cutter—a surgical stapler.

Prozac (fluoxetine)—an antidepressant. Used for treatment of obsessive-compulsive disorder and premenstrual syndrome.

PRP (panretinal photocoagulation).

PRP (proliferative retinopathy photocoagulation).

Pruitt-Inahara carotid shunt—a long polyvinyl tube with an inflatable balloon at each end. The inflated balloon keeps the shunt tube within the vessel; thus no clamps are utilized, resulting in less trauma to the blood vessel. This shunt may also be used in some patients undergoing vascular reconstruction of the leg.

prune-belly syndrome—see *Eagle-Barrett syndrome.*

PS (pulmonary sequestration).

PSA (prostate-specific antigen).

PSA-ACT (prostate-specific antigen bound to alpha-1-antichymotrypsin) —the ratio of PSA-ACT to "free" PSA in serum is indicative of prostate cancer risk. High levels, as revealed by sensitive PSA tests, indicate higher risk for prostate cancer.

PSA4—home blood test to screen for prostate cancer.

PSA (prostate-specific antigen) **index**— see *free/total PSA index.*

psammoma ("sah-mo´mah")—a tumor, especially a meningioma, that contains psammoma bodies.

psammoma bodies—microscopic laminated calcified bodies commonly seen in thyroid and ovarian cancer.

PSC (posterior semicircular canal).

PSC (posterior subcapsular cataract).

PSC (primary sclerosing cholangitis).

PSD (pituitary stalk distortion).

Pseudallescheria boydii—fungus originally identified as one of the agents thought responsible for Madura foot. *P. boydii* is an opportunistic pathogen and has been recognized with increasing frequency as a cause of pulmonary, central nervous system, prostatic, osteomyelitic, ophthalmologic, otitic, and disseminated infections, particularly in patients who are immunocompromised.

pseudodermachalasis—slackening of the skin below the eyebrow, giving the upper eyelid a redundant appearance. "Gravitation of the eyebrow downward caused pseudodermachalasis of the upper eyelids."

"pseudofracture"—see *kink artifact*.

pseudo-Hurler deformity—see *mucolipidosis III*.

pseudomembranous colitis (PMC).

Pseudomonas **exotoxin**—a natural poison from a common bacterium used in the treatment of malignant brain tumors. It is delivered to the tumor site in combination with interleukin 4, a substance to which cancer cells have a receptor. The *Pseudomonas* exotoxin destroys the cancer cell's ability to produce protein and stay alive. Since healthy brain cells do not have interleukin-4 receptors, they are not exposed to the bacterium's toxin.

Pseudomonas maltophilia (Alcaligenes bookeri)—an opportunistic pathogen found in soil, plants, water, sewage, animals, and raw milk. Seen in meningitis, septicemia, pleuritis, infected wounds.

Pseudomonas stutzeri—opportunistic pathogen found in soil but occasionally in sputum specimens, in wounds, ear drainage, and infected eyes; found also on aerosol equipment.

pseudoseizure—an attack resembling an epileptic seizure but having purely psychological causes. It lacks the electroencephalographic characteristics of epilepsy and the patient may be able to stop it by an act of will. Also called *pseudoepilepsy* and *hysterical epilepsy*.

Pseudovent (guaifenesin/pseudoephedrine HCl) **capsules**—a brand name generic expectorant/decongestant.

PSF (posterior spine fusion)—spine surgery.

p.s.i., psi ("sigh") (pounds per square inch)—unit of measurement used in procedures involving pressure. See *Brown-McHardy pneumatic dilator*.

PSIL (percentage signal intensity loss)—MRI term.

P6—acupressure point. See *Neiguan point*.

PSMA (prostate-specific membrane antigen).

psomophagia ("somophagia")—swallowing food without chewing it thoroughly.

psoralen—a light-activated drug used in treatment of psoriasis, and in T- cell lymphoma. See *photophoresis*.

psoralen inactivation technique—used to inactivate a variety of infectious agents including some that are considered more difficult to inactivate than HIV. Involves exposing an active infectious agent to psoralen or one of its derivatives, and thereafter exposing it to ultraviolet light, by which process the psoralen forms chemical bonds with the nucleic acids (DNA or RNA) in the infectious agents.

psoriasis of the penis—can develop from prolonged use of fluorinated steroid creams.

psoriatic onychopachydermoperiostitis—psoriasis condition of the nails consisting of onychopathy, soft tissue thickening, and x-ray evidence of bone erosion and periosteal reaction of the terminal phalanx.

Psorospermium haeckelii—may be confused with helminth eggs in laboratory analysis of feces of individuals who have recently eaten crayfish.

PSP (progressive supranuclear palsy).

PSS (progressive systemic sclerosis). Scleroderma is a form of this disease.

PSV (pressure support ventilation).

PSVT (paroxysmal supraventricular tachycardia).

psychedelic drugs (*not* psychodelic)—refers to certain types of drugs that act on the central nervous system, e.g., LSD, mescaline, etc., producing heightened perception, visual hallucinations, delusions.

PSY Inventory—for assessment of six behavioral characteristics (Sense of Responsibility, Energy and Competitiveness, Obsessive Behavior, Anger and Hostility, Stress-related Disturbances, Time Urgency) in patients who have suffered an acute myocardial infarction.

PTA (percutaneous transluminal angioplasty). Cf. *PTCA, Dotter-Judkins technique.*

PTAH (phosphotungstic acid-hematoxylin)—a histochemical diagnostic stain. See *Mallory's PTAH.*

PTBD (percutaneous transhepatic biliary drainage).

PTC (percutaneous transhepatic cholangiography).

PTC (plasma thromboplastin component)—in bleeding diseases.

PTCA (percutaneous transluminal coronary angioplasty). See *Grüntzig.*

PTDM (post-transplant diabetes mellitus).

PTEN gene—recent findings suggest up to 50% of all endometrial cancers may contain a mutation in this gene.

PTFE (polytetrafluoroethylene)—suburethral sling material used to treat stress urinary incontinence. PTFE does not need pre-clotting, as Dacron does. It is also used as vascular access in hemodialysis.

PTH (parathormone, parathyroid hormone).

PTHC (percutaneous transhepatic cholangiogram).

P-32—a chromic phosphate suspension given via intraperitoneal administration to patients with ovarian cancer. It is used only after a second-look laparotomy has yielded negative findings and its purpose is to attempt to improve survival time.

PTK (phototherapeutic keratectomy).

PTL (pharyngeal lumen airways).

PTLD (post-transplantation lymphoproliferative disorder).

PTMC (percutaneous transvenous mitral commissurotomy).

PTMR (percutaneous transluminal myocardial revascularization).

ptosis ("toe´sis") (noun)—a prolapse or drooping of an anatomic structure, such as the upper eyelid. Cf. *proptosis, phthisis.*

ptotic ("tot´tic") (adj.)—see *ptosis.*

PTRA (percutaneous transluminal renal angioplasty).

p22 phox gene—a gene that appears to provide protection against coronary artery disease by affecting the production of free radicals that oxidize low-density lipoproteins (LDL), the "bad" form of cholesterol that increases risk of heart diseases.

p24 antigen—an HIV core protein that can be detected in HIV-infected blood several weeks before HIV antibodies first appear.

p24 protein—found in the core of the HIV virus and seems to be a relatively stable part of this quickly changing virus.

P300—a test for dementia.

public access defibrillation (PAD).

pubovaginal sling—constructed as part of a one-stage repair of urethral damage.

PUBS (percutaneous umbilical cord blood sampling).

PUD (peptic ulcer disease).

puddle sign—a quick, if unsophisticated, method of differentiating minimal ascites from edema. The patient lies prone for five minutes and then assumes the knee-chest position; dullness on percussion in the periumbilical region indicates ascites rather than edema.

pudendal neurogram (Peds)—used in treating spasticity in plantar flexors in children with cerebral palsy. It is an indirect approach to the assessment of bladder and bowel reflex pathways using sensory evoked potentials from dorsal nerve of the penis or clitoris (a branch of the pudendal).

puerperal abscess—may be caused by *Salmonella bredeney* and group B Streptococcus.

Puestow pancreaticojejunostomy—a procedure performed on patients with obstruction of the pancreatic ductal system resulting in dilated duct, with points of stenosis and distal calculi.

puffer, pink—a patient with early respiratory failure, showing dyspnea but no cyanosis. Cf. *blue bloater.*

puff of smoke (moyamoya)—angiographic diagnosis of bilateral stenosis or occlusion of the internal carotid arteries above the clinoids.

Puig Massana annuloplasty ring—allows for precise final adjustments to ensure atrioventricular competence.

Pulec and Freedman—classification of congenital aural atresia.

Pulmicort Turbuhaler (budesonide)—a once-daily (previously twice-daily) asthma treatment for children and adults. It uses 200 mcg of budesonide inhalation powder.

Pulmo-Aide nebulizer—used to permit easier breathing in patients with allergies, asthma, chronic obstructive pulmonary disease, cystic fibrosis.

pulmonary artery wedge pressure (PAWP).

pulmonary autograft (PA)—the patient's own pulmonary valve used in aortic valve replacement. In the Ross procedure the patient's own pulmonary valve is essentially used as a "spare part" to replace the diseased aortic valve.

pulmonary parenchymal window—a CT setting for examining lung tissue. See also *bone window; brain window; soft tissue window; subdural window.*

pulmonary sequestration—a mass of abnormal lung parenchyma with an anomalous systemic blood supply not communicating with the normal tracheobronchial tree. An intralobar sequestration is contained within the visceral pleura of a lower lobe receiving its blood supply from the abdominal aorta or other thoracic vessel; an extralobar sequestration is a congenital malformation with variable ectopic blood supply.

pulmonary sling syndrome—aberrant left pulmonary artery causing tracheal stenosis and a variety of unilateral aeration disturbances. On x-rays, the left pulmonary artery appears as a small rounded mass between the trachea and esophagus. The left pulmonary artery, as it arises from the right pulmonary artery and hooks around the trachea, can cause compression of the right bronchus with resulting underinflated right lung, but overexpansion of the right lung, or even the left lung, can occur.

pulmonary toilet—postural drainage, percussion, hydration, and other

pulmonary toilet *(cont.)*
means of clearing the respiratory tract.

pulmonary vascular markings (Radiol)—as seen on chest x-ray, the normal radiographic appearance of the branches of the pulmonary arteries and veins about the hila of the lungs.

pulmonary vascular redistribution (Radiol)—on chest x-ray, increased prominence of upper pulmonary vessels and reduced prominence of lower pulmonary vessels at the lung hila in left ventricular failure and other disturbances of circulatory dynamics.

PulmoSphere—particle-processing technology that doubles the quantity of a drug delivered to deep lung using a metered-dose inhaler.

Pulmozyme (dornase alfa)—an aerosolized drug for cystic fibrosis patients. Inhaled once daily, it thins mucus and increases pulmonary function. Pulmozyme is the product of recombinant DNA technology.

Pulsavac III wound debridement system—used to clear excess cement from a surgical site, to wash debris from open trauma fractures, to clear the intramedullary canal for rod or prosthesis placement, or to clean wounds before closure.

pulsed dose therapy—the opposite of a continuous dosing regimen. Medication or treatment is administered in several sessions with longer intervals between. Chemotherapy is an example of pulsed dose therapy. Also called pulse dose therapy, pulse therapy, pulsed therapy.

pulsed dye laser therapy—used for ureteral stone lithotripsy. Cf. *ESWL*. It is said to be a highly effective and safe method to selectively destroy warts without damaging the surrounding skin.

pulse deficit—the arithmetical difference between the apical pulse and the radial or other peripheral pulse. Generally it indicates the number of cardiac contractions per minute that are not sufficiently strong to generate a peripheral pulse.

pulsed electromagnetic therapy—electrically generated magnetic fields for pain relief.

pulsed-field gel electrophoresis—lab test for neurological diseases.

pulsed gradient—MRI term.

pulsed lavage—"The wound was thoroughly irrigated with pulsed lavage and then closed as follows."

PulseDose technology—delivers oxygen in a precise dose with every breath, rather than continuously. Used in DeVilbiss Walkabout portable series.

pulseless electrical activity (PEA)—formerly called *EMD* (electromechanical dissociation). PEA covers EMD, pseudo-EMD, and idioventricular rhythms.

PulseMaster laser—used for laser curettage, or removal of diseased or inflamed soft tissue in the periodontal pocket.

pulse oximetry devices—used extensively in the intensive care unit and operating room to continuously monitor the patient's arterial blood oxygen saturation. They are composed of a sensor which emits two types of light (red and infrared) and a photodetector. The red and infrared light beams are transmitted through the patient's tissue and through arterial blood vessels. When they reach the photodetector on the other side, a computer calculates how much of

pulse oximetry *(cont.)*
each type of light was transmitted. Oxygenated hemoglobin within the arteries absorbs more infrared light, while deoxygenated blood absorbs more red light. These devices can be placed around the patient's finger or over the bridge of the nose, and around the foot or even around the great toe of neonates. Also called *finger oximetry.*

pulse pressure—the difference of the two blood pressure measurements: systolic (the higher number) and diastolic (the lower number). Increased pulse pressure is a predictor of coronary heart disease.

Pulse Pro—heart rate monitor that displays functions on a wristwatch that has most of the features of a normal sport watch. Pulse Pro does not require a chest strap transmitter and is said to be extremely accurate even during vigorous exercise.

PulseSpray—a pulsed infusion system consisting of a syringe and catheter, used to inject thrombolytic agents into a vessel.

PULSES profile—a disability profile:
P   physical condition
U   upper extremity function
L   lower extremity function
S   sensory and communication
     abilities
E   excretory control
S   social support
Scored from 1 (total independence) to 4 (total dependence). A score of 2 represents symptomatology, but no impairment in activities of daily living. A score of 3 means impairment and need for assistance from others.

pulsing current (electrostimulation)—used in nonunion of fractures. When bone is placed in an electromagnetic field, and the field switched on and off, a current in the microampere range is generated in the bone, causing changes in the environment of the cells in the gap region. This leads to bone healing.

Pulsolith laser lithotripter—for non-surgical removal of gallstones and urinary tract stones.

pulsus bisferiens (biferious pulse)—a pulse with two beats, sometimes palpable in combined aortic stenosis and aortic regurgitation.

pulsus paradoxus *(not* paradoxicus). Also, *paradoxical pulse.*

Pulver-Taft weave—a method used in microsurgical tendon transfer.

punctum plug (Oph). See *Freeman punctum plug.*

puncture site complications
arteriovenous fistula
dissection
hematoma
pseudoaneurysm
thrombosis

Punctur-Guard needle—self-blunting needles which reduce the risk of accidental needlesticks.

Puntenney forceps (Oph).

Puri-Clens wound cleanser.

Purlytin (tin ethyl etiopurpurin)—intravenous light-activated drug used with PhotoPoint laser therapy for exudative age-related macular degeneration. Purlytin collects only at the site of abnormal blood vessels.

purse-string mouth—fissures or scarring left by syphilitic lesions around the mouth of neonates with congenital syphilis. Also called *rhagades.*

pursestring or **purse-string suture**—a continuous running suture placed about an opening, and then drawn tight, like a drawstring purse.

Pursuer CBD Helical or Mini-Helical stone basket—an instrument used to trap small stones remaining in the common bile duct (CBD) during laparoscopic cholecystectomy.

pursuit mechanism—the slow, involuntary movement of both eyes as they follow a moving object.

push enteroscope/enteroscopy—diagnostic instrument and treatment procedure for jejunal angiodysplasias and small intestine bleeding sites and lesions. A child-size colonoscope is introduced via the mouth into the upper gastrointestinal tract and advanced to distances beyond the ligament of Treitz.

PUSH (Pressure Ulcer Scale for Healing) **tool**—developed by National Pressure Ulcer Advisory Panel to replace reverse staging of pressure ulcers.

Putti-Platt arthroplasty—for acromioclavicular separation. Subscapularis muscle and capsular repair, for chronic shoulder separation.

PUVA (psoralens, ultraviolet A) **regimen, therapy** ("poo-vah")—used for psoriasis. Ultraviolet A is a longwave ray.

PVA (polyvinyl alcohol) **particles**—an embolic material used in embolization of the potential blood supply to a cranial nerve in interventional radiology procedures of the extracranial head and neck.

PVA (prednisone, vincristine, asparaginase)—chemotherapy protocol for acute lymphoblastic leukemia.

PVB (Platinol, vinblastine, bleomycin)—chemotherapy protocol for germ cell tumors.

PVDA (prednisone, vincristine, daunorubicin, asparaginase)—chemotherapy protocol for acute lymphoblastic

leukemia and non-Hodgkin's lymphoma.

PVE (prosthetic valve endocarditis).

PVG (periventricular gray) **matter**—stimulated with deep brain electrodes to inhibit pain. Cf. *PAG matter.*

PVP (Platinol, VP-16)—chemotherapy protocol for neuroblastoma.

PVP (portal venous-dominant phase) **images** (CT scan).

PVR (postvoiding residual).

PVR (proliferative vitreoretinopathy).

PVS (persistent vegetative state).

PWA (person with AIDS).

pycnogenol—natural supplement being studied as a possible deterrent for heart attacks and strokes. The supplement is made from the bark of pine trees found only in France.

pyknosis—phenomenon where the cell becomes opaque and darkly stained under the microscope, as seen in cell death.

Pylon intramedullary nail system—consists of intramedullary rods and screws for internal fixation of tibial or femoral fractures.

pyloric string sign—an elongated, narrowed pyloric canal; a sign of pyloric hypertrophy which does not change on administration of antispasmodics.

Pylorid (ranitidine bismuth citrate)—drug therapy used in the treatment of duodenal ulcer disease.

Pylori Fiax—objective quantitative IFA (indirect fluorescent antibody) serology assay for *Helicobacter pylori.*

Pylori Stat—rapid EIA (enzyme-linked immunoassay) serology assay for *Helicobacter pylori.*

PyloriTek—test for *Helicobacter pylori.*

pylorus preserving pancreatoduodenectomy (PPPD)—a procedure that

pylorus preserving *(cont.)*
is said to improve upon the standard Whipple procedure. Leaving the pylorus intact results in improved eating habits in postoperative patients and ability to gain weight; no marginal ulceration as is seen in standard Whipple procedure. Transit time is preserved; no dumping, no change in glucose metabolism. After the new procedure, patients are said to have better food intake, increased body weight, no development of gastric or jejunal ulcers, and no clinical signs of digestive disorders such as dumping. Nutrition and digestion are not impeded by the preserved opening mechanism of the pylorus. See *dumping syndrome.*

pylorus-preserving Whipple (PPW) **modification**—used to treat patients with malignant periampullary disease.

pyogenic granuloma—benign polypoid growth containing proliferating capillaries. It may result from trauma and often becomes infected. Also, *granuloma pyogenicum.*

PYP scan (technetium pyrophosphate) —for myocardial infarct imaging.

pyramidal signs (or symptoms)—weakness and spasticity secondary to antipsychotic drugs or chemical imbalances in the brain. When an affected extremity is moved passively, it shows a gradual increase in resistance, then a sudden letting go, resulting in a classic "lengthening and shortening" or "clasp-knife phenomenon." Cf. *extrapyramidal signs, akathisia, tardive dyskinesia.*

pyranocarboxylic acid class—class of drugs chemically different from nonsteroidal anti-inflammatory drugs such as ibuprofen, but exert the same effects in treating inflammation, pain, and fever. Example: etodolac (Lodine, Ultradol).

pyridoxilated stroma-free hemoglobin (SFHb)—artificial blood capable of carrying oxygen, can sustain life at a hematocrit of zero, and is nontoxic to the kidneys.

Pyrilinks-D—a screening urine test that detects bone loss by measuring the rate of bone resorption.

pyrimethamine (Daraprim)—drug used for toxoplasmosis in AIDS patients.

pyrophosphate scan (PYP).

pyrosis—heartburn.

Pyrost—bone replacement material used as a complement to homologous or heterologous bone grafts.

PYtest—urea breath test for *Helicobacter pylori.*

PZT (plumbeous zirconate titanate) **tip** —used with Bovie ultrasonic aspirator.

Q, q

Q-beta replicase—uses an enzyme replicase that makes cRNA from the DNA sequence of interest at a constant temperature detected by ethidium bromide staining of a specimen. See *polymerase chain reaction*.

QCA (quantitative coronary arteriography).

QCT (quantitative computed tomography).

q deletion syndrome—see *13q deletion syndrome* (in the *T*'s).

QDR-1500 or **QDR-2000 Bone Densitometer** (Nuclear Med)—devices that can assess the hip, lumbar spine, and total skeleton. The QDR-2000 includes 5-second scanning capability.

QEEG (quantitative EEG).

Q fever—disease endemic to sheep in the western part of the U.S. It causes flu-like symptoms in humans who are exposed to diseased sheep. These symptoms can be mild, occasionally severe, and can prove fatal. The organism causing Q fever is *Coxiella burnetii*, a rickettsia.

QHS (quantitative hepatobiliary scintigraphy).

q.n.—every night.

q.o.d., QOD—every other day.

QOL, QoL (Quality of Life) **assessment**.

QPD (quadrature phase detector)—MRI term.

QSART (Quantitative Sudomotor Axon Reflex Test).

Qsma (superior mesenteric artery blood flow). Cf. *Rsma*.

Q-switched Nd:YAG laser—used to perform irradiation for postinflammatory hyperpigmentation secondary to granuloma faciale. Also, *Q-switched ruby laser*.

Q-Tc interval—corrected Q-T interval.

QTR (quadriceps tendon rupture)—in the knee.

Q-TWiST (quality-adjusted time without symptoms or toxicity)—a quality-of-life statistical model that discounts survival by time with side effects and symptoms. Originally developed for breast cancer therapies and now applied to AIDS and rectal cancer.

Quad-Lumen drain—perforated drain with a radiopaque stripe, used to monitor closed wound drainage postoperatively.

Quadramet (samarium Sm 153 lexidronam)—drug used in patients with refractory rheumatoid arthritis. Developed originally to treat the severe pain associated with cancers that have spread to bone.

quadrature detector—MRI term.

quadrature phase detector (QPD)—MRI term.

quadrature surface coil system for MR imaging—MRI term.

quadriceps boot (De Lorme boot)—a metal plate that fits over the sole of a shoe and can be fitted with weights of various sizes for therapeutic exercise of the quadriceps muscles.

quadriceps muscle (*not* quadricep)—as in the quadriceps and hamstring muscles. It is one muscle with four heads.

quadriceps tendon rupture (QTR)—in the knee.

quadriplegia—*not* quadraplegia.

Quadripolar cutting forceps—an instrument that limits thermal spread without compromising hemostasis. The forceps is able to dissect, grasp, coagulate, transect, and retract for precise laparoscopic surgery.

quad sets—an exercise to strengthen the quadriceps muscles (for knee pain, as in chrondromalacia patellae). Standing, with the legs straight, tighten the thigh muscles for three seconds, and relax. Do ten of these, and repeat a set of ten about 20 times a day.

QUAD 12000 and **QUAD 7000**—high-field, whole-body, open MRI scanners. The QUAD 12000 does not require the patient to be placed in the traditional tunnel-type MRI scanner and utilizes a magnet with a field strength of 0.6 tesla.

QualiCode *Borrelia burgdorferi* IgG and IgM Western blot kits—in vitro diagnostic tests for the detection of *Borrelia burgdorferi* antibodies for diagnosis of Lyme disease. It is used for patients who have positive or indeterminate ELISA tests.

quality factor—MRI term.

Quality of Life (QOL, QoL) **Assessment**.

Quantiplex HIV RNA Assay—directly quantifies the amount of HIV in the plasma of people infected with the AIDS virus.

quantitative computed tomography (QCT)—using single photon absorptiometry, a noninvasive test for assessment of the skeleton with regard to bone mineral density in osteoporosis, hyperparathyroidism, Cushing's syndrome, and other metabolic diseases known to affect the bones.

quantitative hepatobiliary scintigraphy (QHS).

Quantitative Sudomotor Axon Reflex Test (QSART)—to assess both pre- and post-synaptic activity of the sympathetic sudomotor system. The test is useful in evaluation for reflex sympathetic dystrophy.

Quantum pacemaker.

QuantX color quantification tools (Cardio)—used for transesophageal echocardiography (TEE) imaging on the V5M Multiplane and V510B Biplane TEE transducers. These tools provide numeric and graphic display of color data generated from two user-selectable regions of interest.

QUART (quadrantectomy, axillary dissection, and radiotherapy)—used in treatment of carcinoma of the breast.

Quartet system—used in the diagnosis and treatment of obstructive sleep apnea.

quartz fiberoptic probe.

quaternary ammonium chloride—skin cleansing compound, used in skin preparation prior to surgery.

Quattro mitral valve.

quazepam (Doral)—a benzodiazepine for insomnia, related chemically to Dalmane, Halcion, and Restoril.

Queckenstedt's sign—failure of cerebrospinal fluid pressure to rise and then fall when neck veins are compressed; indicative of a vertebral CSF canal block.

quellung reaction (*not* quelling)—technique for demonstrating the presence of capsular polysaccharide antigen. It is used to diagnose pneumococcal pneumonia.

quench, quenching—a term used when the magnet of the MRI equipment fails or goes down.

Quervain abdominal retractor.

Quervain's disease—see *de Quervain's disease.*

Quervain fracture.

Questionnaire for Identifying Children with Chronic Conditions (QuICCC).

Questus Leading Edge—arthroscopic grasper-cutter.

Questus Leading Edge—sheathed arthroscopy knife.

Quetelet's BMI index—body mass index to assess nutritional status. The formula for BMI is weight/(height) 2.

Queyrat—see *erythroplasia of Queyrat.*

QuickDraw venous cannula—can be placed percutaneously to provide venous drainage in open-chest cardiac procedures, thus eliminating another cannula from the operative field.

QuickSilver—hydrophilic-coated guide wire.

QuickVue Chlamydia test.

QuickVue influenza test—rapid point-of-care test for detection of influenza A and B.

QuickVue one-step *H. pylori* test—uses a smaller blood sample and provides faster results than the original test. *H. pylori* is believed to be associated with over 80% of the cases of peptic ulcer disease.

Quiet interference screw—biodegradable screw that lessens the likelihood of an inflammatory response.

Quikheel lancet—device for obtaining blood sample from the heel of an infant.

quinacrine—a drug used in patients at high risk for repeat pneumothorax; also antimalarial, antihelmintic.

quinapril (Accupril)—once-a-day ACE inhibitor used for hypertension.

Quincke spinal needle.

Quintessence—formulation of essential amino acids which can be used to supplement protein needs (as in low-protein diets used by kidney failure patients) or to enhance nutritional status in individuals with normal protein intake.

Quinton Mahurkar dual lumen catheter—for hemodialysis and peritoneal use. It comes in femoral and subclavian sizes. Also, *Mahurkar dual lumen catheter.*

Quinton PermCath (*not* PermaCath)—a large-bore, double-lumen silicone catheter placed in the internal jugular

Quinton PermCath *(cont.)*
vein and used for long-term vascular access for hemodialysis.

Quinton-Scribner shunt—a vascular shunt used in dialysis patients.

Quinton suction biopsy instrument (Rubin tube)—used in esophageal biopsies.

Quinton tube—used for small bowel biopsy.

quinupristin; delfopristin (Synercid).

Quire mechanical finger forceps—for removal of foreign bodies from the ear.

Quixil (concentrated cryoprecipitated clottable proteins) **spray**—tissue adhesive.

Quixin (levofloxacin ophthalmic solution)—for treatment of bacterial conjunctivitis.

R, r

r—when a lowercase *r* (and sometimes lowercase *rh*) appears before abbreviations or numbers, it often stands for *recombinant*.

RA (rhinocerebral aspergillosis).

RA (rotational atherectomy)—see *high-speed rotational atherectomy*.

RAAA (ruptured abdominal aortic aneurysm).

rAAT—recombinant alpha-1 antitrypsin.

RAB (remote afterloading brachytherapy).

RabAvert (human rabies vaccine)—used in pre-exposure vaccination and post-exposure prophylaxis against rabies.

rabbit nose—habitual repeated wrinkling of the nose by a person with itching of the nares due to allergic rhinitis.

rabbit stools—stools expelled as small pellets. Cf. *ribbon stools*.

rabies vaccine, Rhesus diploid cell strain (RDRV) (adsorbed).

raccoon eyes—discoloration below or around the eyes due to subcutaneous hemorrhage, sometimes seen in basal skull fracture.

racemic ("rah-see′mik") **epinephrine**.

racemic fluoxetine (S-fluoxetine).

rachitic—pertaining to rickets.

rachitic rosary—seen in patients with rickets. So-called because the enlargement of the cartilages at the costochondral junctions has the appearance of a string of beads.

rad (radiation absorbed dose)—see *centigray, gray, joule*.

RAD55 self-irrigating suction bur—for ENT surgery.

RAD40 sinus blade—for ENT surgery.

radial artery graft—tried and abandoned in the 1970s as a coronary artery bypass graft, but recently reinvestigated for the same purpose.

radial head subluxation (RHS) (also called *nursemaid's elbow*)—occurs when the radial head slides under the annular ligament and becomes entrapped. Reduction is achieved through a combination of supination, flexion, and extension, usually with prompt return of function. Recurrent RHS occurs in nearly one-fourth of patients.

radial keratotomy—a procedure for improving vision in myopic patients. Developed by Dr. Fydorov in the

radial keratotomy *(cont.)*
Soviet Union. Radial cuts (8 or 16) are made in the cornea, not quite all the way through. This flattens the shape of the eye, and changes myopia to more normal vision.

Radial Jaw—single-use biopsy forceps.

radial ray defect—see *pouce flottant.*

radial thermokeratoplasty—for correction of hyperopia.

radiation dosages—may be given as rads in a tissue dose, and in roentgens as an air dose. See *centigray; gray; joule.*

radiation-related optic neuropathy (RON).

radical—going to the root or source of a morbid process; directed to the cause, as in "radical excision of a tumor." Also, a fundamental constituent of a molecule; "free radical." Cf. *radicle.*

radical prostatectomy (RP).

radicle—one of the smallest branches of a nerve or a vessel, as in "intrahepatic biliary radicles." Cf. *radical.*

radiculopathy, "salon sink."

radioactive iodinated serum albumin study (RISA).

radioactive seed implants—used to treat early-stage prostate cancer. The implants are tiny radioactive seeds, each one the size of a grain of rice. Each grain is placed at a precise location around the prostate gland and delivers a high dose of radiation to the prostate, while minimizing radiation to nearby organs such as the bladder and the rectum. The procedure is done on an outpatient basis and only takes about an hour to complete. There are said to be few side effects, and the majority of men return to work within five days of treatment.

radioallergosorbent test (RAST).

radiocolloid mapping—see *intraoperative lymphatic mapping.*

radiodermatitis emulsion (RE)

Radiofocus Glidewire *(not* guide wire) —trade name for an angiographic polymer-coated guide wire. It reduces friction and the risk of thrombus formation. The tip of the wire is flexible, to minimize trauma to the vessel.

radiofrequency (RF) **catheter ablation** —a treatment in paroxysmal supraventricular tachycardia when other forms of therapy have not proved effective. Radiofrequency, an electrical current, is delivered via a special type of intracardiac electrode catheter, to the area that is the source of the tachyarrhythmia, e.g., an area of abnormal conduction or impulse formation. This energy heats a tiny bit of tissue, only a few millimeters in diameter and depth, which produces coagulation necrosis. If, on testing, the doctor can reproduce the tachyarrhythmia, further RF current is applied to the tachyarrhythmic focus. The ablation is considered to be satisfactory if the tachyarrhythmia can no longer be induced. Also, *radiofrequency ablation* (RFA).

radiofrequency (RF) **coil; pulse**—MRI term.

radiofrequency percutaneous myocardial revascularization (RF-PMR)—a process that delivers radiofrequency (RF) energy to the oxygen-deprived heart muscle through a catheter, creating small crater-like injuries in the endocardium. It is believed to stimulate the body's healing response and initiate angiogenesis (creation of new vessels).

radiofrequency (RF) **spatial distribution problem**—MRI term.

radioimmunodetection (RAID)—an invaluable method in the management of patients with malignant melanoma, for the entire body can be surveyed with one test.

radioimmunoluminography (RILG)— a system for direct measurement of quantity and distribution of protein in histological specimens.

radioimmunoscintimetry—a means by which surgeons can more readily localize abdominal tumors. A week to ten days prior to surgery, the patient is injected with a monoclonal antibody that is specific to the tumor, and a radioactive substance (marker) attached to the antibody. This enables identification of the tumor intraoperatively with the use of a Geiger counter. Also, *immunoscintimetry*.

radioisotope (see also *technetium*)
Cardiolite (^{99m}Tc sestamibi)
CardioTec (^{99m}Tc teboroxime)
CEAker
Choletec (^{99m}Tc mebrofenin)
fluorodeoxyglucose (FDG)
Hedspa
ImmuRAID (CEA-Tc99m)
indium-111-labeled human non-specific immunoglobulin G (^{111}In-IgG)
iodine 131 MIBG (^{131}I)
iridium 192 (Iriditope) (^{192}Ir)
Macrotec (^{99m}Tc medronate)
nitrogen 13 ammonia (^{13}N)
OncoScint CR103 MOAB labeled with indium 111 (^{111}In)
palladium 103 (^{103}Pd)
ProstaScint (CYT-356 radiolabeled with 111 indium chloride)
Renotec (^{99m}Tc iron-ascorbate DTPA)
rubidium 82 (^{82}Rb)
selenium 75 (^{75}Se)

radioisotope *(cont.)*
specific immunoglobulin G (^{111}In-IgG)
TcHIDA (technetium-HIDA)
Techneplex (^{99m}Tc penetate)
TechneScan MAG3 (^{99m}Tc mertiatide)
technetium ^{99m}Tc albumin
technetium ^{99m}Tc albumin aggregated
technetium ^{99m}Tc albumin colloid
technetium ^{99m}Tc bicisate
technetium ^{99m}Tc colloid
technetium ^{99m}Tc disofenin
technetium ^{99m}Tc etidronate
technetium ^{99m}Tc ferpentetate
technetium ^{99m}Tc furifosmin
technetium ^{99m}Tc gluceptate
technetium ^{99m}Tc glucarate
technetium ^{99m}Tc-GSA (diethylene-triaminepentaacetic acid-galactosyl-human serum-albumin)
technetium ^{99m}Tc iron-ascorbate-DTPA (Renotec)
technetium ^{99m}Tc lidofenin
technetium ^{99m}Tc macroaggregated albumin (^{99m}TcMAA)
technetium ^{99m}Tc medronate (Macrotec)
technetium ^{99m}Tc mertiatide (TechneScan MAG3)
technetium ^{99m}Tc oxidronate
technetium ^{99m}Tc pentetate (Techneplex)
technetium ^{99m}Tc pertechnetate sodium
technetium ^{99m}Tc PIPIDA
technetium ^{99m}Tc pyrophosphate
technetium ^{99m}Tc sestamibi (Cardiolite)
technetium ^{99m}Tc siboroxime
technetium ^{99m}Tc sodium
technetium ^{99m}Tc succimer
technetium ^{99m}Tc sulfur colloid (^{99m}Tc-SC) (Tesuloid)

radioisotope *(cont.)*
technetium ^{99m}Tc teboroxime
(CardioTec)
technetium ^{99m}Tc tetrofosmin
technetium stannous pyrophosphate
(TSPP)
Tesuloid (^{99m}Tc-SC, sulfur colloid)
thallium 201 (^{201}Tl)
xenon 133 (^{133}Xe)

radioisotope stent—a very low-dose
radiation-emitting stent implant designed to prevent or reduce the restenosis of blood vessels following
treatment for coronary artery disease.

radiolabeled peptide alpha-M2—used
in breast cancer imaging and possible therapy.

radiolucent—offering relatively little
resistance to x-rays (by analogy with
translucent).

radiolucent spine frame—a modification of the Relton-Hall spine frame.
Made of strong radiolucent plastic
compounds that achieve x-rays
without metallic shadows that are
common to metal frames. Used in
intraoperative radiography to assess
spinal alignment to prevent overcorrection of the spinal curve and de-
compensation. Recommended to
assist in assessment of hook placement and spine alignment.

**radiolymphoscintigraphy, intraopera-
tive**—combined with blue dye mapping during lymphadenectomy for
melanoma.

radionuclide—radioactive isotope; a
species of atom that spontaneously
emits radioactivity.

radionuclide scan—the introduction
into the body of a radioactive substance whose distribution in tissues,
vessels, or cavities can be detected
and recorded by a device that senses

radiation. The choice of radioactive
substances (radionuclides, isotopes)
is governed by the tendency of certain organs or tissues to take up
(absorb, concentrate) certain elements or compounds. Radionuclides
may be swallowed, inhaled, or injected into a body cavity or into the
circulation. Scanning may be performed immediately after the material is administered (as in studies of
blood flow) or after an interval (as
when absorption or concentration of
a substance in an organ must occur
first). The standard lung scan procedure includes two separate scans of
the lungs, one after inhalation of a
radionuclide and the other after
injection of a second radionuclide
into the circulation. Scanning is done
with a scintillation camera (scinti-
scanner, gamma camera) which creates a picture on film representing
the distribution and intensity of gamma radiation emitted by the patient.

radiopaque—resisting penetration by x-
rays.

RadiStop radial compression system
—for prolonged controlled mechanical compression of the radial artery,
which is becoming an alternative to
the femoral approach for angiography and angioplasty.

Radius enteral feeding tubes.

Radstat—a device and its accompanying
wrist splint that allows selective
compression of the radial artery following catheterization through the
wrist.

RAE endotracheal tubes—both oral
and nasal tubes can be bent to keep
them out of the respective surgical
fields.

RA (rheumatoid arthritis) factor—protein in the blood of most patients

RA (*cont.*)
with rheumatoid arthritis. It is detected by a blood test. Cf. *Rh factor.*

Raf-1—a human protein found to be an autoantigen in Ménière's disease.

Ragnell handheld retractor.

RAI (radioimmunoassay)—used to measure various hormone levels in the blood.

RAID (radioimmunodetection)—used in combination with a monoclonal antibody against carcinoembryonic antigen. See *ImmuRAID.*

Raji cell assay test—for immune complexes.

rake—a bent-tine, forklike retractor.

R-albuterol—a form of albuterol.

rale—a fine crackling, static-like sound heard through the stethoscope, indicating a pathologic condition. Take a lock of hair and roll it between your thumb and index finger near your ear; you've just heard what a crackling rale sounds like. Also, *Velcro rales.*

rale indux—a crepitant rale that is heard in patients with pneumonia at the stage when consolidation begins. Cf. *rale redux.*

rale redux—an unequal subcrepitant sound caused by the passage of air through the fluid in bronchial tubes. This rale is heard when pneumonia is resolving. Also, *rale de retour* (rattle of return).

raloxifene—estrogen-like drug said to provide benefits to the bone and heart health of postmenopausal women.

RAM (rapid alternating movements).

Raman spectroscopy—method of detecting plaque or remote sensing of diseased artery wall in laser angioplasty. Cf. *spectrofluorometry.*

ramipril (Altace)—an antihypertensive belonging to the group of drugs known as ACE inhibitors. See also *fosinopril.*

Ramirez shunt—a vascular access shunt, used in performing dialysis.

Ramsey Hunt (no hyphen) **syndrome** —herpetic eruption of the external ear and ipsilateral facial paralysis, usually with additional symptoms of pain in the affected ear (occasionally with auditory symptoms), oral lesions, reduced tearing, and reduced taste on the anterior two-thirds of the tongue.

Ranawat/Burstein total hip system— porous femoral components for noncemented hip replacement.

Rancho cube—part of an orthopedic apparatus used with the Ilizarov method for leg lengthening. The cube is actually a rectangular pin gripper made from titanium. The cubes come with one to five holes through them to hold the pins and connecting rods of the Ilizarov apparatus. The cubes replace the steel transfixion wires usually used. The advantage of the Rancho cube is that it does not work its way through to the skin surface as the wire can.

Rancho los Amigos cognitive scale in rating posttraumatic amnesia, levels I to VIII.

Level I—no response to any stimulus.

Level II—generalized response, often only to pain, but limited, and inconsistent, nonpurposeful.

Level III—localized response, withdrawal from painful stimuli, and can make purposeful responses. May follow simple commands, but only inconsistently and hesitantly.

Rancho los Amigos *(cont.)*

Level IV—alert, but may be agitated, confused, aggressive, and disoriented. Cannot perform self care.

Level V—confused, with inappropriate response.

Level VI—confused, but with appropriate response.

Level VII—automatic, but appropriate response.

Level VIII—purposeful and appropriate response. Alert, oriented, and can recall past events. Can learn new activities and can perform activities of daily living. Judgment and abstract reasoning are impaired, and there is reduced tolerance to stress; may function at less than optimal level.

Rancho fixation system—modification of the Ilizarov external fixation system that allows the surgeon to build hybrid frames using half-pins or pins and wires.

Rand microballoon—used in microballoon embolization of cerebral aneurysms, arteriovenous malformations, and carotid cavernous fistula occlusion.

randomize—a term used in testing new medications or chemotherapy protocols. Patients are selected at random, rather than in any predetermined manner, to test responses.

Randot ("ran-dot") **test**—not a physician's name; it is a coined word for the random dots that become recognizable as geometric figures when the patient wears a certain kind of eyeglasses. This is a test of binocular depth perception.

Raney clip—used in repair of facial fractures requiring bicoronal incision, to obtain hemostasis of the galea and skin.

Ranfac cholangiographic catheters—LAP-13 for insertion through the lateral port; ORC-B for open procedure, XL-11 for percutaneous or three-puncture technique. Also, *Ranfac laparoscopic instruments.*

range of motion (ROM).

Ranke complex—calcified node, or mass, or granuloma in the chest, from old tuberculosis.

ranolazine—a drug compound for treating angina pectoris.

Rapamune (sirolimus; formerly rapamycin)—immunosuppressive therapy for prophylaxis of renal transplant rejection, liver, bone marrow, and cardiac transplant rejection.

RAP cannula—see *remote access perfusion (RAP) cannula.*

rapid acquisition with relaxation enhancement (RARE)—a version of STIR. See *STIR.*

rapid alternating movements (RAM).

Rapid Drug Screen (trademark)—drugs-of-abuse urine test kit that can be used at home or by businesses.

Rapide suture.

rapid eye movement (REM).

RapidFlap—a cranial fixation device that affixes the bone flap from both sides of the bone.

Rapidgraft—an arterial vessel substitute.

rapid urease test (RUT)—a rapid and accurate test to detect *Helicobacter pylori* in gastric lesions. The test produces a color change in one minute with a specimen of gastric mucosa obtained via endoscopic biopsy. Other tests for *H. pylori* take much longer: Gram stain (1 to 3 hours); culture (4 to 7 days). The RUT allows appropriate treatment to be initiated immediately.

RapiSeal patch—collagen-based bio-degradable patch used to control surgical bleeding in solid organs such as liver and spleen.

Raplon—injectable adjunct to general anesthesia that facilitates endotracheal intubation and provides skeletal muscle relaxation during outpatient surgical procedures.

RAPP (Routine Assessment of Patient Progress)—an assessment instrument for psychiatric inpatients that allows nurses to incorporate both interview and observational data into a comprehensive assessment.

Rapp-Hodgkin syndrome—congenital multisystem disorder characterized by cleft palate and/or cleft lip, partial or complete, and/or absence of teeth, impaired ability to sweat, dysplastic nails, and occasionally other physical abnormalities.

RARE (rapid acquisition with relaxation enhancement) **technique**—MRI term.

Rashkind balloon atrial septotomy—a procedure in which a cardiac catheter with a balloon is inserted; the balloon is inflated, thus enlarging the aperture.

Rashkind cardiac device.

Rashkind double umbrella device—used in reopening a previously occluded ductus arteriosus.

Rasmussen syndrome—chronic idiopathic progressive unilateral hemisphere inflammation.

Rasor blood pumping system (RBPS)—disposable device used in circulatory support and cardiopulmonary bypass. Also an alternative to intra-aortic balloons for acute postoperative cardiac support.

RAST (radioallergosorbent test)
RAST class 0, no likelihood of atopy.

RAST *(cont.)*
RAST 0/I—borderline.
RAST class I response is thought by some to have some significance.
RAST class II and above represents the presence of atopy.
RAST results are reported in units per milliliter (U/ml).

ratbite fever—see *Haverhill fever.*

rating of perceived exertion (RPE)—the patient's assessment of work done on a treadmill test.

ratio
bone and limb growth velocity
C/N (contrast-to-noise)
CT (cardiothoracic)
cup-to-disk
gyromagnetic
helper/suppressor cell
I/E (inspiration/expiration)
L/S (lecithin/sphingomyelin) (in amniocentesis)
M/E (myeloid/erythroid)
RV/TLC (residual volume/ total lung capacity)
S/N (signal-to-noise)
T-lymphocyte subset

rational drug design—use of x-ray crystallography, molecular modeling, or MRI scanning to determine the target molecule of a pathogen, and then use of computers to design an effective drug.

Raulerson syringe—used with guide wire insertion in the Seldinger technique.

Raxar (grepafloxacin HCl)—once-daily quinolone antibiotic, effective against certain respiratory infections.

Rayleigh scattering law (Neuro).

ray resection—resection of a finger or toe, a ray of the hand or foot.

Ray-Tec sponge—x-ray detectable surgical sponge. Cf. *Vistec.*

Ray threaded fusion cage (TFC)—used in lumbar fusion surgery, this

Ray threaded fusion *(cont.)* titanium stabilization device is placed between the vertebrae to maintain the height of the disc space. It has hollow threaded cylinders that are packed with fragments of the patient's bone. The bone then grows through tiny openings in the cylinders to fuse the vertebrae.

Raz double-prong ligature carrier—for performing bladder and bladder neck suspensions.

Razi cannula introducer—used to simplify the procedure and diminish postoperative strokes and memory loss following aortic cannulation.

Raz sling operation—for urinary incontinence. See *vaginal wall sling procedure.*

RBC-CD4—an AIDS drug.

RCA (rotational coronary atherectomy) —see *directional coronary atherectomy* and *radiofrequency catheter ablation.*

rCBF (regional cerebral blood flow)— PET (positron emission tomography) term. See also *rCBV.*

rCBV (regional cerebral blood volume) —PET (positron emission tomography) term. See also *rCBF.*

RCC (renal cell carcinoma).

rCD4 (recombinant CD4)—see *CD4.*

RCP (retrograde cerebral perfusion)— used in cardiac surgery thus: "The Dacron graft was de-aired using RCP, which filled the conduit with dark blood, displacing luminal air."

rCPP (regional cerebral perfusion pressure).

rd (rutherford)—unit of radioactivity.

RDRV (adsorbed)—Rhesus diploid cell strain rabies vaccine. See *HDRV.*

RDS (respiratory distress syndrome).

RDW (red cell diameter width)—a term used in hematology.

RDX coronary radiation catheter delivery system—designed to prevent restenosis in patients who have implanted coronary stents.

RE (radiodermatitis emulsion).

Reactine (cetirizine).

reactive airways disease (RAD)— bronchial asthma.

reactive perforating collagenosis (RPC) —an uncommon disorder in which altered collagen bundles are eliminated through the skin, presenting as cup-shaped epidermal depressions and umbilicated papules or nodules with a central adherent keratotic plug. Both childhood and adult forms are believed to be a cutaneous response to superficial trauma, the adult form always associated with pruritus.

reactive, reparative atypia (Ob-Gyn) —presence of immature cells formed in the process of healing or regrowth of the squamous epithelium. A common finding that often follows treatment of dysplasia and other conditions such as cervical or vaginal infections.

ReAct NMES (neuromuscular electrical stimulation) **device**—used in physical therapy to treat disuse atrophy and other neuromuscular disorders. The system uses Multi-Ply or Soft- EZ reusable electrodes.

reagent—substance involved in a chemical reaction; also a substance used to detect the presence of another substance by chemical means. See *Millon's reagent.* Cf. *reagin.*

reagin—a type of antibody. See *RPR, reagent.*

REAL (Revised European American Lymphoma) **classification of lymphoma**—considers lymphoma in terms of "real" diseases rather than

REAL *(cont.)*
pathologic entities. The major entities are diffuse large B-cell lymphoma, follicular lymphomas, mucosa-associated lymphoid tissue (MALT) lymphoma, peripheral T-cell, small lymphocytic, and mantle cell. Less common are mediastinal large B-cell, anaplastic large T-cell, Burkitt's marginal zone, and peripheral T-cell.

Reality vaginal pouch—reservoir (similar to a diaphragm) placed in the vagina for several hours to collect amniotic fluid. Used to diagnose PPROM (preterm premature rupture of membranes).

real-time color flow Doppler—permits two-dimensional color-coded imaging of blood flow.

real-time position management (REAL) **tracking system.**

real-time ultrasonography—intraoperative scanning technique (frequency around 30 cycles per second [cps]) which permits physiological movement to be observed while it is happening, e.g., it is possible to see a cyst collapsing as its wall is entered. It is used for determining the precise location of tumors of the brain, beneath the cerebral cortex, for removal through very small and accurately placed incisions. It also permits the accurate guiding of biopsy needles, localizing of intracranial cysts, aneurysms or abscesses, or foreign bodies, and makes it possible to position catheters in the ventricles for draining fluids or to measure pressure. In a laminectomy, the spinal cord can be visualized without opening the dura. It is also used for noninvasive exploration of the pelvis and abdomen. It is particularly useful in that the examination can be taped on

magnetic tape and individual frames can be placed in the patient's record. There is no radiation hazard associated with the use of real-time ultrasonography or examination. See *ultrasound.*

Rebel knee orthosis—a pre-sized knee brace designed not to migrate.

Rebetol (ribavirin)—an antiviral drug for severe lower respiratory tract infections.

Rebetron (ribavirin and interferon alfa-2b)—combination drug for the treatment of chronic hepatitis C in patients with compensated liver disease who have relapsed following treatment with interferon alone.

Rebif (recombinant interferon beta)—used to treat multiple sclerosis.

rebound tenderness—test for rebound tenderness; the fingers are pushed into an area far from the area of suspected inflammation and then quickly removed. The rebound of the indented structures causes pain in the area of inflammation.

reboxetine mesylate—selective norepinephrine reuptake inhibitor (NRI) for treatment of depression.

recanalization—see *transcervical balloon tuboplasty.*

Receptin (CD4)—a drug used to treat patients with AIDS.

recession—the moving of the end of an eye muscle (usually the medial rectus or lateral rectus, that adducts or abducts, respectively, the eyeball) and reimplanting it in a slightly different position, for correction of strabismus. Cf. *resection.*

reciprocating saw.

recombinant alpha interferon—see *interferon.*

recombinant alpha-1 antitrypsin (rAAT).

recombinant desulfatohirudin (hirudin)—a direct thrombin inhibitor.

recombinant enzyme replacement therapy—used to treat Pompe's disease, an inherited and usually lethal glycogen storage disease that often afflicts children. In the disease, glycogen accumulates and destroys skeletal, heart, and lung muscle.

recombinant hemoglobin—see *rHb1.1*.

recombinant human erythropoietin (rhEPO)—used to correct the anemia seen with renal failure. Said to be slower in response than packed red cell administration but without adverse reactions of iron overloading and possible viral toxicities.

recombinant human granulocyte colony stimulating factor (r-met HuG-CSF).

recombinant human hemoglobin—see *Optro*.

recombinant human insulin-like growth factor (rhIGF-1).

recombinant human neutral endopeptidase (rNEP).

recombinant immunoblot assay (RIBA)—used in diagnosis of hepatitis C.

recombinant novel plasminogen activator (rNPA).

recombinant platelet-derived growth factor (rPDGF-BB)—stimulates migration and proliferation of fibroblasts and smooth muscle cells and induces the rapid development of granulation tissue.

recombinant prourokinase—can treat stroke for up to 6 hours after symptoms begin, doubling the 3-hour "golden window of opportunity" offered by tPA.

recombinant tissue plasminogen activator (rt-PA).

Recombinate—a recombinant DNA factor VIII used to treat hemophilia.

Because this clotting factor is genetically engineered rather than extracted from human plasma, the risk of HIV contamination is eliminated.

reconstitution—a term used in angiography for maintenance of flow in an artery beyond an area of narrowing or obstruction by establishment of collateral circulation.

reconstruction artifact (Radiol)—error in CT imaging.

reconstruction study—generation of an image by computer processing of scan data. Used in computed tomography scan.

recovery—a term that seems to be replacing "harvest" in the literature in reference to obtaining donor organs for transplantation. See *harvest*.

recruitment—when, in testing hearing, a slight increase in decibel level causes a disproportionate increase in loudness perceived.

rectal endoscopic ultrasonography (REU)—a sonographic transducer is inserted endoscopically to evaluate for possible tumors in the rectum.

rectal linitis plastica (RLP)—a rare colorectal carcinoma with a long delay between onset of symptoms and diagnosis.

rectilinear biphasic waveform for external defibrillation—provides successful defibrillation with less delivered current than conventional monophasic waveform.

Rector-Gordon-Healey-Mendoza-Spitzer type IV renal tubular acidosis—a rare type named for five physicians in different cities who first found and identified it.

recurred (*not* reoccurred)—"The symptoms recurred with the advent of cold weather."

recurrent abdominal pain (RAP).

recurrent respiratory papillomatosis
(RRP)—recurrent benign growths in
the respiratory tract, most common
in the larynx in children. Caused by
HPV (human papillomavirus).

recurrent spontaneous abortions
(RSA).

red cell diameter width (RDW).

**Reddick cystic duct cholangiogram
catheter**—used during laparoscopic
cholecystectomy.

Reddick-Saye screw—inserted through
trocar to provide fixation and traction during laparoscopic cholecystectomy.

Redifurl TaperSeal IAB catheter—for
percutaneous insertion in the femoral artery.

red reflex—an ophthalmologic finding.
When the light from the ophthalmoscope is flashed on the patient's
pupil at a slight angle lateral to the
patient's line of vision and at about
a distance of 12 inches, a bright
orange glow will be noted.

REDS (remote endoscopic digital spectroscopy).

reduced liver transplant (RLT) or **reduced-size liver transplant** (RSLT)
—a segmental liver transplant,
reduced from a larger liver to fit a
smaller recipient, such as a child.
Such transplants can be taken from a
parent or other compatible living
relative. Also called *cut-down liver*.

reduced signal intensity in the center
of the blood vessels on MR angiograms that can mimic intraluminal
thrombus.

reducing substances—positive in stools
of premature infants who are not
properly digesting formula, consists
of various sugars tested by making a
mixture of stool and water and
Clinitest tablet.

Reductil (sibutramine)—drug for the
management of obesity.

reduction columelloplasty (ENT, Plas
Surg)—a procedure for refinement
of the nasal bone or narrowing
splayed medial crura, increasing the
nasolabial angle, modifying the
shape of the nares, and for increasing tip projection.

Redux (dexfenfluramine)—used in the
treatment of obesity. Discontinued
1997. See *Meridia*.

reefing—folding or tucking of skin or
other tissue: "We then performed
arthrotomy, lateral release, and medial reefing of the right patella for
lateral subluxation."

Reese dermatome—a drum-type dermatome that makes grafts from .008
to .034 inch.

**Reese-Ellsworth classification of ret-
inoblastoma**—groups I through V.

Reese's retinal telangiectasia.

Reese stimulator—used in sectioning of
recurrent nerve for spastic dysphonia.

ReFacto—antihemophilic factor (recombinant) used in treating hemophilia
A. It is formulated without human
serum albumin.

refer, referred—also, *referring, refer-
ral,* but *referable.*

reference, ideas of—delusions that
strangers such as radio or television
broadcasters are referring to the patient.

Refinity—brand-name skin products,
including an in-office skin peel treatment.

Refinity Coblation System—wrinkle
reduction procedure.

reflectance-guided laser selection—
used for removal of tattoos. It uses
skin reflectance measurements to determine the optimum laser wavelength to remove various colors in
the tattoo.

reflex—reflected action or movement. Cf. *reflux*.

re-flex (verb)—a hyphen is needed to distinguish *re-flex* (to flex again) from the noun *reflex* (an involuntary action).

reflexes, deep tendon
0   absent
1+   decreased
2+   normal
3+   hyperactive
4+   clonus

reflex sympathetic dystrophy (RSD) —a response to an injury consisting of vasomotor instability, trophic skin changes, swelling, and pain.

ReFlex Wand—disposable surgical device used in the office environment to debulk tonsils without removing them. Also for the treatment of snoring by creating channels in the soft palate for tissue removal and stiffening in a matter of seconds.

Refludan (lepirudin rDNA) **injection** —genetically engineered recombinant form of hirudin for the treatment of heparin-induced thrombocytopenia. Also used as an antithrombotic in the treatment of patients with unstable angina pectoris and/or acute, noncomplete myocardial infarction.

reflux—backward or return flow. Cf. *reflux*.
gastroesophageal
hepatojugular
intrarenal
vesicoureteral

reflux esophagitis, classification— written as grades, with roman numerals:
E-I   erythema, edema
E-II   erosions
E-III   localized deformity
E-IV   stricture

refraction—determination of the refractive errors of the eye for distance and near vision.

Regency SR+ single-chamber, rate-responsive pulse generator.

Regen's flexion exercises (Ortho)— pronounced like "region."

regimen (*not* regime)—a systematic course of therapy, diet, or exercise meant to achieve certain ends. Also, *protocol*.

regime—government or social system; mode of rule or management. Often misused in medicine for *regimen*. Cf. *regimen*.

regional cerebral blood flow (rCBF).

regional cerebral blood volume (rCBV).

regional cerebral perfusion pressure (rCPP).

Registered Health Information Administrator (RHIA)—formerly RRA (Registered Record Administrator).

Registered Health Information Technician (RHIT)—formerly ART (Accredited Record Technician).

Reglan (metoclopramide).

Regnauld-type degeneration—results in first metatarsophalangeal joint space narrowing, loss of joint cartilage, bony spurring, and painful range of motion of the great toe.

Regranex gel (becaplermin)—used for treatment of lower extremity diabetic neuropathic ulcers that extend into the subcutaneous tissue or beyond and have an adequate blood supply. It uses a genetically engineered platelet-derived growth factor (becaplermin) to actively help promote healing.

Regressin—treatment for bladder cancer.

Reichert/Mundinger stereotactic device—used in the treatment of post-traumatic tremor.

Reifenstein's syndrome—partial androgen insensitivity, familial incomplete male pseudohermaphroditism.

Reil, island of—in the brain.

Reinke crystals—crystals contained in interstitial cells (Leydig cells) of human testes. See *Leydig cell.*

Reis-Bückler's corneal dystrophy.

rejection
    acute cellular xenograft
    cellular xenograft
    delayed xenograft (DXR)
    hyperacute (HAR)

Relafen (nabumetone).

relaxation rate; relaxation time—MRI terms.

relaxin (recombinant human relaxin)—used for the treatment of scleroderma.

relaxing incision (or relief incision) an incision made to relieve tension in tissue.

Relay cardiac pacemaker—a dual chamber rate-adaptive pacemaker.

Relenza (zanamivir)—for treatment of uncomplicated acute illness due to influenza types A and B in adult patients and adolescents over 12. The medication is inhaled orally using a handheld breath-activated device called a Diskhaler.

Reliance CM femoral component.

Reliance urinary control insert—a disposable balloon-tipped device that is placed in the urethra and expanded, to prevent urine loss.

ReLibra (testosterone gel)—a once-daily, low-dose, topical testosterone gel to improve libido and well-being in postmenopausal women.

ReliefBand NST (nerve stimulation therapy)—watchlike electronic device for drug-free treatment of nausea and vomiting due to motion sickness, chemotherapy, and pregnancy.

Relpax (eletriptan)—oral drug for the treatment of migraine headaches. It acts on intracranial blood vessels and sensory nerves to relieve pain of migraine attack.

Relton-Hall spine frame.

rem (roentgen-equivalent–man)—unit of measurement of maximum tolerance dose of radiation (for hospital personnel). A permissible dose is 0.1 rem/week, or 5 rems per year. See *gray.*

remacemide—drug used for the treatment of Huntington's disease.

Remeron (mirtazapine)—an antidepressant drug.

Remicade (infliximab)—used for the treatment of moderately to severely active Crohn's disease in patients who have an inadequate response to conventional therapy. It is also indicated for patients with fistulizing Crohn's disease to reduce the number of draining enterocutaneous fistulas. It works by blocking activity of tumor necrosis factor alpha (TNF-alpha), thus reducing intestinal inflammation. In combination with methotrexate, Remicade is now used in the treatment of rheumatoid arthritis. Previously called *Avakine.*

remote afterloading brachytherapy (RAB)—remote-controlled implantation of a radioactive source in a patient for brief treatment without exposing the physician or nurse to radioactivity. The applicator is placed manually, and the radioisotope is administered under computer control by machine, after the physician or nurse has left the treatment room. The most commonly used radioisotopes for this procedure are iridium 192 (^{192}Ir) and cesium 137 (^{137}Cs). Iodine 125 (^{125}I), a low-energy

remote *(cont.)*
radionuclide, may also be used. Cf. *brachytherapy.*

Reminyl (galantamine)—drug used for treatment of Alzheimer's disease.

remnant-like particle (RLP) **lipoprotein**—form of cholesterol that results from metabolism of very low density lipoproteins and chylomicrons, the major triglycerides that carry lipids in the blood. These cholesterol-rich particles are believed to promote plaque formation, which leads to arterial disease and sets the stage for a heart attack.

remote access perfusion (RAP) **cannula**—multifunction catheter used to stop the heart and provide arterial blood flow for the body without need to open the chest. This minimally invasive cardiac surgery is performed through small incisions, or "windows," between the ribs.

remote endoscopic digital spectroscopy (REDS).

remoxipride (Roxiam)—antipsychotic drug that blocks dopamine receptors in order to lower dopamine levels in the brain. (Overproduction of dopamine in the brain is thought to cause psychosis.) Used to treat psychosis and schizophrenia.

REM (rapid eye movement) **sleep**—that period of sleep when the heart rate and respiration are irregular, brain waves are rapid and of low voltage, and dreaming occurs. Cf. *NREM sleep.*

Remune (formerly HIV-1 Immunogen)—used for the treatment of HIV patients.

Renacidin—genitourinary irrigating solution used to dissolve stones.

Renagel (sevelamer HCl)—for reduction of serum phosphorus in patients with end-stage renal disease.

renal cell carcinoma (RCC)—solid renal tumor.

renal helical CT (RHCT)—imaging modality in the evaluation of potential renal donors.

renin levels, serum—elevated in cardiac patients. In addition to cholesterol and triglyceride levels in cardiac patients, you will be hearing about serum renin levels. Studies have shown that elevated cholesterol and triglycerides are not the only factors responsible for an increased risk of heart attacks. It has been found that the risk of heart attack is seven times higher in patients with elevated renin levels. In addition, elevated renin levels may provide the key to the question of why more than half the patients experiencing a myocardial infarction have normal cholesterol levels.

Renova (tretinoin emollient cream)—a prescription skin cream that is said to reduce fine facial wrinkles, brown spots, and surface roughness associated with the natural aging process and chronic sun exposure. It is a reformulation of anti-acne medication Retin-A.

ReoPro (abciximab)—antiplatelet monoclonal antibody that prevents platelet cells from clumping. Used in patients undergoing coronary angioplasty.

repair—see *operation.*

repair chain reaction—involves the use of a polymerase and ligase that is highly specific to detect a known DNA or RNA sequence in a specimen. See *polymerase chain reaction.*

repeated FID (free induction decay)—MRI term.

Repel—bioresorbable barrier film used to prevent postoperative adhesions.

Repela surgical glove—resistant to tear and puncture. Made of Kevlar and Lycra.

reperfusion edema after lung transplantation (Rad)—appears as airspace disease in the middle and/or lower lung zones and is a form of noncardiogenic pulmonary edema.

repetition time (TR)—given in seconds—MRI term.

repetitive strain injury (RSI)—see *carpal tunnel syndrome*.

rephasing gradient—MRI term.

Repifermin (keratinocyte growth factor 2 [KGF-2])—investigational genome-derived therapeutic protein drug for treatment of mucositis associated with bone marrow transplantation.

re-place (verb)—a hyphen is needed to distinguish *re-place* (to place again) from *replace* (to take the place of).

replant splint—designed to treat metacarpal, wrist, and forearm replants. A high-profile crane has constant tension designed for protective extrinsic muscle mobilization.

Replens gel—for vaginal dryness.

RepliCare hydrocolloid dressing material.

Repliderm—a collagen-based dressing for wounds, decubitus or diabetic ulcers, and first- and second-degree burns.

Repliform—for treatment of urinary incontinence and pelvic floor repair.

Replogle tube.

Repose—a surgical system for treating obstructive sleep apnea and snoring. It is a minimally invasive procedure that stabilizes and prevents the tongue from collapsing back and obstructing the airway passage. The procedure does not require incisions and can typically be performed in less than 30 minutes. Recovery time is expected to be much shorter relative to other surgical methods.

Requip (ropinirole hydrochloride)—used to relieve symptoms of restless legs syndrome.

Rescula (unoprostone isopropyl ophthalmic solution) **eye drops**—an intraocular pressure-lowering docosanoid compound for twice daily instillation. Used in lowering intraocular pressure in patients with open-angle glaucoma or ocular hypertension.

resection—excision of a portion of an organ or of a structure. Cf. *recession*.

reservoir—see *device*.

residual—lasting effect of disease or injury.

residual volume/total lung capacity (RV/TLC) **ratio.**

"resigned" person (Psych)—a possible precursor to borderline personality disorder.

resipump—reservoir/pump component of inflatable penile prosthesis.

resolution—the ability of an optical, radiographic, or other image-forming device to distinguish or separate two closely adjacent points in the subject. In computed tomography, resolution is measured in lines per millimeter; the higher the resolution, the sharper and more faithful the image.

Resolve Quickanchor—used for intraosseous screw fixation.

resonators (Plas Surg)—cavities (mouth, nose, throat) that can be used to change the nature of sound produced by the larynx.

ReSound Digital 2000 hearing device —uses digital signal processing circuit technology made by Philips.

RespiGam (immune globulin)—used via an intravenous route of administration to protect against the worst effects of respiratory syncytial virus disease in high-risk children age two and under with bronchopulmonary dysplasia or respiratory problems due to prematurity.

Respiradyne—an electronic instrument that measures pulmonary function.

respirator—see *ventilator*.

respiratory distress syndrome (RDS) —formerly *hyaline membrane disease*. Occurs in the lungs of premature infants due to the lack of surfactant (lubricant). It is this lubricant which helps keep the air sacs in the lungs open on exhalation. Without surfactant, the walls of the air sacs collapse and stick together, making it difficult or impossible to inhale. See *Exosurf, Survanta, lamellar body number density*.

respiratory symptoms (RS)—associated with GERD (gastroesophageal reflux disease).

respiratory syncytial virus (RSV).

respiratory syncytial virus, immunoglobulin (RSV-IG).

respiratory triggering—MRI term.

Respirgard II nebulizer—used to deliver aerosolized pentamidine (Pentam 300, NebuPent). See *NebuPent*.

Respironics CPAP (continuous positive airway pressure) **machine**—device for treatment of sleep apnea and in all-night polysomnogram.

Respitrace machine—used in sleep studies to measure nasal and oral airflow, as well as chest and abdominal respiratory effort.

Respivir (respiratory syncytial virus immune globulin) (name changed to *RespiGam*, 1994)—a drug given intravenously on a monthly basis to premature infants and children with chronic pulmonary disease in order to prevent infection with respiratory syncytial virus.

Response—electrophysiology catheter.

Response GM—a handheld device allowing patients to test their own granulocyte count using a drop of blood.

Res-Q ACD (arrhythmia control device)—a 40-joule implantable cardioverter-defibrillator. Also, *Res-Q AICD* (automatic implantable cardioverter-defibrillator).

Res-Q Micron—an implantable cardioverter-defibrillator used in the management of arrhythmia to prevent sudden cardiac death.

Resten-NG—a gene-targeted therapeutic drug to prevent restenosis following balloon angioplasty.

Reston—foam wound dressing; also hydrocolloid dressing material.

Restore—a close tolerance dental implant system that uses an external hex-based screw system. The term *close tolerance* means that the oral surgeon is able to select an implant that matches the space almost exactly, allowing for a stable fit.

Restore ACL guide system—used in total knee replacement. It includes a tibial guide, a StraightShot graft passer, and an Advantage screw.

Restore alginate wound dressing.

retained bladder syndrome—a condition resulting from the urinary bladder being left in, even when a supravesical urinary diversion is done, e.g., in cases of neurogenic bladder or interstitial cystitis.

Retavase (reteplase)—a "clot-buster" thrombolytic agent.

Retcam 120—a digital camera that takes pictures of the back of the eye.

Retcam *(cont.)*

It is used to follow up premature infants for possible retinopathy of prematurity, which usually strikes in the fourth to tenth week of life and can be treated with laser surgery if diagnosed early.

rete *("ree-tee")* **ridges** (Path)—epidermal projections into dermal tissue.

retention sutures (also, *stay sutures*)—heavy nonabsorbable sutures to reinforce wound closure where there is likely to be unusual postoperative stress.

RET gene test for familial medullary thyroid carcinoma.

Rethi incision (Plas Surg)—a surgical incision in the nose. "Correction was achieved by inserting a columella strut and a tip graft through a Rethi incision."

reticent—reserved, quiet, not inclined to speak out. Dictators use it incorrectly thus: "We discussed having an upper GI and barium enema, which she was reticent to get." Of course, what is meant is *reluctant*.

reticular—pertaining to or resembling a net. Do not confuse with *Roticulator*.

reticulation artifact (Radiol)—a cobweb pattern sometimes seen if film emulsion shrinks because of variation in processing temperature.

reticulose—antiviral drug used in treating HIV opportunistic infections.

retina—innermost, or third tunic, of the eye, that receives the image formed by the lens, and is the immediate instrument of vision.

retinal commotio (concussion)—usually a result of trauma to the eyeball.

retinal detachment—pathological condition where the retina, or part of it, becomes separated from the choroid.

Surgical correction includes cryotherapy (cold), diathermy (heat), photocoagulation (laser), and scleral buckling. These therapies induce a sterile inflammatory reaction that causes retinal re-adherence. See *pneumatic retinopexy; rhegmatogenous retinal detachment; Schepens-Okamura-Brockhurst technique for retinal detachment repair.*

retinal pigment epithelial (RPE) **depigmentation**.

retinal tear; retinal hole—injuries, disease, or degeneration may cause small holes or tears in the retina, allowing the vitreous humor from the large chamber in the back of the eye to seep in between the retina and the choroid, causing the two layers to separate, reducing the blood supply to the retina, and resulting in retinal detachment.

Retin-A Micro (tretinoin gel)—gentler form of tretinoin, said to minimize the irritation commonly experienced by patients using the higher strength acne treatment Retin-A.

retinopathy—any disorder of the retina.
arteriosclerotic
central serous
chloroquine
circinate
diabetic
hypertensive

retinopathy of prematurity (ROP), **posterior**—treated by argon laser photocoagulation.

retinopexy—see *pneumatic retinopexy.*

retinoschisis—splitting of the sensory layers of the retina, usually due to aging.

retractor
Airlift balloon
Alm self-retaining
Bennett bone

retractor *(cont.)*
  bent malleable
  Berkeley-Bonney
  Bookwalter
  Breisky-Navratil
  Buck-Gramcko
  Eccentric "Y"
  Echols
  Elite Farley
  EndoRetract
  eXpose (trademark)
  FlexPosure endoscopic
  Fujita snake
  Fukushima cranial
  Gazayerli endoscopic
  Gilvernet
  Goligher
  Harrington
  Hays
  Henning meniscal
  Hohmann
  Jarit P.E.E.R.
  Laparolift Airlift balloon
  Lone Star
  Magrina-Bookwalter vaginal
  malleable
  Mark II Chandler
  Mediflex-Gazayerli
  Mini-Hohmann
  Miskimon
  Navratil
  Nevyas drape
  Omni
  Omni-Tract adjustable wishbone
  Penfield
  Pitie-Salpetriere saphenous vein
    hook
  Protractor
  Quervain abdominal
  Ragnell handheld
  R-Med miniretractor
  Rosenkranz pediatric
  SaphLITE/SaphLITE II
  Scoville
  Sewell

retractor *(cont.)*
  Spacekeeper
  Space-OR flexible internal
  Tupper hand-holder and retractor
  Upper Hands
  Weitlaner
  wishbone
retrobulbar neuritis—inflammation of the orbital portion of the optic nerve, usually unilateral.
retrograde cerebral perfusion (RCP).
retrolisthesis—the displacement posteriorly of a vertebra on the one below.
retromammary space view (mammography)—for patients with breast implants, the retromammary space view allows for visualization of the posterior border of the implant and the tissue posterior to the implant, not visible with conventional views. A limitation is that the posterior aspect of a retropectoral implant is more difficult to visualize than in prepectoral implants.
retroperitoneoscopy—laparoscopy of retroperitoneal area.
retropubic prostatectomy.
retrospectoscope—a physician's coined term for 20/20 hindsight.
Retrovir (zidovudine, AZT)—used to treat patients with AIDS.
retrovirus—RNA virus. Lentivirus and leukovirus are in this group. Retroviruses were not considered to be pathogenic in humans until the identification of HTLV-I, which causes a leukemia, and HIV. See *HIV.*
Retrox Fractal active fixation lead—consisting of bipolar pre-formed J and bipolar straight lead configurations, allowing atrial and ventricular applications.
REU (rectal endoscopic ultrasonography).

Reuter bobbin tube (ENT)—a tube that looks like a sewing machine bobbin (the round kind).

Reuter suprapubic trocar and cannula system—used in transurethral resection of the prostate.

Reveal insertable loop recorder—an implantable heart monitor manufactured by Medtronic. It is inserted under the skin in the chest area, allowing patients to bathe, swim, and engage in other activities that may be difficult or impossible with an external monitoring device.

Reveal Plus insertable loop recorder—implantable heart monitor with autoactivation capabilities. The recorder continuously monitors the heart's electrical activity and records ECG information in up to a 12-minute "loop," replacing old ECG data with new data.

ReVele—oncology imaging product for use in patients with metastatic breast and prostate cancer.

Reverdin-Green osteotomy—of the metatarsal head.

reverse anorexia syndrome (Psych)—a condition seen in male bodybuilders who feel they are too small, often resulting in (or sometimes a result of) anabolic steroid abuse. The opposite of anorexia nervosa in women, this condition may be due in large part to sociocultural factors evidenced in the gym subculture, bodybuilding magazines and movies starring bodybuilders.

reversible ischemic neurological deficit (RIND)—an episode that may last several hours, longer than a transient ischemic attack.

reversible obstructive airway disease (ROAD)—used synonymously with *asthma*.

Reversionex (HE317)—an immune system regulator for the treatment of HIV/AIDS. It may be used as adjunctive therapy in combination with existing antiretroviral treatments to enhance the immune system's response to HIV.

Revex (nalmefene HCl)—an opioid antagonist for use with overdose.

Rev-Eyes (dapiprazole).

Revia (naltrexone hydrochloride tablets)—used for treatment of alcoholism after detoxification.

Revised European American Lymphoma classification of lymphoma—see *REAL*.

RevitaLase erbium cosmetic laser.

Revo retrievable cancellous screw—acts as a suture anchor in rotator cuff repair.

Revo rotator cuff repair system—used for arthroscopic and open rotator cuff repair.

Rey and Taylor Complex Figure Test—a neurological test.

Rey Auditory Verbal Learning Test.

Reye's syndrome—a rare, but often fatal, disease in children, marked by edema of the brain, fatty infiltration of the liver, unconsciousness, and seizures. Seen after viral illnesses such as chickenpox and influenza. Thought possibly related to the administration of aspirin during these illnesses.

RF (radiofrequency) **coil; pulse**—MRI terms.

RFA (radiofrequency catheter ablation)—used for recurrent tachyarrhythmias.

RF-PMR (radiofrequency energy in percutaneous myocardial revascularization).

RG-83894—see *AIDS vaccine*.

RGO (reciprocating gait orthosis).

RG 12915—antiemetic given to cancer patients who have experienced severe nausea during a prior cycle of chemotherapy.

RGP (rigid gas permeable) **contact lens** (Oph).

r-gp160—a potential vaccine for HIV.

RG-201—antifungal compound used to treat *Pneumocystis carinii* pneumonia.

rhabdomyolysis (disintegration or dissolution of muscle)—newly recognized as a complication following cocaine use.

rhagades (rag'-ah-dez)—fissures or scarring in the skin around the mouth or anus. White linear scars at the corners of the mouth can be a sign of congenital syphilis. See *purse-string mouth.*

rhBMP-2 (recombinant human bone morphogenetic protein)—used in conjunction with a lordotic threaded interbody fusion cage.

rHb1.1 (recombinant hemoglobin)—a genetically engineered hemoglobin that is used as a blood substitute in order to prevent transmission of infectious diseases through transfusions.

RHCT (renal helial CT) **imaging.**

rhegmatogenous retinal detachment —caused by a retinal tear.

rheography, light reflection—imaging procedure that detects deep vein thrombosis using near-infrared light. The light is beamed from diodes to a depth of 1-2 mm into the skin. In the absence of disease, dorsiflexion of the foot will empty the venous plexus of the calf, reduce the amount of light absorbed, and result in an increase in signal. In chronic venous insufficiency, light absorption is reduced to 10-15 seconds. In deep vein thrombosis, light absorption is reduced to less than 10 seconds, showing significantly reduced venous emptying.

rhEPO (recombinant human erythropoietin)—used to correct the anemia seen with renal failure. Said to be slower in response than packed cell administration, but without adverse reactions of iron overloading and viral toxicities. Administered intravenously or subcutaneously.

Rhesus diploid cell strain rabies vaccine (RDRV) (adsorbed).

rheumatic fever diagnosis—see *Jones criteria, revised.*

rheumatoid factor (RH factor, *not* Rh)—an abnormal protein in the blood of most patients with rheumatoid arthritis. Testing for RH factor helps to diagnose this disease.

Rh factor (Rhesus)—an antigen, genetically determined, which is found on the surface of erythrocytes. Incompatibility of the antigens in a mother and fetus is the cause of ery*throblastosis fetalis.* See *RhoGam.*

RH factor (rheumatoid)—see *rheumatoid factor.* Not to be confused with *Rh* (Rhesus) *factor.*

RHIA (Registered Health Information Administrator)—formerly RRA (Registered Record Administrator).

rhIGF (recombinant human insulin-like growth factor)—now mecasermin.

rhinocerebral aspergillosis (RA)—fatal complication common in bone marrow transplantation patients.

Rhinocort (budesonide).

Rhinocort Aqua (budesonide) **nasal spray**—a water-based corticosteroid for once-daily administration in the treatment of seasonal and perennial allergic rhinitis in adults and children over age six.

rhinolaryngostroboscopy (RLS)—used in the diagnosis of laryngeal disorders.

Rhinoline endoscopic system.

Rhino Rocket—nasal packing in a disposable plastic applicator, used for control of postoperative bleeding and for epistaxis.

Rhinotherm—treats nasal congestion and rhinorrhea with hyperthermia, using water-saturated pressured air at 110°F directly to the nasal passages.

Rhino Triangle—polypropylene hip abduction brace for treating hip dysplasia in toddlers up to $2^{1}/2$ years of age.

RHIT (Registered Health Information Technician)—formerly ART (Accredited Record Technician).

Rhizopus nigricans—an allergen.

rhizotomy, functional posterior (including the S2 dorsal rootlet)—procedure for treatment of spasticity in children with cerebral palsy.

Rhodes Inventory of Nausea and Vomiting—an eight-item pencil and paper form that measures the prevalance and amount of distress caused by nausea with or without vomiting.

Rhodococcus equi—aerobic, grampositive coccobacillus infecting horses, swine, and cows that has also been reported in immunocompromised human patients, such as those having undergone organ transplantation or who have HIV disease.

RHS (radial head subluxation).

rHuEPO or EPO (recombinant human erythropoietin)—see *epoetin alfa*.

ribbon stools—stools of greatly narrowed diameter, often due to partial obstruction of the lower bowel by a tumor. Cf. *rabbit stools*.

ribonuclear protein (RNP)—results of ENA testing.

RICE (rest, ice, compression, elevation)—an acronym for basic treatment of most sprains, strains, and other closed soft-tissue injuries, particularly of the extremities. Also used in instructions to patients who have undergone orthopedic surgery or arthroscopy.

Rice-Lyte—an over-the-counter solution containing rice and electrolytes, for controlling infant diarrhea.

Richards hydroxyapatite PORP and TORP prostheses—made of a biocompatible material for ossicular reconstruction.

Richards Solcotrans Plus—see *Solcotrans Plus*.

Richter's hernia—a type of hernia in which only part of the circumference of the bowel passes through the defect; may develop in a trocar site following laparoscopy.

Rickham reservoir—used in obtaining serum methotrexate levels.

Ridaura (auranofin)—used for treatment of rheumatoid arthritis.

RIDD (recombinant interleukin-2, dacarbazine, DDP [cisplatin])—chemotherapy protocol.

ridges, rete ("ree-tee") (Path)—epidermal projections into dermal tissue.

Rid Mousse (pyrethrum extract)—for treatment of head and body lice.

Riedel's struma (*not* stroma)—thyroiditis in which the gland is slowly replaced by hard, dense, fibrous tissue which is difficult to distinguish from cancer. Surgery may be necessary to relieve tracheal compression.

Riester otoscope.

rifabutin (Mycobutin)—used to treat MAC infection in HIV patients.

rifalazil—can potentially shorten antituberculosis therapy by as much as two months.

rifapentine (Priftin)—for treatment of pulmonary tuberculosis. The drug

rifapentine *(cont.)*
reduces the number of treatments required to cure TB.

Rifater (rifampin, isoniazid, and pyrazinamide)—combination regimen for multidrug-resistant tuberculosis.

rifaximin—a broad-spectrum antibiotic for the treatment of hepatic encephalopathy, prophylaxis prior to bowel surgery, and in the treatment of diverticular disease and Crohn's disease.

Right Angle—right angle ArthroWand.

Right Clip—applier used for minimally invasive surgery. It has a right angle that allows for better visualization and manipulation of vessels.

Rigiflex TTS balloon catheter—a through-the-scope catheter with a balloon at the tip that is inserted through the patient's mouth, into the GI tract. Dilates a stenosis in the ileum or colon resulting from Crohn's disease. Also called *Microvasive Rigiflex TTS balloon*.

RigiScan—device for real-time evaluation of penile tumescence and rigidity in erectile dysfunction.

Rigler's sign—visualization of both sides of the intestinal wall on radiography; the bowel wall is outlined very clearly as if etched by a pencil because the gas in the peritoneal space outlines the outside wall. Normally, only the inside of the bowel wall can be seen on a plain film. Rigler's sign is symptomatic of bowel obstruction with pneumoperitoneum.

rigor—rigidity, stiffness (as in *rigor mortis*). Cf. *rigors*.

rigors—chills. Cf. *rigor*.

RIGS/ACT (adaptive cellular therapy)—products for treating patients with advanced carcinoma.

RIGScan and **RIGScan CR49**—used with Neoprobe's RIGS technology for surgical detection of metastatic colorectal cancer.

RIGS system—consists of cancer-specific targeting agents, such as RIGScan CR49, handheld gamma detectors, and methods for their use. A cancer patient is injected before surgery with a low-level radioactive cancer-specific targeting agent. During the operation the surgeon uses the RIGS gamma radiation-detecting probe to locate tissue that contains a significant amount of the radioactive targeting agent.

Riley-Day syndrome (familial dysautonomia)—symptoms include abnormal gastrointestinal motility, ataxia, extremely labile blood pressure, insensitivity to pain, and spinal deformity.

RILG (radioimmunoluminography).

Rilutek (riluzole)—used for treatment of amyotrophic lateral sclerosis.

Rimadyl (carprofen)—a nonsteroidal anti-inflammatory drug.

rimantadine HCl (Flumadine)—an antiviral drug used to prevent infections by influenza type A viruses.

rimexolone (Vexol)—a corticosteroid used post eye surgery.

RIND (reversible ischemic neurological deficit).

Ringer's lactate—see *lactated Ringer's solution*.

Ringer's solution—a physiologic salt solution used for irrigation in surgery. See *lactated Ringer's solution*.

ring forceps *(not* Ring forceps)—also called *sponge forceps*.

ring fracture—encircles the foramen magnum; may be considered a basilar or occipital fracture.

Ring hip prosthesis.

Ring–McLean sump tube—"The tract was dilated to 12 French, and a 12 French Ring–McLean sump tube was placed."

Rinne ("rin-nay") **test**—a test for conductive hearing loss, using air and bone conduction. A tuning fork is stroked or tapped and held close to the external auditory meatus until it is no longer heard. Then the base of the tuning fork is placed near the mastoid bone. If the patient cannot hear it on the mastoid bone, the test is considered normal (positive). If the patient can hear it better by bone conduction, the Rinne is negative, and the patient has a conductive hearing loss.

RinoFlow—micronized nasal irrigation system for treatment of rhinosinusitis.

rippling muscle disease—a rare disease that is usually inherited. May be triggered by an autoimmune phenomenon.

Ripstein procedure—for rectal prolapse.

RISA (radioactive iodinated serum albumin) **study**.

Risperdal (risperidone).

risperidone (Risperdal)—antipsychotic for treating schizophrenia. It is said to be the broadest and safest treatment for this disorder, treating both the "positive" and "negative" symptoms. Previous antipsychotics such as Haldol (haloperidol) treat only the "positive" manifestations. See *negative symptoms of schizophrenia*, *positive symptoms of schizophrenia*.

Risser localizer cast—used in treatment of scoliosis.

Risser sign—indication of skeletal immaturity.

Risser table—used in making an orthosis or body brace. It is a tubular steel frame that supports the shoulders and hips of the patient but permits the technologist ready access to the rest of the torso.

Ritalin (methylphenidate)—CNS stimulant for attention-deficit/hyperactivity disorders and narcolepsy.

ritonavir (Norvir)—a protease inhibitor of HIV-1 infection.

Rituxan (rituximab)—for the treatment of relapsed or refractory low-grade or follicular CD20-positive, B-cell non-Hodgkin's lymphoma.

rivastigmine—an acetylcholinesterase inhibitor that slows effects of Alzheimer's disease in some patients.

Rivas vascular catheter—long-term implantable catheter.

Rizaben (tranilast)—for prevention of restenosis following coronary angioplasty.

Riza-Ribe needle—used with R-Med plug to effect laparoscopic closure of trocar defects.

rizatriptan benzoate (Maxalt).

RLP (rectal linitis plastica) **colorectal carcinoma**.

RLP (remnant-like particle) **lipoprotein**.

RLS (rhinolaryngostroboscopy) **system**.

RLT (reduced liver transplant).

R-Med mini-retractor—used for evaluation of lateral pelvic fossa and posterior surface of the ovaries during diagnostic and operative laparoscopy and mini-laparoscopy.

R-Med Plug—used with Riza-Ribe needle for closure of laparoscopic trocar defects.

RM (Reichert/Mundinger) **stereotaxic system**—used in performing stereotaxic craniotomy. Also for 3-D stereotaxic treatment planning for convergent beam irradiation and radioactive seed implantation.

RMP-7—used for the treatment of brain tumors.

rNEP (recombinant human neutral endopeptidase).

RNP (ribonuclear protein)—result of ENA testing.

rNPA (recombinant novel plasminogen activator)—possible treatment for patients who have had heart attacks or other blood clot-based disorders.

ROAD (reversible obstructive airway disease)—another term for *asthma*.

Robaxacet (methocarbamol and acetaminophen)—for relief of musculoskeletal pain.

Robert Jones bulky soft dressing with Hemovac drainage.

Robicsek vascular probe (RVP)—intravascular flexible surgical probe. Has different sizes of bulbs at the end of the probe and has a flexible one-piece construction without a metal stylet to be removed.

Robin's ("ro-banz") **syndrome**—see *Pierre Robin syndrome, micrognathia-glossoptosis syndrome*.

robin's egg–blue gallbladder—the color of a normal gallbladder, as seen on laparoscopy. An alternative finding when cholecystitis is suspected.

Robodoc—a computerized "surgical assistant" developed in Sacramento, California. It is used to drill the femur cavity for hip replacement surgeries.

Robotrac passive retraction system—mounted on the operating room table, this apparatus holds all types of retractors in a fixed position until repositioned, thus allowing surgical assistants to perform other duties.

ROC (receiver operating characteristic)—MRI term.

ROC and **ROC XS suture fasteners**—used in treatment of female urinary incontinence. These polymer-based devices are used to attach the sagging bladder neck or uterus to the pubic bone.

Rocabado technique—for manipulative (physical) therapy.

Rocephin IM (sterile ceftriazone sodium)—used for treatment of bacterial infections, including those of the lower respiratory tract, the skin, and the urinary tract.

Roche-Microwell Plate Hybridization Method—a test useful in diagnosing *Mycobacterium tuberculosis*.

Rochester bone trephine—a long tube with jagged cutting edges at the distal end; used to remove a dowel of cancellous bone from the iliac crest and insert it into the foot during arthrodesis to correct hallux valgus.

Rochester HKAFO—a hip-knee-ankle-foot orthosis which has separate hip and knee joint locks. For ambulation in children with cerebral palsy and myelomeningocele.

rockerbottom foot—congenital vertical talus foot deformity.

Rockey-Davis incision (*not* Rocky).

RODEO (rotating delivery of excitation off-resonance)—3-D MRI technique.

Roeder loop—the most commonly used slipknot in laparoscopic surgery. Originally developed for tonsillectomy but modified by Semm for use in laparoscopic surgery.

roentgen-equivalent–man—see *rem*.

roentgen knife—not a knife, but a type of stereotaxic radiosurgical device used in surgery to reach deep-seated tumors or arteriovenous malformations in the brain. See *Gamma Knife*.

roentgen stereophotogrammetric analysis (RSA) (Ortho)—allows 3-D measurement of relative implant movement and sometimes measure-

roentgen *(cont.)*
ment of wear. Now being used to assess aseptic prosthetic loosening.

rofecoxib oral medication—said to be as effective in relieving pain and inflammation as the maximum doses of nonsteroidal anti-inflammatory drugs (such as aspirin and ibuprofen), without GI side effects.

Roferon-A (interferon alfa-2a)—a drug used to treat leukemia, carcinoma, AIDS, and Kaposi's sarcoma.

Rogaine (minoxidil)—hair regrowth product available over the counter. Now for the minus—when you stop using it, the hair falls out.

Roger's ("ro-zhay") **disease**—see *maladie de Roger*.

rogletimide—a chemotherapy drug for women with metastatic breast cancer with positive estrogen and progesterone receptor status.

Rogozinski spinal fixation system—system of rods, hooks, and screws used to provide sacral fixation. Provides two points of spinal fixation combined with cross-linking to create strong, stable fixation. Also called *Richards Rogozinski spinal fixation system*.

Roho mattress—air-filled device that helps prevent pressure sores (decubitus ulcers).

ROI (region of interest).

Rokitansky-Aschoff sinuses—small outpouchings of the gallbladder mucosa extending through the lamina propria and muscular layer.

Rokitansky's disease—see *Budd-Chiari syndrome*.

rolandic epilepsy (also *jacksonian*)—see *jacksonian seizure*. Note: The adjective *rolandic* is not capitalized.

rolfing—a type of massage therapy.

rollerball endometrial ablation—an alternative to hysterectomy in a select group of patients with menorrhagia. It uses a rollerball electrode to coagulate the endometrium during a brief outpatient procedure with a short recovery.

Rolyan Firm D-Ring wrist support—see *Firm D-Ring*.

Rolyan Gel Shell splint—a hand splint with a gel pad that applies gentle pressure on the incision site of a carpal tunnel release to help desensitize the area and prevent hypertrophic scar formation.

ROM (range of motion).

Romano surgical curved drilling system—used to drill curved holes, particularly in the bones of the foot and ankle.

Romazicon (flumazenil)—a benzodiazepine antagonist.

Romberg test—for differentiating between peripheral and cerebellar ataxia. The patient stands with feet together, first with the eyes closed, then with the eyes open. The examiner evaluates the amount of body swaying. Some swaying is normal. If the Romberg is positive or equivocal, the patient may be asked to hop in place on one foot and then the other.

"romi" (rule out myocardial infarction)—medical slang used as a verb, as in "The patient was romied." It means a myocardial infarction was ruled out.

RON (radiation-related optic neuropathy).

R on T phenomenon—premature ventricular contractions coming so closely together that ventricles are stimulated in their resting period, which can lead to fatal ventricular

R on T phenomenon *(cont.)* tachycardia or fibrillation. The name reflects the appearance on the electrocardiogram.

Roos test—a maneuver performed to detect thoracic outlet syndrome.

rooting reflex—An infant will turn its head toward the stimulus when its cheek is gently touched (as if it is searching for food).

root signs—signs of compression or injury of spinal nerve roots, such as absence of deep tendon reflexes in a patient with a slipped intervertebral disk.

ROP (retinopathy of prematurity).

ROPA (Regional Organ Procurement Agency)—matches potential donors and recipients for organ transplants.

ROPE (respiratory ordered phase encoding)—a respiratory compensation technique—MRI term.

ropinirole (Requip)—used in treatment of patients with Parkinson's disease.

ropivacaine (Naropin)—anesthetic for advanced pain relief administered via spinal canal.

roquinimex (Linomide)—imunomodulator for HIV; may be used in bone marrow transplant for leukemia.

Rorschach test (Psych)—ink blot test.

Rosai Dorfman disease—sinus histiocytosis of uncertain origin, characterized by massive lymphadenopathy, increased erythrocyte sedimentation rates, and elevated serum immunoglobulins.

Rösch—see *Gianturco-Rösch Z stent.*

rose bengal—a dye, used as a stain to demonstrate the presence of abrasion of the corneal surface in Sjögren's syndrome—"dry eye."

Rosedale Psychiatric Home Care Scale—a 10-item rating scale that identifies essential elements for psychiatric nursing care within the home.

Rosenkranz pediatric retractor system—for use in open heart surgery.

Rosen needle (ENT)—used in ear surgery. "The tube was positioned in place with a Rosen needle."

Rosenthal fibers—seen in pilocytic astrocytoma.

Rosenthal needle—used for bone marrow biopsy and aspiration.

rosettes, Homer-Wright—sometimes seen on histologic examination of medulloblastomas.

Rosomoff cordotomy—a percutaneous radiofrequency cervical cordotomy.

Ross aortic valve replacement procedure—combines use of the patient's own pulmonary valve in the aortic position with use of a homograft to replace the pulmonary valve and right ventricular outflow tract. The patient's own pulmonary valve is essentially used as a "spare part" to replace the diseased aortic valve.

Rossavik growth equation (or model)—equation using fetal growth curves to compare a fetus's growth in the third trimester with its own pattern in the first and second trimesters. Helps to differentiate between fetuses that achieve their growth potential and those with growth failure who are at a greater risk for fetal compromise or postnatal complications.

Rossiter system—unique, inexpensive stretching program that reduces pain in individuals in such diverse occupations as assembly-line worker, computer operator, and musician—any job or activity that requires repetitive tasks. Employees undergo training in powerful two-person stretches, done at the job site, to

Rossiter *(cont.)*
relieve chronic pain, tingling, stiffness, and numbness.

Ross procedure—uses the pulmonary valve from the right side of the heart to replace a defective aortic valve on the left side. To replace the relocated pulmonary valve, surgeons implant a pulmonary valve taken from the hospital's tissue bank of donated human valves. The native pulmonary valve is an ideal substitute because it is about the same size and shape as the aortic valve and is able to close tightly even under high pressure.

Ross pulmonary porcine valve—stentless pulmonary heart valve designed by Dr. Donald N. Ross for pediatric patients. Because it is stentless, it does not require any artificial material, such as a sewing ring, to immobilize tissue.

Rotablator—a high-speed, elliptical, rotating abrasive bur used in percutaneous coronary rotational atherectomy. Resulting particles that are small or smaller than red blood cells wash out downstream from the site of the lesion.

Rotablator RotaLink (and **RotaLink Plus**) **rotational atherectomy device**—for removal of plaque from a coronary artery using a high-speed diamond-tipped burr.

ROTACS guide wire—used to prevent restenosis, or occlusion, of an artery post angioplasty.

Rotalok cup—uncemented acetabular component.

Rotamune—vaccine for the prevention of rotaviral gastroenteritis in infants.

RotaShield—vaccine for the prevention of rotaviral gastroenteritis in infants.

rotating frame of reference—MRI term.

rotational coronary atherectomy—see *directional coronary atherectomy.*

rotavirus—a group of viruses involved in acute gastroenteritis in infants.

Rotazyme diagnostic procedure—an enzyme immunology kit from Abbott Labs for rotavirus antigen in stool and liver aspirates.

Roth-Bernhardt disease—see *meralgia paresthetica.*

Roth Grip-Tip suture guide (Urol).

Rothman Gilbard corneal punch.

Rothmund-Thomson syndrome—oculocutaneous disorder seen with linitis plastica (a gastric carcinoma), and characterized by skin changes including atrophy, telangiectasias, alterations in pigmentation, and sparse or absent eyelashes and eyebrows. Some patients are also found to have cataracts, bone defects, dystrophic nails, and small stature.

Roth retrieval net—gauze-covered net for polyp retrieval.

Roth's spots—small hemorrhages, round or oval lesions with small white centers. May be seen in the ocular fundi in cases of subacute bacterial endocarditis.

roticulating endograsper—a surgical instrument used in minimally invasive surgeries.

Roticulator stapler—*not* reticulator, as sometimes dictated.

Roto-Rest bed.

Ro 24–7429—a TAT gene inhibitor to be used in trials with human patients with HIV.

Rous sarcoma virus—oncogenic retrovirus.

Routine Assessment of Patient Progress (RAPP).

Rouviere, node of.

Roux-Y ("roo-Y") **chimney**—surgical technique. "Transjejunal approaches

Roux-Y chimney *(cont.)*
have been used to examine patients following Kasai procedures, to dilate stenotic hepaticojejunostomies in a retrograde manner, to place a U tube percutaneously, to perform percutaneous hepaticojejunostomy, and to accomplish intermittent biliary access in patients with Roux-Y chimneys brought up to the skin." Also, *Roux-en-Y anastomosis.*

Rovsing's sign—indicative of acute appendicitis. Pain elicited in the lower right abdomen at McBurney's point when the corresponding point in the lower left is pressed.

Rowasa enema—for ulcerative colitis, proctosigmoiditis, proctitis.

Rowe disimpaction forceps (Oral Surg).

Roxicodone (oxycodone HCl).

Roy-Camille plates—used in screw placement in lower cervical spine.

RP (radical prostatectomy).

RPC (reactive perforating collagenosis).

rPDGF (recombinant platelet-derived growth factor).

RPE (rating of perceived exertion).

RPE (retinal pigment epithelium) **dropout**; **clumping**.

RPM (real-time position management) **tracking system**—used in electrophysiologic procedures for real-time visualization of catheters. It assists physicians in precisely manipulating catheters within the heart during procedures.

RPR (rapid plasma reagin)—a test for syphilis, faster than the VDRL, and macroscopic rather than microscopic. See *reagin.*

RPR-CT (rapid plasma reagin circle-card test)—for syphilis. Cf. *RPR.*

RRA (registered record administrator)—see *RHIA.*

RRFs (ragged-red fibers)—a hallmark of mitochondrial encephalopathies.

RRI (recurrent respiratory infections).

RRP (recurrent respiratory papillomatosis).

RS (respiratory symptoms).

RSA (recurrent spontaneous abortions).

RSA (roentgen stereophotogrammetric analysis).

rCD4 (recombinant soluble CD4, Receptin)—a drug for AIDS patients.

Rsch-Uchida (yes, Rsch)—transjugular liver access needle-catheter.

RSI (rapid sequence induction) **orotracheal intubation**—said to have a higher success rate, fewer complications, and produce better patient outcome than noninduced orotracheal intubation and blind nasotracheal intubation. Emergency medicine physicians prefer RSI orotracheal intubation as the method of choice for trauma airway management in the helicopter.

RSI (repetitive strain injury).

RSLT (reduced-size liver transplant).

Rsma (superior mesenteric artery resistance). Cf. *Qsma.*

RSR (reduced sewing ring)—see *Carpentier-Edwards Perimount RSR pericardial bioprosthesis.*

RSV (respiratory syncytial virus).

rt-PA (recombinant tissue plasminogen activator).

Rubens flap—used for breast reconstruction after mastectomy. It is a modification of the deep circumflex iliac artery-iliac crest flap in that there is no bony transfer. The name of the flap is derived from the appearance of the female form in

Rubens *(cont.)*

paintings by Peter Paul Rubens, which shows an area of particular fullness at or just above the iliac crest. This technique is used in patients who have had a previous abdominoplasty and have few other tissues available for an autologous graft except a fullness above the iliac crest region as a result of the abdominoplasty. See *breast reconstruction donor sites.*

rubitecan (RFS2000)—antineoplastic drug derived from the *Camptotheca acuminata* tree that has been shown to stop or reduce pancreatic tumor growth. It is currently being studied as a tumor suppressor in hematologic, ovarian, colorectal, breast, and lung cancers.

RU-486—previous name of *Mifegyne (mifepristone).*

Ruiz-Cohen round expander—a device used for acute intraoperative arterial elongation, which is a reliable method of repairing a small arterial defect as opposed to using an interposition vein graft. The interposition vein graft has been shown to have a higher incidence of thrombosis than the Ruiz-Cohen round expander. However, a vein graft is still the technique of choice for large arterial defects.

Ruiz microkeratome—disposable instrument used to create the corneal flap during a LASIK procedure for vision correction.

Rule of Nines—formula by which the percentage of body surface which has been burned is determined. The head is figured at 9%, as is each arm. Each leg is 18% (2 x 9), as are the anterior trunk and the posterior trunk. This all adds up to 99%. The perineum is figured at 1%. See also *Berkow formula.*

Rumi uterine manipulator and injector.

ruptured abdominal aortic aneurysm (RAAA).

rush immunotherapy—consists of a number of injections given over a short time to densensitize a person to certain allergens, such as dust mites, cat dander, or certain plants.

Russel (one *L*) **gastrostomy kit.**

Russell-Taylor (R-T) **nail.**

Russell traction—used as a temporary measure to stabilize femoral fractures until the patient can be taken to surgery.

Russian forceps.

RUT (rapid urease test).

rutherford (rd) **unit**—a unit of radioactivity; abbreviated *rd.*

Rutkow sutureless plug and patch—repair for inguinal hernia using a simple mesh plug made of preformed polypropylene mesh that maintains a permanent open cone-like shape. It requires no suturing.

Rutzen ileostomy bag.

RVH (right ventricular hypertrophy).

RV/TLC (residual volume/total lung capacity) **ratio.**

RWECochG (round window electrocochleography)—a test for assessing children with cochlear implants for residual hearing in low frequencies.

Rx5000 cardiac pacing system.

RX Herculink 14—pre-mounted stent system for treatment of malignant obstructions of the biliary duct.

RX stent delivery system—a rapid exchange technology that allows cardiologists and catheter lab personnel to decrease their radiation exposure

RX stent *(cont.)*
due to the reduced need for fluoroscopy during placement and catheter exchanges.

Rye histopathologic classification—of Hodgkin's disease.

Ryna-12 S (phenylephrine tannate/pyrilamine tannate) **suspension**—for symptomatic relief of the coryza and nasal congestion associated with the common cold, sinusitis, allergic rhinitis, and other upper respiratory tract conditions.

Rythmol—see *propafenone*. Note the spelling of this drug is *Ry*, not *Rhy*, although it affects the rhythm of the heart.

S, s

SAANDs (selective apoptotic antineoplastic drugs).

SAARD (slow-acting antirheumatic drug)—utilized to slow the progression of rheumatoid arthritis. Examples: antimalarial agent, gold salts, penicillamine, sulfasalazine, methotrexate.

SAB (stereotactic aspiration biopsy).

Saber 30—bisector ArthroWand.

Sable—balloon catheter used in angioplasty procedures.

Sabouraud's medium—culture medium for growing fungi.

Sabreloc spatula needle.

sabre shin deformity—in congenital syphilis, the leading edge of the tibia bows forward.

Sabril (vigabatrin).

saccade—series of involuntary, abrupt, rapid small movements or jerks of both eyes simultaneously in changing the point of fixation.

saccadic pursuit—following movements of the eyes.

saccadic slowing (Oph, Neuro).

sacculotomy—see Fick sacculotomy.

SACH (solid-ankle, cushioned heel) heels—for orthopedic appliances.

Sacks-Vine PEG (percutaneous endoscopic gastrostomy) tube, or Sacks-Vine feeding gastrostomy tube.

sacral insufficiency fracture (SIF)—usually present as nonspecific pelvic or low back pain, often overlooked in the elderly.

sacralization—abnormal bony fusion between the fifth lumbar vertebra and the sacrum.

sacral nerve stimulation (SNS) therapy—implantable device for patients with urge incontinence, resulting from neurological conditions such as spinal cord injury, stroke, spina bifida, or multiple sclerosis. The pulse generator is implanted in the abdominal wall, and a wire lead is attached to a nerve near the sacrum.

sacrospinous colpopexy—gynecologic procedure for restoring vaginal support in women with vault prolapse, massive vaginal eversion, or procidentia.

saddle coil—MRI term.

saddle embolus—a blood clot lodged at the bifurcation of an artery, thus blocking both branches. Also called *pantaloon embolus* or *straddling embolus*. "Significant past history includes a history of saddle embolus."

saddle leather friction rub—observed on heart examination.

Sade modification of Norwood procedure—for hypoplastic left-sided heart syndrome. See *Fontan, Gill/Jonas.*

Sadowsky hook wire—used in breast surgery.

SAE (subcortical atherosclerotic encephalopathy).

SAECG (or **SAEKG**) (signal-averaged electrocardiogram).

Saethre–Chotzen ("say-ther-cho-tzen") **syndrome**—form of familial craniofacial anomaly in which there may be cranial synostoses and other anomalies.

Saf-Clens chronic wound cleanser.

SafeTap tapered spinal needle.

Safety AV fistula needle—for use in hemodialysis.

Saf-Gel hydrogel dressing—for wound hydration.

SAF (self-articulating femoral) **hip replacement.**

SAFHS (sonic-accelerated fracture-healing system) **therapy**—ultrasound therapy which accelerates healing of Colles' fractures and tibial diaphysis fractures.

Saf-T E-Z set—translucent needle shield to protect against accidental needlesticks.

SAF-T shield—postoperative eye protection.

"sagging brain"—spontaneous intracranial hypotension, the result of a hole or tear in the sac around the spinal cord that causes fluid to leak into surrounding tissues. Such tears are not uncommon following spinal taps and other forms of neurosurgery and can also occur with rupture of a benign cyst at the juncture of the sac and a surrounding nerve.

sagittal orientation (Radiol).

sagittal roll spondylolisthesis (Ortho).

sagittal T1-weighted image—MRI term.

SAH (subarachnoid hemorrhage).

Sahara Clinical Bone Sonometer—portable device for estimating bone strength using ultrasound measurements; it transmits high-frequency sound waves through the patient's heel for about 10 seconds and automatically analyzes results.

Sahli needle—used for bone marrow biopsy and aspiration.

SA-IGIV (*Staphylococcus aureus* immune globulin intravenous [human]).

SAIL protocol—for reducing polypharmacy in physician practice. Protocol for each patient should consist of:

Simplicity: Prescribe as few medications as possible, adjusting dosages and individual medications so that fewer meds need to be taken per day and cost to the patient is as low as possible.

Adverse effects: Be constantly aware of possible reaction to or interaction between prescribed medications.

Indications: Be certain that indications for any medication are clear.

Lists: Maintain a precise and current list of all drugs taken by the patient, making sure that the patient and all treating physicians are aware of all meds being taken.

sail sign—anterior and superior elevation of the fat pad in the elbow joint. The sail sign is highly suggestive of intra-articular fracture.

Saizen (somatropin of rDNA origin)—injectable for treatment of pediatric growth hormone deficiency.

SAL (suction-assisted lipectomy).

SAL (suction-assisted lipoplasty).

salaam activity—a form of seizures.

Salagen (pilocarpine hydrochloride)—tablets for treatment of symptoms of radiation-induced xerostomia.

SalEst system—a test that identifies pregnant women at risk for preterm labor. A saliva sample is checked for estriol level. An elevated estriol level could be a warning sign that preterm labor and delivery may occur within 2-3 weeks.

saline-enhanced MR arthrography of shoulder—used as an inexpensive alternative to gadopentetate dimeglumine.

Salix lozenges (sorbitol lozenges)—saliva substitute for relief of dry mouth and throat related to xerostomia and hyposalivation associated with surgery or radiation, Sjögren syndrome, and Bell's palsy.

salmeterol (Serevent)—a long-acting twice-daily bronchodilator delivered via oral inhalation, with 50 mg dose said to last up to $11^1/2$ hours, making it ideal for noncompliant patients and those with nocturnal asthma.

Salmon's law—a method of locating the internal opening of an anal fistula.

salmon-patch hemorrhages (Oph)—usually found in patients with sickle cell disease, occurring in the mid-peripheral part of the fundus of the eye. They are initially red but often turn a salmon color after several days.

Salmon-Rickham ventriculostomy reservoir (Neuro).

"salon sink" radiculopathy—a neurologic condition, presenting as pain, tingling, and weakness radiating from the neck to the upper extremities, caused by compression of a nerve root in the cervical spine when leaning the head back (hyperextension) for shampooing in hair salons. People most at risk are those suffering from preexisting injuries or arthritis of the cervical spine.

saloon door approach—in MIDCAB (minimally invasive direct coronary artery bypass) procedures, a technique in which the intercostal muscles are incised laterally and the adjacent cartilages folded back. It disconnects rather than removes the fourth and fifth costal cartilages and thus helps prevent skeletal defects that occur with complete removal.

SALT (skin-associated lymphoid tissue).

Salter fracture

    I fracture through the plate only

   II fracture through the growth plate and through a portion of the metaphysis

  III fracture through the growth plate and through the epiphysis

  IV fracture through the growth plate, the metaphysis, and the epiphysis

   V a crushing fracture injury of the growth plate

  VI fracture of the perichondrial ring surrounding the epiphysis

Salter osteotomy.

saluresis—excretion of sodium and chloride ions in the urine.

saluting—repeated rubbing of the nose upward to scratch an itchy nose and open the obstructed airway (seen in patients with allergies). Also called *allergic salute*.

Salyer modification—of Obwegeser's mandibular osteotomy.

Salzmann's nodules—in the cornea.

Salz nuclear splitter—used to fracture the nucleus in phacoemulsification (refers to vitreous loss in an extracapsular cataract extraction).

SAM (scanning acoustic microscope).

SAM (subcutaneous augmentation material).

SAM (systolic anterior motion)—as seen on 2-D echocardiogram.

samarium Sm 153 lexidronam (Quadramet).

same-day microsurgical arthroscopic lateral-approach laser-assisted (SMALL) fluoroscopic diskectomy.

"sammoma"—see *psammoma*.

Sampaolesi line (Oph).

SampleMaster biopsy needle—used with INRAD HiLiter ultrasound-enhanced stylet.

Sam splint—foam pad with aluminum center which is invisible on x-ray, waterproof, and reusable.

Sandifer syndrome—rare manifestation of gastroesophageal reflux in children that is associated with abnormal movements and postures of the head, neck, and trunk; treated with Nissen fundoplication and a Heineke-Mikulicz pyloroplasty.

Sandman—a line of sleep disorder diagnostic systems.

Sandostatin LAR Depot (ocreotide acetate for injectable suspension)—designed to prevent diarrhea associated with the chemotherapy drug Camptosar (innotecan), which is indicated as second-line treatment of metastatic colorectal cancer.

Sandoz suction/feeding tube.

Sand process (Dr. Bruce Sand)—uses a holmium laser-based system for collagen shrinkage to correct ophthalmic conditions.

sandwich—see *Marlex methylmethacrylate*.

sandwich treatment—combination of two or more therapies.

Sanger-Brown syndrome.

sanguineous—bloody.

S-A (sinoatrial) **node.**

Sanorex (mazindol).

SANS (Stoller afferent nerve stimulation)—used for the treatment of urge incontinence syndrome. It stimulates the sacral region of the spine that controls bladder function. This reconditions the nerves, suppressing overactivity and restoring normal reflex control.

Santorini plexus—a network of veins in the region of the prostate gland.

Santyl (collagenase)—enzymatic debriding agent.

SaO$_2$ (arterial oxygen saturation)—the percentage of hemoglobin in the arterial blood that is saturated with oxygen. Normal values are 95% to 100%.

SAP (superabsorbent polymer).

SaphFinder surgical balloon dissector—used with EndoSaph in saphenous vein harvesting for CABG procedures.

SaphLITE/SaphLITE II retractor system—stainless steel device for retraction of subcutaneous tissue to afford exposure and visualization of the saphenous vein during saphenous vein harvesting procedures.

SAPHtrak balloon dissector—used to remove the saphenous vein in a minimally invasive procedure. The balloon is inserted through a 1 to 3 cm incision and then inflated, separating the natural tissue planes to create a subcutaneous space along the length of the saphenous vein. Upon removal of the balloon, this "dissected" space can be insufflated with gas to create a surgical working space.

saquinavir (Invirase)—a protease inhibitor which is an addition to the combination therapies for HIV/AIDS that are a great improvement over the modes of therapy used in the past.

sargramostim (Leukine)—granulocyte/macrophage colony-stimulating factor (GM-CSF) used in autologous bone marrow transplantation and to treat Kaposi's sarcoma and CMV retinitis. See *GM-CSF.*

Sarns aortic arch cannula.

SAS (sleep apnea syndrome).

SASMA (skin-adipose superficial musculoaponeurotic) **system**—a face-lift technique said to achieve more lasting results than other techniques.

Sassone score—a system of scoring the appearance (in transvaginal ultrasonography) of ovarian and adnexal masses to distinguish between malignant and benign masses. The score is based on characteristics of the mass: wall structure, presence of septa, loss of echo behind the structure on ultrasound, and echogenicity.

satellite lesion—a smaller lesion, near the primary lesion; accompanying, nearby, subordinate lesions. "There was an indurated, excoriated rash which had no satellite lesions or any appearance of tinea." "Examination reveals an erosive vaginal lesion at 6 o'clock, consistent with herpes, and several satellite lesions which are also erosive, ulcerative lesions."

Saticon vacuum chamber pickup tube —for video camera used in arthroscopy. Cf. *Circon, Newvicon, Vidicon.*

SatinCrescent tunneler, SatinShortcut, SatinSlit keratome—ophthalmic products, satin finish.

Sattler veil—see *bedewing of cornea.*

satumomab pendetide (OncoScint CR/OV)—a monoclonal antibody-based imaging agent used to detect abdominal and pelvic metastases in patients with known colorectal (CR) or ovarian (OV) carcinomas. OncoScint is not used as a screening agent for patients with suspected carcinomas and is used only to reveal metastases not detected by other types of tests. Indium 111, the radioactive imaging agent, is combined with a monoclonal antibody that reacts specifically with the antigen TAG-72 found on the surface of cells of colorectal and ovarian adenocarcinomas. The patient is given OncoScint CR/OV intravenously over five minutes, and then a nuclear scan is used to detect areas of uptake which indicate metastases. This information permits the physician to more accurately plan medical or surgical care. However, OncoScint CR/OV is not useful in detecting hepatic metastases.

saturation—see SaO_2 (arterial oxygen saturation).

saturation recovery technique—MRI term.

Saturn Splint—splinting device for noninvasive treatment of carpal tunnel syndrome.

saucerize—to create a saucer-shaped excavation surgically.

Sauflon PW (lidofilcon B)—soft, extended-use hydrophilic contact lens for aphakia in children.

sausaging of a vein—refers to a narrowing of the vein so that it looks like a string of sausages.

Sauvage graft—filamentous velour Dacron arterial graft material.

Sauve-Kapandji procedure—for reconstruction of distal radioulnar joint. Also called *Kapandji-Sauve procedure.*

Save-A-Tooth—tooth preserving system that can keep a knocked-out tooth alive for up to 24 hours.

SAVVI (not an acronym)—synchronous pacemaker that needs only a single lead. It is used for patients with acquired, congenital, or postoperative atrioventricular block.

Savvy vaginal gel—a contraceptive gel that also prevents transmission of sexually transmitted diseases.

SB Charité III intervertebral dynamic disc spacer—vertebral disk prosthesis for patients with single-level degenerative disk disease for whom back pain, rather than leg pain, is the major complaint.

SBE (small bowel enteroscopy).

SBE (subacute bacterial endocarditis).

SBGM (self blood glucose monitoring).

SBP (spontaneous bacterial peritonitis).

SBSP (simultaneous bilateral spontaneous pneumothorax).

SBRN (sensory branch of the radial nerve).

SCAD (spontaneous coronary artery dissection).

SCA-EX and **SCA-EX ShortCutter catheters with rotating blades**—used for directional coronary atherectomy.

scale—see *classification, score, test.*
Abbreviated Injury Scale
ADAS (Alzheimer Disease Assessment Scale)
Adolescent and Pediatric Pain Tool (APPT)
AIMS (Abnormal Involuntary Movement Scale)
ALS (amyotrophic lateral sclerosis) Functional Rating (ALS-FRS)
ASIA impairment scale
Bayley Scales of Infant Development

scale *(cont.)*
Behavioral Pathology in Alzheimer's Disease Rating
Bethesda rating (for Pap smears)
Brazelton Neonatal Assessment
Cattell Infant Intelligence
CIWA-A (Clinical Institute Withdrawal Assessment–Alcohol)
Dementia Rating (DRS)
Dubowitz scale for infant maturity
Dumas-Duport glioma pathology grading
FACT (Functional Assessment of Cancer Therapy)
Flint Colon Injury Scale (FCIS)
French (sizing)
Glasgow Coma Scale
Glasgow Outcome Scale (GOS)
House-Brackmann facial weakness
HSC (Hospital for Sick Children) pain
Karnofsky rating
Kurtzke Disability Status Scale (KDSS)
Mitsui
Montefiore Organic Brain Scale
Obsessive Compulsive Drinking (OCDS)
Outerbridge
Past Feelings and Acts of Violence (PFAV)
Pressure Ulcer Scale for Healing (PUSH) Ttool
Q-TWiST (time without symptoms or toxicity)
Ranchos los Amigos cognitive
Self-Regard Questionnaire
SHRS (St. Hans Rating Scale for extrapyramidal syndromes)
Suicide Risk (SRS)
Tanner Developmental
Unified Parkinson's Disease Rating
Vineland Social Maturity
visual analogue

scale *(cont.)*
WAIS (Wechsler Adult Intelligence
Scale)
Wechsler Memory Scale
Zung Depression Scale
scalloping of vertebrae (Radiol)—
sometimes seen on x-ray of patient
with sickle cell anemia.
scalp electrode—EKG lead attached to
scalp of infant about to be delivered
to evaluate intrauterine heart rate.
scalp pH—blood sample taken from
scalp of infant about to be delivered
to evaluate intrauterine oxygenation.
scan, scanner—see also *operation* or
procedure.
Aloka scanner
ATL real-time Neurosector scanner
biphasic helical CT
BladderScan
B-scan
Bruel-Kjaer ultrasound scanner
Cardiolite scan
CardioTek scan
cine CT scanner
contrast material enhanced scan
coronary artery (CAS)
CT (computed tomography) scan
CT/T 8800 scanner
Denver Developmental Screening
DermaScan
DEXA (dual energy x-ray absorp-
tiometry) scan
EMI scanner
Evolution XP scanner
FONAR-360 MRI
F-scan
gallium scan
General Electric CT-T scanner
Gyroscan ACS NT MRI
HIDA or TcHIDA scan
Imatron ultrafast CT scanner
indium 111 scintigraphy
Lumiscan 150 scanner
MAA lung

scan *(cont.)*
Max FiberScan laser system scanner
medronate
mPower PET
MUGA (multiple gated acquisition)
"open sky" MRI
PET (positron emission tomography)
PIPIDA, or TcPIPIDA
PYP (pyrophosphate) scan
QUAD 12000 and QUAD 7000
MRI scanner
radionuclide scan
sector echocardiography
sector scanner
serial scans
sestamibi stress scan
Skinscan
Softscan
Somatom DR 1 (2, 3) CT scanner
SPECT (single photon emission CT)
spiral XCT (x-ray computed tomography) scanner
stacked scans
teboroxime scan
TechneScan MAG3 scan
technetium scan
3-Scape Real-Time 3D Imaging
ThromboScan
TransScan TS2000 electrical
impedance breast scanning system
T-Scan 2000
TSPP rectilinear bone scan
unenhanced scan
Vision 1.5-T Siemens MRI
V/Q (ventilation/perfusion) scan
xenon 133 (^{133}Xe) scan
Scanmaster DX x-ray film digitizer—
digitizes x-ray film, allowing the
image to be viewed on a computer
monitor. This permits radiologists to
make clinical diagnoses directly from
the monitor, bypassing the need to
examine the original film.
scanning acoustic microscope (SAM).

Scanning-Beam Digital X-ray (SBDX) —a low-radiation fluoroscopy system used in the diagnosis and treatment of cardiovascular disease.

Scan-O-Grams of lower extremities.

scaphocephaly (sagittal synostosis)—an abnormally long and narrow skull in a newborn, as a result of premature closure of the sagittal suture. It is treated with sagittal craniectomy and biparietal morcellation. See also *craniosynostosis, endoscopic strip craniectomy,* and *helmet-molding therapy.*

Scaphoid-Microstaple system—a simple staple device used for osteosynthesis.

scapholunate arthritic collapse—see *SLAC wrist.*

scarf osteotomy bunionectomy—used for correction of hallux valgus deformity of the great toe.

SCARMD (severe childhood autosomal recessive muscular dystrophy).

scatoma—stercoroma; tumorlike mass in the rectum formed by an accumulation of fecal material. Cf. *scotoma.*

SCC (small cell carcinoma) **of the lung.** Also, *squamous cell carcinoma.*

sCD4 (soluble recombinant human CD4)—see *CD4.*

sCD4-PE40—a drug used to treat patients with AIDS.

Schantz screw (Ortho)—"Good exposure was obtained by inserting a large Schantz screw in the greater trochanter region and retracting the trochanter bone with a T-handled universal chuck."

Schepens-Okamura-Brockhurst technique—for retinal detachment repair.

Scheuermann's disease—osteochondrosis of vertebral epiphyses in the young.

Scheuermann juvenile kyphosis.

Schiek back support—a belt that assists in maintaining proper alignment of the lower back.

Schiller test—when iodine is painted on the cervix, healthy tissue is stained but cancerous tissue is not.

Schinzel acrocallosal syndrome—rare disorder inherited as an autosomal recessive genetic trait and characterized by craniofacial abnormalities, absence or underdevelopment of the mass of white matter that unites the two halves of the brain, additional fingers and/or toes, loss of muscle tone, and mental retardation.

Schiötz tonometry—measures intraocular pressure. See *applanation tonometry.*

Schirmer's test—a strip of filter paper or soft tissue paper (called *tear strips*) placed between the eyelids to determine the quantity of tear production. Used in the diagnosis of Sjögren's syndrome and one of its elements, keratoconjunctivitis sicca, also known as *dry eye.*

schizencephaly—a developmental disorder of cortical migration often associated with epilepsy. Patients with this disorder have significant neurological impairment and often paresis and subnormal intelligence.

schizophrenia—see *negative symptoms of schizophrenia, positive symptoms of schizophrenia.*

Schlemm's canal—in the inner scleral sulcus, against the sclera, a large vessel filled with aqueous humor, closely resembling a large lymphatic channel.

Schlesinger's solution—a morphine solution used for palliative purposes in patients with advanced carcinoma.

Schmidt's elastic–Giemsa stain.

schneiderian papilloma, inverted—an epithelial neoplasm of the nasal wall of uncertain etiology. It has a tendency to recur and has a propensity to be associated with malignancy. Another attribute is its destructive capacity. It appears in men more often than in women, whites more than blacks, and in the sixth and seventh decades of life.

schneiderian respiratory membrane —lines the lateral nasal wall, turbinates, and paranasal sinuses. (Victor Conrad Schneider, late 1600's.)

Schneider Wallstent—see *Wallstent*.

Schober test—measures lumbar flexion for evaluation of spondylitis. Measurements are given in degrees, with normal being 20° or more.

Scholten endomyocardial bioptome and biopsy forceps—used in heart transplantations.

Schönlein-Henoch purpura—a kidney disease with urticaria, erythema, arthritis, arthropathy. Also, *Henoch-Schönlein purpura*.

Schuco nebulizer—used in pediatric settings to produce moist nebulized air as an adjunct to therapy for respiratory problems.

Schuco 2000—a self-contained, portable nebulizer for aerosolization therapy at home or elsewhere.

Schüffner's dots—cytoplasmic stippling.

Schuknecht classification of congenital aural atresia—type A, atresia limited to the fibrocartilaginous part of the external auditory canal; type B, narrowing and sometimes tortuosity of both fibrocartilaginous and bony parts of the external auditory canal; type C, totally atretic canal but well-developed pneumatization of the temporal bone; and type D, total atresia with reduced pneumatization of the temporal bone.

Schuknecht cochleosacculotomy—for treatment of progressive endolymphatic hydrops (Ménière's disease). Involves the placement of an endolymphatic shunt to control a chronic state of excessive accumulation of endolymph.

Schulman's syndrome—seen in a list of conditions that may respond to pentoxifylline therapy; no description given.

schwannoma—see *neurilemmoma*.

Schwartz test—for patency of the deep saphenous veins.

SCID (severe combined immunodeficiency disease). See *bare lymphocyte syndrome, Swiss-type SCID, x-linked SCID*.

scintigraphy, quantitative hepatobiliary (QHS).

scintillating scotoma—flashing lights and expanding circles of light, seen in migraine headache and in disorders of the occipital lobe of the brain. See *fortification spectrum*.

scintimammography (SMM)—screening technique for detection of carcinoma of the breast, using technetium ^{99m}Tc sestamibi (Cardiolite). Is said to be more sensitive than conventional mammography for detecting carcinoma and may reduce the number of mammographically indicated biopsies of the breast that yield negative results for carcinoma.

scintirenography (Urol).

scirrhous ("skir-us")—refers to a hard cancer, e.g., scirrhous carcinoma of the breast. Cf. *serous*.

scissors—face-lift, rhinoplasty, rhytidectomy, and platysma Kaye face-lift scissors. See *device*.

scissors gait (Ortho, Neuro).

SciTojet—needle-free injector for use with human growth hormone.

SCIWORA (spinal cord injury without radiographic abnormality) **syndrome** —occurs when the elastic ligaments of a child's neck stretch during trauma. As a result, the spinal cord also undergoes stretching, leading to neuronal injury or, in some cases, complete severing of the cord.

SCLC (small cell lung carcinoma, or cancer)—see *NSCLC*.

sclera (pl., sclerae)—the tough white tissue that covers the so-called white of the eye.

scleral buckling procedure—used as treatment for primary retinal detachment. Silicone sponge, solid silicone, or fascia lata are attached to the sclera or buried in it. The sclera indents (or buckles) toward the center of the eye. Subretinal fluid is drained, and the retina is reattached (after the fluid has been drained or resorbed) and is in contact with the pigment epithelium. The buckling element can be applied locally or can encircle the eye, as appropriate. Cf. *pneumatic retinopexy,* a newer procedure.

scleral expansion band (SEB)—device used to correct presbyopia. It consists of four segments that are implanted just below the surface of the sclera.

scleroderma (*n*ot scler*a*derma)—a form of progressive systemic sclerosis, a disease of no known cause, no means of treatment, and no cure. It can be manifested by a small area of dry, hard skin or it can be what is called a "diffuse systemic sclerosis," usually affecting the arms and hands. The skin becomes hard and thickened, making it difficult to use the hands. This process can also affect internal organs—lungs, GI tract, kidneys.

This disease is not what one would call an equal opportunity disease; 80% of its victims are women.

ScleroLaser—a laser system used for photothermolysis of leg telangiectasias. It avoids laser exposure to surrounding tissue.

ScleroPLUS HP—a laser system used to treat leg veins plus other vascular conditions such as facial spider veins, port wine stains, hemangiomas, rosacea, stretch marks, angiomas, scars, and warts.

sclerosing encapsulating peritonitis— occurring in a cirrhotic patient with *Listeria* peritonitis and an indwelling peritoneovenous shunt. Treated by repeated operative interventions for removal of the fibrinopurulent exudate encasing the small bowel.

Sclerosol (sterile aerosol talc)—used for treatment of malignant pleural effusion.

sclerotherapy—see *EVS*.

sclerotome—see *Lundsgaard*.

sclerouvectomy, partial lamellar (Oph) —used to remove a uveal tumor and leave intact outer sclera and sensory retina.

SCNB (stereotaxic core needle biopsy) —for breast microcalcifications.

SC-1 needle—used to reposition a subluxated lens in intraocular surgery.

SCOOP 1—a transtracheal oxygen catheter with an opening at the distal tip for oxygen flow. Also, *SCOOP 2*—a catheter with distal and side openings.

scope—see *endoscope*.

Scopette device—used to reduce genital prolapse during urodynamic evaluation.

scorbutic white line—radiologic finding in scurvy.

score—see also *classification, index, scale, test.*
Agatston
APACHE II, APACHE III
Apgar
AUA BPH
Baylor bleeding
"bother"
Braden
cardiac morbidity
Champion Trauma Score
Cockcroft-Gault equation
Cooperman event probability
Detsky modified risk index
Dripps-American Surgical
   Association
Duke treadmill exercise
Eagle equation for cardiac morbidity
Esterman visual function
Glasgow Coma
Gleason
Goldman cardiac risk index
Hughston knee
Injury Severity Score
International Prostate Symptom
   Score (IPSS)
Knee Society Score
Kurtzke disability
LAP (leukocyte alkaline
   phosphatase)
Lysholm knee
McGill pain
Mississippi 3-class scoring system
modified Rodnan total skin-thick-
   ness
Penetrating Abdominal Trauma
   Index (PATI)
PULSES profile
Sassone
Selvester QRS
SmartScore
Tegner activity
treadmill duration (TDS)
scoring incision—in surgery. "This allowed a vertical scoring incision posteriorly, as well as another scoring incision along the bone ridge, permitting swiveling of the cartilage to a more midline position."
Scorpio total knee system.
Scotchcast 2 casting tape (Ortho).
scotoma—an area of depressed vision in the visual field surrounded by an area of more normal vision. Examples: Bjerrum's, scintillating, Seidel's. Cf. *scatoma.*
scotopic sensitivity screening, whole-field (Oph)—may be of value in field-based screening for glaucoma.
Scoville retractor—double-hinged for spinal surgery retraction.
screen craze (Radiol)—a filigree pattern or cobweb appearance on the radiograph, produced by cracked old intensity screens.
"scrim"—ENT slang for speech or auditory discrimination.
Scully Hip S'port—a functional hip support that can be applied in multiple configurations to treat a wide range of hip injuries.
Sculptor annuloplasty ring—combines the features of flexible, rigid, and adjustable rings to adapt to the natural geometry of the annulus.
scurf—flaky material seen usually around the eyelashes but also other parts of the body.
scybalous ("sib-uh-lus") **stool**—hard, dry fecal matter. "He was taking laxatives and enemas, with production of scant, scybalous stools."
scyphoid ("si´foid")—cup-shaped. Cf. *xiphoid.*
SD antigens (serologically determined).
SDAP (single donor apheresis platelets).
SDAT (senile dementia of Alzheimer type).

SD Plasma—designed to eliminate the risk of viral transmission during blood plasma transfusion. While screening of donor transfusions has improved the safety of blood transfusions, SD Plasma reduces the risk of blood-borne viruses from donors who test negative but have been recently infected.

Sea-Band acupressure wristband—said to control nausea and vomiting in some pregnant women.

seabather's eruption (Derm)—itching and rashes appearing on protected and unprotected skin within hours of exposure, believed to be due to contact with larvae of the thimble jellyfish. May also be accompanied by headaches, fever, chills, nausea, and fatigue. Symptoms usually subside within 12 days.

sea-blue histiocyte syndrome—one of the reasons for liver transplant in children.

seabuckthorn seed oil—extracted from the seabuckthorn plant and used for centuries by Tibetan and Mongolian physicians to treat diseases of the GI system. This nutritional supplement is said to work by providing damaged cells in the GI tract the necessary nutrients to repair themselves, including vitamins, fatty acids, flavonoids, and carotenoids.

Sea-Clens wound cleanser.

sea fan—in patients with sickle cell retinopathy. Major nutrient arterioles and draining venules grow in neovascular patches or channels, which develop slightly dilated aneurysmal tips resembling the typical fan shape of *Gongonia flabellum* (sea fan).

sea fronds—description of neovascularization seen on eye examination.

seagull bruit.

SEA (side entry access) **port**.

Seasonale—oral contraceptive product, referred to as the "four-month pill." As opposed to women taking an oral contraceptive 21 consecutive days and having 13 menstrual periods a year, the Seasonale regimen involves taking "the pill" for 84 consecutive days and having four menstrual periods a year.

SeaSorb alginate wound dressing.

seat belt fracture—see *Chance fracture*.

seat belt sign—abrasion across the abdomen following trauma in an automobile accident in which the lumbar vertebrae are fractured from extreme forward flexion. See *Chance fracture*.

sebaceous miliaria—nonfollicular pustulosis of the newborn caused by *Malassezia furfur* yeasts. Cf. *Malassezia furfur pustulosis*.

Sebastiani syndrome—a form of hereditary thrombocytopenia associated with giant platelets.

second impact syndrome—seen in sports medicine. This syndrome affects patients with a previous head injury who are not fully recovered when they experience a second head trauma. Thought to be caused by a temporary inability of the brain to control vascular constriction following head injury, even a slight second injury can cause brain swelling and possible death.

second-look laparotomy—reoperation, for further investigation.

secretin—a human polypeptide hormone secreted by the mucosa of the duodenum and upper jejunum. Secretin has recently been approved for use in the treatment of autism, but its effectiveness is questionable.

sector scan echocardiography—see *two-dimensional echocardiography.*

Secu clip ("C-Q")—clip used in tubal ligation.

secundum atrial septal defect (ASD).

Secur-Fit HA (hydroxyapatite) hip system.

sediment—see *spun urine sediment.*

sed rate (sedimentation rate)—a good indicator of the possible presence (or absence) of generalized systemic illness. When the brief form *sed rate* is dictated in a report, it may be typed as dictated or written out. One would certainly never type *sed rate* if *sedimentation rate* were dictated.

SeedNet system—minimally invasive cryotherapy that permits controlled coverage of a target area in the prostate with IceSeeds, using ultrathin needles, effecting rapid destruction of cancerous tissue.

"see-pap"—see *CPAP.*

SeeQuence disposable contact lens.

Segard (afelimomab)—for the treatment of sepsis and septic shock.

SEG-CES (segmented cement extraction system)—removes cement in a femoral revision procedure.

segments, middle cerebral artery
  M_1 sphenoidal
  M_2 insular
  M_3 opercular
  M_4 cortical

Segond fracture—bony avulsion of the rim of the lateral tibial plateau indicating an injury to the anterior cruciate ligament.

Seguin's sign—involuntary contracture of muscles just prior to an epileptic seizure.

Segura CBD (common bile duct) basket—for use in retrieving gallstones from the common bile duct. See *Insurg laparoscopic instrumentation.*

Seidel humeral locking nail.

Seidel intramedullary fixation.

Seidel test—used with fluorescein dye to locate wound leaks.

SE (spin-echo) image—a magnetic resonance image obtained by the spin-echo technique; with this technique, T2 is determined indirectly, as a function of TE, the echo time.

Seitzinger tripolar cutting forceps—a multiple-function endoscopic instrument; it permits the surgeon to grasp, coagulate, and transect tissue with a single insertion of the instrument. These forceps can be used in a variety of laparoscopic procedures, e.g., colectomy, laparoscopically assisted vaginal hysterectomy (LAVH), oophorectomy, myomectomy, lysis of adhesions, ureterosacral nerve ablation, and Nissen fundoplication.

SELCA (smooth excimer laser coronary angioplasty).

SelCID—drug for treatment of Crohn's disease.

Selecta 7000 laser—for the performance of selective laser trabeculotherapy as a new treatment option for open-angle glaucoma in patients who have not improved with medical and argon laser therapy.

selective apoptotic antineoplastic drugs (SAANDs).

selective estrogen receptor modulator (SERM) class of drugs.

selective tubal assessment to refine reproductive therapy (STARRT) falloposcopy system.

selective tubal occlusion procedure (STOP) contraceptive device.

selegiline—used in treating a number of chronic, intractable neurologic conditions, such as Parkinson's disease.

Seldinger gastrostomy needle.

Selecor (celiprolol).

selective excitation; **irradiation**—MRI terms.

Select joint—orthosis for ambulation in children with cerebral palsy and myelomeningocele.

selenium-75 (^{75}Se)—radioisotope used in pancreatic scan.

self-aspirating cut-biopsy needle—see *PercuCut cut-biopsy needle.*

self-blood glucose monitoring (SBGM) —a more precise method than urine tests in keeping blood glucose levels under control. The blood glucose meter has a lancing device and is used together with reagent strips. One such meter is the Accu-Chek III. It uses a Chemstrip bG reagent, so the color reading can be checked against the digital reading. It also has a memory that holds the last 20 test values with the date and time of each test so they can be compared. Other such meters are *Medisense Pen 2* and *Companion 2.*

self-limiting (or **self-limited**)—said of a disease such as the common cold that typically runs its course and resolves spontaneously without complications or sequelae, even when left untreated.

Self-Regard Questionnaire—a quantitative rating scale to measure stress-personality interactions, expected to be used by clinicians.

Sellick maneuver—pressure on the cricoid during anesthesia induction/intubation. Used to prevent aspiration of stomach contents. Pressure is maintained until the anesthesiologist inflates the cuff on the endotracheal or nasoendotracheal tube.

Selverstone clamp (*not* Silverstone).

Selvester QRS scoring system—a method of measuring the ischemic risk region and infarct size as calculated from the standard 12-lead EKG.

SEM (scanning electron microscope).

sEMG (surface electromyography)— measures the electrical activity of muscles and uses computerized biofeedback therapy to treat patients with chronic pain or injuries. A computer translates information from surface electrodes placed on the muscles into a display on a computer screen. Through the display people learn to identify tensed muscles and learn to relax them.

seminal vesiculography (SVG)—evaluation of the distal male reproductive tract.

Semmes-Weinstein nylon monofilaments—used in determining cutaneous pressure thresholds. Color-coded filaments of different weights are placed, with enough pressure to just bend the fibers, on each phalanx of the fingers, radial and ulnar side, and along the nerve distributions. The patient is not allowed to watch the application of the fibers. A delayed response of more than three seconds is abnormal. The report is coded with colored pencils corresponding to the color-coded, weighted fibers.

Semm hysterectomy—see *CASH.*

Semont maneuver—used in the treatment of benign paroxysmal positional vertigo. This is a procedure whereby the patient is rapidly moved from lying on one side to the other. Also called the *liberatory maneuver.*

Semprex-D (acrivastine)—a combination antihistamine and decongestant used to treat seasonal allergy symptoms.

Senning intra-atrial baffle—for repair of transposition of the great vessels.

Senographe 2000D—digital mammography imaging system.

Sensability—lubricated plastic sheet that a woman holds over her breast to more easily feel for lumps during self-examination.

Sensamide (metoclopramide)—an antiemetic and a radiation sensitizer for patients with inoperable non-small cell lung carcinoma (or cancer).

Sens-A-Ray—digital dental imaging system that utilizes existing x-ray source and replaces traditional x-ray film with a sensor unit that digitizes and transfers images to a computer, providing instant images on a monitor.

Sense-of-Feel prosthesis—an artificial foot which uses a pager-sized pressure transducer to send signals to the residual leg, enhancing balance and a more natural gait and possibly helping to reduce "phantom" pain.

SensiCath optical sensor—used with the OnLineABG blood gas monitoring system.

sensitize—to introduce radioactive material into a fluid, tissue, or space for purposes of performing a radioactive scan; essentially the same as *label*. Cf. *label*.

Sensi-Touch anesthesia delivery system. Also called *Sensi-Touch anesthesia needle*.

sensorimotor skills—alertness, responsiveness, interest in surroundings. *Not* sensory-motor.

sensorineural (*not* sensory neural).

sensory branch of the radial nerve (SBRN).

sensory integration (SI)—a method of treatment in physical and occupational therapy, often in conjunction with NDT (neuro-developmental techniques) and myofascial release.

sensory nerve action potential (SNAP).

Sensory Organization Test (SOT)—used in conjunction with computerized dynamic posturography.

Sentinel implantable cardioverter-defibrillator—used for treatment of cardiac arrhythmia.

sentinel loop—an isolated, gas-filled, distended loop of small bowel that represents paralytic ileus.

sentinel lymph node (SLN)—the node identified as most likely among the 25 or 30 nodes in the axillary basin to contain metastatic disease. Also defined as an enlarged lymph node in the left supraclavicular fossa containing cancer metastatic from the stomach; called *Virchow's* or *Troisier's node*.

sentinel pile—a hemorrhoid or hemorrhoid-like nodule of tissue that forms below an anal fissure.

sentinel skin paddle—a small portion of skin placed over a muscle pedicle graft to facilitate postoperative monitoring by capillary refill.

SEP (somatosensory evoked potential)—used to monitor spinal cord function in spinal injury, and in spinal cord monitoring in surgery. See also *SSEP*, which is synonymous.

SEPA—a dermal absorption enhancer that can accelerate the passage of pharmaceutical agents through the skin.

SEPA/ibuprofen—an ibuprofen gel formulation that delivers ibuprofen directly through the skin into sore muscles.

SEPA/minoxidil—a once-a-day application for hair growth.

Sepracoat coating solution—liquid hyaluronic acid used as prophylaxis against the future development of

Sepracoat *(cont.)*
adhesions by keeping exposed tissues moist before and during surgical procedures.

Seprafilm (sodium hyaluronate and carboxymethylcellulose)—a bioresorbable membrane developed as a temporary physical barrier between tissue surfaces and the site of direct surgical trauma in abdominal and pelvic surgeries. It prevents adhesions from forming after surgery.

Sepramesh—a prosthetic surgical mesh designed to be sutured in place along the abdominal wall to support and strengthen hernia repairs, especially incisional hernias. It contains a bioresorbable barrier that separates the mesh from underlying tissue and organ surfaces to minimize tissue attachment to the mesh.

SEPS (subfascial endoscopic perforator surgery).

sepsis syndrome—an acute systemic illness characterized by hypotension, coagulopathies, and multiorgan failure. The term includes a broad group of patients with systemic inflammatory response syndrome (SIRS), sepsis, septic shock, and/or multiorgan dysfunction syndrome (MODS).

Septopal implant—gentamicin-impregnated PMMA beads on surgical wire, similar to *Septacin implant.*

Septra—see *TMP-SMZ, Bactrim.*

sequela (pl., *sequelae; usually* used in the plural)—a persistent effect of an illness or injury, such as paralysis after a stroke.

sequence—a technique for noninvasive exploration of the biliary tract.

Sequential Multiple Analyzer (SMA).

Sequestra 1000—a blood processing system used to conserve blood during major surgery and perform autotransfusion. It separates blood components such as platelets and plasma prior to surgery for use during the operation. Separated platelets may be used to make "platelet gel," which reduces bleeding and facilitates healing when applied to surgical wounds.

SER (somatosensory evoked response).

Serenoa repens extract (Permixon)—phytotherapeutic agent for benign prostatic hypertrophy. It is an extract of the saw palmetto (*Serenoa repens*).

Serevent (salmeterol)—inhalation aerosol to treat asthma symptoms.

SER-IV (supination, external rotation-type IV fracture).

serial scans—a series of scans made at regular intervals along one dimension of a body region.

SERM (selective estrogen receptor modulator)—a class of drugs including tamoxifen and raloxifene and used in the treatment of cancer and osteoporosis, respectively.

sermorelin acetate (Geref)—given intravenously to assess the ability of the pituitary gland to secrete growth hormone.

seroconversion symptoms—response to a viral illness, including HIV. The symptoms feel like a case of the flu and occur approximately three weeks after exposure.

Seroma-Cath—wound drainage system used to treat postoperative seromas which can be a complication of mastectomy, axillary dissection, abdominoplasty, and some other procedures.

seromuscular intestinal patch graft—used in repair of radiation-induced vesicovaginal and rectovaginal fistulas.

seromuscular *(cont.)*

A segment of intestine is removed and repaired by end-to-end anastomosis. The removed segment is opened, the muscular surface denuded, and the patch applied over the debrided fistulous tract of bladder or rectum.

Seroquel (quetiapine fumarate)—antipsychotic medication.

Serostim (somatoprin of rDNA origin)—an injectable drug used for the treatment of cachexia and body wasting in AIDS patients. It is a mammalian cell-derived recombinant human growth hormone.

serotonin type-3 receptor antagonists—a class of drugs used to treat chemotherapy-induced nausea and vomiting. See *ondansetron*.

serous ("se´rus")—pertaining to serum, resembling serum, or containing serum (as in serous cystadenoma). Cf. *scirrhous*.

SERPACWA (Skin Exposure Reduction Paste Against Chemical Warfare Agents)—developed by the U.S. military to reduce absorption of chemical warfare agents through the skin.

serpiginous—snake-like.

Serratia liquefaciens—formerly classified as *Enterobacter liquefaciens*. It has been isolated from the intestinal tract, respiratory tract, blood, and urine.

Serratia marcescens—an organism that frequently figures in nosocomial infections, mainly in immunocompromised individuals. It causes infections in much the same areas as *E. coli* and is the cause of gram-negative ulcers in infectious keratitis.

sertindole—used to treat psychotic disorders.

Sertoli-cell-only syndrome—characterized clinically by aspermia and histologically by complete loss of the epithelium in the testicular tubules.

sertraline (Zoloft)—an antidepressant (a 5HT blocker) which inhibits the uptake of serotonin in the brain.

serumcidal—see *cidal*.

serum p24 antigen concentration—a marker used to monitor HIV serum levels.

Servo pump—used in cases of hydrocephalus to control intracranial pressure at desired levels.

Serzone (nefazodone)—an antidepressant.

sestamibi stress test—using radioactive imaging agent ^{99m}Tc sestamibi (Cardiolite) to show areas of myocardial infarction in a stress test.

sestamibi Tc-99m SPECT with dipyridamole stress test—used to predict the extent of perfusion abnormalities that occur during coronary occlusion and may facilitate estimation of the total myocardium in jeopardy from a stenotic lesion.

SET three-lumen thrombectomy catheter—Its tip delivers a high-pressure saline stream that microfragments clots. The clot fragments then move through the outflow lumen into a collection bag.

setting sun sign—with increased intracranial pressure or irritation of the brain stem, deviation of the eyes downward so that white sclera is seen above the iris.

sevelamer HCl (Renagel).

7C Gold test—proprietary urine test that measures neuronal thread protein, which is selectively increased in the brain and spinal fluid of an individual with Alzheimer's disease. The test provides rapid results and is easy to read.

17B-Estradiol—seven-day transdermal hormone replacement therapy patch.

severe childhood autosomal recessive muscular dystrophy (SCARMD)—may be caused by a deficiency of the adhalin gene, which has been isolated and found on chromosome 17. When adhalin is absent, muscle cells are more prone to damage, and as the cells break down, the muscles begin to waste away. SCARMD is rare in the U.S. but more common in some Middle Eastern countries.

Sewell retractor (ENT).

sexually transmitted disease (STD).

Sézary syndrome—exfoliative erythroderma, manifested by hyperkeratosis, edema, alopecia, and pigment and nail changes.

SF₆ (sulfur hexafluoride)—a gas used in pneumatic retinopexy.

SFA (subclavian flap aortoplasty).

S-fluoxetine (racemic fluoxetine)—used in an attempt to prevent migraine headache attacks.

SFS (small fragment system)—see *Alphatec.*

SGA (small for gestational age).

Sgambati's reaction or **test** ("zgahm-bah-tee")—a lab test for peritonitis. When the patient's urine is combined with nitric acid and chloroform, a resulting red tint is a positive sign of peritonitis.

SGOT—see *AST.*

SGPT—see *ALT.*

Shade UVAGuard—broad-spectrum sunscreen lotion containing Parsol 1789. See *Parsol 1789.*

SHAFT syndrome—factitious disorder in which a patient manipulates the surgeon to perform operations to fulfill his or her psychological needs. The acronym describes patients who are **s**ad, **h**ostile, **a**nxious, **f**rustrating, and **t**enacious.

shagreen lesions of the optic lens.

Shah permanent tube—a middle ear ventilating tube used in patients with otitis media.

shaken baby syndrome—see *shaken impact syndrome.*

shaken impact syndrome—the newer name for *shaken baby syndrome.* Caregivers, by violently shaking an infant, cause permanent neurological damage by the abrupt acceleration and deceleration of the brain against the cranium, resulting in intracranial hemorrhage.

shake test—tests the maturity of fetal lungs. See *foam stability test.*

Shaldon catheter.

Shapshay/Healy—20 cm phonatory and operating laryngoscope.

sharp and blunt dissection—a surgical term referring to separating or cutting apart tissues with sharp instruments (scalpel, scissors) where necessary and with blunt instruments or fingers where possible. Separation of structures and development of tissue planes by blunt dissection is less traumatic and causes less bleeding.

Sharpey's fibers—collagenous fibers of a tendon, ligament, or periosteum buried in the subperiosteal bone.

Sharplan SilkTouch flashscan surgical laser—now approved for use in hair transplantation.

"sharps"—operating room slang for suture needles, scalpel blades, hypodermic needles, cautery blades, and safety pins, all of which require special handling to avoid injury to healthcare personnel and to reduce their risk of acquiring bloodborne infections. Sometimes a "sharps count" is dictated at the end of an operative report.

SharpShooter—used for "inside-out" tissue repair technique of meniscus suturing.

Sharrard-type kyphectomy (Ortho).

Shaw I and **Shaw II scalpel**—a Teflon-coated hemostatic scalpel used in hot conization of the cervix.

Shaw scalpel—an electrical scalpel. A dictator mentioning this instrument will usually give settings in degrees of temperature.

Sheehy syndrome—rapidly advancing sensorineural hearing loss in younger age groups.

sheet sign—psychological despair in AIDS patients shown by their hiding under bedcovers and refusing human contact.

Shepherd internal screw fixation—for sagittal split ramus osteotomy.

Shepherd technique—for intraocular lens insertion using a 3-4 mm incision and closure with suture knots covered with conjunctiva.

Sherpa guiding catheter—directs balloon catheters rapidly into coronary arteries or other sites where obstructions are treated.

Sherwood intrascopic suction/irrigation system for laparoscopic procedures—allows surgeon to use suction/irrigation and electrocautery without removing the irrigator from the cannula during the cauterization.

Shiatsu therapeutic massage—see also *Ohashiatsu massage.*

shifting dullness on percussion—indicates the presence of ascites. The abdomen is percussed with the patient lying in the supine position, then with the patient lying on each side. If the area of dullness shifts, this indicates the presence of ascitic fluid, rather than edema or cyst.

shift to the left (white blood cells)—means there are increased numbers of immature neutrophils which may indicate presence of infection. The term refers to a white blood cell differential counted manually; the technician uses a diagram which places the younger, developing cells on the left side of the page. A rise in the number of these cells, a shift to the left, is a sign of the body's reaction to an infection, or of leukemia. See *shift to the right.*

shift to the right—means that there are increased numbers of older neutrophils present in the blood. Cf. *shift to the left.*

Shikani middle meatal antrostomy stent—a temporary stent to be placed following endoscopic sinus surgery. May be removed after mucosal layer heals in 10 to 14 days.

shim coil; shimming—MRI terms.

shin splints—painful spasm of shin muscles due to strain, usually as a result of running.

Shirley wound drain.

Shirodkar cervical cerclage procedure.

shock blocks—blocks placed under the foot of a bed to elevate it manually for a patient in shock.

shocky—in shock, or showing signs (tachycardia, pallor, diaphoresis, restlessness) suggestive of shock.

shoelace technique—a surgical technique for delayed primary closure of fasciotomy. Skin staples spaced approximately 2 cm apart function as eyelets for a Silastic vessel loop that serves as the lace. The shoelace technique involves running a Silastic vessel loop through skin staples placed at the skin edge along the initial fasciotomy incision. Daily tightening

shoelace *(cont.)*
of the shoelace permits gradual reapproximation of the skin edges while compartment edema resolves. Closure using a simple suture or Steristrip is then possible after 5-10 days. This allows for gradual closure of open fasciotomy wounds, avoiding the morbidity and cost associated with skin graft or secondary closure.

shoe, WACH (wedge adjustable cushioned heel)—a cast shoe used in orthopedics.

Shohl's solution—used in treatment of renal tubular acidosis.

short arc progressive resistive exercises.

short-bore magnet—MRI term.

ShortCut knife—an ophthalmic knife with a unique rounded tip and short length for intraocular incisions. Also, *A-OK ShortCut knife.*

shorthand vertical mattress stitch—rapid skin everting suture technique.

short inversion time inversion recovery (STIR) (MRI term)—a pulse sequence sensitive enough to detect a broad range of pathologic conditions.

short-limb dwarfism—form of dwarfism in which the extremities are abnormally short, as differentiated from the true, or normal, dwarf, in which the only abnormality is the small size.

short-rod/two-claw technique—spinal instrumentation used to treat thoracic or lumbar spine wedge compression or burst fractures. Although not indicated in every situation, advantages include decreased pain and stiffness and elimination of the need for instrumentation removal.

short TR/TE (or T1-weighted)—MRI terms. TR (repetition time); TE (echo time).

short wavelength autoperimetry (SWAP)—a test for glaucoma. Different intensities of blue light are flashed across a screen, and the patient presses a button every time a blue light is seen. It is hard for a patient with glaucoma to see the blue light since nerve fibers most sensitive to the color blue are the first to be affected by glaucoma. SWAP test is able to spot glaucoma three to four years before white-light testing, allowing stabilization with eye drops or surgery. This test is usually advised for anyone in a high-risk category: over 40; African-American; family history of glaucoma. It is typically given in conjunction with white-on-white testing.

shotty nodes—as in B-B shot. Not to be confused with "shoddy," as in "shoddy merchandise."

Shouldice hernia repair—used for either direct or indirect hernias; a variation of the Halsted-Bassini repair.

SHRS (St. Hans Rating Scale for extrapyramidal syndromes)—a scale for rating tardive dyskinesia.

Shuffors internal screw fixation—used in sagittal split ramus osteotomy.

shunt
Allen-Brown vascular access
Anastaflo intervascular
Buselmeier
Cordis-Hakim
coronary anastomotic
Denver pleuroperitoneal
Gibson inner ear
Gott
Holter
House and Pulec otic-periotic
Kasai peritoneal venous
LeVeen peritoneal
MBTS (modified Blalock-Taussig)

shunt *(cont.)*
mesocaval (MCS)
Orbis-Sigma cerebrospinal fluid
PFTE (polyfluorotetraethylene)
Pruitt-Inahara carotid
Quinton-Scribner
Ramirez
T-AnastoFlo
Thomas vascular access
TIPSS (transjugular intrahepatic
portosystemic)
Torkildsen
transjugular intrahepatic
portosystemic
ventriculoperitoneal (VP)
ventriculosubarachnoid (VS)
Vitagraft arteriovenous
Warren splenorenal
Winters
Shur-Clens wound cleanser.
Shur-Strip (Deknatel)—a sterile wound
closure tape.
Shutt Mantis retrograde forceps—
used in ipsilateral approach to anterior horn of meniscus in arthroscopic
knee surgery.
Shwachman syndrome—pancreatic
exocrine insufficiency and cyclical
neutropenia with growth retardation,
steatorrhea, and abnormalities in
bones and joints, often giving rise to
profound short-stature deformities
and sometimes fatal infections and
visceral hemorrhages.
SI—see *International System.*
SI (sensory integration).
SIADH (syndrome of inappropriate antidiuretic hormone secretion).
SI (sacroiliac) **belt**—see *SI-LOC.*
Sibley-Lehninger—test for serum aldolase.
sibrafiban—oral glycoprotein IIb/IIIa
receptor antagonist said to be the
first oral treatment for recurrent
heart disease.

SIBS (social interaction between siblings) **interview**—a new instrument
to assess sibling relationships in antisocial youth.
SIBS (surgical isolation bubble system).
sick building syndrome—nausea, headache, and some other symptoms experienced by people who work in
some new buildings in which windows cannot be opened. Apparently
caused by many of the chemicals
found in carpeting and furniture.
Sickledex—a screening test for sickle
cell disease.
sickle knife (ENT)—"The periorbita
was opened with a sickle knife in a
posterior-to-anterior direction" (in
an endoscopic orbital decompression
for Graves' disease).
sick sinus syndrome—referring to the
sinoatrial node.
SICOR—a computer-assisted cardiac
catheterization recording system that
automatically calculates, displays,
and reports all hemodynamic parameters, valve areas and shunts, and
then prints a report immediately after
catheterization.
side-biting clamp.
Side Branch Occlusion system—minimally invasive procedure used in
treatment of peripheral vascular disease. Fiberoptic visualization allows
the vascular surgeon to work inside
of saphenous vein, removing vein
valves and sealing off the side
branches.
side-cutting spatulated needle—comes
in one-fifth circle and one-third circle
and is threaded with 4-0 cable-type
Supramid Extra suture material.
side-cutting Swanson bur—used in
revision of total wrist arthroplasty
and other procedures.
side entry access (SEA) **port.**

Side-Fire reflecting dish—used with Surgilase Nd:YAG laser to perform prostate resection in benign prostatic hypertrophy. It consists of a Teflon-coated light guide with a solid gold reflecting dish crimped to the end of a light guide. The gold reflecting dish enables a more precise energy delivery system to the prostatic tissue by deflecting energy at right angles. Solid gold is used because of its high reflectivity and low absorption of laser energy. The device has a venturi aperture that helps to prevent debris adherence on the dish with resultant distortion of the reflecting surface during lasing. Continuous irrigant keeps the reflecting gold dish cool during lasing and prevents distortion and melting of the delivery system.

siderotic nodules in the spleen (Radiol)—seen on x-rays; also called *Gamna-Gandy nodules* or *bodies*. See *Gamna-Gandy bodies*.

SieScape imaging—ultrasound imaging technology that provides panoramic views of ultrasound images in real time. Radiologists are able to view one image rather than having to piece together a series of separate smaller pictures.

sievert (Sv) ("see´vert")—the SI unit of radiation absorbed dose equal to 1 gray (Gy) or 1 joule (J) per kilogram, or 100 rem.

SIF10 Olympus enteroscope.

"sigh"—see *p.s.i.*

Sigma—method used in testing serum CPK. See also *Oliver-Rosalki*.

sigmaS—a serum tumor marker used to distinguish between early and advanced stages of breast cancer. (No space in sigmaS.)

Sigmodontine rodents—vectors of hantaviruses associated with hantavirus pulmonary syndrome.

sign
absent bow-tie
Aaron's
accordion
alien hand
Allis's
Apley
Aufrecht's
Babinski
banana
Bard's
Battle's
blue dot
Blumberg's
Boas
bow-tie
Branham's
brim
Brockenbrough-Braunwald
Brudzinski's
Carabello
Chadwick's
chandelier
Collier's
Courvoisier's
Cullen's
Dalrymple's
Dance's
David Letterman
de Musset's
doll's eye
Dorendorf's
double anterior horn
double-bubble
double PCL (posterior cruciate ligament)
drawer
echo
Ewart's
extrapyramidal
fabere

sign *(cont.)*
  fadir
  Fajersztajn's crossed sciatic
  fat pad
  Federici's
  Finkelstein's
  flipped meniscus sign
  fragment-in-notch
  Froment's
  frontal release
  Galeazzi
  Gauss'
  Goodell's
  Gowers
  Griesinger's
  Hamman's
  Hitzelberger's
  Hoehne's
  Homans'
  Hoover
  impingement
  Jackson's
  Jacquemier's
  Joffroy's
  Lasègue's
  lemon
  linguine
  long tract
  Macewen's
  main d'accoucher
  McCort's
  McMurray
  Moebius'
  Mulder
  mute toe
  Nicoladoni-Branham
  obturator
  oil drop change
  Ortolani's
  parrot's
  Phalen's
  Pinard's
  Pins'
  pivot-shift
  puddle

sign *(cont.)*
  pyloric string
  pyramidal
  Queckenstedt's
  Rigler's
  root
  Rovsing's
  sail
  seat belt
  Seguin's
  setting sun
  sheet
  soft neurologic
  Spurling's
  steeple
  Stellwag's
  string
  target
  tenting
  Terry fingernail
  Terry-Thomas
  Tinel's
  Trousseau's
  Unschuld's
  Valleix
  vital
  von Graefe's
  Weill's

SignaDress—hydrocolloid dressing material.

Signa I.S.T. MRI **scanner.**

signal amplification technique—amplifies a secondary probe attached to the sample via a synthetic DNA probe to isolate a particular DNA or RNA sequence in a specimen. See *polymerase chain reaction.*

signaling, myocardial adrenergic.

signal intensity—in magnetic resonance imaging, the strength of the signal or stream of radiofrequency energy emitted by tissue after an excitation pulse.

signal-to-noise ratio (S/N)—MRI term.

signet-ring pattern—a cellular change wherein the cell has a ring-like configuration, as seen in gastric carcinoma.

Sigvaris compression stockings—for treatment of venous disease in ambulatory patients.

SIHC (surgically implanted hemodialysis catheter).

SIL (squamous intraepithelial lesions).

Silastic bead embolization—used as therapy for some types of arteriovenous fistulae fed by several small arteries in areas not amenable to surgical repair, or if the vessel is not a critical artery which may be obliterated without fear of causing distal ischemia. See *Gianturco coil,* used for the same purpose.

Silastic silo reduction of gastroschisis —see *Silon tent.*

silent—without symptoms or signs, as in silent gallstones, silent myocardial infarction.

"silent" areas of the brain—seizures starting from a focus in these areas produce no aura. See *"eloquent" areas.*

"silent epidemic"—predicted by epidemiologists when, around the year 2030, 20 percent of the population will be over 65. The epidemic referred to is Alzheimer's and other dementing diseases.

silent prostatism—a condition in which progressive obstruction occurs slowly, without symptoms, and the patient presents without urinary complaints. The presence of benign prostatic hypertrophy may be suspected if there is azotemia and if ultrasound shows bilateral hydronephrosis.

Silhouette—therapeutic massage system.

silicon—a chemical element present in sand and various types of rock. Cf. *silicone.*

silicone—an organic compound used in the manufacture of various medical devices such as breast implants, catheters, drains. Cf. *silicon.*

silicone flexor rod—placed in the sheath of the flexor tendon for reconstruction of a finger.

silicone ring.

Silipos Distal Dip—prosthetic sheath/liner which reduces friction and pistoning of an extremity prosthesis.

Silk guide wire (Cardio).

Silk Laser aesthetic carbon dioxide laser system for laser skin resurfacing. See *2040 erbium laser.*

SilkTouch laser—used for hair transplantation. It creates holes in the skin that are small enough to transplant a single hair.

SI-LOC—a type of sacroiliac belt designed to stabilize the SI joint and pubic symphysis after fractures of the pelvic ring. The belt prevents the innominates from being pushed away from each other, pressing the joint surfaces firmly together.

Silon tent—used in an operative procedure for gastroschisis. The tent is placed over the abdominal opening and the intestines are gradually reduced back into the abdomen by ligating the top of the tent progressively. See also *Silastic silo.*

Silon wound dressing—transparent, nonadherent dressing used for partial-thickness wounds such as donor sites and second-degree burns.

Silsoft extended wear contact lenses— used in treating pediatric aphakia.

Silverlon wound packing strips—sterile, nonadherent wound dressing

Silverlon *(cont.)*
with silver for protection against microbial contamination. It is used to control local wound bleeding and nasal hemorrhage; to encourage draining and wicking of fluids from a body cavity, infected area, or abscess; and to remove necrotic tissue from ulcers or other infected wounds when used as a wet-to-dry packing.

Silverstein facial nerve monitor.

Silverstein stimulator probe—used to determine nerve stimulation.

Silverstone—see *Selverston clamp.*

silver wire effect—effect created by narrowing of arterioles in the retina.

Simal cervical stabilization system.

Simdax (levosimendan)—injectable for treatment of congestive heart failure.

simkin analysis (not named for a person). It is **sim**ulation **kin**etics analysis to determine serum acetamino- phen levels.

Simplex-P bone cement.

Simplicity spirometer—for measuring lung capacity and performance.

Simpson atherectomy catheter—used for atherectomy in atherosclerotic peripheral vascular disease (removal and retrieval of atheroma).

Simpson Coronary AtheroCath (SCA) system—a catheter system with a small rotating blade inside used for directional coronary atherectomy.

Simpson peripheral AtheroCath—see *Simpson atherectomy catheter.*

Simpulse system—high-pressure, high-volume pulsed lavage used in joint replacement procedures.

Simulect (basiliximab)—two-dose, high-affinity monoclonal antibody used for prevention of acute rejection episodes in renal transplant recipients.

simultaneous volume imaging—MRI term.

simvastatin (Zocor)—used to lower levels of LDL in patients with hypercholesterolemia which has not responded to dietary measures. Other therapeutic actions include raising levels of HDL and lowering triglyceride levels. This drug belongs to the class known as HMG-CoA reductase inhibitors.

Sinding Larsen–Johannson disease—of the patella. (Sinding Larsen *and* Johannson.)

Sine-U-View nasal endoscope—provides optically precise images when doing sinus surgery.

sine-wave pattern—indicative of hyperkalemia, seen on electrocardiogram. (Pronounced like *sign-wave.*)

Singer-Blom valve—used for esophageal speech in patients who have had laryngectomies.

singer's node—not an eponym, but a small white nodule which is often seen on the vocal cords of singers, or others who use their voices excessively.

Singh–Vaughn–Williams classification of arrhythmias.

single breath-hold sequence—on CT scan.

single-chain antigen-binding (SCA) **proteins.**

single-contrast arthrography—for evaluation of ligamentous injuries of the knee.

Single-Day Baxter infuser—used for postoperative pain control in forefoot operations. It functions by continuous infusion of anesthetic into the malleolar internal space.

single donor apheresis platelets (SDAP).

single-field hyperthermia combined with radiation therapy (radiation oncology)—a technique used for recurrent or advanced carcinoma of

single-field *(cont.)*
the breast. Using ultrasound technology, the tumor is superheated to the point of cell destruction. It can be used for local or regional control of recurrent, previously treated breast cancers.

single-lung transplant (SLT) recipient.

single photon emission computed tomography (SPECT).

single shot fast spin echo (SSFSE)—magnetic resonance imaging of fetal anatomy.

single slice fast dynamic in vivo sequence—MRI term.

SingleStitch PhacoFlex lens—a silicone intraocular lens which folds for easy insertion through the small incision used for cataract surgery. The tiny opening can then be closed with one stitch (hence, SingleStitch).

single-stripe colitis (SSC)—a single stripe of ulcerated mucosa seen on colonoscopy is diagnostic of colitis.

Singulair (montelukast)—a nonsteroidal that blocks leukotrienes to prevent asthma attacks. A once-a-day pill indicated for adults and for children over the age of two.

singultus—hiccups. "The patient was observed to have multiple episodes of singultus during his emergency room stay."

sink-trap malformation—a condition resulting in redundancy and obstruction of an interposed colon segment used to replace an esophagus that has been rendered unusable by the ingestion of a caustic substance.

Sin Nombre virus (SNV)—the cause of Hantavirus pulmonary syndrome.

sinoatrial node (SA or S-A node)—the pacemaker of the heart and what is referred to in "sinus rhythm." See

Flack's node and *Koch's node* (which are synonymous).

Sinskey hook (Oph).

Sinu-Clear procedure—an outpatient procedure using a patented laser delivery system in combination with warmed irrigating fluid to safely remove nasal polyps and diseased sinus tissue.

Sinuscope or SinuScope—a rigid-rod lens optics system for ENT diagnosis and procedures.

SinuScope rigid rod lens optics—used in otolaryngology endoscopic procedures.

Sippy diet—named for Dr. Bertram Welton Sippy, who wrote on gastric and duodenal ulcers.

sirolimus (Rapamune).

SIRS (systemic inflammatory response syndrome).

SIRS/sepsis (systemic inflammatory response syndrome)—sepsis as a result of confirmed infectious process.

SISCOM (Subtraction Ictal SPECT coregistered to MRI)—imaging approach used to pinpoint location of seizure onset by electronically superimposing SPECT images over an MRI of the patient's brain. Surgeons can utilize the new approach in the operating room, in conjunction with other tools, to further confirm location of a seizure prior to removal.

SISI (short increment sensitivity index)—used in hearing test.

Sister Mary Joseph node—lymph node near the umbilicus. Named for the nurse who first observed that when she found such a node, the patient always had pancreatic carcinoma.

site—place or position, as "The site of the abscess was located quickly." Cf. *cite*.

SiteGuard MVP—transparent adhesive film dressing.

SiteSelect—percutaneous breast biopsy system from Imagyn Medical Technologies.

sitostanol ester margarine—a margarine that contains sitostanol ester, a cholesterol blocker.

situ—see *in situ*.

SI (syncytium-inducing) **variant of HIV** —see *nonsyncytium-inducing*.

Sivash prosthesis—total hip prosthesis that does not require use of cement.

sivelestat—neutrophil elastase inhibitor for treatment of acute lung injury and respiratory distress syndrome.

6-AN protocol—topical cream (Derm).

SJM-Seguin annuloplasty ring—a ring with variable flexibility. It is sufficiently rigid in its anterior region to maintain intercommissural distance, yet sufficiently flexible in its posterior region so as not to interfere with left ventricular function and to permit the natural three-dimensional annular mobility, thereby remodeling the mitral valve, correcting dilatation, and preserving physiologic annular function.

Sjögren's syndrome ("sho-grenz")— symptom complex marked by keratoconjunctivitis sicca.

SjO2 (oxygen saturation in the internal jugular vein)—measured by an intravenous catheter in the internal jugular vein. Used to assess cerebral perfusion in head-injury patients.

skeletal targeted radiotherapy (STR) —a radionuclide, holmium-166, linked to a drug that targets the bone in patients with Ewing's sarcoma. By injecting STR into the blood, the radiation can localize in tumors in the bone, thus delivering more radiation to the areas of bone that are directly affected by tumor than the rest of the skeleton.

skeletonize—in Webster's, meaning "to produce in or reduce to skeleton form." Rarely found in medical dictionaries, although doctors use the word in dictation.

Skelid (tiludronate disodium)—a bisphosphonate that controls abnormal bone growth in patients with Paget's disease without interfering with the normal process of bone formation.

SKF (skilled nursing facility).

skier's tear—a rupture of the ulnar collateral ligament of the thumb.

skier's thumb—rupture of the adductor pollicis tendon after forced abduction, an injury from ski poles during falls.

Skil saw—an electric saw you will run into (figuratively speaking) in orthopedic surgery transcription in reference to the etiology of an injury.

Skimmer RRP laryngeal shaver—used to reduce an exophytic mass in the larynx.

skin depth—MRI term.

Skindex, revised—a 29-item quality-of-life questionnaire administered to dermatology patients.

Skin Exposure Reduction Paste Against Chemical Warfare Agents (SERPACWA).

skin fold (skin crease) artifact (Radiol)—a common finding on x-rays of patients with a large body habitus. Skin folds can mimic the streaks of atelectasis on a chest film. Prior studies, follow-up examination with repositioning, and/or clinical correlation may be required to make the differentiation.

skin graft—see *graft, skin.*

skin lesion artifact (Radiol)—Occasionally an astute radiologist will recognize that the pattern of an artifact could be caused by a skin lesion such as a melanoma in the worst possible case. Radiologists usually rule out artifacts with other views, but if they remain, in a case like this they would say "clinical correlation recommended."

Skinlight erbium:YAG laser—used for skin resurfacing, reportedly more gentle than the CO_2 laser, causing less thermal damage and a shorter recovery time.

Skinny dilatation catheter—used in cardiac catheterization. *Skinny* is a trade name.

Skinny needle—see *Chiba needle.*

Skinscan—microprocessor-driven device used for aesthetic laser surgery. It ensures consistent, precise treatment for soft tissue applications, particularly on face.

Skin Skribe—a skin marker used in surgery.

SkinTegrity hydrogel dressing.

Skinvisible—hypoallergenic hand lotion provides a skin barrier that protects against the transmission of nosocomial infections and absorption of noxious chemicals.

skip metastasis—development of recurrent nodal disease in the regional axillary basin when no sentinel nodes have been previously identified.

"skir-us"—phonetic rendering of scirrhous.

Skoog release—of Dupuytren's contracture.

SK-SD, SKSD (streptokinase-streptodornase)—skin test for immune function.

SKY—epidural pain control system.

Skylight—gantry-free nuclear medicine gamma camera.

skyline view of patella (Radiol)—study of the knee region in which the patella is visualized above the distal femur and appears like a rising (or setting) sun.

SLAC (scapholunate arthritic collapse) **wrist**—in which a fracture/deformity has healed in a rotated position and eroded the radioscaphoid joint.

Slant lens—a single-piece intraocular lens with a design which incorporates slanted haptics and a low profile for easy insertion through the longer scleral tunnel and more acute angle of entry now used in intraocular lens surgery. *Slant* is a trademark. Also, *Cilco Slant haptics lens.*

SLAP (superior labrum [or labral] anterior posterior) **lesion**—"He has a SLAP lesion where the labrum is detached superiorly. We used a bur in order to get down to good bloody bone in that area, in an attempt to get the SLAP lesion to heal down to bloody bone."

Slattery-McGrouther dynamic flexion splint.

sleep apnea—disorder associated with snoring, irregular heartbeat, and wakefulness in which soft tissues in the throat can obstruct breathing. In severe cases, this can cause death.

sleep deprivation—lack of total sleep, rapid eye movement (REM) sleep, or nonrapid eye movement (NREM) sleep. Fatigue, irritability, difficulty remembering, difficulty in concentrating, and problems with muscle coordination may be manifestations of sleep deprivation. On the average, adults require from 6 to 9 hours of sleep per night, with older people

sleep deprivation *(cont.)*
thought to require less than younger ones.

Sleeping Buddha—marketed as an herbal alternative to prescription sedatives but found by the FDA to contain an unlabeled prescription drug ingredient, estazolam, which is a sedative of the benzodiazepine family known to have serious side effects, including potential for fetal damage if consumed by pregnant women.

sleeve pneumonectomy—an operative procedure to treat proximal tumors of the lung.

slice fracture—a spinal fracture that goes through the disk or through the vertebral body.

slice profile—MRI term.

slim disease—the term used for AIDS in some countries in Africa because of the great loss of weight seen in this disease. Cf. *wasting syndrome.*

sling
Straight-In male
Stratasis urethral
SurgiSis sling/mesh
Suspend
triangular vaginal patch
UltraSling

sling and swathe—used for immobilization of fractured humerus if comminution is not extensive.

sling ring complex—used to describe tracheal stenosis caused by a combination of a fixed, complete cartilaginous ring and pulmonary sling syndrome. See *pulmonary sling syndrome.*

Slinky catheter—PTCA (percutaneous transluminal coronary angioplasty) catheter for use in invasive catheterization procedures.

slipped upper femoral epiphysis (SUFE)—the most common hip disorder in adolescents.

slip-ring CT technology.

slit-lamp biomicroscopy—allows well-illuminated microscopic examination of eyelids and anterior segment of the eyeball in a three-dimensional cross-section view. See *Haag-Streit slit lamp.*

Slo-phyllin Gyrocaps (theophylline)—for bronchial asthma.

sloughed urethra syndrome.

slow-channel blocking drugs—another name for calcium channel blockers.

SLRT ("slert") (straight leg raising test) (or tenderness).

SLS (Spectranetics laser sheath).

SLS (Spectranetics laser sheath) **laser**.

SLT (single-lung transplant) **recipient**.

Sly disease—a form of mucopolysaccharidosis, with onset at the age of one to two years, manifested by cardiac anomalies, mental retardation, short stature, pectus carinatum, and facies seen in Hurler's syndrome.

slump test—assesses the mobility of the pain-sensitive structures in the vertebral canal. It tests cervical/trunk flexion, straight leg raising, and ankle dorsiflexion. When all components are in place, with the nervous system at full stretch, the cervical flexion is released. Response is deemed positive or negative based on this release.

SMA (superior mesenteric artery).

SMAC (Sequential Multiple Analyzer plus Computer) ("smack")—automated serum chemistry panels (profiles) comprising multiple tests.

SmartBeam—high-resolution, intensity-modulated radiotherapy treatment (IMRT).

SmartNail—see *Bionx SmartNail.*

Smart Scalpel—a closed-loop surgical system for efficient excision of diseased tissue, leaving adjacent healthy tissue intact.

SmartScore—uses high-speed CT images to provide evaluation of heart disease risk.

SMA-6 (Sequential Multiple Analyzer) —test for sodium, potassium, chloride, bicarbonate (CO_2), BUN, and creatinine.

SMA-12 (Sequential Multiple Analyzer) —test for calcium, phosphorus, glucose, BUN, uric acid, cholesterol, total protein, albumin, total bilirubin, alkaline phosphatase, LDH, and AST (SGOT).

SMA-20 (Sequential Multiple Analyzer) —automated serum chemistry panels (profiles) of 20 tests: glucose, BUN, creatinine, sodium, potassium, chloride, calcium, phosphorus, uric acid, cholesterol, total protein, bilirubin, alkaline phosphatase, LDH, AST (SGOT), ALT (SGPT), direct bilirubin, triglycerides, albumin, iron.

small bowel enteroscopy (SBE)—a technique used to visualize the small bowel in patients with idiopathic gastrointestinal bleeding.

small bowel transit time (Radiol)—on upper GI series, the time required for swallowed contrast medium to pass through the small bowel and appear in the colon.

Small-Carrion penile prosthesis— *Small* is an eponym, not a size.

small cell lung carcinoma (or **cancer**) (SCLC).

SMALL (same-day microsurgical arthroscopic lateral-approach laser-assisted) **fluoroscopic diskectomy**—a surgical alternative to open surgical diskectomy.

small for gestational age (SGA).

small patella syndrome—a rare autosomal dominant disorder. Characterized by patellar aplasia or hypoplasia and abnormalities of the pelvic girdle.

SmallPort needle—a phacoemulsification needle used in cataract extraction to remove the nucleus and polish the capsule. It has a smaller opening at the tip than other phacoemulsification needles.

Sm (Smith) **antigen**—in systemic lupus erythematous.

SMAP (systemic mean arterial pressure).

SMART (sperm microaspiration retrieval technique)—infertility procedure.

SMART (surgical myomectomy as reproductive therapy).

SmartBrace—a brace used to treat repetitive stress injuries of the wrist.

"smart" defibrillator—a semiautomatic defibrillator that can be used by emergency medical technicians. It automatically checks impedance to determine loose leads and analyzes the rhythm. If ventricular fibrillation or ventricular tachycardia is detected, the system recommends a shock. This may be repeated as often as necessary. The system will not charge if ventricular fibrillation or ventricular tachycardia are not detected.

SmartKard digital Holter system— directly outputs ECG data from Holter recorder to any Hewlett-Packard laser printer, saving time and eliminating expense of a computer system.

SmartMist—asthma management system designed to improve the effectiveness of metered-dose inhalers.

SmartNeedle—hooked to a Doppler that emits an audio signal that helps locate femoral, subclavian, or inter-

SmartNeedle *(cont.)*
nal jugular vessels for catheterization.

SmartWrap elbow brace—used to treat repetitive stress injuries of the elbow, often referred to as epicondylitis or tennis elbow.

SMAS ("smass") (superficial musculoaponeurotic system)—a term referring to a layer of the face, used in plastic surgery in rhytidectomies.

smasectomy—rhytidectomy technique, coined from SMAS (superficial musculoaponeurotic system).

SMF (streptozocin, mitomycin, fluorouracil)—chemotherapy protocol.

smile (or smiling) **incision.**

Smith-Lemli-Opitz syndrome—autosomal recessive disorder characterized by multiple congenital anomalies, including microcephaly, mental retardation, unusual facies, and genital abnormalities.

Smithwick hook.

SMM (scintimammography).

SMo (stainless steel with molybdenum)—used in orthopedic appliances. It causes minimal tissue reaction.

SMO (supramalleolar orthosis)—allows for plantar flexion and dorsiflexion in orthosis for ambulation in children with cerebral palsy and myelomeningocele.

SmokEvac electrosurgical probe—see *Nezhat-Dorsey Trumpet Valve.*

SmokEvac—trumpet-valve smoke evacuator for laparoscopic surgery.

"smooth brain" (lissencephaly)—syndrome in which the organized "layered" structure of normal brains is lost, resulting in severe neurological dysfunction. All humans born with type 1 lissencephaly suffer from severe mental retardation, and most experience recurrent seizures.

SMPV (superior mesenteric-portal vein).

SMV (superior mesenteric vein).

SMZ/TMP (sulfamethoxazole and trimethoprim)—agents combined in Bactrim and Septra, trade drugs for use against urinary tract infections, and now also used against *Pneumocystis carinii* pneumonia.

SNA, SNB—measurements in orthodontics. S stands for sella, N for nasion (nasal point), A and B are reference points.

SNAP (sensory nerve action potential) (Neuro).

snap gauge band (Urol)—a band made of elastic fabric and Velcro. It has three snaps, designed to open at progressively higher degrees of penile rigidity. Used to test for organic vs. psychogenic impotence. See *Dacomed snap gauge.*

snare resection (band and snare)—technique for cutting tissue in the esophagus.

Sneddon syndrome—livedo reticularis and cerebrovascular lesions involving all the extremities and the trunk, worsening in cold weather and during the acute phase of neurological complications.

Snellen chart—a test for visual acuity, using progressively smaller letters or symbols.

SnET2 (tin ethyl etiopurpurin)—a drug used in photodynamic therapy for treatment of cutaneous carcinomas and AIDS-related Kaposi's sarcoma.

SNHL (sensorineural hearing loss). Note: *Not* sensory neural.

sniff test—forced rapid inspiration under fluoroscopic visualization to detect paralysis of one or both diaphragms. (*Not* an eponym.)

Sn-mesoporphyrin (SnMP)—decreases plasma levels of bilirubin in prema-

Sn-mesoporphyrin *(cont.)*
ture infants with hyperbilirubinemia.
It is given intramuscularly in dosages
calculated by body weight within 24
hours of birth. It is used in conjunction with standard phototherapy. Also
known as *tin-mesoporphyrin* (*Sn*,
chemical abbreviation for *tin*).

SNOCAMP—acronym for report for-
mat required by some managed care
entities to justify reimbursement:
S Subjective
N Nature of presenting problem
O Objective
C Counseling and coordination
of care
A Assessment
M Medical decision making
P Plan

snowball opacities (Oph).

snowbanks (Oph)—aggregation of inflammatory cells seen on the anterior
inferior retina, characteristic of pars
planitis.

snowstorm shadow—on chest x-ray,
one of the indications for diagnosis
of neurogenic pulmonary edema.

Sn-protoporphyrin—a drug for neonates that decreases elevated bilirubin levels faster than phototherapy
by inhibiting an enzyme necessary
for the production of bilirubin.

S/N ratio (signal-to-noise)—used in
MRI scans.

snuffbox—see *anatomical snuffbox*.

snuffles—*not* a mispronunciation of
sniffles, but actually a medical term
for a hemorrhagic nasal discharge,
generally associated with congenital
syphilis in infants.

SOAE (spontaneous otoacoustic emission).

soaker catheter—used for pain management of large surgical incisions.
The catheter distributes fluid in the
same way a soaker hose saturates a
lawn, allowing delivery of local
anesthetic without the undesirable
effects of narcotic pain relievers.

SOAP (Subjective, Objective, Assess-
ment, Plan) **note**—refers to a format
setup of clinic, hospital, and physi-
cian chart notes or progress notes.
Paragraph headings of the report are
usually presented vertically:
SUBJECTIVE:
OBJECTIVE:
ASSESSMENT:
PLAN:
or may be abbreviated vertically:
S:
O:
A:
P:

**Soave abdominal pull-through proce-
dure**—surgery for Hirschsprung's
disease. This procedure does not require pelvic dissection. The aganglionic rectal musculature is not removed; instead, the rectal mucosa is
removed, and the normal ganglionic
segment is then brought down
through the rectal muscular cuff.

Social Adjustment Scale—assessment
inventory used to evaluate patients
with traumatic brain injury. Evaluates function in categories of work,
social and leisure, extended family,
marital, parental, and family unit
roles.

SODAS (spheroidal oral drug absorption system)—trademark system that
controls release and absorption rate
of a drug.

SOD (sphincter of Oddi) **dysfunction**.

Sodium Sulamyd (sulfacetamide sodium)—topical ophthalmic antibiotic
in eye drops and ointment.

sodium tetradecyl sulfate (Sotradecol)
—for bleeding esophageal ulcers.

Soehendra dilator—used to dilate the cystic duct.

Soemmering's area or **ring**—an oval yellowish spot located exactly in the center of the posterior part of the retina.

Sofamor spinal instrumentation device—allows 3-D correction of the spine to treat spinal deformity, trauma, or degenerative disease.

Sof-Gel palm shield—a soft splint with a self-contained gel that prevents skin breakdown associated with neuromuscular and skeletal tightness of the hands.

SofSorb absorptive dressing.

SoftCloth absorptive dressing.

SoftForm facial implant—constructed of ePTFE (expanded polytetrafluoroethylene) and similar to Gore-Tex but shaped in tubes rather than solid strips.

Softgut—a surgical chromic suture.

SoftLight—laser hair removal system, combining a low-energy laser with carbon-based activating lotion to prevent hair growth without affecting the surrounding tissue.

Soft N Dry Merocel sponge—a fiber-free material that is used in wound dressings to keep the patient dry.

soft neurological signs—nonlocalizable (focal) signs. Cf. *localizing or focal neurological signs*.

Softscan—laser scanner used in superficial skin resurfacing.

Soft Shield collagen corneal shield—used for lubrication and protection.

soft tissue shaving cannula (liposhaver)—an alternative to conventional liposuction.

soft tissue window—CT setting for best visualization of nonosseous anatomy. See *bone window, brain window, pulmonary parenchymal window,* and *subdural window*.

Soft Torque uterine catheter—radiopaque tip for fluoroscopic visualization for accurate placement of the catheter and injection of contrast, dye, or washed sperm.

Soft Touch cup (Ob-Gyn)—a disposable, truncated cone-shaped plastic cup constructed of semirigid polyethylene, used for vacuum-assisted deliveries.

Soft-Vu Omni flush catheter—for improved abdominal aortography and studies of iliac arteries and arteries of lower extremities.

Sof-Wick dressings; drain sponges.

Solagé ("so-la-JAY") (mequinol; tretinoin)—topical solution for treatment of solar lentigines.

Solarese (3% diclofenac gel)—topical treatment for actinic keratosis.

solar keratosis—horny skin growth in some individuals, caused by overexposure to sunlight.

Solcotrans closed vacuum-drainage system—for postoperative use following total hip replacement.

Solcotrans drainage/reinfusion system—used as a blood-saving system, especially in spinal fusion procedures.

Solitaire needle—slightly curved needle used for closure following small-incision cataract surgery.

Solo catheter with Pro/Pel coating (Cardio).

SoloPass—a combination stent and catheter used in endoscopic bile duct procedures.

SoloSite—a nonsterile hydrogel that provides moist wound healing.

SoloSite wound gel—clear wound gel that is noncytotoxic and appropriate for use with chronic wounds.

soluble CD4—a drug used to treat AIDS.

Soluset—a volume control device for administering intravenous solutions.

solution—see *medication*.

Solvang graft—a tip graft to the nose.

SomaSensor—a rectangular plastic pad placed across the patient's forehead. This sensor uses an infrared light source directed through the patient's scalp, skull, and brain to continuously measure cerebral oxygen content. The sensor is attached to the Somanetics INVOS cerebral oximeter, which provides a computerized output of the O_2 saturation in both numerical and graphic form. This device is used during anesthesia and in the critical care unit. It has an advantage over pulse oximetry in that it provides accurate readings during periods of hypotension and even cardiac arrest.

somato-emotional release (SER)—use of therapeutic visualization and dialogue techniques to treat posttraumatic stress disorder. Often used in conjunction with CST (craniosacral therapy).

SomatoKine (IGF-BP3 complex)—used for the treatment of wasting conditions associated with chronic disease, e.g., gastrointestinal damage or dysfunction, AIDS, cancer, osteoporosis.

somatomedin C—now *mecasermin*, previously known as *insulin-like growth factor*.

somatomedin levels—drawn for growth hormone testing.

Somatom Plus-S CT Scanner.

SOMATOM Volume Zoom—computed tomography system that aids physicians in monitoring progression of coronary artery disease and evaluating graft patency following bypass surgery.

somatosensory evoked potential (SEP).

somatosensory evoked response (SER).

somatropin (Nutropin).

Somavert (pegvisomant for injection)—treats acromegaly by blocking the effects of excessive growth hormone production by a pituitary tumor.

Somer uterine elevator.

Somjee-Crabtree temporal bone support clamp—for holding temporal bones during dissection. It is structurally very different, more practical, and effective for securing the bone than the temporal bone-holding bowl which has been in use.

Somnoplasty system—minimally invasive radiofrequency-based devices used for ablation of excess tissue in the upper airway in order to reduce or eliminate habitual snoring.

Somogyi units—results of serum amylase testing expressed in Somogyi units.

"somophagia"—see *psomophagia*.

Sonablate 200 system—for the treatment of benign prostatic hyperplasia utilizing high-intensity focused ultrasound technology.

"sonameter"—see *centimeter*.

Sonata (zaleplon)—nonbenzodiazepine sedative/hypnotic for treatment of general insomnia.

Sonazoid—ultrasound contrast agent with cardiology and potential radiology applications, including heart and liver imaging.

Sonde enteroscope—used in intraoperative enteroscopy in localizing small-intestinal bleeding sites, providing complete visualization of the small-bowel mucosa without enterotomy, while avoiding the trauma that can be caused by push endoscopy.

Sondergaard's cleft—the interatrial groove.

Sones catheter.

Sones selective coronary arteriography.

sonic-accelerated fracture healing system (SAFHS).

sonicator (Cardio)—a device that uses sound waves to create a disruption. "A sonicator was used to produce microbubbles in the contrast medium that was injected into both coronary arteries."

Sonic hedgehog (Shh)—protein that is active in promoting the survival of specific neurons from the midbrain, striatum, and spinal cord in vitro. It has implications for treatment of certain neurologic diseases.

Sonksen-Silver visual acuity cards—to test visual acuity in children ages 3 and up or those with communication problems.

SonoCT real-time compound imaging—compiles up to 9 times the information of conventional ultrasound. It offers multiple lines of sight and has the ability to visualize pathologies such as breast lesions.

SonoHeart—handheld digital echocardiography system that provides two-dimensional and PowerMap directional color Doppler images on demand. Allows trained clinicians to instantly assess and document left ventricular function, chamber size, source of murmurs, wall thickness, valve regurgitation, and cardiomyopathies.

sonohysterography—a technique in which the uterus and endometrial cavity are examined by vaginal ultrasound after instillation of fluid into the uterine cavity. Can be performed in the office without need for anesthesia.

SONOLINE Sierra—ultrasound imaging system.

sonolucent—offering relatively little resistance to ultrasound waves (as air or fluid) and hence generating few or no echoes. Cf. *radiolucent; translucent.*

Sonoprobe SP-501 system for endoscopic procedures.

sonopuncture—stimulation of acupuncture points with sound waves.

SonoSite 180—hand-carried ultrasound system designed to augment routine bimanual pelvic exams, assess pelvic pain or abnormal bleeding, and aid in basic fetal assessment, using either transabdominal or intravaginal imaging, all at point of care.

Sonotron—a pulsed radiofrequency therapeutic device used in treating carpal tunnel syndrome and other repetitive stress conditions.

Soothe-N-Seal—a cyanoacrylate adhesive product for the treatment of canker sores. It provides immediate pain relief with a protective barrier against irritation from ingestion of food and liquids.

Sophy programmable pressure valve —used in neurosurgery in the management of hydrocephalus.

Soprano—a cryoablation system.

SorbaView—composite wound dressing.

Sorbie Questor elbow system—for reconstruction of the elbow joint damaged by rheumatoid, degenerative, or post-traumatic joint diseases.

sorbitol (Salix).

Sorbsan topical wound dressing—used to treat decubitus ulcers.

"sore-a-len"—see *psoralen.*

Soriatane (acitretin)—used for treating psoriasis.

SOT (Sensory Organization Test).

sotalol (Betapace)—used to prevent or treat life-threatening arrhythmias.

Sotradecol (sodium tetradecyl sulfate).

souffle ("soo´f´l")—a soft blowing sound heard on auscultation.

southern access—posterior access in operative therapy of fracture dislocation of the hip, appropriate for certain fractures, depending on where the fracture line is.

Southwick osteotomy.

SPA (sperm penetration assay).

Spacekeeper retractor—used in saphenous vein harvesting procedures.

Spacemaker balloon dissector—used in subfascial endoscopic perforator surgery (SEPS). It is a nondistensible balloon filled with saline used to create large laparoscopic working space within the extraperitoneal pelvic region, eliminating risks associated with entry into and closure of the peritoneum.

Space-OR flexible internal retractor —used for retraction of organs and tissues in abdominal surgery.

Space*Saver volumetric pump—infusion pump for delivery of total parenteral nutrition.

sparfloxacin (Zagam)—used to treat community-acquired pneumonia, acute bacterial exacerbations of chronic bronchitis, and acute maxillary sinusitis.

sparrow-picking technique—an acupuncture technique where an herb is placed on the tip of the acupuncture needle or used in a stick form and passed over a tender joint. See *moxa* and *moxibustion*.

SpaTouch PhotoEpilation system— laser/light hair removal device.

spatulated half-circle needle (Oph).

SPE (streptococcal pyrogenic exotoxin).

specialized tissue aspirating resectoscope (STAR). See *OPERA STAR.*

SPECT (single photon emission computed tomography)—a cardiac imaging technique using thallium and a single gamma camera or scintillation camera which moves in a series of positions around the chest of the patient, receiving radionuclide signals from many angles. This provides a three-dimensional image and helps to localize regions of poorly perfused myocardium by eliminating image overlap. Also useful in neurologic diagnosis, especially in assessing stroke prognosis.

spectacular shrinking deficit syndrome (Neuro)—profound hemispheric ischemia that resolves rapidly over hours to days, usually leaving patients with minimal residual effects.

Spectracef (cefditoren pivoxil)—broadspectrum cephalosporin antibiotic for the treatment of respiratory tract infections. It is used to treat acute exacerbations of chronic bronchitis, sinusitis, pharyngitis, and skin and skin-structure infections.

spectral Doppler (Radiol).

Spectranetics laser sheath (SLS)—an excimer laser device to assist in removal of larger-sized pacemaker and implantable cardioverter-defibrillator leads.

Spectraprobe-Max probe (Cardio).

spectrofluorometry—an investigational method to detect and identify bacteria using fluorescence spectroscopy. Expected to provide rapid identification of bacteria without the need for culturing with antigens. Compared with the nonresonance Raman spectroscopy, it is a very sensitive tech-

spectrofluorometry *(cont.)*

nique. This process is expected to have great impact on the diagnosis and treatment of otitis media, where the often empiric choice of an antibiotic to which the bacteria is resistant can mean prolonged disease and increased morbidity. The only method currently available for accurate identification of bacteria is tympanocentesis, which requires the insertion of a needle through the tympanic membrane and is mildly painful. Tympanocentesis may not be readily available in the primary care office, but spectrofluorometry can be used in a physician's office and is noninvasive.

Spectrum tissue repair system—used for arthroscopic or open suturing of knee and shoulder soft tissue.

SpectRx (capital R)—measures LDL and HDL cholesterol levels. This will replace fingerstick and blood drawing. It works by shining a low-power red light beam into the eye. The light beam "scatters" the LDL and HDL particles in the aqueous, and, by a technique called photon correlation spectroscopy, it is possible to count these particles.

Speculite—a tiny bar light attached to a speculum and used in speculoscopy as an adjunct to a Pap smear.

speculoscopy—a visual cervical screening exam used as an adjunct to a traditional Pap smear. The procedure combines 4-6 times magnification, an acetic acid wash of the cervical area, and a small disposable blue-white light source called Speculite. This aids in exposing potentially abnormal cervical areas. Studies have shown that Pap smear alone detected 31% of early precancerous changes, but Pap and speculoscopy together found 83%.

speech mapping of the brain.

speech reception threshold (SRT).

Speed test (J. Spencer Speed)—used to assess biceps tendon for inflammation, SLAP lesion, and avulsion. Resistance is applied to the arm with the shoulder at 90° of forward elevation and forearm in full supination. The test is positive when pain in the shoulder is experienced.

Speedy balloon catheter—used in percutaneous transluminal coronary angioplasty.

Spence, tail of—also called *tail of the breast*. It is the tail-like segment of mammary gland tissue that extends to the axillary region.

SPEP ("S-PEP") (serum protein electrophoresis).

sperm aspiration—technique for obtaining sperm directly from the testicle of a man who has no sperm in his ejaculate.

Sperma-Tex preshaped mesh—knitted polypropylene monofilament mesh used for the repair of inguinal hernia defects.

SpermCheck test—to check for sperm antibodies.

SP-501 Sonoprobe endoscopy system.

SpF Spinal Fusion Stimulator (trademark)—an adjunct to spinal fusion to increase probability of fusion success and to increase the rate of healing after spinal fusion. Implanted cathodes produce a direct current which initiates an electrochemical reaction and stimulates osteogenesis. This process is called *osteoinduction* by the manufacturers.

SPGR (spoiled gradient-recalled) (echo sequences)—MRI term.

sphincter of Oddi dysfunction (SOD).

sphincterotome, Wilson-Cook (modified) wire-guided.

sphincter-saving procedure—used in resection of rectal cancer. Sphincter preservation is the goal of preoperative irradiation of locally advanced rectal cancer in combination with chemotherapy.

Sphrintzen syndrome—velocardiofacial syndrome, caused by a deletion on chromosome 22.

Sphygmocorder—consists of a mercury sphygmomanometer, an occluding cuff, an inflation source, a stethoscope, a microphone capable of detecting Korotkoff sounds, a camcorder, and a display screen, used for recording blood pressure without the intervention of a human observer.

SPI-Argent II—peritoneal dialysis catheter designed to exit site infections.

spica bandage.

spica cast.

spicules of periosteal new bone, irregular perpendicular.

Spiessel lag screws, position screws, internal screw fixation—used in sagittal split ramus osteotomy.

spiking fever—a fever characterized by recurrent, sudden brief elevations that look like a row of spikes on a temperature graph.

spinal cord injury without radiographic abnormality (SCIWORA) syndrome.

spinal cord stimulation—see dorsal column stimulator.

spinal myeloscopy—fiberoptic endoscopic examination of the epidural space for examination and treatment of pain due to inflamed lower back nerves and/or pain after lower back surgery. By applying fluid under pressure, along with manipulation of the myeloscope, nerves can be released from scar tissue, and local anesthetic and steroid can be injected directly onto damaged nerve roots to reduce inflammation and speed the healing process.

SpinaLogic 1000—a bone growth stimulator used for nonoperative treatment for failed spinal fusion surgery, nine months post-surgery. It is a noninvasive, portable, battery-operated, low-energy magnetic field bone growth stimulator.

spin density; spin echo—MRI terms.

spin-echo image (SE)—an MRI image obtained by the spin-echo technique. With this technique, T2 is determined indirectly, as a function of TE (echo time).

spin-lattice relaxation time—MRI term.

spin-warp imaging—MRI term.

SPIO (superparamagnetic iron oxide) oral contrast agent.

SPIR (selective partial inversion-recovery)—prepared T2-weighted fast spin-echo acquisition on MR imaging; fat suppression images.

spiral band of Gosset—the second palmar layer in the hand. Sometimes referred to in dictation of operative procedures for Dupuytren's contracture.

spiral CT—reportedly shows better resolution of tumors and anatomic structures than conventional angiograms. Also called helical CT.

spiral XCT (x-ray computed tomography) scanner.

spiral x-ray computed tomography (SXCT).

spiramycin—for cryptosporidial diarrhea in AIDS patients.

SpiraStent—a ureteral stent designed to facilitate urine flow and relieve obstruction of the ureter.

SpiroFlo—bioabsorbable prostate stent for treatment of temporary urethral obstruction.

spirometer—see *incentive spirometer.*

spirometric gating (or guidance)—in helical CT technology.

Spirulina Pacifica—a nutritional supplement made from microalgae.

Spitz-Holter valve—an old type of valve for ventriculoatrial shunting in hydrocephalus.

Spivack valve—a technique used in performing a Depage-Janeway gastrostomy.

SPLATT (split anterior tibial tendon transfer)—a surgical technique used to correct equinovarus deformity due to cerebral palsy or brain injury. The anterior tibial tendon is split and the lateral part is transferred through the cuboid and then sutured on itself, with the foot in an everted and dorsiflexed position.

splenic perfusion measurement by dynamic CT scan—used in evaluation of portal hypertension.

spline—see *Calcitek spline.*

splint
  acrylic wafer TMJ (temporomandibular joint)
  air (also inflatable)
  AirFlex carpal tunnel
  birdcage
  Brooke Army Hospital
  buddy
  Budin toe
  Bunnell active hand and finger
  Bunnell finger extension
  Bunnell knuckle-bender with outrigger
  Carpal Lock cock-up
  Delbet

splint *(cont.)*
  Denis Browne clubfoot
  Denver nasal
  DonJoy knee
  Doyle Shark nasal
  eZY WRAP
  Firm D-Ring wrist support (Rolyan)
  Flexisplint
  Friedman Splint brace
  HIPciser abduction
  HVO (hallux valgus orthosis)
  Hydro-Splint II
  inflatable
  Joint-Jack finger
  Liberty One
  Link Stack Split
  MindSet toe
  outrigger
  plaster
  polyvinyl-alcohol
  Radstat wrist
  replant
  Rolyan Gel Shell
  Sam
  Saturn Splint
  shin
  Slattery-McGrouther dynamic flexion
  Sof-Gel palm shield
  Stader's
  sugar-tong plaster
  synergistic wrist motion
  talipes hobble
  Thomas
  Thumz'Up functional thumb
  turnbuckle functional position
  Versi-Splint

splinter hemorrhage—a short linear hemorrhage under a fingernail or toenail, longitudinally oriented and looking somewhat like a splinter; often due to trauma but sometimes a sign of infective endocarditis.

splinting—stiffening of muscles to avoid pain in a part or extremity. Examples: "She is splinting rather markedly, and on this basis appears to be short of breath." "This may be associated with a certain amount of splinting and a reluctance to take deep inspirations."

splinting therapy—used not only to facilitate activities of daily living, such as maintaining function in the hand or elbow, but also to correct orthopedic problems and assist in postoperative rehabilitation after replant, flexor tendon, and rheumatoid arthritis reconstruction surgery.

Splintrex—instrument used for rapid removal of wood or metal splinters; consists of forceps and a loupe.

split-flap technique—in vaginal surgery.

split sheath catheter.

split spinal cord malformation (SSCM)—identified in infants by a screening MR imaging study, with type I or II defined by CT myelography. It should be surgically treated when diagnosed.

SP (stump pressure) **measurement**.

spondylodiskitis—inflammation of the vertebra and disk, the etiology of which is not well understood but believed to be an expression of the inflammatory disease encountered in ankylosing spondylitis.

spondylophyte impaction set—used for correction of bony impingements of neural structures.

sponge
Helistat absorbable collagen hemostatic
K-sponge
Lapwall laparotomy
Merocel
peanut

sponge *(cont.)*
pledgets
Protectaid
Ray-Tec x-ray detectable surgical
Sof-Wick
Taka microneurosurgical
Vistec x-ray detectable
Weck-cel

sponge and needle counts—a phrase used in operative reports to indicate that no foreign material or object has been inadvertently left inside the patient in the surgery. It is standard practice for sponges, needles, and certain other articles to be counted before the beginning of surgery and again just before the surgeon begins to close the wound. Usually two persons perform the counts together for greater security. The surgeon does not begin closure of the wound until the sponge and needle counts are reported correct.

sponge dissector (dissecting sponge)— used in surgery. Also called *peanut* or *cherry*. Cf. *spud dissector*.

spontaneous bacterial peritonitis (SBP).

spontaneous coronary artery dissection (SCAD).

spontaneous otoacoustic emission (SOAE)—used in studies of comparative hearing.

spoon forceps.

sporadic (nonfamilial) **clear cell carcinoma**—the most common type of kidney cancer. The gene responsible is the same as the cause of the inherited cancer syndrome called von Hippel-Lindau (VHL) disease.

Sporanox oral solution (itraconazole) —an antifungal drug used in treatment of painful and debilitating fungal infections (such as thrush) of the mouth and esophagus. It is used to

Sporanox *(cont.)*
treat histoplasmosis, blastomycosis, aspergillosis, and cryptococcal meningitis in AIDS patients.

Sporicidin—a glutaraldehyde-phenate cold sterilizing solution for disinfecting surgical instruments, endoscopes, respiratory therapy equipment.

SportsFit thumb orthosis—low-profile orthosis used to protect a thumb joint from sudden forceful motions that could cause injury.

spotting—scanty vaginal bleeding, menstrual or otherwise.

SPPS (single photon planar scintigraphy).

SprayGel adhesion barrier system—reduces or eliminates adhesions following gynecological surgery.

spreader graft—insertion of a piece of cartilage, as between the anterior margin of the nasal septum and the upper lateral cartilage, to reestablish appropriate width (in this case, of the middle third of the nose). May also be called *batten graft.*

spring fixation—the use of springs after lumbosacral fusion to hold graft material in place.

Sprint catheter with Pro/Pel coating (Cardio).

S protein—see *protein S.*

SPTL-1b vascular lesion laser—used for selective photothermolysis of port wine stains, hemangiomas, facial spider veins, scars, angiomas, warts, stretchmarks, rosacea, and other vascular abnormalities.

spud dissector—used in surgery.

spun urine sediment—urine specimen centrifuged to concentrate sediment (cells, casts, crystals, and other formed elements) before microscopic examination. "Spun urine sediment demonstrated 15-20 white cells."

Spurling's sign or **test**—for nerve root compression. To conduct this test, the examiner approaches the seated patient from above and, with both hands, presses down on the patient's head, with added pressure on the spinal nerve roots. Pain indicates impingement on the nerve root by a herniated disk.

spurring (Radiol)—formation of one or more jagged osteophytes, as in osteoarthritis.

Spyglass angiography catheter.

SQS-20 subcuticular skin stapler—uses absorbable staples that result in less scarring. Places staples just below the epidermis for better cosmetic result.

squalamine—an angiogenesis inhibitor used for treatment of advanced ovarian cancer and non-small cell lung carcinoma (or cancer). Named for the shark genus *Squalus*, squalamine is derived from shark liver.

squamous cell carcinoma (SCC).

squamous intraepithelial lesion (SIL)—squamous intraepithelial lesions on Pap smear, reported as low grade or high grade.

square knot—an easy and reliable knot used for tying most suture materials, including surgical gut, collagen, silk, cotton, and stainless steel sutures. May also be indicated in Ethilon (nylon), Ethibond (polyester), and Prolene (polypropylene) sutures.

Squirt wound irrigation system—for large-volume irrigation of a wound site.

Srb's syndrome—costosternal malformation present from birth; named for Srb J. Ueber (no vowel in *Srb*).

S-ROM femoral stem prosthesis.

SRP (surgical reversal of presbyopia)—allows a patient to focus and read by

SRP *(cont.)*

expanding the diameter of the eye overlying the ciliary muscle, increasing the distance between the ciliary muscle and the edge of the crystalline lens, thus allowing the ciliary muscle to exert more force on the lens. Four polymethylmethacrylate segments are inserted around the circumference of the eye and expand the area around the lens, allowing the muscles more room in which to work and enabling the eye to once again focus on small objects such as words on a page.

SRS (stereotactic radiosurgery).

SRT (speech reception threshold).

SRT (smoke removal tube) **vaginal speculum**—used in laser surgery.

SSBE (short-segment Barrett's esophagus).

SSC (single-stripe colitis).

SSCM (split spinal cord malformation).

SSD (shaded surface display)—MRI term.

SSEP (somatosensory evoked potential). See also *SEP,* which is synonymous.

SSFP (steady state free precession)—MRI term.

SSFSE (single shot fast spin echo)—MRI term.

S660 small vessel stent—coronary stent system specifically developed for stenting of vessels that are 2.2 to 2.9 mm in diameter.

S670 coronary stent—over-the-wire stent for maintaining patency of coronary vessels after angioplasty procedures.

SSKI (saturated solution of potassium iodide).

S-sleep (synchronized sleep).

SSP (stereotaxic surface projection).

SSRO (sagittal split ramus osteotomy).

S.S.T. small bone locking nail—used as an intramedullary nailing device for the forearm or fibula.

STAAR implantable contact lens (ICL)—a permanently implanted contact lens that is inserted through a microincision in the eye and placed behind the iris and in front of the patient's natural lens to correct mild to severe myopia and hyperopia.

STAAR Toric—implantable contact lens.

Staarvisc (sodium hyaluronate)—viscoelastic solution for use in numerous ophthalmologic surgical procedures, including anterior segment surgery, cataract removal, and intraocular lens implant procedures.

Stability total hip system—made of titanium Porocoat in one piece to reduce fretting.

Stableloc—external wrist fixation system.

stacked scans—in computed tomography, a series of scans without intervals of unexamined tissue between them. Same as *contiguous images.*

Stader's splint—a metal bar with pins at right angles to the bar; the pins are driven into the fragments of the fractured bone, and the bar holds the pieces in alignment.

Stadol, Stadol NS (butorphanol tartrate)—synthetic analgesic to treat migraines. Previously available only by injection for moderate to severe pain as a preoperative and postoperative medication. Now available as a nasal spray, hence the *NS* in the trade name. One metered spray is the equivalent of a 1 mg dose.

STAE (subsegmental transcatheter arterial embolization).

stages of labor—first stage, dilatation of the cervix until it is fully dilated and flush with the vagina; second stage, expulsion of infant; third stage, expulsion of placenta and membranes and contraction of the uterus.

staging—see *classification*.

Stahl ("stall") **ophthalmic calipers**—used in measuring orbital implants.

"stalk-section effect" (Neuro).

STA-MCA (superficial temporal artery–middle cerebral artery) **bypass procedure**.

Stamey needle—a single-prong ligature carrier used in the Stamey bladder suspension procedure.

Stamey-Malecot catheter (Urol).

Stamey test—used in evaluating patients thought to have renovascular hypertension. The prognosis after corrective surgery is better in patients with a positive Stamey test. In the test a differential ureteral catheterization is done in which urinary flow rate and creatinine or PAH (para-aminohippuric acid) concentrations are measured from each kidney on diuresis. Patients with renal hypertension caused by obstruction of the renal artery will have a significantly decreased flow rate and a significantly increased creatinine or PAH concentration on the same side, as compared with the normal kidney on the other side.

Stamm gastrostomy.

Stammberger antrum punch (ENT).

stamp graft, transplanted—a technique that makes endoscopic mucosal grafting possible and offers a potential breakthrough in the management of laryngotracheal stenosis.

Stanmore shoulder arthroplasty.

stapedectomy—see *laser stapedectomy*.

Staphylococcus aureus Immune Globulin Intravenous (Human) (SA-IGIV)—purified immune globulin G (IgG) derived from pooled adult human plasma used to treat *S. aureus* infections.

Staphylococcus aureus septicemia—seen in AIDS patients.

Staphylococcus epidermidis—skin flora (formerly *Staph. albus*).

stapled lung reduction—procedure for treatment of diffuse emphysema.

stapler
Auto Suture Multifire Endo GIA 30
Auto Suture Premium CEEA
EEA
Endo-GIA suture
Endo-Hernia
Endopath EMS hernia
ILA
Multifire Endo GIA
Multifire GIA
PolyGIA
Premium CEEA circular
Proximate flexible linear
Proximate linear cutter
Roticulator
SQS-20 subcuticular skin
Surgeons Choice
TL-90 (Ethicon)

STAR (specialized tissue aspirating resectoscope)—used in endometrial resection/ablation procedures. See *OPERA STAR*.

stare, thyroid—see *Collier's sign*.

star figure—a star-shaped folding or pleating of the retina due to edema.

Stargardt's dystrophy—prolongation in dark adaptation, possibly a result of vitamin A deficiency.

Starlix (nateglinide)—monotherapy drug for type 2 diabetes, or combination therapy when administered with metformin.

STARRT (selective tubal assessment to refine reproductive therapy) **falloposcopy system**—used for diagnosis of proximal tubal occlusion.

starry-sky pattern—"There was a starry-sky pattern with phagocytosis of tumor cells."

START SMART Program—for patients about to begin assisted reproductive technology techniques. It emphasizes the A, R, and T of Assisted Reproductive Technology: Asking questions of doctors and nurses, Reading and Researching the course of treatment prescribed, and Talking to doctors and nurses throughout the treatment process.

stat or **STAT** (L., *statim*)—immediately. Often used in a request for an emergency lab report or x-ray, or a rush report from Transcription, in which case it means "I need it yesterday." Dictionaries show a period after *stat* because it is an abbreviation, but most medical personnel do not treat *stat* like an abbreviation and do not place a period after it. Often it appears in all caps.

Statak—soft tissue attachment device for use as alternative to conventional transosseous techniques.

Statham electromagnetic flow meter—flow measurements in blood vessels.

statin drugs—a class of cholesterol-lowering drugs that have also been found to protect against stroke and death from cardiovascular disease. Statin drugs are also called *reductase inhibitors* (e.g., simvastatin).

StatLock Universal Plus—used for suture-free anchoring of percutaneous drainage catheters.

Stat 2 Pumpette—disposable I.V. pump that maintains flow rate under changing conditions.

status post—the condition or fact of having sustained an injury or illness or having undergone a surgical procedure, as in *status post appendectomy.*

stavudine (Zerit)—the fourth drug approved by FDA for AIDS and HIV-positive patients who are unresponsive to or intolerant of Retrovir (zidovudine) treatment.

Stayoden 9000F TENS—see *TENS.*

stay sutures—see *retention sutures.*

STD (sexually transmitted disease).

steady state free precession (SSFP)—MRI term.

STEAM (stimulated echo acquisition mode) **sequence**—on MR spectroscopy.

Steell—in Graham Steell murmur.

steel-winged butterfly needle.

Steeper Powered Gripper—electric terminal prosthetic device that allows grasping, picking up, and holding a wide variety of objects.

steeple sign—on chest x-ray.

steerable guide wire system—used in invasive radiological vascular procedures.

Steffee plates and screws—used in lumbar fusion.

Steida process—the lateral bony process which is an extension of the talus of the ankle.

Steinhauser lag screws, position screws, or internal screw fixation—used in sagittal split ramus osteotomy.

Steinmann pin—threaded and non-threaded.

steinstrasse (Ger., stone street)—urinary sand and stone fragments which result from extracorporeal shockwave lithotripsy of kidney stone.

Steis needle—used for bone marrow biopsy and aspiration.

Stela electrode leads—vitreous carbon-tip pacing electrodes.

Stellwag's sign—infrequent blinking in patients with Graves' disease.

stem cell—see *hMSCs* and *HSC*.

stem cell autograft—used to create new skin around cornea scarred by chemical burns or congenital defect of the iris. Damaged skin can lead to rejection of a corneal transplant. Once the stem cells are growing and creating new skin, a routine corneal transplant can be carried out.

stem-cell marrow harvesting—for autologous frozen stem-cell marrow storage. This is done in patients with acute lymphoblastic leukemia while in relative remission, for use in relapse when an HLA-matched compatible donor is not available.

Stemgen—stem cell factor.

Stenotrophomonas (formerly *Xanthomonas*) *maltophilia*—a cause of urinary tract infection.

Stensen's duct.

stent—see also *tube*.
Acculink self-expanding
ACS OTW HP coronary
ACS RX Multi-Link coronary
AneuRx
AngioStent cardiovascular
Atkinson tube
balloon-expandable
Bard Memotherm colorectal
Bard XT coronary
Beamer injection
BeStent
BeStent2 laser-cut
BioSorb resorbable urology
CardioCoil coronary
Cragg Endopro System I
CrossFlex LC coronary
crutched-stick-type biliary duct
digestive-respiratory fistula (DRF)
Double J indwelling catheter

stent *(cont.)*
Double J ureteral
Dumon tracheobronchial
Elastalloy Ultraflex Strecker nitinol
Endocare Horizon prostatic
EndoCoil biliary
endoscopic biliary endoprosthesis
EsophaCoil self-expanding
  esophageal
expandable esophageal (EES)
expandable metallic
Fader Tip ureteral
Focustent coronary
gfx (trademark) coronary
Gianturco expandable (self-expanding) metallic biliary
Gianturco-Rösch Z-stent
Gianturco-Roubin flexible coil
Gianturco-Roubin (GRS)
Guidant Multi-Link Tetra coronary
Harrell Y
Hepamed-coated Wiktor
Hood stoma
InStent Carotid Coil
IntraCoil nitinol
IntraStent DoubleStrut biliary
  endoprosthesis
INX stainless steel
IRIS coronary
KISS (Kidney Internal Splint/Stent)
Lubri-Flex
Megalink biliary
Memotherm nitinol
metallic
MINI Crown
MPD (main pancreatic duct)
Multi-Flex
NexStent carotid
NIR Primo Monorail coronary
NIR with SOX coronary
nitinol mesh
OmniStent
ostiomeatal
Palmaz balloon-expandable
Palmaz Corinthian biliary

stent *(cont.)*
 Palmaz-Schatz coronary and biliary
 Palmaz-Schatz (PSS)
 Paragon coronary
 Percuflex Plus ureteral
 ProstaCoil
 radioisotope
 RX Herculink 14
 Schneider Wallstent
 self-expanding
 Shikani middle meatal antrostomy
 SoloPass
 SpiraStent ureteral
 SpiroFlo prostate
 S660 small vessel coronary
 S670 coronary
 Strecker
 Stryker
 Symphony
 Talent LPS endoluminal stent-graft
 T–Y
 Ultraflex
 UroCoil
 UroLume urethral
 UroLume Wallstent
 VascuCoil peripheral vascular
 Vistaflex
 Wallstent
 Wiktor balloon expandable coronary
 Wiktor GX
 XT radiopaque coronary
 Z
Stenver's views (Radiol).
step-oblique mammography—involves obtaining additional images at stepped increments in obliquity, usually 15° increments, beginning from the view in which a radiographic density is seen and proceeding toward the view in which the density is not seen.
step-off—a gap between bone fracture fragments.
stepping of vessels—abrupt change in the direction of retinal vessels passing over the brim of an abnormally deep optic cup.
Sterecyt (prednimustine)—antineoplastic for malignant non-Hodgkin's lymphoma.
stereognosis—relates to the ability to perceive, recognize, and understand the form of objects only by touching and manipulating them; a test of the function of the parietal lobes of the cerebral cortex.
stereognosis tests—Seddon coin, Moberg pick-up, Downey object recognition, Ayres tactile discrimination tests.
StereoGuide—stereotactic needle core biopsy.
stereolithography—for assessment and surgical planning in treating congenital aural atresia. Fabricates a precision model of the temporal bone from CT imaging and 3-D image reconstruction.
StereoPlan—stereotactic surgery planning software used in neurosurgery.
stereotactic aspiration biopsy—used to biopsy nonpalpable nodules of the breast.
stereotactic core needle biopsy (SCNB)—minimally invasive procedure for tissue diagnosis of nonpalpable breast lesions.
stereotactic needle biopsy—a nonsurgical breast biopsy.
stereotactic pallidotomy—performed for treatment of Parkinson's disease. The neurosurgeon destroys a portion of the globus pallidus, thereby decreasing a patient's muscle rigidity from Parkinson's disease.
stereotactic percutaneous lumbar discectomy (Neuro)—use of stereotactic equipment for precise insertion of the Nucleotome probe and aspiration of the herniated disk.

stereotactic radiosurgery (SRS)—uses a noninvasive (no pins in the scalp) relocatable system for precise localization of a tumor during radiosurgery. See *fractionated stereotaxic radiation therapy; LINAC radiosurgery.*

stereotactic tractotomy—a psychosurgical technique to relieve intractable depression, anxiety, or obsessional states.

stereotactic vs. stereotaxis—often used interchangeably, although *stereotactic* is preferred. *Stereotaxis* is the general term referring to the field. Etymology: Greek *stereos*, solid or three-dimensional; *taxis*, an arrangement; Latin *tactus*, to touch.

stereotaxically guided interstitial laser therapy—to perform in situ ablation of a tumor. A potential alternative to surgical lumpectomy for treatment of breast cancer.

stereotaxic core needle biopsy (SCNB).

stereotaxic surface projection (SSP).

stereotaxy—the use of the Leksell stereotaxic device, modified for use with the CT scanner, for localizing areas of the brain for implanting radioactive sources, or implanting brain electrodes.

Steri-Drape—a plastic incise drape.

sterilely *(not* sterilly or sterily)—performed in a sterile manner.

Steri-Oss dental implant device—for use with threaded and cylindrical implants. Also, *Steri-Oss type 2210 endosteal dental implant.*

steroid—adrenocortical steroid.

steroid-eluting electrode—pacemaker electrode that reportedly increases electrical efficiency when delivering impulses in the pacing range, allowing more of each electrical impulse to reach the inner heart wall.

stethodynia—chest pain.

Stewart-Treves syndrome—lymphangiosarcoma.

St. George total elbow prosthesis.

St. Hans Rating Scale (SHRS)—for extrapyramidal syndromes.

Stickler's syndrome (Oph).

stick tie—in some operating rooms a suture ligature (or transfixion suture), in others a long strand of suture clamped on a hemostat.

Stifcore aspiration needle—used to obtain gastric or bronchial biopsies.

Stilling–Türk–Duane syndrome—see *Duane's syndrome.*

Still's disease—juvenile rheumatoid arthritis.

Stimate nasal spray (desmopressin acetate)—used for treatment of patients with hemophilia A and type I von Willebrand's disease.

Stim Plus—a battery-operated, handheld microcurrent stimulator designed to detect and treat areas of injury. It can also be used to locate and stimulate traditional acupuncture trigger points.

stimulated echo artifact (MRI)—produced by inadequate tuning of fast imaging sequences.

STING (subureteric Teflon injection)—used for treatment of vesicoureteral reflux in children.

STIR (short inversion time inversion-recovery) **sequence**—MRI term.

St. Jude 4F Supreme—fixed-curve electrophysiology catheters.

St. Jude Medical Port-Access—a mechanical heart valve system used to perform a minimally invasive mitral valve repair and replacement using small incisions ("ports") between the ribs instead of opening the thoracic cavity.

stockinette (stockinet)—a knitted, elastic material, used for wrapping over dressings.

stockings or **hose**
Jobst
Sigvaris compression
T.E.D. (thromboembolic disease)
thigh-high antiembolic

Stoller afferent nerve stimulation (SANS).

Stomeasure—part of the Montgomery tracheal cannula system. Allows accurate measurement of the patient's tracheostomy stoma.

StoneRisk profile—diagnostic tests that measure risk factors for the five major classifications of kidney stones. The StoneRisk test analyzes the composition of a kidney stone.

STOO Series Ten Thousand Ocutome —a probe and vitreous cutter.

stooling—defecation. Used generally of infants not yet toilet-trained.

STOP (selective tubal occlusion procedure)—nonsurgical permanent contraception device for women. The implantable device is a small metal coil that is placed through a hysteroscope and deployed into each fallopian tube. The nonsurgical procedure may be performed in the physician's office under local anesthesia (cervical block).

Stoppa operation—preperitoneal prosthetic mesh repair of hernia via laparoscopy.

Storz Calcutript—see *Karl Storz Calcutript.*

Storz cholangiograsper—a cholangiocatheter grasper.

Storz infant bronchoscope.

Storz radial incision marker—used in cataract surgery.

Stoxil (idoxuridine).

STR (skeletal targeted radiotherapy).

strabismus—the deviation of one eye from parallelism with the other. Types: A-pattern, concomitant, incomitant, nonconcomitant.

straddling embolus—same as *saddle embolus.*

Straight-In male sling system—minimally invasive surgery that uses a transperineal approach to bolster the urethra by placing a sling below it. The sling is held in place with bone screws attached to the descending rami of the pubic bone. It replicates lost natural support and helps restore voiding function.

Straight-In surgical system—used for performing open or laparoscopic bladder neck fixation procedures to treat stress urinary incontinence in women.

StraightShot arterial cannula—allows surgeon to incise and cannulate the aorta in one easy step.

strandy infiltrate (Radiol)—pulmonic infiltrate that appears as strands or streaks of increased density on chest x-ray.

strangury—slow, painful urination, caused by spasm of the urinary bladder and urethra. "He has no dysuria, but does have some chronic urinary urgency and frequency. There is no strangury."

Strata hip system.

Stratasis urethral sling—surgically implanted to provide pubourethral support in the treatment of stress urinary incontinence.

StrataSorb composite wound dressing.

Stratus cardiac toponin I test—provides stat assessment of myocardial damage.

Strecker stent—a tantalum-metal mesh, self-expanding stent that may be used in biliary tract or coronary

Strecker *(cont.)*
arteries. It is placed on a balloon catheter and inserted and positioned endoscopically. Covered with a gelatinous layer which dissolves in one to two minutes, the stent then expands and remains expanded due to special memory metal fibers in the stent.

Streptase (streptokinase).

strep throat—streptococcal infection of throat. *(Not* strept throat.)

streptococcal pyrogenic exotoxin (SPE).

streptococcus A infection—not a new infection, but much in the news because of heavy media coverage of a few severe cases of flesh-eating bacteria or necrotizing fasciitis. Group A strep can be spread by foods, surgical instruments, coughs, or handshakes. The infection is virulent in the victim and spreads through the body with astonishing speed, resulting in severe toxic shock syndrome or necrotizing fasciitis. Infection may enter the body via a bruise, chickenpox blister, sore, surgical wound, or other injury. The bacteria multiply rapidly, with the patient exhibiting swollen lymph nodes, rising fever, and excruciating pain at the site of infection. Readily cured with penicillin in its early stages, the infection may be irreversible in as little as four days. In the U.S., the infection affects about 10,000 to 15,000 people each year and leads to 2,000 to 3,000 deaths. In about 5 to 10% of those affected, it leads to necrotizing fasciitis, a gangrenous-type condition in which muscle and fat are broken down by the infection, necessitating surgery and even amputation. Approximately 20 to 30% of those with necrotizing fasciitis die. According to the CDC, the infection affects mostly adults and usually those with other medical or surgical problems. See *"flesh-eating"* bacteria; *necrotizing fasciitis*; and *toxic shock syndrome.*

Streptococcus milleri—a recently identified microaerophilic gram-positive organism; thought to be a significant pathogen in childhood appendicitis.

Streptococcus mitis—an organism seen in subacute bacterial endocarditis, in the upper respiratory tract, and in the eye. "Culture of the anterior chamber, vitreous, and the intraocular lens revealed no growth, but culture of the en bloc lens capsule revealed coalescent growth of *Streptococcus mitis* on chocolate agar."

streptogramin—see *Synercid.*

streptokinase (Kabikinase, Streptase) —a thrombolytic agent used in treatment of massive pulmonary emboli, deep vein thrombosis, and peripheral artery occlusion.

streptokinase-streptodornase (SK-SD) —skin test for immune function.

stress cystogram (Radiol)—study of the bladder to demonstrate stress incontinence. Contrast medium is instilled into the bladder and films are taken while the patient coughs and bears down.

stress-injected—sestamibi-gated SPECT with echocardiography.

stress perfusion and rest function—by sestamibi-gated SPECT.

stress perfusion scintigraphy.

STRETCH cardiac device.

striatal nigral degeneration—a form of atypical parkinsonism. The name comes from the corpus striatum adjacent to the foramen of Monro.

string of beads appearance (Radiol)— sometimes seen on angiography of patients whose renovascular hypertension is secondary to fibromuscular dysplasia.

string phlebitis—a variant of Mondor's disease occurring in pregnancy and which may appear in the axillary area, antecubital fossa, and groin.

string sign—long, severe stenosis of the distal segment of the internal carotid artery. See *myositis ossificans; pyloric string sign.*

strip-biopsy—used in obtaining large particle biopsies in the GI tract.

stroma-free hemoglobin (SFHb) **solution**—for blood transfusions.

Stromagen—an infused autologous adult mesenchymal stem cell product used in breast cancer patients on high-dose chemotherapy.

Stromectol (ivermectin)—antiparasitic medicine used to treat infection with nondisseminated intestinal threadworm (strongyloidiasis).

Strong-Campbell Vocational Interest Inventory (SCVII).

strontium chloride Sr 89 (Metastron) —long-acting injectable radioactive drug for relief of metastatic bone pain. This radiopharmaceutical is said to provide an average of six months' pain relief with a single injection, with no narcotic side effects.

Strother acrochordonectomy—a procedure for removing acrochordons (flesh-toned skin tags) without anesthesia or cryosurgery. A surgical clamp is applied to the base of the lesion and left in place for approximately 15 minutes, following which the clamp is removed and the lesion is excised using fine, delicate scissors.

struma—see *Riedel's struma.*

Stryker drain (Ortho).

Stryker leg exerciser—device that provides continuing passive motion to the leg to help restore a patient's range of motion postoperatively.

Stryker microdebrider—see *Hummer.*

Stryker stent.

STT (scaphotrapeziotrapezoid) **arthrodesis**—used in treatment of Kienböck's disease. See *Kienbock's disease.*

St. Thomas' solution—one of the most widely used solutions for donor heart preservation for transplant procedures. Named for its origin at St. Thomas' Hospital.

Stuart factor—see *blood coagulation factors.*

Stulberg hip positioner—attaches directly to operating table to convert for hip replacement surgery.

stump pressure—pressures measuring retrograde flow.

sty, stye—see *hordeolum.* Some might think that there is a differentiation— that *stye* is a hordeolum and that *sty* is an enclosure for pigs, but dictionaries list both spellings for *hordeolum.*

Stylet—internal esophageal MRI coil; used to image health conditions related to the esophagus and aorta from inside the body.

Stylus cardiovascular sutures—stainless steel needles used during coronary artery bypass grafting, peripheral graft implantation, and valve replacement procedures.

subarachnoid hemorrhage (SAH).

subclavian flap aortoplasty (SFA)—a technique used to correct aortic coarctation in children.

subclavian steal syndrome (Radiol)— cerebrovascular insufficiency caused

subclavian steal *(cont.)*
by obstruction of the subclavian artery proximal to the vertebral artery, reversing the blood flow through the vertebral artery. The subclavian artery thus, in effect, "steals" cerebral blood, causing cerebral or brain stem ischemia.

sub-Coblation—nonablative Coblation technique that shrinks tissue by reducing the level of radiofrequency applied.

subcortical atherosclerotic encephalopathy (SAE).

subcortical dementia—any of a group of dementias thought to be caused by lesions affecting subcortical brain structures more than cortical ones, and characterized by memory loss with slowness in processing information or making intellectual responses. Included are multi-infarct dementia and dementias that accompany Huntington's chorea, Wilson's disease, and paralysis agitans.

subcu or subQ—could mean either *subcutaneous* or *subcuticular. Subcutaneous* is the deeper layer, and *subcuticular* the more superficial layer. This may help in determining which is meant.

subcutaneous augmentation material (SAM)—facial implant material made of expanded polytetrafluoroethylene and used in plastic and reconstructive maxillofacial surgery. See also *Gore-Tex SAM facial implants.*

subcutaneous emphysema (Radiol)—air or gas in subcutaneous tissues as evidenced on an x-ray.

subcutaneous fat lines (Radiol)—the edges or borders of the subcutaneous fat layer as seen on an x-ray.

subcutaneous injection artifact (Radiol)—occurs in a study such as an in-travenous pyelogram, if the contrast agent is accidentally injected subcutaneously instead of intravenously. The arm will opacify instead of the kidneys. This is a very rare error.

subdural window—CT setting used when a subdural hematoma is suspected.

subepithelial hematoma of the renal pelvis (Antopol-Goldman lesion).

suberosis—extrinsic allergic alveolitis caused by exposure to oak bark or cork dust.

subfascial endoscopic perforator surgery (SEPS)—treatment for chronic venous insufficiency.

Subjective, Objective, Assessment, and Plan—see *SOAP.*

Sub-Microinfusion catheter—low-profile catheter with ability to navigate within the cerebral vasculature for precise delivery of agents. It has radial infusion ports which provide mixing of blood and contrast media, an important key to excellent visualization.

submucosal saline injection technique—for treatment of early duodenal cancers and adenomas.

suboptimal films—not as good as might have been expected; usually referring to technical factors in an x-ray study, such as positioning, film quality, and patient cooperation.

subperiosteal corticotomy.

subplatysmal face-lift technique—a deep plane rhytidectomy using tissue mobilization, advancement, and repair.

Sub-Q-Set—see *CSQI.*

subsegmental transcatheter arterial embolization (STAE).

subset—as in "T-cell subset studies," a group within a group (T-4 cells, T-8 cells).

subtraction films (Radiol)—a method to visualize the arteries and veins on x-ray. A scout film is taken first, before the dye is injected. The scout negative is made into a positive (darkens it). Then the angiogram is taken (this is a negative). Then a scout positive is taken and put under the dye-injected negative (the patient, not the film, has had the dye injection), which screens out the bone, so that all that is then visible are the arteries and veins.

Subtraction Ictal SPECT Co-registered to MRI (SISCOM) **imaging system**.

subureteric Teflon injection (STING).

suburethral sling procedure—made of PTFE (polytetrafluoroethylene) and used to treat stress urinary incontinence.

Suby's solution G—used as an irrigant to dissolve some types of kidney stones. Also referred to as *Suby G*.

succimer (Chemet)—a drug to treat lead poisoning in children. A chelating agent which forms a water-soluble complex when it encounters lead in the bloodstream. This complex is then excreted by the kidneys. Can be given orally, lasts 19 days, and is monitored by serum lead levels.

succussion splash—a splashing sound heard when a patient's body is shaken. It indicates the presence of fluid and air in a body cavity, usually the stomach or chest.

Sucraid (sacrosidase)—oral solution used in sucrase deficiency, a genetic disease.

sucralfate (Carafate)—medication used for coating duodenal ulcers.

suction-assisted lipectomy (SAL)—a procedure in which fat is removed by a suction device, rather than by sharp dissection.

suction-assisted lipoplasty (SAL).

Suction Buster catheter—a combination duodenal decompression tube and feeding tube with multiple holes down the side of the tube. Also called *Moss Suction Buster tube*.

Sudan stain—an iodine compound used as a test for stool fat. It colors the droplets of fat, thus making them visible under the microscope. If there is excessive fat in the stool (steatorrhea), it may indicate liver disease, small bowel malabsorption problems, or pancreatic problems. If, on the other hand, the stool fat is extremely low, that may mean a vitamin D deficiency (since vitamin D is fat soluble).

Sudeck's atrophy—acute osteoporosis.

SUDS HIV-1 (single-use diagnostic system for HIV screening)—can be performed in a healthcare setting without special equipment.

SUFE (slipped upper femoral epiphysis).

sugar-tong plaster splint—used for immobilization in Colles' fracture.

Sugiura esophageal varices procedure—esophageal transection with paraesophagogastric devascularization.

Suh ventilation tube (ENT).

SUI (stress urinary incontinence).

Suicide Risk Scale (SRS)—assesses past history of suicide attempts, present suicidal ideation, and feelings of hopelessness or depression.

Sulamyd (sulfacetamide sodium)—a sulfonamide used for treatment of conjunctivitis. See *Sodium Sulamyd*.

Sular (nisoldipine) **tablets**—a calcium channel blocker, used to lower blood pressure. Taken as a single dose in 24 hours.

Sulfamylon (mafenide acetate)—adjunctive topical antimicrobial agent to control bacterial infections when

Sulfamylon *(cont.)*
used under moist dressings over meshed autografts on excised burn wounds.

sulfur hexafluoride (SF_6)—a gas used in pneumatic retinopexy.

sulindac (Clinoril)—a nonsteroidal anti-inflammatory drug used to treat osteoarthritis, rheumatoid arthritis, bursitis, and gout, as well as to prevent colorectal adenocarcinoma in patients with multiple polyposis. Sulindac is being tested to see if it helps reduce colon cancer in patients without the hereditary disorder.

sumatriptan (Imitrex)—for relief of migraine. See *Imitrex*.

summation gallop (S3 and S4)—in cardiac examination.

summation shadow artifact (Radiol) (also called *superimposition* or *construction artifact*)—superimposition of pulmonary vessels on end and/or bony shadows, which may mimic a lesion. Different views can resolve the issue. This artifact occurs frequently.

Summit LoDose collimator.

sump syndrome—cholestasis in patients who have undergone choledochoduodenostomy (CDS). It occurs when ingested food particles lodge between the CDS and ampulla of Vater.

sundown syndrome—complex of symptoms such as disorientation, agitation, and emotional stress which appear in elderly patients about the time of sunset. The hypothesized causes include decreasing light levels which increase disorientation in patients whose sight is already impaired, dehydration, or progressive fatigue. The patient afflicted with this syndrome is termed a *sundowner*, a pejorative term.

Sundt-Kees clip—for clipping aneurysms.

Sunna circumcision—female genital mutilation consisting of removal of prepuce and/or tip of clitoris. (*Sunna* in Arabic means "tradition.") See also *clitoridectomy* and *infibulation*.

sunrise view of the patella (Radiol).

sunset eyes—an abnormal appearance of the eyes in which the pupils lie at or below the level of the lower lids; seen in infantile hydrocephalus and due to retraction of the upper lids.

superabsorbent polymer (SAP)—a promising embolic material that may be used in place of the other particle embolic materials.

Superblade—a small blade used in ophthalmology.

superconducting magnet—MRI term.

superficial musculoaponeurotic system (SMAS).

Superglue (cyanoacrylate)—a tissue adhesive.

superimposition artifact (Radiol)—see *summation shadow artifact*.

superior mesenteric vein (SMV).

superior vena cava (SVC) **syndrome**.

supernate—the liquid material that rises to the top, after the solid material, or sediment, has settled to the bottom. Also, *supernatant*. Cf. *infranate*.

Super-9 guiding cardiac device.

supernumerary—more than the usual number, as of digits, or parathyroid glands.

superparamagnetic iron oxide (SPIO) contrast medium.

Super PEG tube—percutaneous endoscopic gastrostomy tube. *Super* is a trade name.

Super Pinky—a pink rubber ball with attached elastic headband. The ball is applied over the closed eyelids to lower intraocular pressure prior to surgery on the eye.

SuperQuad assistive device—a walking cane with a quad base and a lower hand grip designed to reduce the amount of effort and strength required to stand up.

SuperStitch—for use in suturing vascular puncture sites.

"super stress test"—cardiac test used to detect T-wave alternans in order to identify patients at high risk for sudden cardiac death. Similar to an exercise stress test.

SuperVent—aerosol solution for treatment of cystic fibrosis.

Supprelin (histrelin acetate)—used to treat children with precocious puberty.

suppressor cell, or **T-8 suppressor cell**—lymphocytes, part of the immune system. These are different from the T-4 lymphocytes attacked by the virus, but they need to interact with T-4 cells for the immune system to function correctly. Also called *cytotoxic cells.*

supraglottoplasty—a procedure to treat severe laryngomalacia.

Supramid suture—a multiple monofilament nylon stranded suture in a nylon sheath, used for intestinal anastomoses.

suprasellar—above the sella turcica.

supratentorial symptoms—a way for physicians to indicate confidentially that there might be a functional overlay to an illness. The tentorium lies at the base of the cerebrum in the brain; hence, by definition, activity the patient can control is above this point. It can also be used in a somewhat pejorative sense or whenever physicians want to indicate among themselves, without being understood by laymen reading the record or overhearing, that the patient might have an element of hypochondriasis to his complaints.

supratip nasal tip deformity—the characteristic rounded shape of a baby's nose; also called the *universal nose of childhood.*

supraventricular tachycardia (SVT) or **tachyarrhythmia**.

Supreme electrophysiology catheter.

suramin—an old drug now used to treat HIV-associated malignancies.

surcingle ("sur-single")—a girdle; also a band, belt, or girth passing over a horse's back or saddle. See *Von Lackum surcingle.*

SureBite biopsy forceps—a flexible tube with a cup biopsy tip for gastrointestinal biopsies.

SureCell Chlamydia test kit.

SureCell herpes (SC-HSV) **test kit**.

Sure-Closure—a skin-stretching system used to approximate wounds or incisions that might normally require grafting or that have a high probability of separating. Currently used in podiatric surgery, particularly on the bottom of the foot.

SureCuff—tissue in-growth cuff that provides catheter fixation.

SurePress compression dressing or **wrap**.

SureSite—transparent adhesive film dressing.

Suretac—bioabsorbable shoulder fixation device.

SureTrans—autotransfusion system for orthopedics.

surface coil—in magnetic resonance imaging, a simple flat coil placed on the surface of the body and used as a receiver.

surface electromyography (sEMG).

surfactant—a combination of the phospholipids, lecithin and sphingomyelin, which coat the alveoli. In

surfactant *(cont.)*

premature infants, surfactant levels are so low and the resulting surface tension of the alveoli so high that the lungs collapse with each breath. Surfactant derived from amniotic fluid (Human Surf) or from cows' lungs (Infasurf) can be used to correct the deficit.

surfactant, heterologous—surfactant derived from sources other than human, including bovine or porcine sources. Surfactants reduce surface tension of pulmonary fluids and contribute to the elasticity of the lung and are important in treatment of conditions such as cystic fibrosis.

surfactant, homologous—surfactants derived from human sources, the only source at this time being amniotic fluid collected from uncomplicated term pregnancies. It is the only surfactant replacement that contains all the surfactant proteins. Disadvantages of human-derived surfactants are the limited supply and the risk of transmission of viral agents.

Surfaxin (lucinactant)—pulmonary surfactant used in treatment of full-term infants with meconium aspiration syndrome (MAS).

Surfit ("sure-fit") adhesive.

surf test—medical slang for surfactant test of amniotic fluid.

Surgeons Choice—the trade name of the ILA surgical stapling system. (Note that there is no apostrophe used.) See *ILA stapler.*

surgeon's knot (also *friction knot*)—used in tying Vicryl and Mersilene sutures.

surgical gut—catgut, an absorbable suture. May be made from the serosal layer of beef intestine or the submucosal layer of sheep intestine.

surgical isolation bubble system (SIBS)—used to maintain sterile operative field.

surgically implanted hemodialysis catheter (SIHC)—a dual lumen central venous catheter.

Surgical Navigation Network—Windows NT image-guided surgery software platform.

Surgical No Bounce Mallet—designed to allow easier orthopedic prosthesis installation, resulting in less trauma to the patient and less fatigue to the surgeons. (Note: *not* Surgicel.)

Surgical Nu-Knit—absorbable hemostatic material (like a loosely knitted fabric, but thicker and more closely woven than Surgicel), oxidized regenerated cellulose.

surgical reversal of presbyopia (SRP)—a procedure using the scleral expansion bands.

Surgical Simplex P—radiopaque bone cement.

Surgicel—an oxidized regenerated cellulose product that will be absorbed by body tissues; used for hemostasis. Cf. *Surgical Nu-knit.*

Surgicel Nu-Knit—absorbable hemostatic agent.

Surgidac—braided polyester suture material.

Surgidine—a germicidal solution. "The left leg was prepared with Surgidine and draped."

Surgifoam absorbable gelatin sponge—sponge for obtaining hemostasis during surgical procedures when control of bleeding by other means is ineffective or impractical.

Surgilase CO_2 laser—a laser using gold as an additional catalyst, allowing more controlled tissue effects and a higher peak power.

Surgilase 150—high-powered CO_2 laser with three operating waveforms: SurgiPulse, PowerPulse, and continuous wave.

Surgilav machine—used in washing the acetabulum or other operative area in orthopedic surgery.

SurgiLav Plus—hydrodebridement portable system for cleaning debris and necrotic tissue from chronic wounds.

Surgilene—a monofilament polypropylene suture material.

Surgilon—braided nylon suture material.

Surg-I-Loop—silicone loops, available in a variety of widths and colors, used during surgery to provide retraction, occlusion, and identification of veins, arteries, and nerves.

Surgiport—disposable surgical trocar and sleeve to be used during endoscopic procedures and laparoscopic surgery.

Surgi–Prep (Betadine, povidone-iodine) —surgical preparation solution.

Surgipro—a prolene mesh used in hernia repairs.

SurgiScope—uses robotic arm with MR and CT interactive guidance to plan and perform brain surgery, allowing smaller incisions and reducing risk to patient.

SurgiSis sling/mesh—for reinforcement of soft tissues where weakness exists. It is intended for colon and rectal prolapse repair, reconstruction of the pelvic floor, bladder support, tissue repair, and sacrocolposuspension. Also used for pubourethral support for the treatment of urinary incontinence due to hypermobility and intrinsic sphincter deficiency.

Surgitron—portable radiosurgical unit; it has four therapeutic currents, as well as bipolar capabilities for microsurgical procedures.

Surgiview—multiuse disposable laparoscope.

Surodex (dexamethasone)—corticosteroidal anti-inflammatory used as an intraocular injection after cataract surgery.

sursumduction—upward movement of only one eye in testing for vertical divergence. Also, *supraduction, superduction, supravergence, sursumvergence.* Cf. *circumduction.*

Survanta (beractant; modified bovine surfactant extract)—used to treat respiratory distress syndrome in premature infants. See also *Exosurf, RDS, surfactant.*

survivor's guilt—a phenomenon that afflicts those who live through devastating circumstances, such as epidemics, or who simply outlive peers or spouses. If the spouse became demented and had to be institutionalized, the guilt is especially intense and a cause of depression.

Susac's syndrome—microangiopathy of the brain, branch retinal artery occlusions, and hearing loss in young women between the ages of 21 and 41. It is self-limiting, most often one to two years in duration, but about half of the patients will have residua, including total deafness.

Suspend sling—surgical implant device for the treatment of stress incontinence in women.

Sustain—HA (hydroxyapatite) biointegrated dental implant system.

sustention (postural) **tremor**—a tremor of a limb that increases when the limb is stretched.

Sustiva (efavirenz)—non-nucleoside reverse transcriptase inhibitor said to reduce HIV levels in blood to unde-

Sustiva *(cont.)*
tectable levels when taken in standard triple-drug therapy.

Sutralon—nonabsorbable synthetic polyamide suture used in general soft tissue approximation and/or ligation, including use in cardiovascular, ophthalmic, and neurological procedures.

SutraSilk—nonabsorbable silk suture used in general soft tissue approximation and/or ligation, including cardiovascular, ophthalmic, and neurological procedures.

Suturamid suture material.

suture—a quick-reference list of suture material, technique, and type. The burgeoning field of laparoscopic and other minimally invasive surgeries may bring with it a number of new suture and knot techniques, as surgeons develop intracorporeal suturing methods. Tying sutures long distance by means of instruments viewed through a scope or video camera is a skill in itself and far removed from the suturing of open procedures. Examples:
Aberdeen knot
Acier stainless steel
Ailee
ArthroSew
baseball stitch
Biosyn
Bondek absorbable
braided Mersilene
braided Nurolon
bridle
bunching
catgut
collagen
convertible slip knot
coupled
crossed-swords technique
Dacron
Dafilon surgical

suture *(cont.)*
Deklene
Deknatel
Dermalene
Dermalon
Dexon Plus
Dexon II
DG Softgut
double-armed
Endoknot
Endoloop
Ethibond
Ethiflex
Ethilon monofilament nylon
funicular
Gambee
gift wrap technique
Gillies horizontal dermal
guy
Herculon
interrupted near-far, far-near
Krackow
Maxon polyglyconate monofilament
Mersilene
Mersilk braided silk
Monocryl (polyglecaprone 25)
Nurolon
out-in-out technique
Panacryl absorbable
PDS (polydioxanone) II Endoloop
Perma-Hand braided silk
Pilot
Polydek
polyglactin
Polysorb
Prolene
Pronova nonabsorbable
pursestring or purse-string
Rapide
retention
Roth Grip-Tip
Sabreloc (spatula needle)
Sepramesh
shorthand vertical mattress
Softgut

suture *(cont.)*
  stay
  stick tie (suture ligature or trans-
    fixion suture)
  Stylus cardiovascular
  SuperStitch
  Supramid
  Suretac
  surgical gut
  Surgidac braided polyester
  Surgilene
  Surgilon
  Sutralon
  SutraSilk
  Suturamid
  Sutureloop colposuspension
  swaged-on
  Synthofil
  Teflon
  Tevdek
  Thiersch
  Ti-Cron
  transfixion
  Tycron
  undyed braided polyglycolic acid
  Vicryl Rapide
  wing
  Z-stitch
"sutured in place, shield-shaped tip graft" (ENT)—sounds poetic? At least alliterative. Included because it's the kind of expression, dictated rapidly, that can become unintelligible unless one knows it. The tip referred to is the tip of the nose.
suture ligature—see *stick tie* and *transfixion suture.*
Sutureloop—ready-to-use needle/colposuspension suture suitable for use with various procedures and needles. It consists of two USP Novafil sutures with prethreaded Teflon pledgets. A radiopaque clip is applied to each pledget to enable postoperative x-ray visualization of buttress position.

Suture Strip Plus—a stretch wound closure strip.
Suture/VesiBand organizer—attaches to drape or skin within the sterile field to eliminate entanglement of multiple sutures and silicone bands.
SVC (superior vena cava) **syndrome**—caused by obstruction of the SVC due to a variety of malignant and benign entities.
SVG (seminal vesiculography).
SVR (systemic vascular resistance).
SVT (supraventricular tachycardia, or supraventricular tachyarrhythmia).
swaged-on (rhymes with "wedged") suture. The suture and needle are fused together. Also called *atraumatic suture.*
swamp-static artifact—see *tree artifact.*
Swan-Ganz catheter—used to monitor pulmonary capillary wedge pressure.
swan-neck catheter.
Swanson PIP joint arthroplasty—"A Swanson PIP joint arthroplasty of the right ring finger and extensor pulley reconstruction, for boutonnière deformity, was performed, using a Swanson prosthesis."
Swanson Silastic implant (Ortho).
SWAP (short wavelength autoperimetry).
Swartz SL Series Fast-Cath introducer.
sweat chloride levels—an elevated level of chloride in perspiration is a sign of cystic fibrosis. One method of measurement is the pilocarpine iontophoresis method.
Swede-O-Universal braces (Ortho).
"sweetheart"—operating room slang for Harrington retractor, so-called because the tip of the blade is somewhat heart-shaped. See *Harrington retractor.*
Sweet Tip pacing lead—with screw-in tip for permanent implantation. It is

Sweet Tip *(cont.)*
used for either atrial or ventricular applications. Also, *Sweet Tip Rx pacing lead.*

Swenson papillotome—used to perform a papillotomy during an endoscopic transpapillary catheterization of the gallbladder in patients with symptomatic gallstones.

Swenson pull–through procedure—for Hirschsprung's disease.

swimmer's view (Radiol)—an oblique view of the thoracic spine in which the arm nearer to the x-ray source hangs at the patient's side and the opposite arm is upraised.

SwingAlong walker caddie—attachment to a walker to hold additional objects such as trays, hooks, and dinnerware.

swing test—measures heart rate variability in patients with congestive heart failure.

Swiss lithoclast—intracorporeal lithotripter for endoscopic stone disintegration.

Swiss-type SCID (severe combined immunodeficiency disease)—caused by lymphoid stem-cell defect.

Swivel-Strap brace (Ortho)—wraps anatomically and allows counterrotation.

Swiss ball therapy—therapeutic exercises using a heavy-duty vinyl ball. It helps to increase range of motion, strength, endurance, motor skills, and balance and is useful in treating upper body ailments.

SWJ (square-wave jerks) (Neuro).

sword-fighting—refers to the placing of laparoscopic or thoracoscopic ports too close together, which interferes with maneuverability of the instruments. Also called *fencing-in.*

SXCT (spiral x-ray computed tomography).

Syed-Neblett brachytherapy method.

Sygen (ganglioside)—a drug designed to promote nerve growth following spinal cord injuries.

Symbion J-7-70-mL-ventricle—total artificial heart.

Syme amputation—ankle disarticulation. "The patient should consider talking with other amputees about the likelihood of a below-knee amputation prosthesis, as I don't feel that a Syme amputation would be indicated in this patient."

Symlin (pramlintide)—for use in type 1 and insulin-dependent type 2 diabetes. It works by making insulin take up glucose more efficiently.

Symmetra ^{125}I **brachytherapy seed**—for treatment of prostate cancer.

symmetrical phased array—term used in B-scan, Doppler, and color Doppler imaging. See *B-scan.*

Symmetry EndoBipolar generator.

Symphonix Vibrant soundbridge—a transducer surgically implanted in the middle ear to enhance hearing, with an external component worn behind the ear.

Symphony stent—a self-expanding nitinol stent used in diseased arteries of the legs, usually in conjunction with balloon angioplasty.

Synagis (palivizumab)—used for prevention of serious lower respiratory tract disease caused by respiratory syncytial virus (RSV) in pediatric patients at high risk for RSV disease. Synagis is administered by IM injection once per month during anticipated periods of RSV prevalence in the community (usually beginning in October and lasting through March or April). High-risk children include premature infants and children with bronchopulmonary dysplasia.

Synarel (nafarelin acetate)—nasal spray used in treatment of endometriosis.

SynchroMed infusion system—an implanted programmable pump and catheter used to deliver morphine into the epidural space. It is used to treat cancer patients with unrelieved pain. This pump can also deliver chemotherapy drugs, clindamycin (to treat osteomyelitis), and baclofen (to treat chronic muscle spasticity).

synchronized sleep (S-sleep, or non-REM [NREM] sleep)—precedes desynchronized sleep and is the time when the muscles begin to relax, when fatigue is relieved. There are also changes in electrical activity on EEG. Cf. *REM* and *desynchronized sleep*. See *polysomnogram*.

synchronous airway lesions (SALs)—associated with laryngomalacia, requiring epiglottoplasty.

syncytial ("sin-sish-al") **knot formation**—a placental layer which proliferates and folds on itself, producing tangles of tissue.

syncytium-inducing (SI) **variant of HIV**—causes a more rapid decline in CD4 cells and progression to AIDS than does the nonsyncytium-inducing variant. See *nonsyncytium-inducing*.

syndactyly—a congenital anomaly in which the webbing between two (or more) digits extends to fusing the fingers to each other.

syndrome
Aarskog
abdominal compartment (ACS)
abdominal cutaneous nerve
   entrapment
ablepharon macrostomia (AMS)
acute compartment
acute tumor lysis (ATL)
adult respiratory distress (ARDS)

syndrome *(cont.)*
ALCAPA (anomalous origin of left
   coronary artery from the
   pulmonary artery)
alien hand
anserine bursitis
anticonvulsant hypersensitivity
antiphospholipid antibody (APS)
apallic
apple peel
Baastrupi's
Baller-Gerold
bare lymphocyte
Bartter's
Bazex
beat knee
Beckwith-Wiedemann
Behçet's
Blackfan-Diamond
Bland-Garland-White
Bloodgood's
Bloom
Blue Angel
blue diaper
blue rubber-bleb nevus
blue toe
blue velvet
Boerhaave's
Bowen Hutterite
BPTI (brachial plexus traction
   injury)
brain death
Brett's
bronchio-oto-renal (BOR)
Brown's
Brown's tendon sheath
Brueghel's
Budd-Chiari
buried bumper
burning mouth (BMS)
burning vulvar
calciphylaxis
capillary leak
carpal tunnel (CTS)

syndrome *(cont.)*
  cast
  cat's cry
  cauda equina
  Cheatle's
  Chilaiditi
  chronic fatigue
  chronic fatigue immune dysfunction
  chronic intestinal pseudo-obstruction
  Cobb's
  Coffin-Lowry
  compartment
  Cooper's
  corneal exhaustion
  Cotton-Berg
  CPD (chorioretinopathy and
    pituitary dysfunction)
  CREST
  cri du chat
  Crigler-Najjar
  CRST
  CTS (carpal tunnel)
  cubital tunnel
  Cushing's
  cyclic vomiting
  Dandy-Walker
  de Clérambault
  delayed pulmonary toxicity (DPTS)
  de Morsier's
  de Morsier-Gauthier
  Denys-Drash
  DiGeorge
  DIMOAD
  DOOR (deafness, onychodystrophy,
    osteodystrophy, retardation)
  double whammy
  Duane's retraction
  dumping
  dysplastic nevus
  Eagle-Barrett
  EEC
  Ehlers-Danlos
  empty nest
  empty sella

syndrome *(cont.)*
  eosinophilia-myalgia (EMS)
  failed back surgery (FBSS)
  false memory
  familial visceral neuropathy
  FAMMM (familial atypical multiple
    mole melanoma)
  fat embolism (FES)
  Fechtner
  fetal hydantoin
  fibrocystic breast
  fish-odor (primary trimethyl
    aminuria)
  Fitz-Hugh and Curtis
  Fleischner's
  Fournier's
  fragile X
  Funston's
  GALOP
  Garcin's
  Garin-Bujadoux-Bannwarth
  gas-bloat
  Gastaut's
  GEMSS (glaucoma, lens ectopia,
    microspherophakia, stiffness of
    the joints, and shortness)
  Gerstmann's
  Gianotti-Crosti's
  Gilles de la Tourette's
  Gitelman
  Goldenhar
  Greig cephalopolysyndactyly
  Guillain-Barré
  half base
  Halbrecht's
  Hamman-Rich
  Hantavirus pulmonary (HPS)
  Harada's
  heart and hand
  HEE (hemiconvulsion, hemiplegia,
    epilepsy)
  HELLP
  hemolytic uremic (HUS)
  Henoch-Schönlein

syndrome *(cont.)*
HPRC (hereditary papillary renal
  cancer)
HVS (hyperventilation)
ICE (iridocorneal-endothelial)
impaired regeneration (IRS)
insulin resistance
Ivemark's
Jackson-Weiss
Jaffe-Campanacci
Janus (Brett's syndrome)
Jerusalem
Josephs-Blackfan-Diamond
Juberg-Marsidi
Kasabach-Merritt
Kaznelson's
Kearns-Sayre-Shy
Klinefelter's (XXY)
Klippel-Feil
Koerber-Salus-Elschnig
LADD (lacrimoauriculodentodigital)
Landry-Guillain-Barré-Strohl
laparoscopic surgeon's thumb
large vestibular aqueduct
late luteal phase dysphoric disorder
  (LLPDD)
Laurence-Moon-Biedl
lazy leukocyte (LLS)
Lejeune's
Lennox-Gastaut
LEOPARD
Leriche
Lesch-Nyhan
Li-Fraumeni (LFS)
locked-in
locker-room
Löffler's (Loeffler's)
loin pain hematuria
"lottery fantasy"
Louis-Bar's
Lowe's
Lown-Ganong-Levine
lymphadenopathy (LAS)
Maffucci's
Marcus Gunn's jaw-winking

syndrome *(cont.)*
Marshall's
MAS (meconium aspiration)
Mayer-Rokitansky-Kuster-Hauser
  (MRKH)
McCune-Albright
medial tibial stress (MTSS)
Meige's
Meigs'
MELAS
MEN (multiple endocrine neo-
  plasia)
MEN I (type I)
meningococcal supraglottitis
Menke's steely hair
minor vestibular adenitis
micrognathia-glossoptosis
Mirizzi's
monosomy 7
Mouchet's
MRKH (Mayer-Rokitansky-Kuster-
  Hauser)
mucocutaneous lymph node
  (MLNS)
multiple endocrine neoplasia type 2b
multiple evanescent whitedot
multiple organ dysfunction (MODS)
multiple organ failure (MOF)
Munchausen
myalgic encephalomyelitis (ME)
myelodysplastic (MDS)
Myhre
nephrotic
nerve root compression
Nezelof
Norrie neurodevelopmental disorder
Ogilvie's
oligoteratoasthenozoospermia
organic brain
os trigonum
otospongiosis/otosclerosis
ovarian hyperstimulation (OHSS)
ovarian remnant
painter's encephalopathy
pallid infantile

syndrome *(cont.)*
- Parinaud's oculoglandular
- Penderluft
- Peutz-Jeghers
- PHACE
- Phocas
- Pierre Robin
- pigment dispersion (PDS)
- Plummer-Vinson
- POEMS
- Poland's
- postviral fatigue
- P pulmonale
- presumed ocular histoplasmosis (POH)
- prune-belly
- pulmonary sling
- Ramsey Hunt
- Rapp-Hodgkin
- Reifenstein's
- respiratory distress (RDS)
- retained bladder
- reverse anorexia
- Reye's
- Riley-Day
- Robin
- Rothmund-Thomson
- Saethre-Chotzen
- Sandifer
- Sanger-Brown
- SAS (sleep apnea)
- Schinzel-type acrocallosal
- Schwachman's
- SCIWORA (spinal cord injury without radiographic abnormality)
- sea-blue histiocyte
- Sebastiani
- second impact
- sepsis
- Sertoli-cell-only
- Sézary
- SHAFT (sad, hostile, anxious, frustrating, tenacious)
- Sheehy

syndrome *(cont.)*
- SIADH
- sick building
- sick sinus
- SIRS/sepsis (systemic inflammatory response)
- Sjögren's
- sloughed urethra
- small-patella
- Smith-Lemli-Opitz
- "smooth brain" (lissencephaly)
- Sneddon
- spectacular shrinking deficit
- Sphrintzen
- Srb's
- Stewart-Treves
- Stickler's
- Stilling-Türk-Duane
- subclavian steal
- sump
- sundown
- sundowner
- superior vena cava (SVC)
- Susac's
- systemic capillary leak (SCLS)
- systemic inflammatory response (SIRS)
- Takatsuki
- talar compression
- tarsal tunnel
- Terson
- tethered cord
- 13q deletion
- thoracic endometriosis (TES)
- 3M (Miller, McKusick, and Malvaux)
- Tillaux-Phocas
- Tolosa-Hunt
- tooth and nail
- Tourette's
- transient bone marrow edema
- translocation Down
- trisomy-D
- tumor lysis (TLS)
- Turner's

syndrome *(cont.)*
UGH+
Unverricht-Lundborg
Usher's
VACTERL
VATER
venous leak
vestibular adenitis
Vogt-Koyanagi-Harada
vulvar vestibulitis
wasting
white clot
white dot
Winchester
Wiskott-Aldrich
WPW (Wolff-Parkinson-White)
XXY (Klinefelter's)
Yentl syndrome
Yunis-Varon
Zollinger-Ellison (ZES)
synechialysis (Oph).
Synercid (quinupristin; dalfopristin)—the first injectable antibiotic in a distinct class of antibacterials known as streptogramins. It is used for the treatment of bloodstream infections due to vancomycin-resistant *Enterococcus faecium* and skin and skin-structure infections caused by methicillin-susceptible *Staphylococcus aureus* or *Streptococcus pyogenes.*
synergistic wrist motion splint.
Synergraft—tissue-engineered replacement heart valves.
Synergy neurostimulation system—implantable dual channel therapy designed to aid in management of chronic intractable pain in trunk or limbs.
synovial frost (Ortho).
Syn-Rx (pseudoephedrine HCl/guaifenesin)—14-day regimen for treatment of sinusitis.

Synsorb Cd—treatment for *C. difficile*-associated diarrhea (CDAC).
Synsorb Pk—potential treatment for prevention of hemolytic uremic syndrome.
Syntel latex-free embolectomy catheter—balloon embolectomy catheter used on patients with latex allergies.
Synthaderm—synthetic (polyurethane) occlusive wound dressing used on ulcerations, usually on the lower extremities.
Synthes CerviFix system—used for stabilization and promotion of fusion of the cervical spine and occipital-cervical junction.
Synthes compression hip screw—American version of the German AO hip compression screw.
Synthes dorsal distal radius plate—for fixation of fractures, osteotomies, and carpal fusions involving the distal radius; applied to the dorsal aspect.
Synthes drill.
Synthes mini L-plate (Hand Surg).
Synthes transbuccal trocar (Oral Surg).
Synthofil suture—nonabsorbable polyester braided and coated suture for skin closure and cardiovascular and arterial surgery.
syntonic—characterized by normal emotional response. "His affect was generally appropriate, and mood syntonic."
Synvisc—an elastoviscous hyaluronan preparation with similar properties to healthy human synovial fluid. Injected into the knee joint, it helps to protect and lubricate joints affected by osteoarthritis.
Syringe Avitene—an endoscopic delivery system for Avitene, a collagen hemostat. Note that *Syringe* is part of the trade name.

system—see *device*.

systemic and topical hypothermia.

systemic capillary leak syndrome (SCLS)—a rare condition characterized by unexplained episodic capillary hyperpermeability due to a shift of fluid and protein from the intravascular to the interstitial space. This results in diffuse swelling, weight gain, and renal shut-down. The disease evolves into multiple myeloma in some patients.

systemic lupus erythematosus (SLE) —an inflammatory disorder of the connective tissues, characterized by a "butterfly" erythema over the malar area and the bridge of the nose, arthralgias. It may include renal involvement, recurrent pleurisy, splenomegaly, and involvement of other body systems. It is thought to be an autoimmune disorder. It is seen predominantly in young women but is also seen in children. Also called *disseminated lupus erythematosus*. See also *Farr test*.

systemic mean arterial pressure (SMAP).

systemic vascular resistance (SVR).

System·S soft skeletal implant—used in hand arthroplasty.

systolic anterior motion (SAM) on **2-D echocardiogram.**

Szabo-Berci needle drivers—designed for use with Karl Storz endoscopes for advanced suturing techniques.

T, t

T (tesla)—SI unit of magnetic strength (used in MRI). The term *gauss* was formerly used.

TAAA (thoracoabdominal aortic aneurysm) **surgery**.

TAB (tumescent absorbent bandage)—a post-tumescent wound dressing to keep the patient dry.

TAC (transient aplastic crisis).

TAC ("tack") (triamcinolone cream)—used in the treatment of psoriasis and other dermatological conditions.

TACE (transcatheter arterial chemoembolization)—the most common non-surgical treatment for hepatocellular carcinoma.

Tachyarrhythmia Detection Software —provides fully automatic detection and treatment of life-threatening arrhythmias.

tacrine (Cognex)—a treatment to improve cognitive performance in Alzheimer's disease. It prevents destruction of acetylcholine, a neurotransmitter in the brain. See *velnacrine*.

tacrolimus (Prograf)—antibiotic which suppresses the action of lymphocytes and prevents rejection of a newly transplanted liver. It is said to be significantly more effective than cyclosporine and to cause fewer side effects. Tacrolimus is also an immunosuppressive drug used for the treatment of psoriatic arthritis.

Tactilaze angioplasty laser catheter— vaporizes atherosclerotic plaque by means of an angioplasty catheter threaded through the artery.

tactoid bodies—fibrillary aggregates which can be seen in neurofibromas representing rounded aggregates of collagen and cell processes, and probably represents a degenerative change.

TAE (transcatheter arterial embolization).

tag (Nuclear Med)—to label, i.e., to render a substance radioactive by incorporating a radionuclide in it; also, to cause a tissue or organ to take up radioactive material. Cf. *label, sensitize*.

Tagarno 3SD cine projector—for angiography.

tag image file format (TIFF).

TAG (tissue anchor guide) **system**.

tail—slender appendage, as in tail of Spence, tail of the breast. Cf. *cauda*.

tail of breast—in mammography, a wedge-shaped zone of breast tissue extending toward the axilla. Also known as the *axillary tail of Spence*.

tail of Spence—also called *tail of the breast*. It is the tail-like segment of mammary gland tissue that extends to the axillary region.

tailor's bunion—a name from the distant past when tailors sat cross-legged on the floor to do their sewing, and thus developed bunions on the fifth metatarsal (rather than the first metatarsal where they usually occur).

Taka microneurosurgical sponge—developed by Dr. Takanori Fukushima.

Takatsuki syndrome (Neuro).

Takayasu's arteritis—arteritis involving the aortic arch and its branches.

Take-apart scissors and forceps.

takeoff of a vessel (Radiol)—in angiography, the commencement (or origin) of a vessel as it branches off from a larger vessel.

talcosis—intravascular, perivascular, and alveolar granulomatous inflammation in which foreign bodies (talc and sometimes starch) can be identified. This talcosis is found in almost all I.V. drug abusers. It may cause abnormalities in pulmonary function.

talc poudrage and **talc slurry**—used to perform pleurodesis.

Talent LPS endoluminal stent-graft system—used for the treatment of abdominal aortic aneurysms.

talipes hobble splint—see *Denis Browne clubfoot splint*.

TAM (total active motion).

Tamiflu (oseltamivir phosphate)—investigational medication found to be safe and effective in preventing influenza in elderly and high-risk patients.

tamoxifen citrate (Nolvadex)—chemotherapy drug.

T-AnastoFlo shunt—disposable shunt for preventing ischemia by providing the flow of blood or cardioplegia solution distal to an anastomosis site during the construction of coronary artery bypass grafts.

"T and C"—slang for Tylenol and codeine. When a physician dictates, "The patient was given T and C for pain," one should transcribe, "The patient was given Tylenol and codeine for pain."

Tandem cardiac device.

tandem mass spectrometry—screening blood test for newborns that scans for over 25 genetic diseases.

tangential cut—a cut which is slightly off center, or glancing.

tangential speech—rambling, tending to go off on tangents.

Tanne corneal punch.

tanned red cells (TRC) **test**.

Tanner Developmental Scale—stages secondary sexual characteristics on a scale of I to V, I indicating no development, V indicating full development; "breasts Tanner stage II," for example. Also, *Marshall and Tanner pubertal staging*.

Tanner mesher—a device used to mesh skin in preparation for grafting; permits the skin to stretch, thus covering a greater area. See also *Tanner-Vandeput mesh dermatome*.

Tanner-Vandeput mesh dermatome — an instrument that cuts small parallel slits in split thickness skin grafts,

Tanner-Vandeput *(cont.)*
permitting the graft to expand two to three times its original size. When the graft is applied, the slits expand and become diamond-shaped areas which then epithelialize from the surrounding skin edges.

Tanner-Whitehouse bone age reference values for North American children.

tantalum bronchogram (using powdered tantalum).

tantalum mesh, plate, ring, wire. Tantalum is not an alloy; it is biologically inert, having great tissue acceptability and high tensile strength. In plate form it is used for skull plates.

Tao (troleandomycin).

tap—see *glabellar tap*.

TAP (tumor-activated prodrug)—technology used with proprietary antibodies for drug research.

tape
Cath-Secure hypoallergenic
Dacron
Elastikon elastic
Hy-Tape
lap
MaxCast
Microfoam surgical
Scotchcast 2 casting
Shur-Strip
Transpore surgical

taper—to reduce the dose of a medicine gradually; to change size gradually.

TAPET (tumor amplified protein expression therapy)—drug delivery that uses genetically altered strains of *Salmonella* as a vehicle for the delivery of antineoplastic drugs to tumor sites with minimal effect on healthy tissue.

TAPP (transabdominal preperitoneal) hernia repair.

TARA (total articular replacement arthroplasty) **prosthesis**—see *Townley TARA prosthesis*.

tardive dyskinesia (Psych)—involuntary tics, which may consist of continuous chewing motions or darting movements of the tongue, jerky dancing motions, or slow writhing motions of the hands or arms, secondary to long-term administration of antipsychotic drugs. Symptoms usually resolve on discontinuing the drug or reducing the dosage. See *extrapyramidal signs*. Cf. *pyramidal signs, akathisia*.

tardy palsy—referred to in electromyograph reports and nerve conduction velocities, with reference to carpal tunnel syndrome. Example: "Impression: Slowing of ulnar nerve, slowing across the elbow, consistent with a tardy palsy."

targeted cryoablation devices—used to treat liver and other cancers.

target lesion—a skin lesion consisting of concentric rings of erythema. For example, target lesion (of Lyme disease). See *erythema migrans*.

target sign—a test for cerebrospinal fluid leak. If a cerebrospinal fluid leak is suspected, examination of the bloody fluid placed on porous paper will show a clear halo around the inner bloody residue if positive.

Target Tissue Cooling System (TTCS) —allows for the use of a cooling medium (such as water) on human tissue during the application of laser energy. The cooling of the target tissue prevents thermal damage, and the coolant facilitates the establishment of a photo-acoustic effect which aids in the removal of tissue.

Targis microwave catheter-based system—nonsurgical, catheter-based transurethral thermoablation system to treat benign prostatic hypertrophy.

Targocid (teicoplanin).

Targretin (bexarotene) **gel 1%**—topical therapy for treatment of cutaneous lesions in patients with stage IA, IB, or IIA cutaneous T-cell lymphoma (CTCL) who have not tolerated other therapies or who have refractory or persistent disease.

Tarlov ("tar-loff") perineurial cyst.

tarsal cyst—see *chalazion*.

tarsal tunnel syndrome—a group of symptoms caused by compression of the posterior tibial nerve, or the plantar nerves, in the tarsal tunnel, resulting in pain, numbness and paresthesias of the plantar aspect of the foot. "The left medial great toe pain was suggestive of tarsal tunnel syndrome." Cf. *carpal tunnel syndrome*.

Tart cells—named for the patient in whom the cells were discovered. They can be seen in some cases of rheumatoid arthritis or serum sickness.

TASH (transcoronary ablation of septal hypertrophy).

Tasmar (tolcapone)—for use in conjunction with levodopa/carbidopa in both nonfluctuating and fluctuating Parkinson's disease. Tasmar is the first of a new class of Parkinson's disease drugs called COMT inhibitors that enhance the effectiveness of levodopa by blocking one of the main enzymes responsible for breaking down levodopa in the blood stream before it reaches the brain.

TAT (thrombin-antithrombin III complex) **inhibitor**—a drug to treat HIV-positive patients.

Taussig-Bing anomaly—a congenital defect of the heart, characterized by complete transposition of the pulmonary artery in association with a ventricular septal defect. Symptoms may include cyanosis, dyspnea on exertion, severe pulmonary hypertension, systolic murmur, loud pulmonic second sound, and polycythemia. Incomplete bundle branch block or right ventricular hypertrophy may also be present.

Taut catheters—several different types of catheters utilized for intraoperative cholangiography.

Taut cystic duct catheters—used in operative cholangiography.

Taxol (paclitaxel)—a cytotoxic agent, now found to be beneficial in the treatment of carcinoma of the ovaries.

Taxotere (docetaxel)—a taxoid administered intravenously for the treatment of non-small cell lung and breast cancer.

Taylor pinwheel—used in sensory examination in neurologic testing.

tazarotene (Tazorac).

Tazidime (ceftazidime).

Tazocin—European name for U.S. drug Zosyn.

Tazorac (tazarotene topical gel)—for treatment of stable plaque psoriasis and mild to moderately severe facial acne vulgaris.

TBB (transbronchial biopsy).

TBNA (transbronchial needle aspiration).

TBSA (total body surface area).

TBT (transcervical balloon tuboplasty).

TCA (tricyclic antidepressant).

TCCB (transitional cell carcinoma of the bladder).

TCCO (transcranial cerebral oximetry).

TCD/CBDE (transcystic duct/common bile duct exploration)—performed via laparoscopy.

TCD (transcranial Doppler) **measurements**.

TCD (transcranial Doppler) **velocities**.

T-cell—thymus-derived lymphocyte, a part of the immune system. See *B-cell, T-4, T-8*.

T-cell function test—can detect lack of T4-helper (CD4) cell activity in fighting infection before counts actually start to diminish. It gives clinicians more information on their patients' actual immune status and aids in making the timing of antiviral treatment more effective.

TcHIDA ("tek-high-dah")—see *HIDA, PIPIDA*.

Tc 99m or ^{99m}**Tc** (technetium). See *medications* and *technetium*.

TCN-P (triciribine phosphate)—chemotherapy drug.

TCP (total cavopulmonary connection) —the Fontan procedure preferred over atriopulmonary (AP) connection in recent studies. Patients having TCP are shown to recover with less exercise intolerance, perfusions, arrhythmia, thrombus, and protein-losing enteropathy (PLE) than patients having AP.

TCP/IP (transmission control protocol/ Internet protocol)—computer telecommunications term, also used in teleradiology.

TCPM pneumatic tourniquet system— for orthopedic procedures.

TCR (tear clearance rate) (Oph).

TCR (T-cell receptor) **peptide vaccine** —used in treatment of multiple sclerosis. It works by reducing specific T-cell populations in cerebrospinal fluid.

TCu380A IUD (intrauterine device).

T-cuts—for corneal astigmatism.

TDD (thoracic duct drainage).

TDP (torsades de pointes).

TDR (thymidine deoxyriboside).

TDS (treadmill duration score).

TE (echo time)—in magnetic resonance imaging, the interval between the first pulse in a spin-echo examination and the appearance of the resulting echo.

TEA (transluminal extraction atherectomy).

tear—see *Mallory-Weiss tear, retinal tear*.

tear clearance rate (TCR) (Oph).

tear strips—see *Schirmer's test*.

tease—gentle freeing of tissues in surgery.

Tebbetts rhinoplasty set—designed for open and closed rhinoplasty procedures. Includes an osteotome, alar stabilizing jig, speculums, and retractors.

teboroxime scan—a cardiac scan using radioactive imaging agent ^{99m}Tc teboroxime (CardioTec) to show areas of myocardial infarction. Used for emergency scans, it clears rapidly from the blood to allow subsequent scans, if necessary.

TEC (transluminal extraction catheter).

TEC (thiotepa, etoposide, carboplatin) —chemotherapy drug for malignant glioma.

TECAB (totally endoscopic coronary artery bypass).

TECA (technetium albumin) **study.**

teceleukin and interferon alfa-2a— chemotherapy drug for metastatic renal cell carcinoma and malignant melanoma.

TechneScan MAG3—renal diagnostic imaging agent that uses technetium ^{99m}Tc mertiatide to determine kidney function.

technetium—an element, an isotope of which Tc 99m (^{99m}Tc) is used as a diagnostic aid in liver, brain, lung,

technetium *(cont.)*
and kidney scans. See *medications*; *radioisotopes*.

technetium glucarate—a nuclear "hot spot" imaging agent for the early and rapid diagnosis of acute myocardial infarction.

technetium GSA (diethylenetriamine-pentaacetic acid-galactosyl-human serum-albumin)—imaging agent for liver scintigraphy. May be used for perioperative assessment of hepatectomy.

technetium macroaggregated albumin (Tc 99m MAA, or ^{99m}Tc-MAA)—predictor of gastrointestinal toxicity in hepatic artery infusion.

technetium pertechnetate (Tc 99m)—a tracer used in radionuclide studies for active gastrointestinal bleeding; this material labels red blood cells. If bleeding occurs in a period of up to 24 hours that the labeled red blood cells remain in the circulating blood, the tracer will extravasate and accumulate at or near the site. It is also used to demonstrate the presence of a Meckel's diverticululm.

technetium sulfur colloid (^{99m}Tc-SC) (Tesuloid)—a tracer used in radionuclide scans for active gastrointestinal bleeding. This material is cleared from the blood and concentrated in the reticuloendothelial system with a half-life of less than $2^{1/2}$ minutes. If GI bleeding occurs during this time, the tracer will accumulate at the bleeding site.

Techni-Care surgical scrub.

technique—see *operation*.

Techstar and **Techstar XL**—percutaneous vascular surgery system.

Techstar percutaneous closure device —also referred to as *Perclose closure device* (the manufacturer).

T.E.D. (thromboembolic disease) **stockings** or **hose**—antiembolism stockings. Trademark *T.E.D.* has periods.

TEE (transesophageal echocardiography)—see *Acuson V5M*.

TEF (tracheoesophageal fistula).

Teflon-coated hollow-bore needle (ENT)—used in ear surgery.

Teflon paste injection for incontinence—a procedure in which injection of a Teflon paste (Polytef, Ethicon) into the periurethral tissues at the bladder neck is done on an outpatient basis to restore urinary control in incontinent women, particularly the elderly. The injection works by adding bulk to these tissues, compressing the urethral lumen and increasing the resistance to the outflow of urine.

Tegaderm transparent dressing—a waterproof dressing for wound and I.V. site coverage. Made by 3M.

Tegagel—hydrogel dressing and sheet.

Tegagen HG—alginate wound dressing.

Tegagen HI—alginate wound dressing.

Tegapore—contact-layer wound dressing.

tegaserod (Zelmac)—drug treatment for irritable bowel syndrome in patients whose primary symptom is constipation.

Tegasorb dressing—a hydrocolloid wafer dressing used in treatment of wounds, e.g., pressure ulcers (decubitus ulcers). These dressings are permeable to moisture vapor and to oxygen, so they permit oxygen exchange; but they are impermeable to bacteria, so they prevent contamination. These dressings are contraindicated in the presence of infection.

Tegner activity score—done pre- and postoperatively for knee reconstruction surgery.

Teichholz ejection fraction—used in echocardiogram.

teicoplanin (Targocid)—an antibiotic that is given to patients who have an infection resistant to vancomycin. Administered once a day IV or IM.

T-8 cell—also called suppressor/cytotoxic cell. See *suppressor cell*.

Tekna mechanical heart valve.

TeleCaption decoder—allows hearing-impaired or deaf persons to read program captions on television.

telecurietherapy—radiotherapy.

telemedicine—a live, two-way audio/video exchange of medical information, education, and surgery procedures.

telepathology—transmission and interpretation of tissue specimens via remote telecommunication, generally for the purpose of diagnosis or consultation but also for continuing education.

teleradiology—the transmission of images from a local (transmitting) site to a remote (receiving) site for interpretation at the remote site.

Telescopic Plate Spacer (TPS)—expandable titanium spacer intended to replace one or two vertebral bodies that must be removed due to cancer, thus avoiding the destabilization of the spine that occurs due to corpectomy.

telesensor—"Star Trek" technology today, consisting of miniature computerized devices the size of a computer chip which attach to the body to sense vital signs and electrical conductivity of the skin and transmit the information to geographically distant receiving stations. Telesensors are developed for applications in medicine as well as the military.

Teletrast—an absorbable surgical gauze which contains a plastic thread that has been impregnated with barium sulfide, thus making it radiopaque. Among other applications, it is used in microvascular decompression to displace a vessel that is compressing the trigeminal nerve.

Teller acuity card (TAC)—used for acuity measurement in examination for macular heterotopia and for macular fold.

telogen—the resting phase of hair growth. See *anagen*.

telomerase—an enzyme that causes cancer cells to multiply out of control. Now used to retard the aging process at the cell level.

teloxantrone HCl—drug used in treating patients with solid tumors when other chemotherapy is ineffective.

TEM (transanal endoscopic microsurgery).

temafloxacin (Omniflox) broad-spectrum oral antibiotic for respiratory, genitourinary, and skin infections.

Temodar (temozolomide)—oral medication used for treatment of recurrent glioblastoma multiforme (an aggressive brain tumor). Temodar is one of several drugs in a new class of compounds known as *imidazotetrazines*.

TEMP (tamoxifen, etoposide, mitoxantrone, Platinol)—chemotherapy protocol used to treat breast carcinoma.

temporal arcade.

temporal instability—MRI term.

temporomandibular joint (TMJ).

T.E.N.—see *Vivonex T.E.N.*

Tenckhoff—peritoneal dialysis catheter.

Tender Touch Ultra cup (Ob-Gyn)—a disposable, truncated, cone-shaped plastic cup constructed of silicone elastomer (a soft, pliable plastic), for vacuum-assisted deliveries.

tendinitis—*not* tendonitis.
tendo Achillis (or Achilles tendon).
tendon—the fibrous cord by which a muscle is attached. Cf. *tenon*.
10-EDAM—see *EDAM*.
Tendril DX—implantable pacing lead with a tip electrode that releases steroid upon entering the heart tissue. The steroid reduces inflammation, allowing for a lower voltage stimulation threshold.
Tendril SDX—steroid-eluting, active fixation pacing lead with a diameter of 6.2 French (less than 1/10 inch), allowing a less traumatic insertion procedure.
tenidap (Enable)—first in a class of antiarthritics called cytokine modulators. It blocks prostaglandins, which maintain inflammation and increase the erosive effects of chronic arthritis.
teniposide (Vumon)—chemotherapy drug for refractory childhood acute lymphoblastic leukemia.
Tennant nuclear ball rotator (Oph).
Tennison-Randall repair—for cleft lip.
Tennis Racquet catheter—used in angiography. This is a trade name, and the catheter does look like a tennis racquet.
tenon (not tendon)—a projecting member in a piece of wood or other material for insertion into a mortise to make a joint. See *mortise*. Cf. *tendon*.
TENS (transcutaneous electrical nerve stimulation)—a nondrug, noninvasive, nonaddictive alternative for control of pain. It appears to enhance the concentration of beta-endorphins significantly. The TENS system consists of a small battery-powered stimulator with lead wires that attach to two or more surface electrodes. See *AdvanTeq II TENS, Eclipse*

TENS, Maxima II TENS, Stayoden 9000F TENS, and *PENS*.
Tensilon test—for myasthenia gravis.
tension-free vaginal tape (TVT) **procedure**.
tenting of hemidiaphragm—on chest x-ray, a distortion of the diaphragm by scarring, in which an upward-pointing angular configuration (like a tent) replaces all or part of the normal curved contour of a hemidiaphragm.
tenting sign—a simple test for severe dehydration; a pinched fold of skin will stay tented up.
10-20 System—see *International 10-20 System*.
Tenzel calipers—modification of Jameson calipers. Used to measure the eyelid crease.
TEOAE (transient evoked otoacoustic emission).
TEP (tracheoesophageal puncture).
TEP (totally extraperitoneal) **hernia repair**—identical to the TAPP (transabdominal preperitoneal) technique, but takes place in the preperitoneal space.
Tequin (gatifloxacin)—quinolone antibiotic for treatment of community-acquired respiratory tract infections.
terahertz waves—new imaging technology that can peer inside living and inanimate objects and provide 3-D images.
terazosin (Hytrin)—an antihypertensive used for the symptoms of benign prostatic hyperplasia (or hypertrophy).
terbinafine (Lamisil).
terlipressin (Glypressin)—used to treat bleeding esophageal ulcers.
terminal sedation (TS)—palliative option for the terminally ill, along with VSED (voluntarily stopping eating and drinking), undertaken at the

terminal sedation *(cont.)*
request of a mentally competent patient who is suffering consistent intolerable pain. See also *PAS, VAE,* and *VSED.*

teroxirone (alpha-TGI)—chemotherapy drug given intraperitoneally for advanced malignancies of the abdominal cavity.

"terrible triad" of the shoulder—concomitant presentation of rotator cuff tear, brachial plexus injury, and anterior shoulder dislocation. This combination of injuries most often occurs in patients over age 40.

Terrien's degeneration—marginal thinning and degeneration of the upper nasal quadrants of the cornea.

Terry fingernail sign—see *Terry nails.*

Terry keratometer—enables surgeons to measure astigmatism while the patient is still on the operating table after surgery, and while the final wound closure is being accomplished.

Terry-Mayo needle (Urol)—a heavy, small Mayo needle.

Terry nails—white opaque ground-glass appearance of the nails proximally, with a normal pink area distally. Seen in cirrhosis of the liver and certain other liver diseases. "Terry nails are present, and he has some clubbing."

Terry-Thomas sign—see *David Letterman sign.*

Terson syndrome—characterized by vitreous hemorrhage with intracranial hemorrhage. Can include perimacular retinal folds. Previously described only in association with *shaken baby syndrome.*

tertiary contractions—on upper GI series, aberrant contractions of the esophagus, occurring after the primary and secondary waves of normal swallowing.

tertipara—a woman who has given birth three times (para 3).

Terumo dialyzer—for hemodialysis.

Terumo guide wire—used to pass strictures encountered during ERCP.

Terumo SteriCell processor trypan blue—dye exclusion test to measure bone marrow viability.

TES (thoracic endometriosis syndrome).

TES (*Toxocara* excretory secretory) **antigen.**

tesla (T)—SI unit of magnetic strength (used in MRI). The term *gauss* was formerly used.

TeslaScan (mangafodipir trisodium)—hepatocyte-specific MRI contrast medium used for the detection and characterization of liver lesions.

Tesla system—imaging technique that facilitates brain scans on small babies, visualizing structures of the brain that were previously indiscernible.

test or **assay**—a quick-reference list of laboratory, neurologic, orthopedic, and other specialty tests. See also *classification, index, scale, scan, score.*

Access Ostase serum-based
AccuPoint hCG Pregnancy Test Disk
acoustic stimulation
Actalyke activated clotting time (ACT)
Adams
adenovirus
Ad7C cerebrospinal fluid
Advanced Care cholesterol
Affirm one-step pregnancy
Affymetrix GeneChip lab analysis
agarose gel electrophoresis (AGE)
agglutination

test *(cont.)*
air conduction
AlaSTAT latex allergy
Alatest latex-specific IgE allergen
Alberts' Famous Faces Test
Alexagram breast lesion diagnostic
alkaline phosphatase antialkaline
  phosphatase (APAAP) antibody
Allen's circulatory
Allen picture visual acuity
alpha-fetoprotein (AFP)
alpha-2 antiplasmin functional
  assay
alternans noninvasive cardiac
  diagnostic
Amplicor *Chlamydia* Assay
Amplicor CT/NG
Amplicor *Mycobacterium
  tuberculosis*
Amplified *Mycobacterium tuber-
  culosis* Direct (MTD)
Amsler grid
Ana-Sal saliva-based HIV
anticytoplasmic antibody
antiendomysial antibody IgA
Apo E
applanation tonometry
apprehension
Apt-Downey alkali denaturation
arginine tolerance (ATT)
AUA symptom index
auramine-stained buffy coat smear
Autoclix blood glucose
Autolet blood glucose
AutoPap
Aware AccuMeter rapid HIV
BAEP (brain stem auditory evoked
  potential)
BAER (brain stem auditory evoked
  response)
Bang's horseshoe-crab blood
Bard BTA Test
Barlow hip dysplasia
BDProbeTec ET system
Bender Gestalt Test

test *(cont.)*
bentonite flocculation
benzalkonium chloride patch
Berens 3-character (eye)
Berkson-Gage breast cancer
  survival rates
Bielschowsky's head tilt
BiliCheck
Bing auditory acuity
Biocept-5 pregnancy
Biocept-G pregnancy
Bioclot protein S assay
Biosafe PSA4
BioStar strep A 01A
Bladder Tumor Assay
Blessed Information Memory
  Concentration
bone conduction test
Bonney
BRACAnalysis comprehensive gene
  test
branched chain DNA assay
breath hydrogen excretion
breath pentane
Brief Neuropsychological Mental
bronchoprovocation
Bruininks-Oseretsky Test of Motor
  Proficiency
BTA stat Test
buccal smear
buffy coat smear
B-VAT (Baylor Visual Acuity Test)
CA15-3 RIA
"cake mix" kit for hematopoietic
  progenitor assay
caloric test of vestibular function
capillary blood sugar
capillary electrophoresis
carbolfuchsin stain, Tilden's
Cardiac T Rapid Assay
carotid sinus massage
carpal compression
C-cholyl-glycine breath excretion
cell assay
Chemstrip bG

test *(cont.)*

ChemTrak *Helicobacter pylori*
Cherry-Crandall serum lipase
Cholestech LDX system with the
  TC and Glucose Panel
CholesTrak home cholesterol
chromohydrotubation
CIE (countercurrent immunoelectrophoresis)
CIWA-A (Clinical Institute Withdrawal Assessment–Alcohol)
Clancy circumduction-adduction
  shoulder maneuver
clonogenic assay
CLOtest (*Campylobacter*-like
  organism)
coin test
cold water calorics
ColoCARE
colorectal cancer screening
Colorgene DNA Hybridization
complement fixation
concealed straight leg raising
C1q assay
Confide HIV
Copalis ToRC total antibody assay
copper-binding protein (CBP)
corneal impression (CIT)
Coulter HIV-1 p24 antigen assay
cover-uncover
cracker
cribogram
cross-chest adduction
cross-cover
cryocrit
C-terminal assay
CTFC (corrected TIMI frame
  count)
C-urea breath excretion
C-urinary excretion
Cybex
dark-field microscopy
DDT ([fluorescein] dye disappearance test)
Denver Developmental Screening

test *(cont.)*

DFA (direct fluorescent antibody)
Diagnex Blue
digital movement analysis (DMA)
dipyridamole thallium stress
direct fluorescent antibody (DFA)
Directigen latex agglutination
Dix-Hallpike
DNA ploidy analysis
DNA sequencing
Doppler Perfusion Index (DPI)
Downey texture discrimination
DPPC (dipalmitoyl phosphatidyl-
  choline)
Draw-a-Bicycle (DAB)
Draw-a-Flower (DAF)
Draw-a-House (DAH)
Draw-a-Person (DAP)
DR-70 blood
duck waddle
duction
Dunlop synoptophore
Durkan CTS (carpal tunnel syn-
  drome) gauge
dye exclusion
EAST
EIA, EIA-2 (enzyme-linked
  immunoassay)
electrotransfer
ELISA (enzyme-linked immuno-
  sorbent assay)
Ellestad treadmill stress
EMIT (enzyme-multiplication
  immunoassay)
Entero-Test
Envacor
EP (evoked potential)
Equate Legionella water
ER (evoked response)
ergonovine maleate
estrogen receptor
ETCO$_2$
ExacTech blood glucose meter
exercise tolerance
EZ-Screen Profile

test *(cont.)*

fabere
Factor III multimer
factor V Leiden mutation
fadir
Fagan
Farr
Fastex proprioceptive and agility
FDT (fluorescein disappearance)
fecal occult blood (FOBT)
F_ECO_2
FEF_{25-75}
fern
fetal fibronectin (fFN)
Fick cardiac output
finger-to-nose (F to N)
Finkelstein's
Fisher's exact
5'nucleotidase
FlexSure HP (*Helicobacter pylori*)
flocculation flow cytometry
Flu-Glow
FLU-OIA rapid
Fluor-i-Strip
fluorescein dye disappearance (DDT)
fluorescein uptake
fluorescent cytoprint assay
foam stability
Folstein's Mini-Mental Status Test
forced oscillation technique (FOT)
free beta
free PSA (prostate-specific antigen)
free/total PSA (prostate-specific antigen) index
FTA-ABS test (fluorescent treponemal antibody absorption test for syphilis)
Functional Capacity Evaluation (FCE)
Functional Intact Fibrinogen (FiF)
gait and station
galvanic body sway (GBST)
Galveston Orientation and Amnesia Test (GOAT)

test *(cont.)*

Gastroccult
GeneAmp PCR
GenESA System pharmacological stress
GGTP liver function
glabellar tap
glial fibrillary acidic protein (GFAP)
Gluco-Protein
glycosylated hemoglobin
Gomori (or Grocott) methenamine silver (GMS)
gonioscopy
Goodenough
GRASS
Gravindex pregnancy
guaiac
Guthrie LEAP assay
Hallpike caloric stimulation
Hallpike-Dix maneuver
halo
Halstead-Wepman Aphasia Screening Test
Heartscan heart attack prediction
heavy metal screening
heel-to-shin
heelstick hematocrit
Heinz body
Helisal rapid blood
HemaStrip-HIV 1 and 2
hematopoietic progenitor clonogenic assay
Hemoccult Sensa system
Hemoccult II
Hemochron high-dose thrombin time (HiTT)
HemoCue
Heprofile ELISA
HercepTest
Heritage Panel
Herp-Check
High-Risk Hybrid Capture II HPV
histoculture drug response assay (HDRA)

test *(cont.)*

Histoplasma capsulatum polysac-
  charide antigen
HIV phenotype
HIVAGEN
homogeneous gene assay system
horizontal adduction
Hpfast agar gel
H reflex electrodiagnostic
HRL color vision
H-SLAP (human stromelysin aggre-
  gated proteoglycan)
Hybritech Tandem PSA ratio
  (free PSA/total PSA)
Hycor rheumatoid factor (RF) IgA
  ELISA autoimmune
HZA (hermizona)
ice water calorics
I-HAST (In-Home Alzheimer's
  Screening Test)
iliopsoas
immunobead assay
ImmunoCard STAT! Rotavirus
ImmunoCyt
Incomplete Sentence Blank Test
  (ISB)
indirect fluorescent antibody (IFA)
Inform HER-2/neu gene-based
ink potassium hydroxide
Intercept oral fluid drug
intracavernous injection
intraoperative endoscopic
  Congo red
INVOS 2100 breast cancer
Ishihara color vision
islet cell antibodies screening (ICA)
Isletest and Isletest-ICA
Jaeger's
Jamar grip
k82 ImmunoCap blood
KetoSite
Kleihauer-Betke
Kleihauer
Krimsky's
Kruskal-Wallis

test *(cont.)*

Kveim
Lachman
lamellar body number density
Landolt's ring
LAP (leukocyte alkaline
  phosphatase)
latex agglutination
LDL Direct
leucine aminopeptidase
Lezak's Malingering Test
lift-off
ligase chain reaction
Limulus amoebocyte lysate (LAL)
litmus
liver function (LFT)
Liver Panel Plus 9
Lp(a)
LRUT (locally made rapid urease)
Maddox rod
MAIPA (monoclonal-antibody-
  specific immobilization of
  platelet antigens) assay
Mancini plates
Mantoux tuberculosis
Master's two-step
maternal serum alpha-fetoprotein
  (MSAFP)
Matritech NMP22 test for bladder
  cancer
Mayo Clinic system test for
  primary biliary cirrhosis
McNemar's
MCT (Motor Control Test)
mental status
Mentor BVAT
MEP (multimodality evoked
  potential)
MHA-TP (microhemagglutination
  test for Treponema pallidum)
Micral chemstrip
Micral urine dipstick
Microflo test strip for glucose mon-
  itoring
Micro-monitor

test *(cont.)*

    microsomal TRC (tanned red cells)
    Mini-Mental State Examination
       (MMSE)
    Minnesota Multiphasic Personality
       Inventory (MMPI)
    Minnesota Test for Differential
       Diagnosis of Aphasia
    Miraluma
    Mississippi Scale for Combat-
       Related Posttraumatic Stress
       Disorder (PSD)
    Miyazaki-Bonney
    modified rapid urease (RUT)
    Moire topographic assessment
    monoclonal antibody-based enzyme
       immunoassay
    Monojector blood glucose
    Motor Control Test (MCT)
    multiple sleep latency (MSLT)
    MultiVysion PB assay
    MycoAKT latex bead agglutination
       for *Mycobacterium* detection
    Myers-Briggs Personality Inventory
    Nardi (morphine-prostigmine)
    NAT (nucleic acid testing)
    Naughton cardiac exercise treadmill
    Neurobehavioral Cognitive Status
    N-geneous HDL cholesterol
    N High Sensitivity CRP (C-reactive
       protein) assay
    NicCheck-I
    NMP22
    nuclear contour index (NCI) on
       blood lymphocytes
    nucleic acid sequence-based
       amplification assay
    nucleic acid testing (NAT)
    Nymox urinary
    O&P (ova and parasites)
    octopus peripheral vision
    octopus visual field
    Oliver-Rosalki serum CPK
    ophthalmodynamometry
    ophthalmoscopy

test *(cont.)*

    Opus cardiac troponin I assay
    OralScreen 3-panel oral fluids
    OraSure
    OraTest
    Ortho HCV 2.0 ELISA
    osmolality
    Ostase biochemical marker of bone
       turnover
    Osteo-Gram
    Osteomark
    Osteomark NTx Assay
    otoacoustic emission (OAE)
    Ouchterlony double diffuse
    ox cell hemolysin
    oxytocin challenge (OCT)
    pad urinary incontinence
    PainBuster disposable infusion pain
       management kit
    PapNet
    Paragon immunofixation
       electrophoresis
    PASAT (paced auditory serial
       addition task)
    past-pointing
    patellar apprehension
    Pathfinder DFA
    Patrick's (fabere)
    PCR (polymerase chain reaction)
    peak expiratory flow rate (PEFR)
    PEFR (peak expiratory flow rate)
    pentagastrin stimulated analysis
    periodic acid-Schiff (PAS)
    Persantine thallium stress
    Phadiatop
    PharmChek
    PHA skin
    Phalen's
    pilocarpine iontophoresis
    pivot-shift
    Polateset vision
    polymerase chain reaction (PCR)
    positive acetowhite
    posteromedial pivot shift
    PPD skin

test *(cont.)*
  PPL skin
  PRA (plasma renin activity)
  Preadmission Acuity Inquiry (PAI)
    tool
  preimplantation genetic diagnosis
  Premier Type-Specific HSV-1
    ELISA
  Premier Type-Specific HSV-2 IgG
    ELISA
  Preven emergency contraceptive kit
  PreVue Lyme disease
  PRIME-MD (computerized version
    of Primary Care Evaluation of
    Mental Disorders)
  prostate-specific antigen (PSA)
    free/total index
  Protocult
  PSA (prostate-specific antigen)
    index
  PSA4 home blood
  PSY Inventory
  P300 dementia
  Pylori Fiax assay
  Pylori Stat assay
  PyloriTek
  Pyrilinks-D urinary assay
  PYtest
  Q-beta replicase
  QSART (quantitative Sudomotor
    Axon Reflex Test)
  QualiCode *Borrelia burgdorferi* IgG
    and IgM Western blot kits
  Quantiplex HIV RNA assay
  Queckenstedt
  quellung reaction
  Quetelet's BMI index
  QuICCC (Questionnaire for Identi-
    fying Children with Chronic
    Conditions)
  QuickVue *Chlamydia*
  QuickVue influenza
  QuickVue one-step *H. pylori*
  radioallergosorbent (RAST)
  Raji cell assay

test *(cont.)*
  Randot
  Rapid Drug Screen
  rapid plasma reagin (RPR)
  RAPP (Routine Assessment of
    Patient Progress)
  RAST test for measuring atopy
  recombinant immunoblot assay
  refraction
  Reitman-Frankel SGOT and SGPT
  renin
  repair chain reaction
  RET gene
  Rey and Taylor Complex Figure
    Test
  Rey Auditory Verbal Learning Test
  Rhodes Inventory of Nausea and
    Vomiting
  RIGScan CR49 test for colorectal
    cancer detection
  Rinne
  RISA (radioactive iodinated serum
    albumin)
  Roche-Microwell Plate
    Hybridization Method
  roentgen stereophotogrammetric
    analysis (RSA)
  Romberg
  Roos
  Rorschach
  Rotazyme diagnostic
  RPR (rapid plasma reagin)
  RPR-CT (rapid plasma reagin
    circle card test)
  RUT (rapid urease test)
  SalEst system
  Schiller
  Schirmer's
  Schwartz
  scotopic sensitivity screening,
    whole-field
  sed rate (sedimentation rate)
  Seidel
  self-blood glucose monitoring
    (SBGM)

test *(cont.)*

Sensory Organization Test (SOT)
SEP (somatosensory evoked
  potential)
SER (somatosensory evoked
  response)
serum protein electrophoresis
7C Gold urine
Sgambati's test for peritonitis
shake
short wavelength autoperimetry
Sibley-Lehninger serum aldolase
SIBS (social interaction between
  siblings) interview
Sickledex
Sigma CPK
signal amplification technique
simkin analysis
Skindex questionnaire, revised
slit-lamp
slump
SMAC
SMA-6
SMA-12
SMA-18
SMA-20
Snellen chart
sniff
Sonksen-Silver acuity cards
SpectRx
Speed
Stamey
StoneRisk profile
straight leg raising (SLRT)
Stratus cardiac toponin I
streptokinase-streptodornase
  (SK-SD)
Strong-Campbell Vocational Interest
  Inventory (SCVII)
"super stress test"
surf (surfactant)
sweat chloride
tandem mass spectrometry
tanned red cells (TRC)
T-cell function

test *(cont.)*

Teller acuity cards
Tensilon
tenting
Tes-Tape urine glucose
TestPackChlamydia
thallium stress
Thayer-Martin gonorrhea
Thematic Apperception Test (TAT)
ThinPrep and ThinPrep 2000
Thompson
Thorn
Thrombus Precursor Protein (TpP)
thyrocalcitonin for pheochromo-
  cytoma
thyroperioxidase antibody
thyroxine radioisotope assay
  (T_4RIA)
tilt
tine
Titmus
T-lymphocyte subset ratio
Toxocara ELISA
TpP (thrombus precursor protein)
Tracer Blood Glucose
Trail Making Test
treadmill
Triage cardiac system
T.R.U.E. (thin-layer rapid use epi-
  cutaneous) allergen patch
T water fructose intolerance
tyramine test for pheochromo-
  cytoma
tyrosine tolerance
Tzanck
UBT breath
Uni-Gold *H. pylori*
uPM3 urine
upper limb tension (ULTT)
Uricult dipslide
Uriscreen
Urocyte diagnostic cytometry
van den Bergh's
VDRL
Velogene rapid MRSA assay

test *(cont.)*
    Velogene rapid TB assay
    Velogene rapid VRE assay
    VEP (visual evoked potential)
    VER (visual evoked response)
    vertebral artery
    VEX (vasodilator plus exercise)
      treadmill
    ViraPap
    ViraSTAT immunofluorescence
      assay
    Virgo Anti-Cardiolipin screening kit
    Visidex, Visidex II
    visual field
    Visual Neglect
    von Kossa calcium
    Wada
    Weber
    Well-Cogen latex agglutination
    WEST (Weinstein Enhanced
      Sensory Test)
    Westergren sedimentation rate
    Western blot electrotransfer
    Wilcoxon rank sum
    wing
    Wirt stereo
    Wisconsin Card Sorting
    Wood's light
    Worth four-dot (W4D)
    Wroblewski serum LDH
    Yergason
    zona hamster egg
    ZstatFlu

testicular interstitial fluid (TIF).

Testoderm patch—for men with testosterone deficiency.

Testoderm TTS (testosterone transdermal system)—used for the treatment of men with testosterone deficiency. It is a thin, clear patch that can be placed on the arm, back, or upper buttocks and delivers a 5 mg dose of testosterone through the skin over a 24-hour period.

TestPackChlamydia—a quick office test for *Chlamydia* based on enzyme-linked immunosorbent assay. No spaces in trademark.

TET (tubal embryo transfer).

tethered cord syndrome—seen when an area of the spinal cord is firmly caught up in scar tissue or between vertebrae.

tetracycline—a common oral antibiotic that can also be given by intrapleural injection to sclerose lung tissues and reduce the chance of repeat pneumothorax.

tetralogy of Fallot ("fal-lo")—complex of four congenital cardiac anomalies: pulmonary stenosis, ventricular septal defect, dextroposition of the aorta, and right ventricular hypertrophy. Cf. *Fallot's pentalogy, Fallot's trilogy.* See also *pink tetralogy of Fallot.*

Tetrax interactive balance system—used for posturography evaluation of central and peripheral neurologic disturbances.

"tet spell"—medical slang for a "spell typical of tetralogy of Fallot."

Teveten (eprosartan mesylate)—an angiotensin II receptor antagonist used in treatment of hypertension, either alone or in combination with other antihypertensives such as diuretics and calcium channel blockers.

Texas Scottish Rite Hospital (TSRH).

TFC (threaded fusion cage)—see *Ray threaded fusion cage.*

TFC (triangular fibrocartilage).

TFCC (triangular fibrocartilaginous complex)—a structure in the wrist that may exhibit thinning in patients with gymnast's wrist.

TFD (tight fingertip dilated)—as in "The cervical os was TFD."

TFL (tensor fasciae latae).

T-4 cell—the cell specifically attacked by the HIV virus. Called helper/inducer T-cell.

T4, soluble recombinant human—a drug used to treat HIV-positive patients.

TFPI (tissue factor pathway inhibitor).

TGA (transposition of the great arteries).

TGF-B (transforming growth factor-beta)—a protein found to promote bone healing and now used in treatment of nonunion of fractures, as a bone graft material, and to promote ingrowth of tissue into a hip prosthesis.

TGF-Beta 3—used for the treatment of oral mucositis.

T-graft configuration technique—a new technique in coronary artery bypass graft surgery using arteries from both the arm and chest to form a T-shaped conduit around the diseased portions of the heart. It is said to offer patients hope for longer-lasting bypasses with reduced chances for postoperative infections.

THA (total hip arthroplasty).

ThAIRapy Vest—portable device that utilizes high-frequency chest wall oscillation (HFCWO) to provide airway clearance. The vest is linked to an air pulse generator which inflates and deflates the vest from 5 to 25 times per second, gently squeezing the thorax and creating high expiratory air flow within the lungs, moving mucus toward the larger airways for clearance by coughing. See also *ABI Vest Airway Clearance System.*

thalidomide (Thalomid).

thallium SPECT (thallium 201 single-photon emission computed tomographic) **imaging**—evaluates the presence and extent of myocardial perfusion defect. Also used in stroke and other neurological assessment.

thallium stress test—used to reveal the presence and extent of coronary artery disease by comparing blood flow in the heart during treadmill exercise with the blood flow at rest. Thallium is taken up by the heart in direct proportion to the blood flow, and images of areas of the heart showing thallium retention delineate the areas of arterial blockage. The radioisotope used is thallium 201 (Tl-201).

Thalomid (thalidomide)—recently approved by FDA for treatment of debilitating and disfiguring lesions associated with erythema nodosum leprosum (ENL), a complication of Hansen's disease (leprosy). Used to counteract weight loss in AIDS patients.

Thal repair of esophageal stricture.

Thayer-Martin culture medium—used in testing for *Neisseria gonorrhoeae*.

THC:YAG laser (thulium, holmium, chromium: YAG crystal)—performs a sclerostomy to reduce intraocular pressure in uncontrolled glaucoma.

THE (transhepatic embolization).

theca cell—found in the ovary after ovulation, derived from nurse cells surrounding the developing egg.

theca lutein cyst (of the ovary)—caused by high HCG (human chorionic gonadotropin) levels in molar pregnancies.

The Closer—provides minimally invasive closure of an arterial access site in the femoral artery following a diagnostic procedure such as coronary angiography.

thelarche—the beginning of breast development.

Thematic Apperception Test (TAT)—mental status examination.

Theochron (theophylline)—trade name for extended release theophylline.

Therabite jaw motion rehabilitation system—a device designed for patients with reduced jaw movement or jaw hypomobility following surgery and/or radiation treatment. It helps patients open their mouths, encourages healing, improves speech, and promotes better oral hygiene.

Thera-Boot compression dressing or wrap.

Thera Cool cold therapy—used to treat postoperative pain and swelling as well as during rehabilitation.

TheraCys (BCG live intravesical)—injected directly into the bladder to treat patients with recurrent bladder tumors. Contains an attenuated strain of *Mycobacterium* known as bacillus Calmette-Guérin (BCG), after the two French bacteriologists, Albert Calmette and Camille Guérin, who first weakened the bacillus through many series of cultures.

Theradigm-HBV (hepatitis B virus).

Theradigm-HPV—for treatment of cervical cancer associated with human papilloma virus (HPV).

Therafectin (amiprilose HCl)—an oral drug for the treatment of rheumatoid arthritis.

TheraGym exercise balls—used for improving gross motor control, range of motion, muscle tone, and balance by both pediatric and adult orthopedic patients.

therapy—see *operation*.

TheraSeed—an alternative permanent implant with a 17-day half-life. A palladium 103 (Pd-103) active isotope in a titanium capsule, it is used in the treatment of rapidly growing tumors.

Thera-Soft hand/wrist orthosis—used for wrist drop and finger contraction.

TheraSphere—nonsurgical outpatient therapy that uses microscopic glass beads to deliver radiation therapy treatment for inoperable hepatocellular carcinoma.

Theratope-STn—a synthetic therapeutic cancer vaccine that stimulates the patient's immune system to fight disease.

Therex—based on the humanized monoclonal antibody huHMFG1, which targets most common epithelial cancers, including breast, lung, ovarian, gastric, and colorectal.

ThermaChoice uterine balloon therapy—treatment for excessive menstrual bleeding. It can be performed on an outpatient basis under local anesthesia. A balloon catheter is inserted vaginally and inflated with a small amount of sterile fluid, after which a heating element inside the balloon raises the temperature to approximately 87° Celsius for a total of 8 minutes. The result is thermal ablation of the uterine lining.

Therma Jaw (or Thermajaw) **hot urologic forceps**—allows simultaneous tissue sampling and electrocoagulation of a biopsy site, eliminating the need for exchange of instruments through a flexible cystoscope.

thermal quenching—a cooling technique that protects the skin during laser treatments for hair removal or vascular lesions.

thermistor—a type of thermometer that registers very small changes in temperature. "Respiratory parameters were monitored by nasal and oral thermistor and abdominal and chest wall strain gauges."

thermistor-plethysmography (Cardio).

ThermoChem-HT system—used in intraperitoneal hyperthermic chemotherapy (IPHC). It heats fluids (chemotherapy agents) and recirculates them into the peritoneal cavity to treat GI and other cancers within the peritoneal cavity.

thermodilution catheter—specially designed, triple-lumen Swan-Ganz catheter. One lumen is used to inject a cold solution to measure cardiac output. See *thermodilution technique*.

thermodilution technique—to obtain numerical values to calculate cardiac output. Following injection of a cold solution (saline, 5% dextrose in water, or autologous blood) into the right atrium, a change in temperature of the circulating blood can be detected by a temperature-sensitive catheter in the pulmonary artery.

Thermoflex system—a water-induced thermotherapy (WIT) system for the treatment of benign prostatic hyperplasia and associated urinary obstruction.

Thermophore—moist heat pads for external application of heat, to relieve pain.

Thermoscan Pro-1-Instant thermometer—able to obtain a reading in just two seconds using infrared technology. Using a special speculum which fits into the ear canal, the thermometer accurately reflects the body core temperature because of its closeness to the tympanic membrane. An aural temperature reading is unlike oral readings which can be affected by eating, drinking, or smoking.

Thermoskin arthritic knee wrap—a heat retainer with a Trioxon lining used to help ease the pain and discomfort of arthritis sufferers. The heat retainers are also available for the back, hand/wrist, ankle, and elbow areas.

Thermo-STAT—a new armcuff device that speeds delivery of heat to the heart and internal organs of patients who develop hypothermia during surgery.

TherOx 0.014 infusion guide wire—used primarily in percutaneous transluminal coronary angioplasty (PTCA). It also provides site-specific delivery of drugs or fluids into the coronary arteries.

The Sensar—foldable acrylic posterior chamber intraocular lens. The Sensar is delivered into the eye through The Unfolder.

The Unfolder—intraocular lens (IOL) implantation system used to deliver The Sensar foldable acrylic posterior chamber IOL.

THI needle—used in cardiac surgery to express air from the ventricle.

thianamycin—an antibiotic.

Thiersch-Duplay urethroplasty.

Thiersch graft—a delayed pedicle skin graft.

Thiersch suture.

thigh-high antiembolic stockings—see *stockings*.

thin-layer chromatography screen—an analytic technique used to screen serum or urine samples for poisons or drugs of abuse.

ThinLine EZ—a bipolar cardiac pacing lead.

ThinPrep and **ThinPrep 2000**—screening test for cervical cancer, which may replace the conventional Pap smear. The FDA supports the claim that ThinPrep improves the detection of low-grade lesions by 65% and reduces the number of inadequate

ThinPrep *(cont.)*
specimens by more than 50%. It assures uniformity of slide samples.

THINSite dressing—multilayer dressing that has an extremely low profile and will conform to almost any body contour.

THINSite with BioFilm—hydrogel topical wound dressing used to treat pressure ulcers, arterial and venous stasis ulcers, and dermal wounds.

thiopental sodium—general anesthetic agent.

Thioplex (thiotepa).

thiotepa (Thioplex)—an antineoplastic palliative drug used particularly in cases of papillary carcinoma of the urinary bladder, adenocarcinoma of the breast, and adenocarcinoma of the ovary.

third intercondylar tubercle of Parsons (TITP)—frequent and prominent in patients with osteoarthritis of the medial FTJ (femorotibial joints) and prominent tibial spines. TITP is also known as *Parsons knob* or *Parsons tubercle*, depending on size.

third spacing—movement of fluids in the body into the third space (not the vascular space, in the blood vessels, and not inside cells, in the intracellular space). This interstitial fluid can be in one organ or systemic, and can be caused by lymphatic blockage, increased capillary permeability, or lowered plasma proteins.

13-cis-retinoic acid, 13-CRA—see *isotretinoin*.

13q deletion syndrome (46 Dr or 46 Dq)—due to a deletion of the long arms of chromosome 13 (one of the group D chromosomes). The syndrome may include mental retardation and physical retardation, broad nasal bridge, large and prominent low-set ears, facial asymmetry, hypertelorism, ptosis, epicanthus, microcephaly, microphthalmia, imperforate anus, and a number of other anomalies.

Thomas needle—used for bone marrow biopsy and aspiration.

Thomas shunt—vascular access shunt used in performing dialysis.

Thomas splint.

Thom flap—laryngeal reconstruction.

Thompson test—"The Achilles tendon is intact by Thompson test." With the foot at rest, compression of the calf (gastrocnemius) muscle causes ankle flexion if the Achilles tendon is intact.

thoracic duct drainage (TDD)—being evaluated as an adjunct to classical immunosuppression (preoperatively) in the prevention of early rejection of organ transplants.

thoracic endometriosis syndrome (TES)—deposition of endometrial tissue in the pleuropulmonary organs. There is a significant association between the presence of pelvic endometriosis and TES. Chest pain is the presenting symptom, and pneumothorax is the most common manifestation.

thoracic OPLL (ossification of the posterior longitudinal ligament)—a rare entity causing thoracic myelopathy. One of the well-known causes of cervical radiculomyelopathy.

thoracic splenosis—a rarely encountered condition, consisting of multiple pleural-based nodules that are most often identified accidentally on routine chest x-rays. The splenic nodules may mimic neoplasms radiographically.

thoracolumbar "burst" fractures (Ortho).

thoracolumbosacral (TLSO) **brace**.

thoracophrenolaparotomy—minimally invasive surgery involving entry into the thorax and abdomen around the diaphragm.

Thoralon—biomaterial used in Aria coronary artery bypass graft for patients with few or no suitable native vessels.

Thora-Port—used for safe insertion of thoracoscopic instruments.

thorascopic apical pleurectomy—for treatment of SBSP (simultaneous bilateral spontaneous pneumothorax).

thorascopic talc pleurodesis—performed under local anesthesia for treatment of SBSP (simultaneous bilateral spontaneous pneumothorax).

Thoratec ventricular assist device (VAD)—provides mechanical circulatory support via left or right ventricle or both. The patient's blood is diverted from the failing ventricle into the assist device, which pumps the blood back to the body, simulating the function of the heart. Two blood-pumping sacs, one for each side of the heart, are attached to the body and tethered to a machine the size of a ventilator. This is not a permanent solution; what it does is "buy time" until the heart recovers (if it can) or until a suitable donor heart becomes available.

Thorel's bundle—a bundle of muscle fibers in the heart that connects the sinoatrial and atrioventricular nodes.

Thorn test—a test of uric acid excretion, and also a test to help in the diagnosis of Addison's disease.

Thornton double corneal ruler (Oph).

Thornton 360° arcuate marker—used during corneal surgery and during keratotomy for astigmatism.

Thornwaldt cyst (also, *Tornwaldt*)—can be seen on CT scan as a mass high in the nasopharynx, midline between the longus capitis muscles, or just off midline. It may contain only fluid, but sometimes there is a calcification within it.

THORP (titanium hollow-screw osseointegrating reconstruction plate) **system**—screws and plates for alloplastic mandibular reconstruction.

THR (total hip replacement).

threaded interbody fusion cage—hollow cylinder packed with bone graft material and implanted between the vertebrae to facilitate spinal fusion.

threadwire saw—a new device for cutting bone.

3DCE (three-dimensional contrast-enhanced) **magnetic resonance angiography technique** using MR fluoroscopy and 3-D spiral recording of data acquisition—MRI term.

3DFT (three-dimensional Fourier transform)—a less frequently used image reconstruction process in MRI than 2DFT.

3DFT magnetic resonance angiography—noninvasive vascular imaging technique.

3-D gadolinium-enhanced MR angiography—for aortoiliac inflow assessment plus renal artery screening.

3-D IVUS (three-dimensional intravascular ultrasound).

3-D-MSI (magnetic source imaging).

3-Dscope—three-dimensional laparoscope said to cut operative time for complicated laparoscopic procedures by adding the third dimension of depth perception.

3-D SSP (3-D stereotaxic surface projection).

3-D time of flight magnetic resonance angiographic sequences (3DTOF MR angiographic sequences).

3-D TurboFLAIR (fluid-attenuated inversion recovery)—MRI technique that allows for better visualization of tissue structures because the imaging passes are actually interleaved rather than stacked.

3M Clean Seals—a waterproof protection bandage.

3M syndrome—named for last initials of three researchers (J.D. Miller, V.A. McKusick, P. Malvaux) who were among the first to identify the disorder, characterized by low birth weight, dwarfism, abnormalities of the craniofacial area, distinctive skeletal malformations, and/or other physical abnormalities. It is thought to be inherited as an autosomal recessive genetic trait.

three-pillow or **two-pillow orthopnea** —refers to the number of pillows a patient must use to prop up in bed in order to sleep comfortably without difficulty breathing.

3-prong (or three-prong) **rake blade**—a self-retaining retractor blade.

3-Scape real-time 3D imaging—used with Sonoline Elegra ultrasound platform to improve detection and characterization of organ tumors.

thromboelastograph (TEG)—used to confirm coagulopathy such as that which occurs during liver resection. This allows for rapid diagnosis and institution of proper hemostatic treatment for platelet and coagulation factor abnormalities.

thromboembolic disease (TED).

thrombolytic assessment system (TAS) —a system about the size of a desktop calculator. It uses a disposable cord with a test well for a single drop of blood to perform coagulation studies. The card is encoded with the patient's ID number and the coagulation study results. It can also be linked to printers and computers for archiving and future retrieval.

ThromboScan MRU (molecular recognition units)—imaging agent combined with molecular recognition units to produce better scans.

thrombosis—formation or presence of thrombus. See *central splanchnic venous thrombosis* (CSVT); *deep venous thrombosis* (DVT)

ThromboSol—extends the shelf-life of transfusable platelets.

thrombotic thrombocytopenic purpura (TTP)—complication in AIDS patients.

thromboxanes (TxA_1 and TxB_2)—stimulators of platelet aggregation.

thrombus—a clot in the cardiovascular system. See also *thrombosis*.

Thrombus Precursor Protein (TpP)—test for early diagnosis of preeclampsia. Women with preeclampsia have lower levels of TpP in the second trimester, prior to onset of clinical manifestations.

thulium–holmium–chromium:YAG laser (THC:YAG laser).

thumb, gamekeeper's.

thumbprinting (Radiol)—indentations that look like thumbprints, seen radiographically on the surface of the colon in a barium enema. They are indicative of ischemic colitis or of hematoma formation on the bowel wall.

ThumZ'Up—a functional thumb splint consisting of a clear plastic shield over the base of the thumb and an elastic bandage that encircles the wrist and base of thumb. The splint holds the thumb in an upright position, such as when you give the "thumbs up" sign, hence the name. (Note apostrophe in trade name.)

thunderclap headache—a sudden, extremely painful, high-intensity headache (not migraine, tension, or cluster headache). The name is very descriptive. May indicate a brain aneurysm and impending rupture.

Thunder God vine—ancient Chinese remedy under study for its ability to block inflammation in rheumatoid arthritis. Using a very precise molecular target, the herb affects only the inflammation and has very few side effects.

thymic humoral factor—a drug for HIV-positive patients.

thymidine deoxyriboside (TDR)—chemotherapy drug.

Thymoglobulin (antithymocyte globulin [rabbit])—immunosuppressive antibody that can prevent organ loss for kidney transplant recipients.

thymopentin (Timunox)—a drug for HIV-positive patients.

thymostimuline (TP-1)—drug used to treat patients with AIDS.

thyrocalcitonin—test for pheochromocytoma.

Thyrogyn (thyrotropin alfa)—a monoclonal antibody-based therapy used for the treatment of ovarian cancer. May be used for the treatment of gastric cancer.

thyroid stare—see *Collier's sign.*

thyroid storm—episode of heightened thyroid hormone activity due to sudden release of an abnormal amount of hormone into the circulation. A thyroid storm may be induced by stress or infection, or it may occur spontaneously. Symptoms are anxiety, rapid pulse, fear, high fever, restlessness, breathing problems, exhaustion. In severe cases, which may prove fatal, the patient may be delirious and then become comatose. Also, *thyroid crisis.*

thyroperoxidase (TPO)—a thyroid enzyme, present in over 95% of patients with malignant thyroid tumors.

thyroperoxidase antibody test—for thyroid disease.

thyroplasty type I (also called laryngoplasty) (ENT)—used in treatment of unilateral vocal cord paralysis with resulting hoarseness or inaudibility. It involves placing a silicone implant through a "window" made in the thyroid cartilage. The implant pushes the paralyzed vocal cord medially to meet the functioning (moving) cord. The operation is performed under local anesthesia so the patient can phonate during the course of the procedure, and the surgeon can evaluate the quality of the patient's voice and assess the movement of the vocal cords. Thyroplasty types II and III are used to change tension of the vocal cord and the pitch of the voice. These are new procedures. The procedure previously in general use, the injection of Teflon into the vocal cord, is said to still be the treatment of choice for some debilitated or elderly people, but one of its disadvantages is that Teflon has been known to "migrate" and cannot easily be removed.

thyroxine radioisotope assay (T_4RIA).

TI (inversion time)—MRI term.

TIA (transient ischemic attack)—cerebrovascular occlusion, in which the symptoms resolve within 24 hours. Cf. *CVA.*

tiagabine (Gabitril)—add-on therapy used in the treatment of partial-seizure epilepsy.

Tiazac (diltiazem)—a once-daily coronary vasodilator, or calcium channel blocker, used to treat hypertension.

tibial plateau—a flattened surface at the upper end of the anterior aspect of the tibia.

tic—involuntary repetitive muscle movement. See *Tourette's syndrome and Gilles de la Tourette's syndrome*. Cf. *tick*.

Tice (intravesical BCG)—immunizing agent for tuberculosis; antineoplastic used to treat bladder carcinoma.

tick—a small bloodsucking arthropod; the lesion produced by its bite may cause anything from a small papule to a large ulcerating wound, with acute pain and swelling. See *Lyme disease*, which is transmitted by the deer tick. Cf. *tic*.

Ticlid (ticlopidine).

ticlopidine (Ticlid)—a drug used to prevent initial and recurrent strokes in patients with transient ischemic attacks. Because it causes neutropenia and agranulocytosis, it is used only in patients who cannot tolerate aspirin therapy.

Ti-Cron—see *Tycron*.

tidal volume—the amount of air exchanged with each breath. A respiratory response to exercise.

Tielle absorptive dressing.

Tiemann Meals tenolysis knife.

tiered-therapy programmable cardioverter-defibrillator (PCD).

"tie-sis"—see *phthisis*.

TIF (testicular interstitial fluid).

TIFF (tag image file format)—computer graphics format used in teleradiology.

tight asthmatic—an asthmatic with extreme difficulty breathing, that is, with extreme bronchospasm. "Examination revealed a very tight asthmatic, using accessory muscles, and breathing at 28. He had tight inspiratory and expiratory wheezing."

tight fingertip dilated (TFD).

Tikhoff-Linberg shoulder resection—used in bone and soft tissue sarcomas of proximal upper limb that do not involve nearby neurovascular structures. Resection includes distal clavicle, proximal humerus, and part or all of scapula, as well as adjacent muscles, while preserving the function of the forearm and hand. A skeletal prosthesis is used to preserve limb length and stabilize the arm to the chest. A TRAM (transverse rectus abdominis myocutaneous) flap may be used to ensure wound healing.

TIL (tumor-infiltrating lymphocytes).

Tilade (nedocromil sodium)—inhaled drug for reversible obstructive airway disease.

Tillaux-Phocas syndrome—see *fibrocystic breast syndrome*.

tilt-table test (Cardio)—a test to identify and counsel patients who are likely to experience recurrent syncope. The patient is restrained on an electric tilt table. The table is tilted to a head-up position, an I.V. infusion of isoproterenol given, and the test is concluded at the end of a 10-minute head-up tilt or when the patient faints.

tilt test—a commonly used clinical tool for assessment of volume status with orthostatic change in pulse and blood pressure. It is particularly valuable in evaluating patients with hemorrhage, diarrhea, vomiting, and increased insensible fluid losses.

time
  acquisition
  activated coagulation (ACT)
  Duke bleeding
  echo (TE)
  interpulse
  inversion (TI)

time *(cont.)*
  Ivy bleeding
  relaxation
  repetition (TR)
  tincture of (TOT)
time-of-flight echoplanar imaging
  (MRI term)—venous occlusion of
  the structure in question is carried
  out and released to augment blood
  flow and enhance visualization.
time-resolved imaging by automatic
  data segmentation (TRIADS).
TiMesh—titanium mesh bone-plate and
  screw system used for rigid fixation
  of bone fractures.
TIMI (thrombolysis in myocardial infarction).
Timoptic Ocumeter—single-dose eye
  drops for glaucoma.
Timoptic XE (timolol)—an ophthalmic
  gel formulation of this drug used to
  treat glaucoma and previously administered as drops.
Timunox (thymopentin)—a drug used
  to treat HIV-positive patients.
tincture of time (TOT)—as in "Given
  tincture of time, we may soon see a
  resolution of his symptoms." It's a
  physician's way of saying, "Let's
  just wait a bit and see if it doesn't
  clear up on its own." Physicians say
  that aggressive treatment may cure
  only a small number of illnesses,
  and that tincture of time (watchful
  waiting) cures a large proportion of
  curable illnesses.
Tinel's sign—positive if there is tingling
  and numbness at the distal end of a
  limb when percussion is performed
  over the site of a divided nerve. The
  fact that there is some sensation indicates that the nerve has not been
  completely divided, or that there is
  some regeneration of the nerve.

tine test—a tuberculin skin test in which
  a multiple-puncture device is used.
  The blades resemble the tines of a
  fork, hence the name. Not as reliable
  as the Mantoux test, but a good mass
  screening test.
tin-mesoporphyrin—see *SnMP.*
tioconazole (Vagistat)—antifungal vaginal ointment.
TIPS (transjugular intrahepatic portosystemic) **shunt**—a procedure for
  treatment of gastric antral vascular
  ectasia with portal hypertension.
tirofiban (Aggrastat)—a nonpeptide
  platelet IIb/IIIa receptor antagonist;
  platelet aggregation inhibitor for
  acute coronary syndrome, unstable
  angina, myocardial infarction, and
  cardiac surgery.
Tischler cervical biopsy punch forceps.
Tis disease—carcinoma (tumor) in situ
  of the bladder.
Tisseel—"surgical glue" made from
  two naturally occurring compounds
  derived from human blood: fibrinogen (a human blood protein) and
  thrombin (an enzyme). The product
  works by forming a flexible material
  that can stop oozing from small,
  sometimes inaccessible blood vessels during surgery when conventional surgical techniques are not
  feasible.
tissue engineering—creation of tissues
  that can be used to augment a normal tissue, replace abnormal tissue,
  or stimulate the development of normal tissue. New tissue engineering
  technologies are utilizing live cells to
  help heal chronic wounds.
tissue factor pathway inhibitor—important in the coagulation process.
tissue glue or solder—see *protein solder.*

tissue morcellator—instrument used to reduce large organs or tissue masses (enclosed in a specially designed bag) to small pieces for removal through the small incisions created for minimally invasive surgery, such as laparoscopy. Cf. *morselize*.

tissue plasminogen activator (t-PA).

tissue-selective estrogens (Ob-Gyn)—show promise as treatment of osteoporosis in postmenopausal women.

Titanium VasPort (Cardio)—an implantable vascular access device.

titer
anti-RHO-D
antistreptolysin (AST)
antiteichoic acid
HI (hemagglutination inhibition)
microsomal TRC antibody
TRC (tanned red cells) antibody

Titmus test—for stereo acuity. The test pattern can be seen in three dimensions only when both eyes are working together. Cf. *litmus test*.

TITP (third intercondylar tubercle of Parsons).

TI-23—a cytomegalovirus monoclonal antibody used to treat CMV retinitis.

t.i.w.—three times a week.

TJF-100 Olympus endoscope with reusable biopsy channel caps.

TKA (total knee arthroplasty).

TKO-type I.V. (to keep open [the vein])—intravenous infusion given as slowly as possible to keep the blood from clotting in the needle, but not to give the patient significant fluid volume. Also, *KVO-type I.V.* (keep vein open).

TL-90 (Ethicon) **stapler**—used in hepatic resection to minimize the blood loss from the cut surface of the liver as well as time consumed for the procedure. Livers from adults (par-

ents, for example) must be cut down to fit children.

TLC (total lymphocyte count).

TLC (triple-lumen catheter).

TLC G-65 (gentamicin liposome)—a drug used to treat MAI infections in AIDS patients.

T-lens—therapeutic contact lens.

TLI (total lymphoid irradiation)—used previously for cancer, now used with organ transplant patients to suppress T cells and decrease organ rejection. It may even allow transplant patients to avoid taking immunosuppressive drugs.

TLSO (thoracolumbosacral orthosis)—a semirigid plastic jacket (brace) used to treat scoliosis in children. The jacket is worn during the years of growth to prevent or slow further progression of the curve beyond 30°.

T-lymphocyte subset ratio—used to measure an AIDS drug's ability to improve immune function.

TMA (transmetatarsal amputation).

TMA (trimethylamine).

"T-max"—slang for temperature maximum, the highest recorded temperature.

TMJ (temporomandibular joint).

TMJ fossa-eminence prosthesis—used to treat internal derangement, adhesions, perforations, and ankylosis of the temporomandibular joint.

TMP-SMZ (trimethoprim-sulfamethoxazole) (Bactrim, Septra)—antibiotic often used in treating the first episode of *Pneumocystis carinii* pneumonia.

TMR (transmyocardial revascularization)—a holmium laser procedure performed on the beating heart to create pathways within the heart muscle.

TMST (treadmill stress test).

TMS 3-dimensional radiation therapy treatment planning system—provides extremely accurate information allowing for precise delivery of the radiation treatment plan.

TNB (transthoracic needle biopsy).

TNB (Tru-Cut needle biopsy).

TNF (tumor necrosis factor)—a chemical toxin released from a gene (introduced by genetic engineering into human white blood cells) and toxic to malignant tumors. Therapy currently used to treat patients with malignant melanoma. Certain white blood cells known as tumor-infiltrating lymphocytes (TIL), which the body naturally produces to fight malignancies, are removed from the patient's body and genetically altered to include the gene that produces tumor necrosis factor. These cells are then given back to the patient. They migrate to the tumor site and begin manufacturing TNF.

TNK-tPA—a second-generation tissue plasminogen activator (t-PA). Note: While *t-PA* (with the hyphen) is preferred, Genentech, the manufacturer, specifically left out the hyphen in the drug name, perhaps to avoid a double hyphen.

TNM classification of malignant tumors: *T* represents the size of the tumor, *N* the clinical status of the nodes, and *M* metastasis.

T1   Direct extension of primary tumor.

T2   Direct extension of primary tumor to specific organs.

T3   Direct advanced extension of tumor, unresectable.

TX   Direct extension of tumor not assessed.

N0   Regional lymph nodes not involved.

TNM *(cont.)*

N1   Regional lymph nodes involved.

NX   Regional lymph nodes not assessed.

M0   No distant metastases.

M1   Distant metastases present.

MX   Distant metastases not assessed.

Stage I, T1-2, N0, M0—No extension or node involvement.

Stage II, T3, N0, M0—Advanced extension, unresectable.

Stage III, T1-3, N1, M0—Node involvement.

Stage IV, T1-3, N0-1, M1—Distant metastases present.

TNMES (transcutaneous neuromuscular electrical stimulation).

tNOX (quinol oxidase)—an overactive form of an enzyme known as *NOX*. The NOX enzyme is found on the surface of cells and plays a key role in growth of both normal and cancerous cells. Green tea has been found to inhibit the activity of this enzyme.

TNP-470—a fungus-derived drug inhibitor of angiogenesis. It shows promise in investigational treatment of glioblastoma, the most malignant primary brain tumor, as it appears not to have a toxic systemic effect.

Tobi (tobramycin solution for inhalation)—used in the management of cystic fibrosis (CF) patients with *Pseudomonas aeruginosa.*

toborinone—intravenous drug which strengthens the ability of the heart to contract; does not increase the rate of contractions, as vesnarinone does. See *vesnarinone.*

TobraDex (tobramycin, dexamethasone) **ophthalmic suspension, ointment**—combination antibiotic and steroid for topical ophthalmic use.

Todd-Wells guide—used in stereotaxic procedures. Cf. *BRW CT stereotaxic guide*.

toe–in gait—in ambulatory children with congenital clubfeet.

toeing in, toeing out—turning the forefoot in or out in walking.

toe–out gait.

toe–to–hand transfer and **foot-to-hand transfer**—the transplantation of toes to the hand to replace traumatically amputated or congenitally absent digits (e.g., great toe may be transplanted to thumb position).

TOF (time-of-flight) MR angiography.

togavirus—a subgroup of arboviruses (arthropod-borne viruses) that includes viruses carried by mosquitoes and ticks. The togavirus is so-called because it wears a covering (or toga) and is the cause of hemorrhagic fever.

tokos or **tocos**—slang terms for tokodynamometer, a uterine contraction monitoring device. Cf. *Tokos*.

Tokos—former name of Matria, a company that provides remote electronic uterine contraction monitoring services. Cf. *tokos*.

Toldt ligament; **line of Toldt**—see *white line of Toldt*.

tolerogen—a substance that the immune system recognizes as "self," and not a foreign substance. Tolerogens are made by chemically linking fragments of DNA with specific protein molecules which the body already recognizes as "self." Tolerogens have potential in the control of autoimmune diseases such as systemic lupus erythematosus, rheumatoid arthritis, myasthenia gravis, etc.

Tolosa-Hunt syndrome—painful ophthalmoplegia.

tolrestat (Alredase) (Oph)—reduces the complications of diabetes, reducing the cellular damage caused by long-standing insulin-dependent diabetes, especially diabetic neuropathy and retinopathy.

toluidine blue stain.

Tom Jones closure—heavy retention suture closing all layers together (instead of in separate layers) except for the skin.

tomodensitometric examination, abdominal—to measure tissue densities. A technique that might be used to diagnose pheochromocytoma (in an unusual location).

tomography

ACAT (automated computerized axial tomography)

cine CT (computed tomography)

computed (CT)

computed tomographic angiography (CTA)

computed tomography laser mammography (CTLM)

computed tomography angiographic portography (CTAP)

computed tomography laser mammography (CTLM)

computerized axial (CAT)

dynamic computerized

electron beam computed

electron beam (EBT)

FDG (18-fluorodeoxyglucose) positron emission

optical coherence (OCT)

PET with 3-D SSP (positron emission tomography with 3D stereotaxic surface projection)

positron emission (PET)

quantitative computed (QCT)

single photon emission computed (SPECT)

SOMATOM Volume Zoom

tomography *(cont.)*
  spiral x-ray computed (SXCT)
  ultrafast CT electron beam
  ultrasonic
Tomudex (raltitrexed)—a drug used to treat advanced cancer, particularly colorectal cancer.
T1—the time it takes for protons to return to their orientation to a static magnetic field after an excitation pulse (MRI term).
T1FS (T1-weighted fat-suppressed) **images** (MRI term).
T1-weighted fat-suppressed gadolinium-enhanced SE images—MRI term.
T1-weighted gadolinium-enhanced SE images—MRI term.
T1-weighted image—a spin-echo image generated by a pulse sequence using a short repetition time (0.6 seconds or less) (MRI term). Also called *"short TR/TE."*
tonic-clonic seizure—the newer name for *grand mal seizure.*
tonometry (*not* tenometry) (Oph)—measurement of intraocular pressure in the diagnosis of glaucoma. See *applanation tonometry, Schiötz tonometry.*
Tono-Pen tonometer (Oph)—used in measuring intraocular pressure.
tonsil channeling—creation of channels in the tonsils using Coblation Channeling technique as a debulking procedure.
Toomey syringe kit—designed to reduce cross-contamination in office aspiration procedures.
tooth and nail syndrome—ectodermal disorder in which certain primary teeth and/or several secondary teeth may either be absent or widely spaced and misshapen. Certain nails may be absent at birth and then grow

extremely slowly, particularly during the first two to three years of life. The toenails are usually more severely affected than the fingernails. It is inherited as an autosomal dominant genetic trait.
Topamax (topiramate)—antiseizure medication for adults with epilepsy. It is also used for add-on therapy in pediatric patients from 2 to 16 years of age who suffer from uncontrolled partial seizures; for treatment of bipolar disorder; and for migraine headaches.
Topaz CO_2 laser—used in skin rejuvenation procedures.
Topel knot—a twist knot designed for laparoscopic procedures. See also *Aberdeen knot, convertible slip knot.*
Top-Hat supra-annular aortic valve.
Topiglan—alprostadil topical gel used as therapy for erectile dysfunction.
topodermatography—an imaging technique used to identify and evaluate changes of cutaneous lesions in melanoma screening or follow-up of cancer patients.
topotecan (Hycamptin)—used to treat advanced carcinoma of the pancreas, prostate, stomach, or head and neck, and also small cell lung carcinoma, but not leukemia. Previously known as hycamptamine.
Toprol XL (metoprolol succinate).
Toradol (ketorolac tromethamine).
"tor-a-fur"—see *ftorafur.*
TORCH screening (titer)—acronym
  T toxoplasmosis
  O other
  R rubella
  C cytomegalic inclusion disease
  H herpes
    Also:
  TO toxoplasmosis
  R rubella
  C cytomegalovirus infections
  H congenital herpes

Toric intraocular lens—a foldable lens used in cataract surgery that corrects preexisting astigmatism.

Torkildsen shunt procedure—ventriculocisternostomy.

Tornwaldt bursitis.

Tornwaldt (Thornwaldt) **cyst** (ENT)—can be seen on CT scan as a mass high in the nasopharynx, midline between the longus capitis muscles, or just off midline. It may contain only fluid, but sometimes there is a calcification within it.

Toronto parapodium—has one lock for both hip and knee joints. Orthosis for ambulation in children with cerebral palsy and myelomeningocele.

Toronto SPV valve—a stentless porcine heart valve entirely supported by the patient's aorta. Without a stent apparatus to occupy space, larger heart valves can be implanted, thus improving blood flow.

TORP (total ossicular replacement prosthesis)—in otological surgery.

torr—a unit of measurement that relates to pressure in the patient in neurosurgery, when hypothermia and hypotension are used: "The pressure was kept at 70 torr and then dropped to 60 torr."

torsades de pointes ("tor-sahd´duh pwahnt") (Fr., fringe of pointed tips) —very rapid ventricular tachycardia in which there is waxing and waning of amplitudes in the QRS complexes as seen on the electrocardiogram. It could be self-limiting or go on to ventricular fibrillation. *Torsades de pointes* refers to the twisting, torsion, or waving of points in the appearance of the ECG tracing.

torsemide (Demadex, Presaril)—a diuretic to treat hypertension or relieve the edema associated with conges-

tive heart failure or renal or liver disease.

Torula histolytica—the cause of torulosis, the old name for cryptococcosis.

Tostrex—transdermal testosterone gel for treatment of male hypogonadism.

TOT (tincture of time).

total abdominal evisceration (TAE)—a technique for harvesting transplant organs from a dead donor. The kidneys, liver, pancreas, duodenum, and spleen are removed en bloc rather than individually. This harvesting technique is faster, and preliminary reports suggest that there is a lower incidence of loss of function in donor organs removed by this method.

total cavopulmonary connection (TCP)—used in a modified Fontan procedure for surgical correction of a double-inlet left ventricle. Venous blood from the inferior vena cava is channeled directly into the main pulmonary artery via an intra-atrial baffle created with autologous pericardium. Blood from the distal superior vena cava is diverted directly into the right pulmonary artery, and the single ventricular chamber is thus dedicated to systemic circulation. This procedure avoids the prosthetic conduits used in other types of repairs.

total knee arthroplasty (TKA).

totally extraperitoneal (TEP) **hernia repair.**

total lymphocyte count—a quick and inexpensive test that may be a useful indicator of nutritional status and outcome.

total lymphoid irradiation (TLI).

total mesorectal excision (TME)—meticulous surgical dissection of the mesorectal tissues to improve the results of surgery for rectal cancer.

TOTAL O₂ system—a supplementary oxygen system. It provides home oxygen patients with stationary oxygen as well as the ability to fill portable oxygen cylinders for ambulation.

Toupet (partial posterior) **fundoplication**—a posterior, 270° wrap of the esophagus as surgical treatment of severe gastroesophageal reflux disease. It replaces the 360° wrap of the Nissen fundoplication. Results are said to be excellent with fewer complications than the Nissen procedure.

Tourette's syndrome (maladie des tics) —a disorder of tics, throat sounds, generalized jerking movements, and the uncontrollable use of obscene language. Also, *Gilles de la Tourette's syndrome.*

Tourguide guiding catheters—a line of French guiding catheters (sizes 6 through 10) to be used in interventional cardiac procedures, including PTCA, athrectomy, and stenting.

Towne projection in x-rays (Radiol)—occipital view of the skull.

Townley TARA prosthesis (Ortho)—see *TARA prosthesis.*

Townsend knee brace—made of lightweight titanium and graphite.

toxic—showing signs of toxemia or septicemia, such as fever, tachycardia, flushing, and mental confusion.

toxic shock syndrome—not a new infection, but mentioned often in the news in connection with group A streptococcal infections. It was big news during the tampon scare of the 1980s. See *streptococcus A infection; necrotizing fasciitis;* and *"flesh-eating" bacteria.*

Toxocara **ELISA**—test for endophthalmitis.

Toxocara **excretory secretory antigen** (TES antigen)—indicative of *Toxocara* nematodes (on ELISA test).

Toxoplasma gondii—can cause central nervous system toxoplasmosis in patients with AIDS.

t-PA (tissue plasminogen activator) (Activase, alteplase)—given intravenously to dissolve a thrombus.

TPDCV (thioguanine, procarbazine, DCD [mitolactol], CCNU, vincristine)—chemotherapy protocol for brain tumors.

TP-40—chemotherapy drug given intravesically to patients with unresectable superficial bladder carcinoma.

TP10—complement inhibitor; potential treatment to reduce consequences of reperfusion injury and improve postoperative outcomes in infants undergoing cardiac surgery.

T-piece oxygen—administration of humidified oxygen through a tube connected to a T-shaped connector attached to an endotracheal tube.

TPM (total passive motion).

TPN (total parenteral nutrition) **line**.

TP-1 (thymostimuline)—used to treat AIDS.

TpP (thrombus precursor protein)—an in vitro diagnostic test for the risk assessment of blood clot formation.

TPPN (total peripheral parenteral nutrition).

T-PRK (tracker-assisted photorefractive keratectomy).

TR (repetition time)—in magnetic resonance imaging, the interval between one spin echo pulse sequence and the next.

TRA (all-trans-retinoic acid)—a form of vitamin A given orally to patients with malignant solid tumors unresponsive to other chemotherapy.

trabecula (pl., trabeculae)—thin fibrous band of tissue.

trabeculoplasty—brief laser treatment which produces tightening of the outflow mechanism in glaucoma patients by placing a number of pinpoint lesions directly over the drain. Usually performed under topical anesthesia on an outpatient basis. Also, *argon laser trabeculoplasty*.

Tracer Blood Glucose Micro-monitor for self-testing by diabetics.

TracerCAD—a computer program used to create better-fitting limb prostheses.

Tracer—hybrid wire guide for endoscopic surgery.

tracheal tug—downward impulse imparted to the trachea by aortic aneurysm, synchronous with heartbeat.

trachelotomy—incision into, or excision of, the neck of the uterus (cervix uteri); also called *cervicectomy*. Cf. *tracheotomy*.

tracheoesophageal puncture (TEP)—a promising option for post total laryngectomy patients (other than esophageal speech or an artificial larynx). TEP can be performed at the same time as the laryngectomy (primary TEP) or at a later time (secondary TEP). Delaying the procedure would be for poor tissue quality, poor clinical status, or the need for planned postoperative radiation treatment.

tracheostomy, percutaneous dilational (PDT).

tracheotomy—incision of the trachea. Cf. *trachelotomy*.

Trachlight—lighted stylet used in intubation of surgical patients.

track—the path along which something has moved and left a mark, e.g., needle track. This word is not often used in medical dictation. Cf. *tract*.

tracker-assisted photorefractive keratectomy (T-PRK).

Tracker-18 Soft Stream catheter—a microcatheter used to deliver drugs to lyse intracoronary thrombi. The holes in the sides of the catheter deliver a soft stream which does not injure the blood vessel.

tract—a collection of nerve fibers that have a common origin, function, and termination—as in spinal tract; or a group of organs that are arranged serially and together perform a common function—as in gastrointestinal tract; or an abnormal passage through tissue—as sinus tract, fistulous tract. Cf. *track*. See *Bachman tract*.

traction
Bryant's
Buck's
Cotrel
Crutchfield skeletal
halo
halter
Russell's

tract of Lissauer—a white matter tract immediately posterior to the dorsal horn of the spinal cord gray matter through which small nociceptive nerve fibers pass.

Trager therapy—gentle rocking movements used to ease pain and tension in conditions such as Parkinson's disease, irritable bowel syndrome, chronic back pain, and multiple sclerosis.

TRAIDS (transfusion related AIDS, acquired immunodeficiency syndrome).

Trail Making Test—neurological test.

Trak Back—disposable pullback device that provides steady and precise pullback of intravascular ultrasound catheters, facilitating viewing of 3-D-

Trak Back *(cont.)*
like images, in addition to conventional cross-sectional displays.

TRAM (transverse rectus abdominis myocutaneous) **flap**.

tramadol (Ultram)—an analgesic for the management of moderate to moderately severe pain. It is said to be significantly less addictive than codeine and morphine.

transabdominal preperitoneal (TAPP) **hernia repair**—an approach to laparoscopic inguinal hernia repair using balloon distention to permit better exposure and reduce risk of preperitoneal adhesions.

transabdominal thin-gauge embryofetoscopy (TGEF)—fiberoptic endoscope inserted into the uterus to obtain information (in addition to that already provided by transvaginal ultrasound) to aid in diagnosing fetal anomalies.

transanal endoscopic microsurgery (TEM)—a minimally invasive technique for resection of sessile adenomas and some rectal carcinomas.

transaxial fat-saturated 3-D images —MRI term.

transbronchial biopsy (TBB)—histopathological findings of specimens graded on the International Society for Heart and Lung Transplantation system.

transbronchial needle aspiration (TBNA).

transcarotid balloon valvuloplasty—used in infants with congenital aortic valve stenosis. The neck artery is used because it is larger and can be directly repaired, and surgeons are able to avoid losing a leg artery. The procedure is monitored by transesophageal echocardiogram.

transcatheter ablation—used to describe interventional electrophysiology procedures in which direct current or radiofrequency energy is used to ablate (remove) arrhythmogenic areas in the myocardium.

transcatheter arterial chemoembolization (TACE).

transcatheter arterial embolization (TAE)—used to deliver chemotherapeutic agents through the common hepatic artery to liver neoplasms.

transcervical balloon tuboplasty (TBT) —procedure to open blocked fallopian tubes that are the cause of infertility. Anesthesia is obtained with a paracervical block and a catheter is inserted into the blocked fallopian tube under fluoroscopic guidance. Less expensive than standard surgery for blocked tubes or in vitro fertilization. Also called *recanalization*.

transconjunctival approach to orbital tumors.

transcoronary ablation of septal hypertrophy (TASH)—believed to be an effective way to relieve resting left ventricular outflow tract obstruction in hypertrophic cardiomyopathy.

transcranial color-coded sonography —bedside procedure using ultrasound that traces the cerebral blood flow to ascertain the presence and location of an arteriovenous malformation.

transcranial Doppler (TCD) **velocities**.

transcutaneous electrical nerve stimulation (TENS).

transcutaneous neuromuscular electrical stimulation (TNMES).

transcutaneous oxygen level ($TcPO_2$).

TransCyte—a human-based, bioengineered temporary skin substitute for the treatment of burns.

transdermal patch for glucose monitoring—a disposable transdermal patch applied to the skin for 5 minutes; a pocket-sized monitor then reads the patch and indicates the patient's blood glucose level.

Transeal transparent adhesive film dressing.

transesophageal echocardiography (TEE)—a semi-invasive procedure that provides views of the posterior structure of the heart and is the investigation of choice for diagnosis of acute dissection of the aorta, assessment of aortic graft dehiscence, and in search for a potential cardiac source for thromboembolism.

transesophageal pacing system—eliminates the use of drugs in nonexercise stress testing for patients with congestive heart failure and other late-stage cardiovascular diseases.

transfemoral liver biopsy.

transferred immune response—technique of transferring antibodies from cancer cells of one cancer patient to a healthy patient, and then transplanting healthy bone marrow back into the cancer patient.

transferrin (as in ferrous)—a glycoprotein. Also, *iron binding protein*.

transfixion suture—suture ligature; used to suture a large blood vessel closed; secures against slippage of the knot; sometimes called stick tie.

transhepatic embolization (THE).

transhiatal esophagectomy.

transient aplastic crisis (TAC)—an illness in which red cell production virtually stops, and the red blood cell count falls rapidly; a complication of parvovirus B19 infection.

transient bone marrow edema syndrome—a self-resolving condition related to the bone marrow edema pattern seen on MR imaging.

transient evoked otoacoustic emission (TEOAE)—frequently used to determine the physiological condition of the cochlea in studies of comparative hearing.

transient ischemic attack (TIA).

TransiGel—hydrogel-impregnated gauze.

transitional cell carcinoma of the bladder (TCCB).

transjugular intrahepatic portosystemic shunt (TIPS or TIPSS)—a treatment modality for portal hypertension-induced variceal hemorrhage unresponsive to sclerotherapy. Although the procedure has been improved with the use of an expandable Wallstent for better shunt patency, stenosis may still occur in about half of the patients, necessitating shunt revision by stent replacement or angiographic dilation of the shunt or addition of a second one.

transjugular liver biopsy.

translabyrinthine removal of large acoustic neuromas.

translocation Down syndrome—a variation of Down syndrome, caused by an extra twenty-first chromosome that moves from the twenty-first chromosome pair to either the thirteenth or fifteenth pair, resulting in 13/21 or 15/21 translocation Down syndrome. Cf. *trisomy-D syndrome*.

transluminal endovascular graft placement—a procedure in which a compactly folded graft is delivered through a sheath, deployed, and pressed against the vessel by balloon inflation. It is performed to reduce an aortic aneurysm.

transluminal extraction catheter (TEC)—cone-shaped rotating device

transluminal *(cont.)*
with suction that cuts plaque from the lumen and sucks out the pieces.

transmission control protocol/Internet protocol (TCP/IP).

transmyocardial revascularization (TMR).

transnasal endoluminal ultrasonography—a method to study the anatomy of the GI tract.

Transorbent—multilayer dressing that includes an extra soft foam layer to protect and cushion a wound.

transpapillary endoscopic cholecystotomy—drains the gallbladder in acute acalculous cholecystitis. It is done in place of more aggressive percutaneous, laparoscopic, or open cholecystotomy, primarily in patients at high surgical risk.

transparent adhesive film—semi-permeable membrane dressings that are waterproof yet permeable to oxygen and water vapor. These dressings help prevent bacterial contamination and maintain a moist wound environment. They also facilitate cellular migration and promote autolysis of necrotic tissue by trapping moisture at the wound surface. Some newer transparent films are designed simply to keep I.V. sites dry; these have a higher moisture vapor permeability (MVP) and are not used on wounds. See *dressing*.

transplantation—see *orthotopic transplantation*.

transplant rejection classification—The classification system of the International Society for Heart and Lung Transplantation divides acute rejection (AR) into grades: grade AO, none; grade A_{2a}, minimal, mild, with evidence of bronchiolar inflammation; grade intermediate, and

severe acute rejection. It also recognizes four categories of chronic rejection (CR) and inflammation in describing airways and vessels.

transposition of the great arteries (TGA).

transpupillary thermotherapy—ophthalmological treatment of occult wet age-related macular degeneration.

transrectal ultrasound (TRUS)—used in assessing and characterizing the degree of pathology of prostatic abscess.

TransScan TS2000 electrical impedance breast scanning system—real-time noninvasive radiation-free imaging device that maps local electrical impedance properties of breast tissue, using inherent differences between neoplastic and normal tissues.

transthoracic echocardiography (TTE)—evaluates the structure, function, and size of pulmonary and aortic valves.

transthoracic needle aspiration biopsy of benign and malignant lesions.

transthoracic needle biopsy (TNB)—used to diagnose thoracic lesions.

transtracheal oxygen catheter—can replace a nasal cannula for better patient comfort and aesthetics. Inserted at the base of the neck through a small, permanent, surgically created tract into the trachea. The catheter is connected to tubing to a portable oxygen tank.

transtympanic steroid administration—steroids administered directly to the middle ear effective in treating sudden-onset sensorineural hearing loss in patients who have failred to respond to systemic steroid therapy.

transumbilical breast augmentation (TUBA)—an innovative technique using a small incision in the navel as an access point for insertion of saline-filled breast implants.

transurethral balloon Laserthermia prostatectomy—investigational procedure in which the prostate is irradiated with a Prostalase (Nd: YAG) laser system inserted transurethrally through a balloon device. The balloon can be monitored via transrectal ultrasound. See *Prostalase laser system.*

transurethral incision of the prostate (TUIP)—an alternative to transurethral resection of the prostate (TURP). TUIP is nearly as effective in reducing symptoms of benign prostatic hypertrophy and can be done on an outpatient basis. It is limited to patients who have 30 g or less of prostatic tissue to be resected.

transurethral microwave thermotherapy (TUMT)—heats the prostate via a transurethral application. It houses a microwave antenna in a water-cooled sheath, thus protecting prostatic mucosa while delivering deeper heating to obstructing parenchyma. When tissues are heated to greater than 45°C, necrosis occurs, resulting in ablation or resorption of overgrown prostatic tissue.

transurethral needle ablation (TUNA) —procedure for treatment of benign prostatic hypertrophy. Radiofrequency is delivered through side-deploying needles to create coagulative necrotic lesions within the prostate. The prostate then retracts, opening the prostatic urethra.

transurethral ultrasound-guided laser-induced prostatectomy (TULIP) (Urol)—a surgical treatment for benign prostatic hypertrophy. Ultrasound is used to visualize the enlarged prostate, and a 90° angle side-firing laser is used to destroy the obstructing prostatic tissue. Postoperative complications such as hemorrhage are minimal, and most patients go home the next day. See also *transurethral balloon Laserthermia prostatectomy.*

transvaginal sacrospinous culpopexy —a modification of the sacrospinous colpopexy for women with vaginal vault prolapse. See *sacrospinous colpopexy.*

transvaginal suturing (TVS) **system** — a surgical device to correct female stress urinary incontinence.

transvaginal ultrasound (TVS)—may replace endometrial biopsy as the standard diagnostic procedure for vaginal bleeding among postmenopausal women.

transvenous liver biopsy—a faster (takes about 10 minutes to perform), simpler method for obtaining liver tissue that is used when percutaneous liver sampling is contraindicated by bleeding tendency, ascites, pulmonary emphysema, peliosis hepatis, or liver amyloidosis. Under fluoroscopy, a sheathed needle is inserted via the jugular vein down to the hepatic vein, which is pierced to obtain a specimen of liver parenchyma. The procedure produces a smaller specimen but is safer because liver capsule is not pierced and any bleeding is confined to venous bleeding.

transverse magnetization; orientation —MRI term.

transverse rectus abdominis myocutaneous (TRAM) **flap**—used in breast reconstruction. In this technique to

transverse *(cont.)*
    reconstruct the breast, tissue is transferred from the central portion of the abdomen onto the chest wall, or tunneled beneath the skin to the breast. Also called *tummy tuck flap*.

TRAP (tartrate resistant acid phosphatase)—osteoclast marker enzyme used in the diagnosis of histological aspects of heterotopic bone.

trastuzumab (Herceptin).

Trasylol (aprotinin)—a protease inhibitor used for reducing perioperative blood loss and the need for blood transfusions in cardiopulmonary bypass patients in repeat CABG.

Traube's space—the gastric bubble, which causes a different tympanitic note from percussion over the lungs.

TraumaJet—wound debridement system capable of removing contamination, as well as damaged tissue, from a traumatic wound.

traumatic aortic injuries in children—diagnosed by helical CT scan and transesophageal echocardiography. Injuries may include left apical cap, pulmonary contusion, aortic obscuration, and mediastinal widening.

Travasorb MCT—a medium chain triglyceride food supplement.

Travenol infuser—a disposable device for the delivery of continuous parenteral drug therapy to patients who can be ambulatory.

Traverso-Longmire technique—for resection of a malignant tumor of the pancreas.

TRC (tanned red cells) (microsomal TRC antibody titer)—a test used in the study of thyroid antibodies.

treadmill testing—stress testing of cardiac response, in which the patient progressively increases walking speed, and the incline of the treadmill is also increased. The test is continued until signs of ischemia are noted, or when the target heart rate is reached. The test is discontinued when the patient becomes fatigued, short of breath, or notes claudication or vertigo.

treatment—see *medications, operation*.

tree artifact (Radiol)—a tree-shaped spot on a radiograph caused by exposure of undeveloped film to visible light including sparks of static electricity. Also, *crown artifact* and *swamp-static artifact* (the same phenomenon).

trefoil balloon catheter—see *percutaneous transvenous mitral commissurotomy*.

Trelex mesh—used for reinforcement of repair during inguinal herniorrhaphy.

tremor, pill-rolling.

trepopnea ("tree-pop-nee´uh")—preference for the recumbent position, because breathing is easier in that position.

T₄RIA—thyroxine radioisotope assay.

TRIADS (time-resolved imaging by automatic data segmentation) (MRI)—provides variable resolution of an individual's respiratory cycle.

Triage cardiac system—rapid diagnostic test designed to aid in detection of heart attacks.

triamcinolone cream (TAC).

Triangle gelatin-sealed sling material—designed for a less invasive transvaginal procedure to treat female stress incontinence. Triangle material is sealed with an absorbable bovine gelatin that is crosslinked to control the rate of its resorption in the body. This may help to reduce inflammation during the healing process.

"triangle of doom"—see *triangle of pain*.

triangle of pain (also, electric zone; "triangle of doom")—used to describe the triangular area between the gonadal vessels medially and the iliopubic tract laterally. May be dictated in hernioplasty or laparoscopic herniorrhaphy reports. The truly dangerous region is deep to the iliopubic tract where position of nerves cannot be seen or predicted with certainty.

triangular vaginal patch sling—a sling created from the anterior vaginal wall. A procedure for stress urinary incontinence and hypermobile urethra.

TriCitrasol (anticoagulant sodium citrate solution)—anticoagulation therapy.

triceps skin fold—useful in nutritional status analysis.

trichiasis—inversion of the eyelashes so that they rub against the cornea, causing continual irritation of the eyeball.

trichinosis—infection with trichinae; caused by eating undercooked pork and some other meats containing *Trichinella spiralis*. Cf. *trichocyst, trichosis*.

trichocyst—a cell structure which is derived from the cytoplasm. Cf. *trichinosis, trichosis*.

trichosanthin—see *compound Q*.

trichosis—a disease of, or abnormal growth of, the hair. Cf. *trichinosis, trichocyst*.

Trichosporon beigelii—seen in postsurgical soft tissue infections.

trichotillomania—compulsive tugging at one's hair. "Her symptoms included rather depressive features and trichotillomania."

triciribine phosphate (TCN-P)—drug used to treat non-small cell lung carcinoma.

Tricodur Epi (elbow) compression support bandage.

Tricodur Omos (shoulder) compression support bandage.

Tricodur Talus (ankle) compression support bandage.

Tricomin—for treatment of hair loss.

Tricor—see *micronized fenofibrate*.

tricorrectional bunionectomy—bunion repair procedure also used to repair juvenile hallux valgus deformity. The bunion deformity is corrected in all three planes with a distal metatarsal osteotomy involving a transverse V-osteotomy with a long plantar hinge using cannulated bone screws for fixation. Does not interfere with the epiphyseal growth center of the first metatarsal.

tricyclic antidepressant (TCA).

TriFix spinal instrumentation system—pedicle screw fixation system used for stabilization of the spine.

triggering mechanism—a precipitous event or process causing onset of acute disease, e.g., acute cardiovascular disease or sudden death.

trigger point—a localized zone of tenderness, especially in a muscle.

Trileptal (oxcarbazepine)—anticonvulsant medication.

Trilogy acetabular cup—comes in non-holed, cluster-holed, or multi-holed models.

Trilogy DC+—pacemaker used in patients with sick sinus syndrome and intermittent heart block.

Trilogy SR+—single-chamber pacemaker that "learns" the patient's lifestyle and adapts to changes during activity and rest.

Trilucent breast implants—breast implants filled with vegetable oil.

trimethoprim-sulfamethoxazole—see *TMP-SMZ, Bactrim, Septra*.

trimetrexate—an antineoplastic used for various carcinomas and also *Pneumocystis carinii* infection.

trimetrexate glucuronate (NeuTrexin) —an antineoplastic for *Pneumocystis carinii* pneumonia. It is used with concurrent leucovorin (rescue) as a second-line treatment when Bactrim/ Septra therapy has failed. It may also be used to treat a variety of solid tumors.

Tri-Nasal Spray (triamcinolone acetonide)—nasal spray for patients 12 and over with seasonal and perennial allergic rhinitis.

tripe palm—cutaneous marker for internal malignancy which produces a rugose or corrugated thickening of the skin of the palm.

Triphasil (levonorgestrel and ethinyl estradiol)—triphasic contraceptive.

"triple A" (AAA)—medical slang for *abdominal aortic aneurysm.*

triple antibiotics.

triple-dose gadolinium-enhanced MR imaging without MT (magnetization transfer).

triple-H therapy (hypertensive hypervolemic hemodilution) **after subarachnoid hemorrhage**.

tripoding—Gowers' sign, classical sign of Duchenne muscular dystrophy.

Trippi-Wells tongs—used for traction.

triquetrum—the triquetral bone in the wrist, between the pisiform and lunate bones; os triquetrum, also called *triangular bone.*

trisomy-D syndrome—manifested by the following clinical features: apneic spells, apparent deafness, capillary hemangioma, cardiac defects, characteristic dermal pattern, cleft lip and palate, death in early infancy, ear malformation, polydactyly, scalp defects, and severe central nervous system defects. Cf. *translocation Down syndrome, trisomy-G.*

trisomy-G—genetically determined disorder; one of a group of such disorders associated with increased risk of leukemia.

Tritec (ranitidine bismuth citrate)—histamine H_2 antagonist used in combination with clarithromycin to treat active duodenal ulcer associated with *H. pylori.*

Triumph VR pacemaker—a single chamber adaptive rate pacemaker.

TroCam—endoscopic system placing the camera and lighting directly into the surgical field for computerized imaging.

Trocan disposable CO_2 trocar and cannula.

Troisier's node—see *sentinel node.*

troleandomycin (Tao)—antibiotic in the macrolide class of drugs, similar in effectiveness to penicillin and erythromycin but with fewer side effects.

troponin T—see *cardiac troponin T.*

Trousseau's sign—the occurrence of carpal spasm, in latent tetany, when the upper arm is compressed (as with the use of a tourniquet).

Trovan (trovafloxacin)—used for the treatment of bacterial infections, including gram-negative, gram-positive, atypical, and anaerobic bacteria.

Trovan/Zithromax Compliance Pak— specific dual treatment for uncomplicated urethral gonorrhea in males and endocervical and rectal gonorrhea in females caused by *Neisseria gonorrhoeae* and nongonococcal urethritis/ cervicitis caused by *Chlamydia trachomatis.*

Trovert—a growth hormone antagonist used to treat acromegaly and to improve insulin sensitivity in diabetic patients.

troxacitabine (formerly BCH-4556)—anticancer compound for the treatment of leukemia and a variety of solid tumors.

TR/TE, long—see *T2-weighted image.*

TR/TE, short—see *T1-weighted image.*

Tru-Area Determination—wound-measuring device.

Tru-Close wound drainage system—a completely closed wound drainage system with a unique splittable design providing two drains through one exit site. Because the evacuator is never opened or emptied, patients and healthcare personnel are protected from exposure to contaminated body fluids.

Tru-Cut needle—used for liver biopsy.

T.R.U.E. (thin-layer rapid use epicutaneous) **allergen patch test**—a ready-to-apply allergen patch test that can be used for 24 allergens and allergen mixes, capable of detecting up to 85 of the most common substances that cause allergic contact dermatitis.

True-Flex intramedullary nail—fluted titanium nail for fixation of upper extremity fractures.

true vertigo—a feeling that everything is revolving around the patient, or that he himself is revolving. Differentiated from mere dizziness.

TruJect—self-administered autoinjector drug delivery system. Approximately the size of a pen, it is spring-activated and pre-filled to deliver subcutaneous or intramuscular injection of medication with the touch of a button.

Trumpet Valve hydrodissector—see *Nezhat-Dorsey Trumpet Valve hydrodissector.*

truncation band artifact—see *edge ringing artifact, Gibbs phenomenon.*

TruPulse CO_2 laser system—used for skin resurfacing.

Truquant BR—an in vitro test kit for the detection of recurrent breast cancer in women with stage I or stage II disease. The test detects the presence of the CA27.29 antigen, a breast cancer tumor marker, in the blood.

TRUS (transrectal ultrasonography)—to evaluate prostate carcinoma.

Tru-Scint AD—imaging agent for the detection of recurrent breast cancer.

Trusopt (dorzolamide HCl)—2% ophthalmic solution for reduction of intraocular pressure in patients with ocular hypertension or open-angle glaucoma.

TruWave pressure transducer—disposable transducer in a closed, needleless blood sampling system.

TruZone PFM (peak flow meter)—for asthma and emphysema in both children and adults.

TS (terminal sedation).

T-Scan 2000—transpectral impedance scanner that performs electrical mapping of breast lesions in patients who have had ambiguous mammogram results. The device is designed to improve diagnostic accuracy and lower the number of unnecessary biopsies.

TSF (triceps skin fold).

TSH-01—a transdermal tape with natural estrogen and 17 beta-estradiol. Used as treatment for climacteric disturbances and postmenopausal osteoporosis. The base material of the tape is polymer technology that mitigates skin irritation.

T-Span tissue expander.

TSPP rectilinear bone scan (technetium stannous pyrophosphate).

TSRH (Texas Scottish Rite Hospital) **Crosslink**—a spinal instrumentation system used to stabilize the rods used in correction of scoliosis. Also, *Cotrel-Dubousset*.

T-TAC (transcervical tubal access catheter).

TTE (transthoracic echocardiography).

T3 system—a targeted transurethral thermoablation system for treatment of benign prostatic hyperplasia. The system is catheter-based to provide a "nonsurgical," anesthesia-free procedure.

TTP (thrombotic thrombocytopenic purpura).

T2 (MRI term)—the time it takes for protons to go out of phase after having been shifted in their orientation by an excitation pulse.

T-2 protocol—for treatment of Ewing's sarcoma.

T2-weighted fast SE images (MRI).

T2-weighted image (MRI term)—a spin-echo image generated by a pulse sequence using a long repetition time (2 seconds or more). Also called *long TR/TE*.

T2-weighted turbo SE images (MRI).

TUBA (transumbilical breast augmentation).

tube (see also *stent*)
   Abbott-Rawson
   Activent antimicrobial ventilation tubes for myringotomy
   Bivona TTS (tight-to-shaft) tracheostomy
   Blakemore-Sengstaken
   Broncho-Cath endobronchial
   Caluso PEG
   Cantor
   Celestin latex rubber
   Combitube
   Ewald
   fenestrated tracheostomy

tube *(cont.)*
   fil d'Arion silicone
   Flexiflo Stomate low-profile gastrostomy
   germination
   Guibor Silastic
   K-Tube
   Keofeed feeding
   Lanz low-pressure cuff endotracheal
   Mark IV
   MIC gastroenteric
   MIC-Key G gastrostomy
   MIC-Key J gastrostomy
   Micron bobbin ventilation
   MIC-TJ (transgastric jejunal)
   Miller-Abbott
   Molteno seton
   Montgomery Safe-T-Tube
   Moss G-tube PEG kit
   Moss nasal
   Moss Suction Buster
   nasogastric (NG) feeding
   nasojejunal (NJ) feeding
   Newvicon vacuum chamber pickup
   NG (nasogastric) feeding
   Nuport PEG
   Nyhus/Nelson
   Olympus One-Step Button
   ostiomeatal stent
   Pedi PEG
   PEG (percutaneous endoscopic gastrostomy)
   Pitt talking tracheostomy
   Radius enteral feeding
   RAE endotracheal
   Replogle
   Reuter bobbin
   Ring–McLean sump
   Sacks-Vine PEG (percutaneous endoscopic gastrostomy)
   Sandoz suction/feeding
   Saticon vacuum chamber pickup
   Shah permanent
   Suh ventilation
   Super PEG

tube *(cont.)*
  Versatome laser fiber
  Vidicon vacuum chamber pickup
tuber cinereum—part of the hypothalamus.
tuberculosis, classification of:
  TB0—no exposure, no infection.
  TB1—exposed to tuberculosis, infection status unknown.
  TB2—latent infection, no disease (positive PPD).
  TB3—active tuberculosis
    pulmonary—receiving no chemotherapy
    pleural—receiving chemotherapy (date).
    lymphatic—chemotherapy terminated (date).
    bone and/or joint—completed prescribed chemotherapy course.
    genitourinary—incomplete chemotherapy course.
    other locations: disseminated (miliary), meningeal, peritoneal.
  TB4—inactive tuberculosis, healed or adequately treated.
  TB5—possible tuberculosis, status unknown (rule out TB).
tuberculosis tests—see *Amplified Mycobacterium Tuberculosis Direct Test* and *Roche-Microwell Plate Hybridization Method*.
Tubex injector—a closed injection system to protect doctors and nurses against needle-stick injuries.
tubing forceps—used in glaucoma patients for trimming, handling, and insertion of drainage tube into scleral entry site.
tuboplasty—see *transcervical balloon tuboplasty*.
TUIP (transurethral incision of the prostate).
tularemia—a febrile illness, first described in Tulare, California. The

vector (carrier) is thought to be *Ixodes pacificus*, a common deer and cattle tick.
TULIP (transurethral ultrasound-guided laser-induced prostatectomy).
tulip probe.
tulip tip—on end of PEG feeding tube.
tumescent absorbent bandage (TAB) **dressing**.
tumescent technique—a liposuction technique where high-volume, pressurized fluid formula is infiltrated, distending, anesthetizing and exsanguinating the region, allowing for almost bloodless and painless surgical removal of excess fatty tissues during liposuction.
Tum-E-Vac—gastric lavage kit for use in emergency situations.
tummy tuck flap—method of breast reconstruction in which the transverse rectus abdominis muscle (TRAM) flap is used to create a myocutaneous flap which is tunneled beneath the skin to the breast. Similar in procedure to an abdominoplasty, hence the name *tummy tuck flap*. Also called *TRAM flap*.
tumor—see *disease*.
tumor-activated prodrug (TAP).
tumoral calcinosis—a rare systemic disorder characterized by ectopic soft tissue calcification near the joints.
tumor amplified protein expression therapy (TAPET).
tumor blush—vascularization seen on angiography. Increased vascularization is a clue to the presence of a tumor and may represent a malignancy rather than hypertrophy.
tumor-infiltrating lymphocytes (TIL).
tumor lysis syndrome (TLS)—a rare complication following chemotherapy in which massive lysis of malignant cells releasing their intracellular

tumor lysis *(cont.)*
components causes an acute episode of hyperuricemia, hyperkalemia, and hypocalcemia. TLS can lead to renal failure and even death.

tumor marker—a biochemical indicator (CA 15-3, CA 19-9, CA27.29, CA 72-4, DR-70, for example) that, when found in the blood, urine, or serum, indicates the presence of a tumor. Examples of these markers are *carcinoembryonic antigen* (CEA) as a marker for carcinomas of the lung, digestive tract, and pancreas; *prostate-specific antigen* (PSA) for cancer of the prostate; *alpha-fetoprotein* (AFP) for hepatomas and teratomas, Paget's disease of the bone, and Hodgkin's disease. See also *antigen, Bcl-2 oncogene, chromosome 14q tumor marker, CYFRA 21-1, gene, neuron specific enolase,* and *oncogene.*

tumor necrosis factor—see *TNF.*

tumor plop—the sound made by a pedunculated myxoma in a cardiac chamber when the patient is rolled over.

tumor suppressor genes
APC (adenomatous polyposis coli)
DCC (deleted in colon carcinoma)
NF1 (neurofibromatosis)
NF2 (neurofibromatosis)
RB1 (retinoblastoma)
TP53 (p53)
VHL (von Hippel-Lindau)
WT1 (Wilms tumor)

TUMT—see *transurethral microwave thermotherapy.*

TUNA—see *transurethral needle ablation.*

TUNEL stain—terminal deoxynucleotidyl transferase-mediated deoxyuridine triphosphate used to stain the placenta to identify apoptosis (programmed cell death).

tunnel views (Radiol).

Tuohy needle—used to insert a lumbar subarachnoid catheter.

Tupper hand-holder and retractor—provides total accessibility and stability required for meticulous hand surgery.

turbo spin-echo sequences (MRI)—superior to gradient-echo sequences in visualizing the biliary tree.

turbo STIR images—MRI term.

TurboVac 90—suction ArthroWand.

Turco's posteromedial release of clubfoot.

turgor pressure—pressure in capillaries.

turnbuckle functional position splint—designed to reduce wrist flexion contractures. The splint controls wrist-hand angle with a turnbuckle, which can be adjusted in fine increments.

Turner's mosaicism (syndrome).

Turner-Warwick method—uses the right gastroepiploic artery as the vascular supply for a pedicle graft in a bowel reconstruction procedure.

Turner-Warwick urethroplasty.

"turn-up" plasty—a seldom-used procedure that provides a stump for an above-the-knee prosthesis by removing the infected femur, foot amputation, knee disarticulation, and then turning the lower leg up, using the tibia to support the femoral component of a joint replacement.

Turvy internal screw fixation—used in sagittal split ramus osteotomy.

Tutofix—cortical pin for fixation of small and medium fractures. Tutofix pins are produced from bovine compact bone.

Tutoplast—brand name for tissues which have been treated through a process of preservation and viral inactivation and then implanted or re-implanted into the patient. Reportedly shows great promise for bone tumors.

Tuwave—programmed TENS waveform treatment mode used to reduce edema and pain following surgery or trauma. See *TENS*.

TVS (transvaginal ultrasound).

TVT (tension-free vaginal tape) **procedure**—for treatment of female stress urinary incontinence. Prolene mesh tape is woven through pelvic tissue and positioned underneath the urethra, creating a supportive sling. The procedure is performed under local anesthesia, and results of surgery can be assessed before the patient leaves the operating room.

T water test—for fructose intolerance.

twenty-nail involvement (or *20-nail*)—psoriatic involvement of all 20 fingernails and toenails.

2040 crbium SilkLaser—computerized erbium laser used for plastic and dermatological surgery, including incision, excision, ablation, vaporization, and/or coagulation of soft tissue.

2010 Plus Holter system—computerized digital systems for analysis of data collected from Holter monitoring; used for monitoring, analysis, and diagnosis of possible cardiac abnormalities.

20/30 Indeflator inflation device—for inflating and maintaining consistent pressure during surgical procedures.

21-channel EEG (electroencephalogram).

twig—smaller than a branch, e.g., in a vessel or nerve. "There is a possi-

bility that a neural branch or twig was injured, and should the sensory symptoms persist, she was advised to return."

Twin Jet nebulizer—for administration of aerosolized drugs such as pentamidine.

Twisk needle holder, forceps, scissors —a combination instrument used in microsurgery.

2-CdA (2-chlorodeoxyadenosine)—chemotherapy drug used to treat acute myeloid leukemia. Cf. *CDA*.

2C3—anti-VEGF (vascular endothelial growth factor) antibody with the ability to block the binding of a growth factor to receptors found on tumor vasculature, with the effect of inhibiting tumor vessel growth.

Twinrix (hepatitis A inactivated and hepatitis B [recombinant] vaccine)— a combined vaccine against hepatitis A and B.

two-dimensional echocardiography (sector scan)—noninvasive technique for diagnosis, making catheterization unnecessary for some cardiac lesions.

2DFT (two-dimensional Fourier transform)—a mathematical process that creates MRI images from raw data; 3DFT also exists but is used less.

2-D IVUS (two-dimensional intravascular ultrasound).

two-flight dyspnea—difficulty breathing that occurs on climbing two flights of stairs. (But what is a flight? Ten steps? Twenty steps?)

two-layer latex and Marlex closure technique—a simplified wound management technique consisting of a temporary two-layer sandwich of synthetic materials (Esmarch latex rubber bandage and Marlex nonab-

two-layer *(cont.)*
    sorbable synthetic mesh). Effects temporary abdominal wall closure and thus protects the intestine, prevents adhesions, and can be easily revised at bedside.

Two-Photon Excitation (TPE)—light-based technology that uses short pulsed bursts of long-wavelength light for destruction of cancerous and diseased tissues.

two-stage capsulorrhexis—for endocapsular phacoemulsification (Oph).

two-stick or **three-stick technique**—colloquial term for two or three ports (incisions) used during thoracoscopy or other minimally invasive procedure.

"Tyco #3"—medical slang for Tylenol No. 3 (Tylenol with codeine).

Tycron suture—nonabsorbable polyester fiber surgical suture. *Tycron* and *Ti-Cron* are sold by different manufacturers but appear to be the same material.

Tygon tubing—used in venovenous bypass for transplantation of the liver, and for other uses.

Tylok cerclage cabling system.

tylosis—callosities. See *hypertylosis*.

tympanocentesis—see *spectrofluorometry*.

tympanoplasty—see *crowncork tympanoplasty*.

Tyndall effect—see *aqueous flare*.

Typhim Vi—typhoid vaccine.

typhlitis—inflammation of the cecum; also, *cecitis*.

Typhoon microdebrider blade—self-irrigating, disposable cutter blade used in endoscopic sinus surgery.

tyramine test—for pheochromocytoma.

tyrosine tolerance test.

T–Y stent—a tracheobronchial stent which has both T-shaped and Y-shaped sections. Used to maintain a patent airway after burns or trauma.

Tzanck ("zank") **preparation.**

U, u

UAC (umbilical artery catheter).

UBC (University of British Columbia) **brace**.

UBT breath test—noninvasive procedure for diagnosis of *Helicobacter pylori*.

UCBL (University of California Berkeley Laboratory) **orthosis**.

UCLA pouch—for continent urinary diversion, formed from colon.

UC strip—catheter tubing fastener.

UD-BMT (unrelated donor, bone marrow transplantation).

Uendex (dextran sulfate).

UES (upper esophageal sphincter).

UGH+ syndrome—symptoms of uveitis, glaucoma, hyphema, plus vitreous hemorrhage.

UHMWPe (ultra-high molecular weight polyethylene) **ball liner**—Enduron acetabular liner.

Uhthoff's ("oot'-hoff") **phenomenon**; **sign**—nystagmus in patients with multiple cerebrospinal sclerosis.

Uldall *(not* Udall) subclavian hemodialysis catheter.

ulegyria—destruction of the cortex in a deep sulcus of a gyrus.

Ulson fixator system—orthopedic device used for percutaneous pinning and external fixation techniques. It is used to repair Colles wrist fractures, requiring the insertion of two percutaneous pins into the intramedullary canal followed by application of an external Ulson fixator with a clamp assembly.

Ultane—general inhalational anesthetic.

Ultec—hydrocolloid dressing.

Ultima C femoral component—"The femoral canal was then reamed up to a #2 Ultima C size femoral component."

Ultrabrace—a custom-fitted, postop knee orthosis in which patients can ambulate with adjustable dynamic assistance or resistance.

UltraCision ultrasonic knife—ultrasonically activated scalpel used to dissect tissue with simultaneous hemostasis in minimally invasive surgery. Improved healing and reduced tissue injury are the result of minimal thermal injury produced by this instrument compared to the heat-generating electrocautery or laser.

UltraCision *(cont.)*

In addition, there is no smoke, char, or odor. Its use requires no protective eye gear or special safety equipment. See *Harmonic Scalpel.*

Ultradol (etodolac)—an analgesic and nonsteroidal anti-inflammatory drug.

Ultra-Drive bone cement removal system—used in total hip revision to remove old cement without damage to the cortical wall. Ultrasonically tuned tool tips to provide audible and tactile feedback in order to differentiate between cement and bone.

Ultra 8 balloon catheter.

ultrafast CT—see *cine CT.*

ultrafast CT electron beam tomography—computed tomography that is more accurate and rapid than digital fluoroscopy.

UltraFine erbium laser system—used for skin resurfacing.

Ultraflex stent—a self-expanding stent made of an elastic metal, nitinol, which is encased in gelatin and an outer plastic sheath. It is implanted endoscopically over a guide wire. Once in place, the plastic sheath is removed and the stent expands as the gelatin dissolves. It is used to treat esophageal stenosis in patients with unresectable esophageal carcinoma.

Ultraject—contrast media in prefilled plastic syringe, providing accurate dosing and protection against accidental needle-stick injuries.

UltraKlenz wound cleanser.

UltraLite—flow-directed microcatheter.

Ultram (tramadol HCl)—for chronic pain relief.

Ultramark 4 ultrasound.

UltraPulse CO$_2$ laser—used for laser resurfacing treatment of wrinkled, scarred, or sun-damaged skin of the face.

Ultraseed system—ultrasound-guided brachytherapy system for treatment planning of transperineal prostate implantation of radioactive seeds in prostate cancer.

UltraSling—supports the glenohumeral joint in neutral position with 10° of abduction. It is used for postoperative rehabilitation following arthroscopic repair of SLAP (superior labrum anterior posterior) lesions.

ultrasmall superparamagnetic iron oxide (USPIO)—used as an imaging agent for hepatic MR imaging.

ultrasonic aspiration—a safe and effective method for obtaining local control of large neuroblastomas.

ultrasonography—a means of visualizing internal structures by observing the effects they have on a beam of sound waves. The sound used for this procedure is at a higher frequency (pitch) than the human ear can detect. Ultrasound waves pass through air, gas, and fluid without being reflected; however, they bounce back from rigid structures such as bone and gallstones, creating an "echo" that can be detected by a receiver. Solid organs such as the liver and kidney partially reflect ultrasound waves in predictable patterns. Waves are also reflected from the interface between two structures. Ultrasonography might be compared to taking a flash photograph. Light from the flashbulb bounces off the patient and comes back to create an image on film of the surface contours of the patient; however, the echo must be converted electronically to a visible image before it can be interpreted. Sophisticated electronic equipment permits ultrasound scanning of a body region with genera-

ultrasonography *(cont.)*

tion of a two-dimensional picture of internal structures. In practice, the same device that generates the sound waves (called a transducer) also acts as the receiver. Although it emits signals at a rate of 1000 per second, the transducer is actually functioning as a receiver 99.9% of the time.

ultrasound (US)
ADR
Aloka
ATL real-time
BladderScan
B-mode
contrast echocardiography
diathermy
duplex
endoscopic (EUS)
endovaginal (EVUS)
frequency domain imaging (FDI)
gray scale
high-intensity focused (HFU)
NeuroSector
Photopic Imaging
real-time
transcervical tuboplasty
transnasal endoluminal
transrectal
TRUS (transrectal ultrasound)
Ultramark 4

ultrasound biomicroscopy (UBM).

ultrasound diathermy—heats to a tissue depth of 5 to 6 cm and is used to warm areas around tissue interfaces such as joints.

ultrasound-guided anterior subcostal liver biopsy.

ultrasound-guided pseudoaneurysm compression—treatment for catheter-related femoral injuries.

ultrasound transcervical tuboplasty—unblocks obstructed fallopian tubes, without exposing the patient to abdominal surgery, x-rays, or x-ray

dyes. A cervical cannula is positioned, and Doppler ultrasound is used (instead of fluoroscopy) to thread a catheter into the blocked tube, where normal saline is injected to check catheter position. Then a flexible wire is threaded through the catheter to break up the obstruction.

UltraThon—highly effective insect repellant originally developed for use by the U.S. military, now being released to the public in response to serious mosquito and tick-borne diseases in the northeast part of the country. It has a 33% DEET (diethyltoluamide) content in a controlled-release polymer-based cream.

Ultratome—small sphincterotome manufactured by Microvasive.

Ultravate (halobetasol propionate)—topical anti-inflammatory.

Ultravist (iopromide) **contrast agent**—used in CT and angiocardiography.

ULTT (upper limb tension test).

umbilical artery velocimetry—used to determine the gestational age of a fetus. This technique uses a Doppler ultrasound to compare systolic and diastolic blood flow in the umbilical artery. Other techniques used to determine fetal gestational age include mean amniotic fluid index and biophysical profile.

umbilical coiling index—a reference point for diagnosing fetal problems. The normal umbilical cord consists of three intertwining blood vessels in Wharton's jelly, which fall into fixed coils. The average umbilical cord has 11 such coils. However, 5% of umbilical cords are completely straight. This phenomenon has been associated with fetal anomalies, fetal heart rate decelerations, passing meconium, premature labor, and even

umbilical coiling *(cont.)*
fetal death. The umbilical coiling index (expressed as coils/cm) is determined by dividing the number of coils by the length of the umbilical cord. An index of less than 0.1 coils/cm is associated with the above-mentioned fetal problems. A normal value (the mean index) is 0.21 coils/cm.

umbrella cell—found on the surface of the urothelium.

undyed braided polyglycolic acid suture.

unenhanced scan—a scan made without the use of a contrast material.

ungual tuft—tip of the nail.

unicornuate uterus—often found in women with urinary tract anomalies, such as renal agenesis contralateral to the hemi-uterus and ectopic kidney. A rare malformation that is difficult to recognize without invasive procedures. Thus, it is diagnosed only by the presence of gynecological symptoms such as pelvic pain, infertility, or repeated abortion.

Uniflex intramedullary femoral nail system.

Uniflex polyurethane adhesive surgical dressing.

Uni-Gold—*H. pylori* one-step test using only one drop of whole blood, serum, or plasma to test for the presence of IgG antibodies to the bacterium.

Unigraft bone graft material—synthetic bioactive glass material used in the repair of oral defects, including periodontal defects, extraction sites, and augmentation of the alveolar ridge.

Unilab Surgibone—nonantigenic, sterile, specially processed mature bovine bone used instead of autologous or homologous bone for implantation into humans to fill cavities from which tumors or cysts have been removed. There are also specially prepared onlay grafts that have cancellous bone on one side and cortical bone on the other, and also load-bearing cancellous bone blocks and dowels.

UNILINK system—a mechanical anastomotic device, designed for work under the operating microscope, to anastomose small blood vessels.

Unimar J-Needle—a suturing needle for closing deep tissue layers in a small opening into a body cavity.

Uniprost (prostacyclin)—subcutaneous therapy for treatment of late-stage pulmonary hypertension.

UniPuls electro-stimulation instrument—provides full TENS application along with stimulation of acupuncture sites.

Uniretic (moexipril/hydrochlorothiazide) —used for treating hypertension.

UniShaper—a single-use keratome.

uni-tip deformity—often the result of nasal tip surgery in which the domes of the lower lateral cartilages become pinched or over-narrowed and take on a uni-tip shape. The tip of the nose has a normal bidomal shape.

Unitron Esteem CIC (completely-in-the-canal) **hearing aid**.

Unity-C pacemaker—single-pass, rate-adaptive cardiac pacing system.

Univasc (moexipril HCl)—a low-cost single-dose ACE inhibitor used to treat hypertension.

universal donor cells—cells of genetically engineered transgenic animals, such as pigs, the organs of which may be used for xenotransplantation.

Universal fixation screws.

universal vacuum release (UVR).

University of Akron artificial heart—fully implantable artificial heart that does not need to be connected to a machine outside the patient. Contains batteries to provide power and electromagnets to move the blood through its chambers.

University of Wisconsin solution—for donor heart preservation.

Unna boot (Ortho)—see *Unna paste.*

Unna-Flex compression dressing and wrap.

Unna-Pak compression dressing and wrap.

Unna paste—a moist paste impregnated with zinc oxide, calamine lotion, and glycerin. It is applied as a "cast" (Unna boot) and provides topical treatment and compression for venous stasis ulcers.

unreamed femoral nail (UFN)—an intramedullary nail used for repair of pathologic, epiphyseal, subtrochanteric, and ipsilateral fractures of the femoral neck. There is less iatrogenic damage to the vascularization of the bone (than with a reamed femoral nail), the risk of fat embolism syndrome and ARDS is reduced, and the operation is a less time-consuming procedure, associated with less blood loss.

Unschuld's sign—a tendency to have cramps in the calves, an early indication of diabetes mellitus.

Unverricht-Lundborg syndrome—progressive myoclonus epilepsy, a genetic syndrome. The malignant form, associated with progressive dementia may be called *Lafora body disease,* the benign form *Baltic myoclonus.*

UPF prosthesis (Universal proximal femur)—see *Bateman UPF prosthesis.*

upgoing toes—abnormal response to the Babinski test, in which the great toe curls upward when the sole of the foot is stroked. Diagnostic of disorders of the central nervous system.

UPLIFT (uterine **p**ositioning via ligament **i**nvestment **f**ixation and **t**runcation) **procedure**—a laparoscopic procedure that shortens and strengthens the round ligaments to perform uterine suspension.

uPM3 urine test—found to be 80% correct in detecting a gene marker of prostate cancer. The test may eliminate the need for painful prostate biopsy in many cases.

Upper Hands—a self-retaining retractor used in liver transplantation.

upper limb tension test (ULTT)—considered an analog to the straight leg raising test for the lower limb, it assesses pain responses consequent to passive movements of the upper limb and neck.

UPPP (uvulopalatopharyngoplasty).

Uprima (apomorphine)—drug for treatment of male impotence. It is a dopamine receptor agonist that acts on the central nervous system, which then initiates a chain of reactions that result in increased blood flow to the male genital organs.

uptake—in radionuclide scans, the absorption or concentration of a radionuclide by an organ or tissue. Also, *fluorescein uptake.*

urachus, patent—in a neonate, incomplete closure of the umbilicus through which urine escapes; a urachal cyst may form and require surgical treatment.

uracil mustard—chemotherapy drug.

Ureaplasma urealyticum—organism suspected of creating a higher incidence

Ureaplasma urealyticum (cont.)
of infertility in women. It is also a risk factor for respiratory disease in the first three years of life.

Ureflex ureteral catheter—for intravenous pyelogram.

ureteral calculi in pregnancy—may be diagnosed with small instruments and treated without resorting to ionizing radiation, but using only ultrasound monitoring and rigid ureteroscopy.

ureteropelvic junction (UPJ).

ureterorenoscopy—rigid or flexible retrograde, combined with percutaneous resection, used as treatment for transitional cell carcinoma of renal pelvis.

ureteroscopy—with small rigid instruments, such as the Gautier ureteroscope, may be performed on the entire urinary tract even during advanced pregnancy. Stones may be fragmented, extracted, or displaced, and double pigtail ureteral catheters may be applied with only sonographic guidance, at times without use of anesthesia.

urethral and vesical neck damage to women, caused by aggressive transurethral resection of the bladder neck; incontinence procedures (including anterior plication, anterior colporrhaphy, and needle urethropexy); injudicious use of indwelling urethral catheters in neurologically impaired or debilitated patients; invasive tumors (e.g., cervical carcinoma); obstructed obstetrical delivery; pelvic trauma; radiation; and urethral diverticulectomy.

urethral reconstruction complications
detrusor muscle instability
fistula formation
hydronephrosis

urethral reconstruction *(cont.)*
ischemia or sloughing of the flap
urinary incontinence
urinary retention
vesical neck stenosis

urethral surgical reconstruction—used to fashion an unobstructed neourethra and maintain continence.

URF-P2 choledochoscope.

Uricult dipslides—used in testing urine for bacteria.

uridine rescue—a drug regimen which allows larger than usual doses of flurouracil to be given to patients with metastatic colorectal carcinoma.

urinary diversion procedure—for intestinal urinary conduit.

urinary tract anomalies—often associated with unicornuate uterus in women.

Uriscreen—a urine specimen test to detect bacteriuria, especially in pregnancy. It is said to be a reliable alternative to culture screening of all pregnant patients and is estimated to save as much as 80% of all unnecessary cultures.

UroCoil—self-expanding stent used to treat strictures of the male urethra.

Urocyte diagnostic cytometry system —noninvasive test for carcinoma of the urothelium.

urocytogram—study of estrogen effect on desquamated cells from the urogenital tract (used in investigation of precocious puberty).

urofollitropin (Metrodin)—used to induce ovulation in patients with polycystic ovaries who don't respond to Clomid.

urokinase (Abbokinase)—a thrombolytic agent used in treatment of massive pulmonary emboli, deep vein thrombosis, and peripheral artery occlusion. In treating pulmonary

urokinase *(cont.)*
emboli, urokinase is given intravenously. In treating PAO, urokinase is administered directly into the thrombus and surrounding area via a central line with proximal and distal infusion wires. This drug is also being tested for possible use in ischemic or embolic stroke and subclavian vein thrombosis.

Urolase fiber—for visual laser ablation of prostate.

Urologic Targis—a targeted transurethral thermoablation system.

Uroloop—a surgical device that cuts and vaporizes tissue simultaneously.

UroLume endoprosthesis—tiny, expandable wire stent used to open and keep the urethra patent as treatment for benign prostatic hyperplasia.

UroLume urethral stent—used for recurrent bulbomembranous urethral strictures.

Urolume Wallstent—a metallic stent placed in the urinary tract.

UroMax II catheter—a high pressure ureteral balloon catheter.

urothelium—epithelium of the urinary bladder.

UroVive—a self-detachable balloon system for treating urinary stress incontinence. It is a urethral bulking agent consisting of a micro-balloon permanently implanted in a minimally invasive fashion into the urinary sphincter muscle. It is a one-time treatment performed on an outpatient basis.

Urowave—uses microwave thermotherapy to reduce the size and symptoms associated with an enlarged prostate.

Urso (ursodiol)—tablets used for treatment of primary biliary cirrhosis.

ursodeoxycholic acid (ursodiol)—used to dissolve stones. *"To consider use of ursodeoxycholic acid in a person this young would not be appropriate, as he has a high possibility of recurrence, even after dissolution of the stones."* See *Actigall.*

urushiol ("oo-roo-she-all")—that component in poison oak, poison sumac, and poison ivy that causes the contact dermatitis in people who are sensitive to these plants.

USCI cannula.

USCI Goetz bipolar electrodes.

USCI NBIH bipolar electrodes.

Usher's syndrome type 1—congenital nerve deafness and retinitis pigmentosa.

USPIO (ultrasmall superparamagnetic iron oxide)—used as an imaging agent for hepatic MR imaging.

Utah artificial arm—a myoelectric prosthesis for amputations above the elbow; it comes with either a hook or an artificial Myobock hand.

uterine balloon therapy—a procedure using a catheter and balloon to heat the inside of the uterus and destroy its lining to stop excessive menstrual bleeding. An alternative procedure to hysterectomy.

uterine cry—see *cry, uterine.*

uterine positioning via ligament investment fixation and truncation (UPLIFT) procedure.

uterus didelphys—double uterus.

"u-thymic"—see *euthymic.*

"u-thyroid"—see *euthyroid.*

U-Titer—a computer-based assessment technique used in nearly all clinical domains.

Utrata capsulorrhexis forceps—used in small-incision eye surgery. Cf. *Kraff-Utrata tear capsulotomy forceps.*

uveitides—plural form of uveitis.

UVR (universal vacuum release) (Ob-Gyn)—used in vacuum deliveries.

uvulopalatopharyngoplasty (UPPP)—a surgical treatment for sleep apnea in patients who cannot tolerate or do not respond to medical therapies, such as wearing a CPAP (continuous positive airway pressure) or BiPAP (bi-level positive airway pressure) mask during sleep. UPPP involves the removal of the tonsils, adenoids, posterior soft palate, and extra mucosal tissue in the pharynx.

V, v

V (ventricular).

Vabra aspirator—disposable system for endometrial screening.

VAB-6—chemotherapy protocol for testicular cancer.

V.A.C. (vacuum-assisted closure)—assists in wound closure by applying localized negative pressure to draw edges of the wound toward the center. Applied to a special dressing positioned in the wound cavity or over a flap graft, this pressure-distributing wound packing helps remove fluids from the wound and increase blood perfusion.

VAC (vinblastine, actinomycin D, cyclophosphamide)—chemotherapy protocol.

VACA (vincristine, actinomycin D, cyclophosphamide, Adriamycin)—chemotherapy protocol.

VACAD (vincristine, Adriamycin, cyclophosphamide, actinomycin D, dacarbazine)—chemotherapy protocol.

vaccine (see also *medications*)
Acel-Imune
AIDS
AIDSVAX B-B vaccine

vaccine *(cont.)*
DTaP
edible
FluMist flu
Fluogen influenza virus
Gastrimmune (gemcitabine)
gp120
gp160
Helivax
Hib (*Haemophilus influenzae* type B)
HIB polysaccharide
HIV
influenza
Lipomel
L-Vax leukemia
LYMErix recombinant protein
Melacine
M-Vax cancer
Nabi-NicVAX nicotine
NicVAX
Oncophage cancer
Prevnar
RabAvert (human rabies vaccine)
r-gp160
RG-83894
Rhesus diploid cell strain rabies (RDRV) (adsorbed)

vaccine *(cont.)*
rp24
Twinrix (hepatitis A inactivated and hepatitis B [recombinant])
Typhim Vi typhoid
vaccinia
Vaxid
VaxSyn HIV-1
zoster immune globulin (ZIG)

vaccinia vaccine (No, the physician who dictates this is not stammering.)—"The patient received vaccinia vaccine last summer." This is a vaccine used infrequently, generally by those who have contact with smallpox virus in laboratories.

Vac-Lok—a patient immobilization cushion that creates a precise, rigid mold to hold the patient's body in place during imaging procedures. The cushion is radiotranslucent and artifact-free.

VACP (VePesid, Adriamycin, cyclophosphamide, Platinol)—chemotherapy protocol.

Vac-Pak Pad—a pad used for immobilization in total hip surgery.

VACTERL syndrome
V   vertebral or vascular defects
A   anorectal malformation (imperforate anus)
C   cardiac anomaly
TE   tracheoesophageal fistula
R   renal anomaly
L   limb anomaly

Vacurette—suction curet (Ob-Gyn).

Vacutainer—rubber-stoppered vacuum tube to draw blood.

VAD (ventricular assist device)—see *Thoratec ventricular assist device.*

VAD (vincristine, Adriamycin, dexamethasone)—chemotherapy protocol.

VAD/V (vincristine, Adriamycin, dexamethasone, verapamil)—chemotherapy protocol.

VAE (voluntary active euthanasia). See also *PAS, TS,* and *VSED.*

vagal nerve implant—given to a patient with epilepsy that cannot be controlled by drugs or surgery. The implant is placed subcutaneously under the collarbone, and two electrodes from it are placed on the vagal nerve. When patients sense the onset of a seizure, they activate the implant to stimulate the vagal nerve. This appears to interrupt epileptic activity in the brain.

vagal paraganglioma—see *glomus vagale.*

Vagifem vaginal tablets (estradiol hemihydrate)—for relief of postmenopausal atrophic vaginitis due to estrogen deficiency.

vaginal birth after (previous) **cesarean section** (VBAC).

vaginal candle (Oncol)—used in radium insertion.

vaginal construction techniques
Abbe-McIndoe operation, using split-thickness skin grafts
colocolponeopoiesis
Frank nonsurgical perineal autodilation
McCraw gracilis myocutaneous flap
Williams vulvovaginoplasty

vaginal contraceptive film (VCF)—spermicidal contraceptive that begins to dissolve instantly and washes away with the body's natural fluids, thereby not having to be removed.

vaginal flap reconstruction of urethra and vesical neck in women—approaches are 1) anterior bladder flap (Tanagho procedure); 2) posterior bladder flap (Young-Dees-Leadbetter procedure); 3) vaginal flap. Vaginal flap reconstruction is said to be more successful than bladder flap operations.

vaginal flap reconstruction and pubovaginal sling procedure—used to treat women with extensive vesical neck and/or urethral damage.

vaginal interruption of pregnancy, with dilatation and curettage (VIPDAC).

vaginal wall sling procedure—for recurrent stress urinary incontinence in elderly women due to severe genital prolapse. Similar to the Raz procedure, this procedure uses a vaginal wall graft to provide increased urethral compression and stability of the bladder base. Because it results in vaginal shortening, it is not recommended for sexually active women. See also *abdominal sacral colpoperineopexy*, *Raz procedure*, *sacrospinous colpopexy*, and *triangular vaginal patch sling*.

Vagistat (tioconazole)—antifungal vaginal ointment.

vagus nerve stimulation (VNS)—provided by implanted pulse generator in patients with epilepsy and other neurological disorders.

VAI (vincristine, actinomycin D, ifosfamide)—chemotherapy protocol.

Vairox high compression vascular stocking.

valacyclovir HCl—investigational suppressant for HIV-related herpes simplex, herpes zoster, and cytomegalovirus.

valganciclovir—oral drug for the treatment of HIV-related cytomegalovirus infections.

Validyne manometer.

Valle hysteroscope.

Valleix sign—an uncomfortable burning pain that radiates proximally toward the calf upon palpation of the course of the posterior tibial nerve from the proximal aspect of the medial malleolus distally toward the anterior aspect of the calcaneus.

ValleyLab—laparoscopic and electrosurgical instruments.

valley-to-peak dose rate—lowest dose to highest dose.

VALOP-B (etoposide, doxorubicin, cyclophosphamide, vincristine, prednisone, and bleomycin)—chemotherapy protocol.

Valtrac BAR (biofragmentable anastomotic ring).

Valtrex (valacyclovir HCl)—used for treatment of recurrent genital herpes (herpes simplex virus) and for herpes zoster (shingles) in otherwise healthy adults. It is contraindicated in immunocompromised individuals.

valve—see also *prosthesis*.
Bauhin ileocecal
Biocor porcine stented aortic and mitral
Biocor stentless porcine aortic
Capetown aortic prosthetic
CPHV OptiForm mitral
CryoLife-O'Brien
CryoValve-SG
dual switch (DSV)
Freestyle aortic root bioprosthesis
glutaraldehyde-tanned porcine heart
Hall prosthetic heart
Hancock M.O. II Bioprosthesis porcine
Heister
Ionescu tri-leaflet
Kock nipple
Krupin-Denver eye
Medtronic Hancock II tissue
mitral valve homograft
Mosaic heart
Orbis-Sigma cerebrospinal fluid
Quattro mitral
Ross pulmonary porcine
Spitz-Holter
Synergraft

valve *(cont.)*
   Tekna mechanical heart
   Top-Hat supra-annular aortic
   Toronto SPV
   Xenomedica prosthetic
   Xenotech prosthetic
valvotomy—see *percutaneous mitral balloon valvotomy* (PMBV).
VAM (VP-16, Adriamycin, methotrexate)—chemotherapy protocol.
VAMP (vincristine, actinomycin-D, methotrexate, prednisone)—chemotherapy protocol for acute leukemias in children.
Van Bogaert's disease—a rare familial disease, resulting in hepatomegaly secondary to very high concentrations of cholesterol esters.
Vancenase Pockethaler (beclomethasone dipropionate)—an inhaler only about 3″ in size that fits in the pocket and, according to the manufacturer, provides a warmer medication on application.
vancomycin-resistant enterococci (VRE).
vancomycin-resistant *Enterococcus faecium* (VREF) **infection**.
van den Bergh's test—of the concentration of bilirubin in the blood. Normal range: direct bilirubin 0.0 to 0.1 mg per 100 ml of serum; total bilirubin 0.2 to 1.4 mg per 100 ml of serum.
Van Herick (Oph)—as "Anterior chambers were deep by Van Herick."
van Heuven's anatomic classification (Oph)—diabetic retinopathy.
Vaniqa ("van-ih-KA")—prescription cream that stops facial hair growth in women.
Vanlev (omapatrilat)—cardiovascular compound for treatment of hypertension.
van Loonen operating keratoscope.

Vannas capsulotomy scissors.
vanSonnenberg sump—for percutaneous abscess and fluid drainage. (Note: There is no space in *vanSonnenberg*.) See also *vanSonnenberg-Wittich catheter*.
Vantin (cefpodoxime proxetil)—antibiotic used for a shortened five-day course to treat maxillary sinusitis in adults and otitis media in children. It is also used to treat pneumonia and three common respiratory pathogens—*S. pneumoniae*, *H. influenzae*, and *Moraxella catarrhalis*.
VAPE (vincristine, Adriamycin, procarbazine, and etoposide)—protocol for treating bronchogenic small cell carcinoma.
VaporTrode—roller electrode specially designed for electrovaporization of prostate tissue.
variable screw placement (VSP)—used along with slotted plates with transpedicular screws to correct spondylolisthesis.
variable threshold angina—see *mixed angina*.
varicella vaccine (Varivax)—for the prevention of chickenpox. This live attenuated vaccine was developed from an otherwise healthy boy with chickenpox. Protective antibodies produced by this vaccine are believed to be effective for about six years.
varicella zoster virus—see *VZV*.
Varidyne drain (ENT).
VariLift spinal cage—implantable device used for vertebral fusion in the treatment of degenerative disk disease.
Vari/Moist wound dressing—has nonadherent moisture vapor characteristics.
Varivas R—denatured homologous vein harvested after saphenous vein

Varivas R *(cont.)*
stripping and used in various lengths for vascular access and bypass surgeries.

Varivax (varicella vaccine).

vasa deferentia—plural of *vas deferens.*

Vas-Cath—acute and chronic catheters for insertion in subclavian or jugular veins. "An 11.5 French Vas-Cath was then passed through the peel-away sheath and into the inferior vena cava."

Vascor (bepridil).

VascuCoil peripheral vascular stent —a self-expanding nitinol stent used in smaller blood vessels, such as femoral arteries of the thigh, whereas conventional peripheral vascular stents are used only in the large iliac arteries of the pelvic region.

Vascu-Guard—a peripheral vascular patch derived from bovine pericardium. Used in carotid endarterectomy.

vascular and airway modeling—a finding on CT scan.

vascular brachytherapy—used to apply gamma radiation therapy to help prevent reblockage of arteries. It uses a closed-end catheter containing radioactive seeds of IR-192 that can deliver a therapeutic dose up to a diameter of several millimeters.

vascular endothelial growth factor (VEGF) (Ob-Gyn)—known to be particularly responsible for promoting neovascularization in human breast cancer. Also, an angiogenic protein and vasopermeability factor whose intraocular concentrations are closely correlated with active neovascularization in patients with diabetes mellitus, central retinal vein occlusion, retinopathy of prematurity, and rubeosis iridis (Oph).

vascular flasks—"Endoscopic ultrasonogram revealed a well-circumscribed hyperechoic pancreatic tumor, with anechoic areas corresponding to vascular flasks." The term is also used to describe pathologic appearance after pancreaticoduodenectomy.

vascularized fibula graft—insertion of a portion of fibula into an osteonecrotic hip. With blood vessels attached, the fibular bone grows and strengthens the hip, thereby obviating the need for hip replacement.

vascular targeting agent—technology for treatment of solid tumors based on targeting components that deliver a variety of therapeutic agents to the blood vessels supplying tumors. These localized agents then specifically destroy or occlude the tumor vessels.

Vascutek Gelseal—knitted and woven vascular grafts. Also, Vascutek Gelsoft.

vasoactive intestinal polypeptide.

Vasomax—an oral treatment for male erectile dysfunction.

VasoSeal VHD (vascular hemostatic device)—designed to provide an immediate hemostatic seal at the area of arterial puncture site wound by delivering highly purified collagen directly to the surface of the artery. Used during coronary angiography and angioplasty procedures as well as radiologic procedures.

VasoView balloon dissection system.

Vasoview Uniport—endoscopic saphenous vein harvesting system requiring only a single 2-cm incision. All instruments operate through a single multilumen catheter.

VAT (vinblastine, Adriamycin, thiotepa) —chemotherapy protocol.

VATER syndrome
V vertebral and/or vascular defects
A anorectal malformation
TE tracheoesophageal fistula
R radial, ray, or renal anomaly
VATS (videoassisted thoracic surgery)
Vaughn-Williams antiarrhythmic effect.
VAX-D (vertebral axial decompression) **therapy**—for treatment of herniated or slipped disks, sciatica, and degenerative disk disease not responding to standard medical therapy. A special decompression table is used in 30-minute sessions over a period of two months; the procedure stretches the spine and slowly decompresses the injured disk.
Vaxid—DNA-based vaccine for the treatment of B-cell lymphoma.
VaxSyn HIV-1—gp160 vaccine against HIV. See *AIDS vaccine*.
VBAC (vaginal birth after [previous] cesarean section).
VBC (VePesid, BCNU, cyclophosphamide)—chemotherapy protocol.
Vbeam—a pulsed dye laser system used to treat cutaneous vascular lesions.
VBG (vertical-banded gastroplasty).
VBMCP (vincristine, BCNU, melphalan, cyclophosphamide, prednisone)—chemotherapy protocol.
VBMF (vincristine, bleomycin, methotrexate, fluorouracil)—chemotherapy protocol.
VBP (vinblastine, bleomycin, cisplatin)—chemotherapy protocol.
VCAB (ventriculocoronary artery bypass) revascularization procedure.
VCDF (volume-cycled decelerating-flow ventilation).
VCF (vaginal contraceptive film).
VCS clip adapter—tiny metal clips used to join vascular structures without penetrating the lumen.

VCUG (vesicoureterogram).
VCUG (voiding cystourethrogram).
VDRL (Venereal Disease Research Laboratory) **test**—diagnostic test for syphilis. Do not translate *VDRL* in reports.
vectis—a curved lever used for traction on the fetal head during delivery.
vectorcardiography—noninvasive cardiac diagnostic procedure that presents the same diagnostic information as that given by electrocardiography, but in a different form. It gives a three-dimensional picture of the conduction of electrical impulses from the sinoatrial node, across the right atrium to the atrioventricular node, down the bundle of His, through the bundle branches to the apex, and upward into the Purkinje fibers, stimulating the myocardial muscle.
Vector intertrochanteric nail.
Vector and **VectorX large-lumen guiding catheters**—used with interventional technologies such as stents and atherectomy devices.
Vectra vascular access graft (VAG)—for use in renal dialysis patients, primarily as a shunt between an artery and a vein to gain access to the circulatory system in order to remove toxins from patients' blood during hemodialysis.
VED (vacuum erection device)—vacuum constriction device used to treat erectile dysfunction.
VEGF (vascular endothelial growth factor).
Veingard—transparent dressing which is moisture-permeable, waterproof, and sterile. Used over an intravenous site, so the site can be monitored.
vein of Galen—vena cerebri magna, the great cerebral vein, formed by the two internal cerebral veins; named

vein of Galen *(cont.)*
after a second century A.D. Greek physician.

vein of Labbé ("lab-bay").

VeIP (vinblastine, ifosfamide, Platinol)—chemotherapy protocol.

Velban (vinblastine).

Velcro rales.

Veldona—low-dose interferon alfa in lozenge form for oral administration. Used for the treatment of dry mouth and decreased salivary gland function associated with Sjögren's syndrome.

Veley headrest—Light-Veley headrest used in neurosurgical procedures.

velnacrine maleate (Mentane)—for patients with Alzheimer's disease. A derivative of tacrine (Cognex).

velocity encoding—on brain magnetic resonance angiography.

Velogene rapid MRSA assay—gene-based diagnostic assay for rapid identification of methicillin-resistant *Staphylococcus aureus.*

Velogene rapid TB assay—gene-based diagnostic assay for the rapid identification of *Mycobacterium tuberculosis.*

Velogene rapid VRE assay—gene-based diagnostic assay for the rapid identification of vancomycin-resistant *Enterococcus faecalis* and *Enterococcus faecium.*

velolaryngeal endoscopy—endoscopy of the soft palate (velum palatinum) and laryngeal mechanisms.

Velosulin BR insulin—human buffered regular insulin (rDNA origin) injection, indicated for use in external insulin infusion pumps and with U-100 insulin syringes.

Velpeau dressing or bandage—used for treatment of dislocation of the shoulder or other shoulder girdle injuries. It consists of bandaging the arm in such a manner that the injured arm is bent at the elbow over the patient's chest, with the palm of the hand at the uninjured shoulder, taking the weight off the injured shoulder.

VenaFlow compression system—intermittent pneumatic compression system indicated for deep vein thrombosis prophylaxis. Not to be confused with *Venaflo needle.*

Venaflow vascular graft—used to reduce the incidence of hyperplasia.

Vena Tech LGM filter—an inferior vena cava filter used to prevent recurrent pulmonary embolism. Can be placed in the jugular or femoral artery. *LGM* is for *Lehman, Gerofliea,* and *Metais*—the French engineers who developed the filter.

venetian blind artifacts—secondary to interleaving of magnetic resonance images.

venipuncture (*not* veno- or vena-).

venlafaxine (Effexor)—a fast-acting antidepressant in the class of drugs known as phenethylamines.

Venodyne compression system—for deep venous thrombosis (DVT).

venogram (*not* venagram).

veno-occlusive disease (VOD).

venous leak syndrome (Urol)—disorder that interferes with veno-occlusive mechanism of the corpora cavernosa, resulting in failure to trap blood within the penis. It prevents storage of blood so that an erection cannot be maintained.

venous web disease (hepatic)—see *hepatic venous web disease.*

Ventak AICD pacemaker.

Ventak AV III DR—automatic implantable cardioverter-defibrillator system.

Ventak Mini II (and **III**) **AICD** (automatic implantable cardioverter-defibrillator)—a small implantable defibrillator that, with the incorporation of Guidant's TRIAD defibrillation energy delivery system, is used for treating patients with life-threatening rapid heart arrhythmias.

Ventak Prizm—dual chamber physiologically shaped implantable defibrillator.

VentCheck—handheld monitor that verifies and confirms ventilator settings.

venter (noun)—belly, or belly-shaped part. See *ventral*.

Ventex dressing—a two-level wound dressing system for deep wounds, such as those associated with venous ulcers, donor sites, stage II and III pressure ulcers, and abrasions. It controls moderate to heavy exudative drainage. The first layer closest to the skin is a vented transparent film that allows for wound inspection without disturbing new granulation or epithelial tissue. Centrally located vents allow controlled escape of excess exudate. Over this, an outer absorbent dressing is placed, which can absorb more than 15 times its weight in exudate. Its polyurethane backing forms a barrier against bacteria and fluids and seals out the external environment on all four sides. Cf. *Aquasorb*, *Curasorb*, and *ClearSite*.

ventilate (verb)—to express verbally, especially as a release for pent-up emotions. Also, to breathe for a patient either by means of a handheld bag or mechanical respirator.

ventilation—high-frequency jet and high-frequency oscillation assisted respiration for premature infants. See *noninvasive extrathoracic ventilation* (NEV).

ventilation-exchange bougie—an airway device that can be mounted on a fiberoptic laryngoscope for passage through the larynx into the trachea via a laryngeal mask airway. Subsequent removal of the fiberoptic laryngoscope and laryngeal mask airway allows a tracheal tube to be railroaded into position over the ventilation-exchange bougie.

ventilator or **respirator**
ACD (active compression-decompression) resuscitator
BABYbird respirator
BagEasy respirator
Bennett PR-2 ventilator
Bird respirator
Bourns-Bear ventilator
Bourns infant ventilator
cuirass respirator
high-frequency jet ventilator
high-frequency oscillation ventilator
KinetiX ventilation monitor
Monaghan 300 ventilator
MVV (maximal voluntary ventilation)
Porta-Lung noninvasive extrathoracic ventilator (NEV)
portable volume ventilator

Ventra catheter—used for percutaneous thromboarterectomy.

ventral (adj.)—toward the belly, anterior. See *venter*.

ventricular assistance device—see *DMVA*.

ventricular assist device (VAD).

ventricular ejection fraction—portion of the total volume of a ventricle that is ejected during ventricular contraction (systole); usually expressed as a percent rather than a fraction. Determined in multiple gated acquisition scan, or MUGA.

ventricular endoaneurysmorrhaphy—a procedure for the repair of ventricular aneurysm using an elliptical patch graft that both restores normal shape, internal contours, and volume of the ventricle and preserves its external anatomy, permitting revascularization of the anterior descending or other coronary arteries when indicated.

ventriculocisternostomy—Torkildsen shunt procedure.

ventriculoperitoneal (VP) shunt—used in the treatment of normal pressure hydrocephalus. A small catheter is passed into a ventricle of the brain. A pump is attached to keep fluid away from the brain. Another catheter is attached to the pump and tunneled under the skin, behind the ear, down the neck and chest and into the peritoneal cavity.

ventriculotomy, partial encircling endocardial—to relieve ventricular tachycardia in patients with ischemic heart disease.

Ventritex Angstrom MD implantable cardioverter-debrillator.

ventroposterolateral thalamic electrode—see *VPL thalamic electrode.*

Ventureyra ventricular catheter—a process for the prevention and treatment of proximal obstruction in CSF shunts.

venturi mask—used in the administration of oxygen.

VEP (visual evoked potential)—see *brain tests, noninvasive.*

VER (visual evoked response) (Neuro).

Verbatim balloon catheter—so named because the balloon expands precisely to preprogrammed sizes. Used in coronary angioplasty.

Verbrugge bone clamp (Ortho)—used in acetabular fracture repair.

Verdia (tasosartan)—a once-daily antihypertensive medication.

Veress needle (*not* Verres)—used in laparoscopy for insufflation of carbon dioxide.

VeriFlex—cardiac device.

Veripath peripheral guiding catheter—single-lumen guiding catheter used to provide a pathway through which therapeutic and diagnostic devices are introduced into the peripheral vasculature.

Verluma (nofetumomab) **diagnostic imaging agent**—for detection of small cell lung carcinoma (or cancer) throughout the body. It can detect protein found on the surface of most small cell lung carcinomas, and is used as a diagnostic tool on patients who have biopsy-confirmed tumors.

vermian veins—veins of the cerebellar vermis.

Vernier calipers—used to measure the amount of intervertebral disk protrusion present, or for any other fine measurement.

VERP (ventricular effective refractory period).

VerreScope—microlaparoscopic entry and instrument system designed for laparoscopy under local anesthesia (LULA).

Versadopp 10 probe—pen-size ultrasonic Doppler probe.

Versa-Fx—femoral fixation system which requires removal of less bone.

VersaLight laser—for skin resurfacing.

Versalok—a low-back fixation system that uses polyaxial screws rather than set screws or locking nuts.

VersaPoint system—a minimally invasive hysteroscopic fibroid removal device. It utilizes bipolar electrovaporization technology to instantly vaporize tissue upon contact.

Versaport—trocar system requiring a smaller incision site, reducing risk of herniation and improving cosmetic results.

VersaPulse holmium laser (Neuro)—for use in laser nucleotomy. See *laser nucleotomy*.

Versatome laser fiber—a specialized fiberoptic tube used to deliver laser energy.

Versed syrup—used in children to help alleviate anxiety before a diagnostic or therapeutic procedure.

versions—in ophthalmology, binocular voluntary movement of the eyes in conjugate gaze (in the same direction). See also *ductions*.

Versi-Splint—a carry bag with ABS plastic components of splints which can be used to stabilize any joint in an emergency.

vertebral artery testing—performed to assess the relationship between cervical spine movement and symptoms which may be vertebrobasilar in origin. Tests include sustained rotation, left and right; sustained extension; sustained rotation and extension, left and right; and any position that is described by the patient to elicit dizziness.

vertebral body impactor—an instrument used in the management of thoracic and lumbar spine fractures, after first performing hemilaminectomy and resection of the pedicle on the side where there is most compression of the spinal canal. "With the impactor, the bone graft was securely seated."

Vertetrac ambulatory traction system —noninvasive device for relief of low back pain.

vertex—top, generally used alone to refer to the top of the head, as in "vertex presentation," but also used in referring to the top or apex of other organs. Cf. *vortex*.

vertical-banded gastroplasty (VBG).

vertical tripod fixation (VTF)—for transscleration of intraocular lens.

vertigo—see *true vertigo*.

Vesanoid (tretinoin)—a drug derived from vitamin A used to treat refractory acute promyelocytic leukemia.

Vesica—percutaneous bladder neck stabilization kit used in treating stress urinary incontinence.

vesical (adj.)—pertaining to the bladder. Cf. *vesicle*.

vesicant—a drug or agent that causes blistering. "Serious tissue damage can result if vesicants leak from a previously punctured site."

vesicle (noun)—a small blister, a small bladder or sac containing liquid. Cf. *vesical*.

vesicoureterogram (VCUG).

vesicourethral suspension—Marshall-Marchetti-Krantz procedure.

vesnarinone—an oral drug which strengthens the ability of the heart to contract and increases the rate of contractions. See *toborinone*.

vessel-sizing catheters—used to determine size of a stent to be placed or a vena cava filter to be used. They are also used to measure and size stent grafts for procedures involving abdominal aortic aneurysms. The catheters are marked with 2, 11, or 20 platinum bands, depending on need and area to be measured, and dictators may refer to them as 2-band catheters, 11-band catheters, etc.

vestibular adenitis—see *vulvar vestibulitis syndrome*.

vestibular window—opening between the tympanic cavity and the scala vestibuli of the cochlea, into which

vestibular *(cont.)*
the footplate of the stapes fits. Also called *oval window, fenestra ovalis, fenestra vestibuli.*

vestibulodynia—combination of constant vulvar pain of vestibular origin and dyspareunia, affecting women who are older than those with vestibulitis alone. It is associated with human papillomavirus DNA and dysuria. Also called *vulvar vestibulitis syndrome.*

Vestra (reboxetine mesylate)—a selective norepinephrine reuptake inhibitor (selective NRI) antidepressant.

V.E.T. (vacuum erection technologies)—a manual vacuum device used to produce penile erections in patients with erectile dysfunction. The trademark spelling includes periods.

Vexol (rimexolone)—ophthalmic suspension for treating postoperative inflammation after ocular surgery and for treating anterior uveitis.

VEX (vasodilator plus exercise) **treadmill test.**

VFA (vocal fold atrophy).

"V fib" (ventricular fibrillation).

V5M Multiplane transducer—delivers superior image quality by combining higher frequency image quality with penetration appropriate for a complete TEE exam. See *QuantX* and *Doppler tissue imaging.*

V510B Biplane TEE transducers—see *QuantX* and *Doppler tissue imaging.*

VHL (von-Hippel-Lindau) **disease; gene; syndrome.**

VHS variable-angle hip fixation system.

Viadur (leuprolide acetate implant)—once-yearly implant for palliative treatment of advanced prostate cancer.

Viagra (sildenafil citrate)—an oral drug for treatment of erectile dysfunction.

Viasorb wound dressing.

Vibracare—percussor machine for patients with cystic fibrosis. Provides optimal postural drainage. See also *Flimm Fighter.*

Vibram—soled rockerbottom shoe used after foot surgery.

Vibrant D and **Vibrant P soundbridges**—implantable medical prostheses indicated for the treatment of hearing impairment due to sensorineural deafness. The devices convert acoustic sounds to amplified vibrations inside the middle ear.

vibrational medicine—a category of alternative medical practices that encompass homeopathic remedies, flower essences, crystal healing, therapeutic touch, acupuncture, radionics, electrotherapy, herbal medicine, psychic healing, and therapeutic radiology.

vibration-assisted CRP (canalith repositioning procedure). See *CRP.*

vibrissae ("vi-bris'ee")—the hairs that grow in the nostrils.

vibroacoustic stimulation (Ob-Gyn)—application of vibrations against a mother's stomach to help rouse a fetus and aid in external cephalic version. It is performed to reposition the fetus to avoid vaginal breech delivery or cesarean section.

VIC (vinblastine, ifosfamide, CCNU)—chemotherapy protocol.

Vickers ring tip forceps.

Vicoprofen (hydrocodone bitartrate and ibuprofen)—opioid/ibuprofen combination for use as an analgesic.

Vicryl Rapide—a synthetic absorbable suture (polyglactin 910) for short-term wound closure. It is said to have a rapid absorption rate—about seven to ten days.

VID (vitello-intestinal duct)—a patent (clear) VID in neonates can produce a T-shaped prolapse of intestine through the umbilicus.

vidarabine (adenine arabinoside, Ara-A, Vira-A)—an antiviral drug for herpes simplex and herpes zoster infections.

videoassisted thoracic surgery (videothoracoscopy)—minimally invasive surgery of the chest, using techniques similar to laparoscopy.

video densitometry (VD).

videoendoscopic surgical equipment —for minimally invasive surgical approaches, such as removal of a mediastinal cyst between right lower lung vein and right atrium.

videoendoscopic swallowing study (VESS)—used for evaluation of pharyngeal dysphagia, particularly in elderly patients.

VideoHydro laparoscope—contains a port for viewing and one for irrigation and removal of fluid.

videokeratography (Oph)—provides mapping of the corneal structure with a high degree of efficiency.

videolaseroscopy—see *laparoscopic laser cholecystectomy*.

Videx (didanosine, ddI)—initial therapy in treatment of AIDS in patients with no prior history of antiretroviral drug use. Videx taken alone and Videx taken with AZT are thought to be superior to AZT alone.

Vidicon vacuum chamber pickup tube —for video camera used in arthroscopy.

VIE (vincristine, ifosfamide, etoposide) —chemotherapy protocol.

view
Arcelin's
Caldwell
Chausse's

view *(cont.)*
dens
Hughston
Laurin x-ray
Law's
Low-Beer's
Mayer's
outlet
Owen's
retromammary space
Schuller's
Stenver's
sunrise
Towne
tunnel
Waters'

Viewing Wand—a combination of a medical imaging workstation and a probe that allows the surgeon to see the trajectory of the probe relative to the location of a tumor, cyst, or other lesion, as well as the surrounding anatomy.

ViewPoint CK (conductive keratoplasty) **system**—device used to perform conductive keratoplasty, a nonlaser radiofrequency procedure that reshapes the cornea for correction of hyperopia.

vigabatrin (Sabril)—an anticonvulsant for complex partial seizures, for treatment of drug-resistant epilepsy in children and adults, and to reduce intractable infantile spasms.

Vigilon dressing —a synthetic (polyethylene) occlusive dressing, for use on ulcerations. The dressings relieve pain, cause debridement, and stimulate the formation of granulation tissue. "The recipient sites were protected with Vigilon dressing material, then covered with wet Kerlix gauze, and then dry Kerlix gauze."

villose (adj.)—variant spelling of *villous*.

villous—shaggy with soft hairs; covered with villi; "villous adenoma." Also spelled *villose*. Cf. *villus*.

villus (pl., villi)—small vascular protrusion, particularly a protrusion from the surface of a membrane, commonly seen in small bowel. Cf. *villous*.

vilona (inosine pranobex)—used for patients with AIDS.

viloxazine (Catatrol)—an antidepressant used for patients with narcolepsy and cataplexy.

VIMRxyn (synthetic hypericin)—a topical, light-activated therapy for psoriasis, cutaneous T-cell lymphoma, warts, Kaposi's sarcoma, and other specific skin diseases related to viruses and cancer.

Vincasar (vincristine).

Vincent's infection—necrotizing ulcerative gingivitis.

vindesine sulfate (Eldisine)—an alkaloid antineoplastic for a wide range of cancer types.

Vineland Social Maturity Scale—used in psychiatry/psychology evaluation.

vinorelbine (Navelbine)—chemotherapy drug made from a vinca alkaloid extracted from the plant *Vinca rosea* (periwinkle).

violaceous ("vi-o-lay´shus")—violet-colored. Usually refers to lesions on the skin.

Vioxx (rofecoxib)—a pain medication that is said to be easier on the stomach than aspirin. Works well for relief of menstrual and postsurgical pain.

Viozan—investigational inhaled medication for symptoms of chronic obstructive pulmonary disease.

VIP (vasoactive intestinal peptides)—"Elevations of VIP are associated with bronchogenic carcinoma."

VIP (VePesid, ifosfamide [with mesna rescue], and Platinol)—chemotherapy protocol for recurrent testicular carcinoma.

VIP-B (VP-16, ifosfamide [with mesna rescue], Platinol, bleomycin)—chemotherapy protocol.

VIP-DAC (vaginal interruption of pregnancy, with dilatation and curettage).

vipoma—an endocrine tumor that produces VIP. See *VIP* (vasoactive intestinal peptides).

vipoma syndrome—also known as *WDHA* (watery, secretory diarrhea, hypokalemia, and achlorhydria) *syndrome*.

Viprinex (ancrod)—clot-busting drug derived from the venom of Malaysian pit vipers. It may offer a longer treatment window and have fewer risks than tissue plasminogen activator (tPA). The drug must be given to stroke patients within 3 hours of the onset of stroke symptoms.

Viracept (nelfinavir mesylate)—an HIV protease inhibitor used for patients with advanced HIV disease.

viral hepatitides—hepatitis A, B, C.

Viramune (nevirapine)—used for treating patients with HIV.

ViraPap—human papillomavirus detection test used along with the standard Pap smear.

ViraSTAT—an immunofluorescence assay for viral culture of parainfluenza, using fluorescently labeled monoclonal antibodies which are type-specific.

Viratrol—a handheld battery-operated device that delivers a minute charge to prevent oral and genital herpes lesions from forming or to speed the healing process.

Virazole (ribavirin).

Virchow's node—enlarged supraclavicular lymph node; often the first sign of a malignant abdominal tumor. Also called *sentinel* or *signal node*.

Virend—used to treat herpes simplex virus.

virgin—a term used to refer to previously unoperated anatomy, stenosis, or herniation, such as virgin lumbar anatomy, virgin lumbar spinal stenosis, virgin disk herniation.

Virgo anti-cardiolipin screening kit — ELISA test kit used in screening patient serum for the presence of autoantibodies that are typically observed in patients with systemic lupus erythematosus and other connective tissue diseases.

Viringe—a prefilled, needleless, vascular access flush device for both saline and heparin applications.

viroid—a virus-like unenveloped infective RNA particle.

Virtual Hospital Room Communicator—a hardware communications module located at the point of patient care, storing data from a variety of monitoring devices. Captured data is valuable to both providers and payors for clinical, utilization management, and reimbursement purposes.

virtual labor monitor (VLM)—one receiver is attached to the laboring mother's torso; another is fastened to the fetal presenting part, thus allowing the recording of the movement of the fetus down the birth canal. Under development is a VLM with 3D computer graphics simulation.

Virtuoso—a portable three-dimensional imaging system.

virus—not a living organism, but a very small segment of genetic material (DNA or RNA) encased in a protective protein shell. Upon entering a living cell, the virus assumes control of that cell's function and reproduction. The normal operations of the cell are suspended and it becomes a factory for the synthesis of more virus. Finally the cell disintegrates, releasing hundreds of new virus particles, which can then invade other cells. Viral infection typically elicits an acute, self-limited inflammatory response, without suppuration or fibrotic reaction. Viruses show a predilection for skin and mucous membranes, and even those that cause systemic disease often produce eruptions of papules or vesicles (as in measles and chickenpox). Viruses cause the common cold, influenza, measles, mumps, chickenpox, warts, herpes simplex, hepatitis, poliomyelitis, AIDS, and rabies. For quick-reference list, see *pathogen* and individual entries:
adenovirus
AIDS-related virus
Andes
arbovirus
ARV
avian influenza A (H5N1)
baculovirus (genetically engineered)
Bayou
Black Creek Canal
Epstein-Barr (EBV)
gamma-herpesvirus
hepatitis B (HBV)
herpes simplex virus (HSV)
herpesvirus
herpes whitlow
herpes zoster (HZV)
H5N1
HHV-8 (human herpesvirus-8)
HIV (human immunodeficiency)
HIV-1E

virus *(cont.)*
  KSHV (Kaposi sarcoma-associated
    virus)
  HTLV-I retrovirus (human T-cell
    leukemia/lymphoma virus)
  HTLV-III (human T-cell lympho-
    tropic virus)
  human herpesvirus 6 (HHV-6)
  human mammary tumor (HMTV)
  human papillomavirus (HPV)
  human parvovirus B19 (HPV B19)
  Laguna Negra
  Juquitiba
  lentivirus
  leukovirus
  lymphocytic choriomeningitis
    (LCMV)
  McKrae strain of herpesvirus
  MCV (molluscum contagiosum
    virus)
  Nipah
  nonsyncytium-inducing (NSI)
    variant of the AIDS
  oncogenic retrovirus
  picornavirus
  porcine endogenous retrovirus
    (PERV)
  respiratory syncytial (RSV)
  retrovirus
  RNA
  rotavirus
  Rous sarcoma
  Sin Nombre (SNV)
  togavirus
  varicella zoster (VZV)
  West Nile
  zoonotic retrovirus
virus-like infectious agent (VLIA)—a
  microbacterium.
virus-like particle—see *VLP.*
Viruzilin—immunostimulant against
  pancreatic cancer.
Visage Cosmetic Surgery System—
  wrinkle reduction procedure using
  Coblation.

Visa II PTCA catheter.
VISC (vitreous infusion suction cutter).
viscera—plural form of *viscus.*
Viscoat (hyaluronate sodium; chondroitin sulfate sodium)—viscoelastic solution used to coat delicate tissues in
  eye surgery, to reduce risk of tears,
  to prevent further tearing of tissue, to
  prevent vitreous loss. It is indicated
  for use as a surgical aid in anterior
  segment procedures, including cataract extraction and intraocular lens
  implantation. It helps to maintain a
  deep chamber during anterior segment surgery and protects the corneal endothelium and other ocular
  tissues. This solution also maintains
  the normal position of the vitreous
  face, thus preventing postoperative
  flattening of the chamber.
Viscoheel K, Viscoheel N—orthosis
  used to reduce shock load to joints
  and spine, as well as to correct varus
  and valgus position of the heel and
  leg axis.
Viscoheel SofSpot—orthosis used to
  reduce heel spur pain and plantar
  fascial pain.
viscous—thick, not readily flowing. Cf.
  viscus.
viscus (pl., viscera)—an internal organ,
  particularly one in the abdominal or
  thoracic cavities. Cf. *viscous.*
Visi-Black surgical needle—a needle
  with a nonshiny finish and a slim,
  tapered point. The black finish is
  intended to provide greater visibility
  within the operative field.
Visicath—a small endoscopic instrument, which may be used for bedside
  examination of the airway.
Visick (grades I-IV)—grading system
  for postgastrectomy recurrence of
  carcinoma.

Visidex, Visidex II—blood glucose testing strips.

Visijet hydrokeratome—high-energy, supersonic waterjet beam used to cut the cornea, specifically developed to create a LASIK flap in refractive surgery. See *LASIK*.

Visilex—polypropylene mesh specifically designed for laparoscopic hernia repair.

Vision 1.5-T Siemens MRI scanner.

Vision PTCA catheter.

Visipaque (iodixanol) **intravascular injection**—radiographic nonionic isosmolar contrast medium (IOCM).

Visitec circular knife.

Visitec crescent knife.

Visitec EdgeAhead phaco slit knife (Oph).

Visitec stiletto knife (Oph)—used in vitreoretinal surgery. Also, *cannula, cystitome, needle, nucleus hydrodissector.*

Vistaflex—balloon expandable, platinum alloy biliary stent.

Vistec x-ray detectable sponge—a surgical sponge with radiopaque strands running through it for x-ray visualization (just in case the sponge count is incorrect!).

Vistide (cidofovir)—used to treat relapsing cytomegalovirus retinitis via intravitreous injection in AIDS patients.

visual analogue scale—method often used in pain management to rate pain.

visual evoked potential (VEP).

visual field testing—to test the function of retina, optic nerve, and optic pathways when both central and peripheral visual fields are examined.

Visual Neglect Test—to assess neurological deficit following an incident such as a subarachnoid hemorrhage.

The patient is shown a page with 32 lines scattered randomly across it and is asked to cross out each line. If the patient fails to cross out more lines on one side of the page than the other, the side with the most errors corresponds to the side of visual neglect.

Visudyne (verteporfin for injection)—treatment for the wet form of age-related macular degeneration.

Visuflo—a device that blows a stream of filtered, humidified air onto a suture site to remove unwanted blood flow.

Visulas Nd:YAG laser.

visuscope—an instrument for testing the amblyopic eye.

VISX excimer laser—used in laser vision correction procedures to correct astigmatism.

VISX Star S2 excimer laser system—considered safe and effective for treatment of up to 14 diopters of myopia and up to 5 diopters of astigmatism.

VISX WaveScan Wavefront System (Oph)—allows instant measurement of refractive aberrations using highly advanced optics that project light into the eye and analyze the returning wavefront. The system produces a WavePrint, much like a "fingerprint" of the eye.

VitaCuff—a subcutaneous attachable cuff containing silver, for use with central venous catheters, to decrease bacterial infections at the site of entry.

VitaCuff antimicrobial cuff—discourages bacterial migration at the exit site of catheters.

Vitallium—trademark for an alloy used in prostheses and in skull plates. See *McKeever Vitallium cap prosthesis*.

Vitalograph spirometer.

vital signs—pulse, respiration, temperature. Sometimes a physician dictates, "Four vital signs are normal." In that case, blood pressure is the fourth sign.

Vitatron Diamond pacemaker—responds to circulatory needs caused by a patient's emotional state as well as level of physical activity.

Vitatron Diamond II—a dual sensor, dual chamber pacemaker that is designed to improve a patient's exercise tolerance and provide a steady, stable ventricular beat.

Vitatron pacing systems—include the QT sensor and the Activity (ACT) sensor, as well as the Diamond II DDR, the Ruby II DDD, the Topaz II SSIR, and the Jade II SSI.

Vitatron catheter electrode (Cardio).

vitelliform macular degeneration.

Vitesse Cos—laser catheter by Spectranetics containing optical fibers that are "optimally spaced" to improve debulking efficiency (the dissolving of tissue blocking an artery).

Vitesse E-II—eccentric, rapid-exchange coronary catheter.

Vitex (equal amounts of human thrombin and fibrinogen)—a tissue adhesive.

Vitrase—for treatment of vitreous hemorrhage or bleeding into the back portion of the eye.

Vitrasert intraocular implant—a form of Cytovene (ganciclovir) available in a timed-release delivery form implanted in the eye to treat cytomegalovirus.

Vitravene injection (fomivirsen sodium)—ophthalmic antiviral for treatment of CMV retinitis in AIDS patients.

Vitrax—viscoelastic used in ophthalmic surgery.

vitrectomy—surgical procedure used for bleeding inside the eye, usually caused by diabetic retinopathy. The blood-filled vitreous is removed and replaced with a clear solution. See *open-sky vitrectomy*.

vitrector probe—used during cataract surgery to simultaneously aspirate, cut, and irrigate with balanced salt solution.

Vitreon (perfluorophenanthrene)—type of substitute solution for vitreous humor. Used to float and help facilitate removal of a dislocated intraocular lens.

vitreous base—attachment to the ciliary epithelium (near the ora serrata).

vitreous body—a transparent jelly-like mass that fills the cavity of the eyeball.

vitreous cutter—instrument used in eye surgery such as vitrectomy.

vitreous face—anterior surface, that which is behind the lens.

vitreous space—vitreous body or the cavity it occupies.

vitro—see *in vitro*.

Vivelle; **Vivelle-Dot** (estradiol transdermal system)—transdermal patch available in four dosage strengths. It is small, thin, flexible, and translucent, delivering consistent levels of estradiol through the skin and into the bloodstream. It is used for treating symptoms of menopause, vulvar or vaginal atrophy, and hypoestrogenism.

vivo—see *in vivo*.

VLAP (visual laser ablation of prostate).

VLCD (very low-calorie diet)—a specific diet of nonfat milk with vitamins and mineral supplements.

VLDL (very low-density lipoprotein).

Vleminckx's solution ("vlem-inks")—antiseptic used in patients with severe acne.

VLIA (virus-like infectious agent)—a microbacterium.

VLM (virtual labor monitor).

VLP—a virus-like particle believed to be the etiologic agent of enterically transmitted non-A, non-B hepatitis.

V-MAX—virtual reality device that magnifies and makes things clearer for individuals with low vision.

VMP (VePesid, mitoxantrone, prednimustine)—chemotherapy protocol.

VNS (vagus nerve stimulation).

VNUS Closure catheter; radiofrequency generator—a device for shrinking varicose veins to occlusion. Used as an alternative to vein-stripping surgery.

VNUS Restore catheter—partially shrinks over-dilated varicose veins to restore competency of vein valves as a possible treatment for deep vein reflux.

vocal cord—*not* vocal chord.

Vocare bladder system—designed for patients with spinal cord injuries that cause loss of bowel and bladder control. Sensory nerves are severed and electrodes connected directly to nerve roots. The electrodes are also attached to a receiver implanted under the skin. The patient places the stimulator over the receiver, and the bladder is emptied.

VOD (veno-occlusive disease).

Voerner's disease—rare form of hereditary epidermolytic palmoplantar keratoderma, which includes hyperkeratosis of the skin of the palms and soles, with fissuring and marked hyperhidrosis.

Vogt-Koyanagi-Harada disease.

Vogt lines—seen on the cornea in keratoconus.

voiceprints—acoustic spectrographic methods to detect abnormalities in the cries of infants.

Volkmann's contracture—neurovascular contracture of an extremity due to arterial occlusion.

Volkmann's spoon—a small spoon used in removal of pancreatic calculi.

Volk Pan Retinal Lens—for binocular indirect ophthalmoscopy.

Volk QuadrAspheric fundus lens—a diagnostic/therapeutic contact lens with four aspheric surfaces.

Volk SuperPupil NC (non-contact) **lens** —for indirect ophthalmoscopy to view small pupils.

Volmax (albuterol)—oral bronchodilator.

Voltaren (diclofenac sodium)—a nonsteroidal anti-inflammatory drug in delayed-release tablets, used to treat arthritis.

Voltaren eye drops (diclofenac sodium 0.1%)—used to treat photophobia in patients undergoing incisional refractive surgery and following cataract surgery.

volume acquisition—MRI term.

volume analysis—MRI term.

volume element (voxel)—MRI term.

volume rendering of helical CT data.

volumetric segmentation—allows for quantifying the tumor burden in patients with cancer.

voluming artifact (Radiol).

voluntarily stopping eating and drinking (VSED)—undertaken at the request of a mentally competent patient, along with terminal scdation, a palliative option for the terminally ill. See also *PAS*, *terminal sedation (TS)*, and *VAE*.

voluntary active euthanasia (VAE).

Volutrol—control apparatus for intravenous infusion.

volvulated Meckel's diverticulum—a term coined from "volvulus."

Volz total wrist arthroplasty.

Von Frey's test—test of cutaneous sensibility performed with a Semmes-Weinstein pressure anesthesiometer.

von Graefe's sign—in exophthalmos, the upper lid lags behind the lower, exposing the eyeball.

von Hippel-Lindau (VHL) **disease**—an inherited disease in which affected persons are predisposed to develop multiple tumors, including cancers of the kidney, eye, brain, spinal cord, and adrenal gland. The identification of the VHL gene in affected families has led to better management of the disease.

von Hippel-Lindau (VHL) **gene**—identified by researchers at the National Cancer Institute in Bethesda, Maryland, as the gene for von Hippel-Lindau disease. The gene is also involved in clear cell skin cancer, which is not hereditary.

von Hippel-Lindau (VHL) **tumor suppression gene**—leads to identification of proteins that seem to interact with this gene product.

von Kossa staining—demonstrates the presence of calcium in tissues.

Von Lackum surcingle—a traction device using straps that apply contralateral pressure; for correction of scoliosis. See also *surcingle*.

von Recklinghausen's disease—neurofibromatosis.

von Rokitansky's disease—see *Budd-Chiari syndrome*.

von Willebrand's factor (vWF)—antigen levels most elevated in giant cell arteritis, but also found in Sjögren's syndrome, choroiditis, and polymyalgia rheumatica. Elevation of the vWF antigen levels may help in the differential diagnosis of giant cell arteritis. Cf. *giant cell arteritis*; *von Willebrandt's knee*.

von Willebrandt's knee—nothing to do with the knee, but is a group of optic nerve fibers, located in the anterior optic chiasm, that loop forward into the contralateral optic nerve and then back into the appropriate optic tract. Cf. *von Willebrand's factor*.

Voorhees needle (Ob-Gyn). *Not* to be confused with *Veress needle*.

Voptix—a computer program that stores and displays corneal thickness data taken from a variable array of corneal positions.

VOR (vestibulo-ocular reflex).

vortex—a whorled pattern or arrangement, such as is found in fingerprints or the pattern of hair growth at the crown of the head. Cf. *vertex*.

Vortex router (ENT).

Vortex stabilization system—utilizes vacuum-assist technology, enabling physician to immobilize the artery while performing beating-heart bypass.

Voxgram—multiple-exposure hologram of CT image. See *digital holography system*.

Voyager Aortic IntraClusion device—for use in stopped-heart procedures that include CABG, mitral valve replacement, and valve repair; allows performance of four critical functions through a single incision.

Vozzle Vacu-Irrigator—used for controlled irrigation and evacuation of body tissue and fluids in surgery.

VPAP (variable positive airway pressure).

VPCA (vincristine, prednisone, cyclophosphamide, ara-C)—chemotherapy protocol.

VPL thalamic electrode (ventroposterolateral). This is used to alleviate intractable pain by deep brain stimulation, and is internalized in much the same way as a pacemaker. See also *electrode*.

VPP (VP-16 and Platinol)—chemotherapy protocol for small cell lung carcinoma (or cancer).

V/Q (ventilation/perfusion) **scan**. Also, *VQ*. (The *Q* stands for *quotient*.)

VRE (vancomycin-resistant enterococci).

VREF (vancomycin-resistant *Enterococcus faecium*) **infection**.

VS (ventriculosubarachnoid) **shunt**—used in spine surgery.

VSED (voluntarily stopping eating and drinking). Also, *TS (terminal sedation)*.

VSP (variable screw placement).

"V tach" ("vee-tack")—medical slang for ventricular tachycardia or ventricular tachyarrhythmia.

VTED (venous thromboembolic disease).

V3 loop—part of the envelope surrounding the HIV virus. V3 loop vaccines are in the process of development.

VT/VF (ventricular tachycardia/ventricular fibrillation).

vulnerable myocardium—heart wall at risk for injury from infarction.

vulvae—see *kraurosis vulvae*.

vulvar vestibulitis syndrome—a symptom complex associated with a significant long-term history of moderate to severe chronic introital dyspareunia and tenderness of the vulvar vestibule. A treatment program consisting of electromyographic biofeedback-assisted pelvic floor muscle rehabilitation exercises is reported to produce significant decreases in subjective pain. See *vestibulodynia*.

Vumon (teniposide).

vWF (von Willebrand's factor).

VZV (varicella zoster virus)—a virus often found in patients who have had bone marrow transplants.

W, w

WACH shoe (wedge adjustable cushioned heel)—a cast shoe used in orthopedics. (Pronounced "watch.")

Wada test—a test to determine hemispheric dominance.

Wagner's distraction device (Ortho)—increases the length of the femur or tibia.

WAIS (Wechsler Adult Intelligence Scale).

Waldhausen subclavian flap technique—used in repair of coarctation of the aorta.

Wallaby phototherapy system (Peds)—illuminator (light source) box and fiberoptic cable with a panel on the end that can be wrapped around or placed under the baby.

Wallace Flexihub central venous pressure cannula.

Wallace pipette—a one-step procedure to collect cells from the ectocervix and endocervix without the trauma of an endocervical brush or swab and spatula.

Wallach Endocell—a sterile, disposable endometrial cell sampler.

Wallach pencil—a cryosurgery instrument, used for treatment of retinal tears and trichiasis.

wallerian degeneration—reaction resulting from a cut or injury to distal nerve fragments.

Wallstent—a self-expanding arterial stent placed in percutaneous transluminal angioplasty to prevent mural thrombus formation. The Wallstent biliary endoprosthesis is a self-expanding metal stent that may be used in esophageal, biliary tract, or coronary artery stenosis or obstruction. See *Schneider's Wallstent; transjugular intrahepatic portosystemic shunt.*

Walsham forceps—used in repair of facial fractures.

wandering spleen—a rare condition in which the spleen has a long vascular pedicle that allows the organ to move freely in the abdomen. Pedicle may become torsed.

WAP (wandering atrial pacemaker).

Wardill palatoplasty.

Warm 'n Form—lumbosacral corset.

WarmTouch patient warming system —manages patient body temperatures intraoperatively to prevent postoperative hypothermia.

Warren splenorenal shunt.

Wartenberg pinwheel—used in sensory examinations.

Warthin-Starry technique—silver stain used to identify *Helicobacter pylori*.

Warthin's tumor—adenolymphoma. (Alfred S. Warthin, M.D., U.S. pathologist.) Cf. *Wharton's tumor*.

Was-Cath catheter for percutaneous thromboarterectomy.

washerwoman's skin—the macerated appearance of the skin after long immersion in water. Used in autopsy dictation.

Washington regimen—postoperative care following tendon repair.

washout phase—in radionuclide scans, scintiscanning of the lungs at the conclusion of the inhalation phase of a lung scan, after an interval during which all inhaled radionuclide has been exhaled.

wasting syndrome—a life-threatening weight loss, often seen in AIDS.

water brash—regurgitation of excessive saliva from the esophagus, often combined with some gastric juice; heartburn; pyrosis.

Waterfield needle—used for bone marrow biopsy and aspiration.

water hammer pulse—a very rapid upstroke and falloff, indicative of a number of cardiac problems, the common denominator being a low resistance of the runoff of blood.

water-induced thermotherapy (WIT) —treatment of benign prostatic hyperplasia by introducing heated (60°C) water into the prostatic urethra by means of a special heat-transmitting balloon catheter. The precisely controlled heated water destroys a predictable amount of tissue, which is reabsorbed into the body, and the obstructed urethra is reopened. WIT is an outpatient procedure requiring only topical anesthesia. See *Thermoflex system*.

watermelon stomach—gastric antral vascular ectasia (GAVE). It is associated with cirrhosis, scleroderma, and atrophic gastritis. The stomach exhibits prominent erythematous stripes running from the pylorus to the antrum that resemble the stripes on a watermelon. The "stripes" exhibit ectasias and intravascular thrombi, and can cause GI bleeding and anemia. Treatment includes laser or bipolar coagulation to control bleeding.

Water-Pik irrigator—may be used as a verb, e.g., "The canal was Water-Piked, packed with epinephrine-soaked sponges, and then packed with a dry sponge and sucked dry."

watershed region—in anatomy a "continental divide" from which vascular supply (or ascites) can go in either of two directions. Strokes in watershed regions of the brain are more devastating. There is an abdominal watershed and one in the upper pulmonary area which divides tracheal blood supply from retrograde lung supply. Lung transplants usually have the anastomosis in this region, and bronchial dehiscence can result from airway ischemia following disruption of the vascular supply in the watershed area.

water-soluble contrast medium (WSCM).

Waterston method—uses a portion of the transverse and descending colon as an interposition graft to replace an

Waterston *(cont.)*
esophagus destroyed by caustic substance ingestion.

Waters view (Radiol)—occipital film for view of the maxillary sinuses. Named for Charles Alexander Waters, M.D., U.S. radiologist.

Watson-Jones tenodesis—corrects instability arising from injury of both the anterior talofibular ligament and calcaneofibular ligament.

Watzke Silicone sleeve—used in scleral buckling procedures.

wavefront measurement—measures unique optical aberrations in a patient's eye by projecting light into the eye and analyzing the returning wavefront. This allows treatment with a wavefront-guided ablation pattern to reshape the cornea for indications such as myopia, hyperopia, astigmatism, and ocular abnormalities.

wavelet scalar quantization (WSQ).

waves—see *Cannon waves.*

WaveWire—high-performance angioplasty guide wire used to measure blood pressure in the coronary arteries. By taking blood pressure measurements on both sides of a lesion, the cardiologist can determine whether the lesion is significantly affecting blood flow. It may be used in combination with the FloWire Doppler guide wire if a patient has more than one blockage or lesion in an artery.

Wayfarer prosthesis—modifiable foot prosthesis.

WCST (Wisconsin Card Sorting Test).

WDE (wound dressing emulsion).

WDHA (watery, secretory diarrhea, hypokalemia, and achlorhydria) **syndrome**. See *vipoma syndrome.*

wean—to slowly decrease a person's dependence on something—a ventilator, for example; to discontinue a medicine by gradually reducing the dose.

weave—see *Pulver-Taft weave.*

Weaveknit vascular prosthesis—see *Microknit vascular prosthesis.*

Weber test (ENT)—for conducting hearing loss. The Weber test uses bone conduction. The base of the activated (tapped or stroked) tuning fork is placed against the forehead, the vertex of the skull, or the front teeth, and the patient is asked in which ear he hears the sound best. In conductive hearing loss, the sound is referred to the deafer ear. In perceptive hearing loss, the sound is referred to the better ear. See *air conduction, bone conduction*, and *Rinne test.*

Wechsler Adult Intelligence Scale—mental status examination.

Wechsler Memory Scale or **Test**—mental status examination.

Wedeen wire passers—designed with S-curve to pass around bone in orthopedic procedures.

Wedge—electrosurgical resection device used in transurethral resection of the prostate.

wedged hepatic vein pressure (WHVP) **measurement**—used to estimate portal vein pressure.

Weerda distending operating laryngoscope.

Wegener's granulomatosis—systemic vasculitis that can involve any organ system. A newly identified serologic marker, cytoplasmic pattern antineutrophil cytoplasmic autoantibody, makes possible the early diagnosis of Wegener's granulomatosis.

Wehbe arm holder—for operating table.

Wehrs incus prosthesis—used in ear reconstructive surgery.

Weigert stain—see *elastic fibers stain*.

weightbearing, nonweightbearing—terms frequently used in orthopedic dictation (*nonweightbearing extremity, weightbearing crutches*), although they do not appear in medical dictionaries. Many ask whether they should be hyphenated. The trend in language is to combine words without hyphens after compound nouns become common. An architectural term comparable to *weightbearing* is *loadbearing*, and it is treated as one word. Some may wish to hyphenate, as *non-weightbearing, non-weight-bearing*, or *nonweight-bearing*, but it seems simpler and clearer to make *weightbearing* and *nonweightbearing* single words.

Weill's sign—indicative of pneumonia in an infant. During respiration, the subclavicular space on the affected side shows no expansion.

Weir excisions—alar excisions of the nose.

Weitlaner retractor.

Welchol—new name of Cholestagel (colesevelam hydrochloride), for the treatment of hypercholesterolemia.

Wellferon (interferon alfa-n1)—chemotherapy drug also used to treat Kaposi's sarcoma in AIDS patients, and to treat hepatitis C.

wen—a sebaceous cyst or other bland swelling on, in, or under the skin.

Werdnig-Hoffmann disease—infantile motor neuron disease.

Wernicke's area of the brain (in the superior temporal gyrus)—important as the area involved in spoken language.

Wernicke's disease—a vitamin B_1 deficiency disease that causes memory loss.

Wesolowski vascular prosthesis—fine-knit Dacron prosthesis. See *Microknit vascular prosthesis*.

WEST (Weinstein Enhanced Sensory Test)—tests various body parts to determine degree of diabetic neuropathy.

Westergren test—for sedimentation rate.

Westerman-Jensen needle—used for bone marrow biopsy and aspiration.

Western blot (blotting) **electrotransfer test**—a second-line AIDS test, more sensitive, given as a backup when the ELISA test is positive.

WEST-foot—a sensory nerve tester using patented SofTip monofilaments.

West Nile virus—a mosquito-borne encephalitis spread from the northeast area of the United States by birds migrating south. Although most patients suffer only mild flu-like symptoms, the elderly and those with immune deficiencies are extremely vulnerable to more serious infection.

"wet" age-related macular degeneration (ARMD) (Oph)—the more severe type of ARMD. The membrane underlying the retina thickens, then breaks. The oxygen supply to the macula is disrupted, and the body responds by growing new abnormal blood vessels. These begin to grow through the breaks in the membrane behind the retina toward the macula, often raising the retina. These abnormal blood vessels tend to be very fragile and often grow, leak, or bleed, causing scarring of the macula. The damage to the macula results in rapid central vision loss. Once the vision is destroyed, it cannot be restored.

wet field cautery *(not* Wetfield).

wet mount—a method of microscopic examination in which the specimen (a fluid or fluid suspension) is placed on a slide and then covered with a coverslip, rather than drying the specimen. "Wet mounts showed positive trichomoniasis."

wet prep (also *wet mount*). "Wet preps were taken, which were negative for yeast but positive for *Trichomonas*."

wet reading—a term describing a stat (immediate) radiograph film reading. When wet chemistry was in use, a radiologist read a freshly developed wet film in the darkroom when a fast result was needed. Dry chemicals have been used for many years in radiology darkrooms, but convention still calls a stat report a "wet reading."

wet-to-dry dressings—sterile gauze is soaked in sterile normal saline, applied to a wound, and allowed to dry; when removed, it facilitates debridement.

Wharton's tumor (and *duct*)—benign papillary cystadenoma of the submaxillary gland. Cf. *Warthin's tumor*.

wheal *(not* wheel). If you scratch the skin of your forearm with your fingernail, you may find, after a few minutes, a raised area appearing where you made the scratch. It may also become erythematous and may or may not itch. This is a wheal. A wheal may represent a positive reaction in skin tests (such as the tine test for PPD), and the diameter of the wheal is measured to determine whether the response is positive or negative. In tuberculin testing, a wheal of 8 to 10 mm in diameter 48 to 72 hours after injection is considered positive. Cf. *wheal and flare reaction*.

wheal and flare reaction—reaction to a test administered via injection. See *wheal*.

Wheaton Pavlik harness—orthopedic brace for children.

wheat weevil disease—extrinsic allergic alveolitis caused by exposure to wheat flour and weevils.

wheelchair artifact (Radiol)—seen in patients x-rayed in their wheelchairs because they were too ill to lie flat for imaging.

wheelchairs and motorized personal transport systems (Rehab)
Action A4 sports chair
Affiniti Hoveround mobile chair
Amigo mobile chair
Barracuda sports chair
Chairman Corpus motorized chair
Convaid buggies
Cruiser Transport
EZ Rider chair
Hoveround HVR 100 power control programmable chair
Invacare chair
Iron Horse outdoor activity chair
Kid-EXB 2 child's chair for bus transport
Kuschall chair
LaBac adjustable chair system
Mulholland Growth Guidance System
Paraglide chair
Quickie P210/Sunrise chair
Slam'R adjustable chair
Spirea adjustable foldable wheelchair
Supernova Xtreme sports chair
Tarsys tilt and recline system
Viper chair by Radius
Vision/Epic chair
Zippie P500

Wheeless method—for surgical construction of a J rectal pouch.

whiplash technique—for repositioning a catheter with a trocar under fluoroscopy.

Whipple's disease—intestinal lipodystrophy, a rare chronic inflammatory disease, and an intestinal disorder of malabsorption. It primarily affects the small intestine and the mesenteric lymph nodes, but it may affect other organs including the brain, spinal cord, and peripheral nerve plexuses. The onset is usually in middle age and occurs nine times more often in men than in women. Symptoms involve multisystems and may include ataxia, personality changes, seizures, memory deficits, ophthalmoplegia, and hearing loss.

Whipple pancreaticoduodenectomy—used for tumor of the distal common duct or when severe pancreatitis is confined to the head of the pancreas.

whistletip ureteral catheter.

Whitacre spinal needle.

White and Panjabi criteria—for cervical spine x-ray evaluation.

White classification—diabetes mellitus.

white clot syndrome—spontaneous major arterial thrombosis in a patient receiving heparin therapy, usually preceded by thrombocytopenia (low platelet count).

white dot syndrome—see *multiple evanescent white dot syndrome.*

white limbal girdle of Vogt (Oph).

white line of Toldt—lateral reflection of posterior parietal pleura of abdomen over mesentery of ascending and descending colon.

whitlow, herpes—herpetic infection of the fingertips.

Whitnall's ligament—one of the support structures of the eyelid.

whole body hyperthermia—see *hyperthermia, whole body.*

whole body 29FDG scanning.

whole-field scotopic sensitivity screening (Oph)—field-based screening for glaucoma.

Wholey ("wooley") **wire**—used in opening a stenosed vessel. "The subclavian stenosis was crossed with a Wholey wire and a 7F diagnostic catheter."

WHVP (wedged hepatic vein pressure) **measurement.**

Wiberg classification of patellar types (I, II, III) in relation to shapes of the inferior surface of the patella, and in association with chondromalacia patellae.

wick (usually gauze)—used for drainage of a wound. "A large amount of liquid pus was drained from the wound. The wound was packed with $1/_2$" plain gauze. He is to have the wick removed in two days."

Wiener filter (MRI term)—recovers resolution and reduces image noise while improving quantification of regional myocardial perfusion with thallium-201 tomography.

Wiktor balloon expandable coronary stent (Cardio)—compressed stent made of tantalum wire which is inserted over the balloon of a coronary artery catheter and then expanded at the site of the angioplasty. Left in place, the stent remains expanded and prevents re-stenosis of the artery.

Wiktor GX—a coronary stent coated with Hepamed (heparin) to retard clotting. You may also hear it dictated as *Hepamed-coated Wiktor stent.*

Wilcoxon rank sum test—used in legionnaires' disease.

Wilde incision (ENT).
Williams-Beuren syndrome—idiopathic infantile hypercalcemia. Patients have elfin facies, failure to thrive, and sometimes supravalvular aortic stenosis and mental retardation.
Williams cardiac device.
Williams flexion exercises—involving flexion of the neck, trunk, pelvis, and legs. Designed to alleviate lower back pain by stretching the extensor muscles in the lower back and strengthening flexors, such as the rectus abdominis and gluteus maximus.
Williams vulvovaginoplasty.
Will Rogers phenomenon—a higher observed survival for every stage of disease without actually improving overall survival. Based on a comment by humorist Will Rogers, "When the Okies left Oklahoma and moved to California, they raised the average intelligence of both states!"
Wilmington—see *port of Wilmington.*
Wilson-Cook wire-guided sphincterotome (modified)—used in endoscopic procedures.
Wiltse approach—midline or bilateral paraspinal approach used in lumbosacral fusion.
Wiltse pedical screw system—fixation system used for the treatment of severe spondylolisthesis of the L5-S1 vertebra, degenerative lumbar scoliosis, and spinal stenosis when decompression is required.
Wiltse rods—used with bone graft in correcting and stabilizing vertebrae in spondylolisthesis.
WinABP ambulatory blood pressure monitor—stores up to 120 hours of ambulatory BP readings and sends to a Windows-compatible printer in chart or graph form.

Winchester syndrome—rare disorder believed by some scientists to be closely related to hereditary lysosomal storage disorders. Major symptoms may include short stature, arthritis-like symptoms, and eye and skin abnormalities.
windlass effect—creates an intrinsic foot support system that counters the pronatory ground reactive forces on the forefoot during propulsion.
windowed balloon—a shaded balloon (the unshaded portion is the "window") used with photodynamic therapy to deliver laser radiation to a targeted area, such as a portion of the esophagus. See *photodynamic therapy.*
winged scapula—caused by a stretching injury to the long thoracic nerve. This results in weakness of the serratus anterior, with "winging," or wing-like protrusion, of the scapula.
wing sutures.
wink—see *anal wink.*
WinRho SD antibody—used for the treatment of immune thrombocytopenic purpura.
WinRho SDF—an anti-D polyclonal antibody used for the treatment of acute childhood ITP (immune thrombocytopenic purpura).
Winston-Lutz linac (linear accelerator) **method**.
Winters shunt—corpus spongiosum to corpus cavernosum (for priapism).
Wirsung dilatation—actually, dilatation of Wirsung's duct. "There was no bile duct or Wirsung dilatation or vascular invasion." Used on an abdominal CT report in pancreatic metastasis from renal cell carcinoma.
Wirt test—for assessing stereoscopic acuity.

Wishard catheter—a catheter with one hole at the end; used for diagnostic purposes.

wishbone retractor—see *Omni-Tract adjustable wishbone retractor.*

Wiskott-Aldrich syndrome—dysgammaglobulinemia.

Wissinger rod—to correct shoulder instability. "We inserted a Wissinger rod anteriorly, and we looked for the probe as it entered anteriorly."

WIT (water-induced thermotherapy).

Witzel duodenostomy.

Witzel tunnel—for feeding jejunostomy.

Wixson hip positioner—for total hip and revision hip surgery.

Wizard cardiac device.

Wizard microdebrider—self-irrigating debrider used in endoscopic sinus surgery.

wobble board—a physical therapy apparatus used for patient education of proprioception and balance.

Wolfe graft—used in hand surgery.

Wolfe mammographic parenchymal patterns.

Wolff-Parkinson-White syndrome.

Wolvek sternal approximation fixation instrument—used to close a sternotomy incision after cardiopulmonary bypass surgery.

Womack procedure—splenectomy, resection of superior half of the greater curvature of the stomach, devascularization, and transgastric suturing of the varices for portal hypertension-induced variceal bleeding.

Wong-Staal scissors—another innovative way to keep the AIDS virus from replicating, from scientist Flossie Wong-Staal. Working with Arnold Hempel, she fashioned a molecule that cuts up the genes of the virus which control its activities.

Wood's light examination—of skin and hair for evidence of fungal infection.

wood pulp worker's lung disease—extrinsic allergic alveolitis caused by exposure to moldy logs.

Woods screw maneuver (Ob-Gyn)—used in vaginal delivery to deliver the infant's shoulders, sometimes used in conjunction with other maneuvers.

word salad—mixture of words and phrases that lack comprehensive meaning or logical coherence, commonly seen in schizophrenic states.

Woringer-Kolopp disease—manifested in cutaneous lymphoma.

Workhorse percutaneous transluminal angioplasty balloon catheter—used for PTA treatment of obstructive lesions of the iliac, femoral, and renal arteries or synthetic arteriovenous dialysis fistulae; catheters are not designed for use in coronary arteries.

Woronoff's rings—in psoriasis.

Worst gonioprism contact lens—a lens that allows the surgeon to directly examine synechiae (adhesions) which have formed around the haptics of an anterior chamber intraocular lens. The surgeon can then lyse these synechiae without having to cut the haptics of the intraocular lens. The intact intraocular lens can then be removed with less tissue trauma than if the haptics had been cut.

Worth 4-dot test (W4D) (Oph)—combined with stereopsis on the Titmus stereo test, used for evaluating the ability of the two eyes to perceive images simultaneously.

Woun'Dres hydrogel dressing.

Wound-Span Bridge II—trade name for a dressing that holds the ends of a wound together by spanning it rather than pressing on it.

Wound Stick measuring system—includes Wound Stick for measuring and marking the size and depth of a wound, and Wound Stick tunneler for probing the dimensions of an ulcer.

wrap-around ghosting artifact (Radiol)—see *aliasing artifact*. If the field of view (FOV) is too small, some of the radiographic image can wrap around and reappear on the other side of the image. The zebra artifact can occur with interference between the main image and the aliased part in gradient echo sequences.

Wrightlock posterior fixation system —spinal fixation system used for correction of scoliosis and spine instability, consisting of a stainless steel rod and Morse taper locking mechanism.

Wright needle—used to fashion a fascia lata sling to repair ptosis.

Wright peak flow—a metered measurement used in testing pulmonary function. "The lungs are clear to percussion and auscultation. There is no wheezing. His Wright peak flow on three occasions was 525."

Wright's stain—used in the diagnosis of *Pneumocystis carinii* pneumonia. See *GMS*, *Gomori or Grocotti methenamine silver*.

wrinkle artifact—see *kink artifact*.

Wrisberg—see *nerve of Wrisberg*.

Wristaleve—a corrective wrist support to alleviate symptoms of carpal tunnel syndrome.

wrist drop—passive flexion of the wrist due to paralysis of extensor muscles.

Wroblewski method—of testing serum LDH.

WR-2721—see *ethiofos*.

WSCM (water-soluble contrast medium).

WSQ (wavelet scalar quantization).

W-stapled urinary reservoir (or ileal neobladder)—a procedure for providing post total cystectomy patients with an orthotopic neobladder (rather than ileal diversion). A portion of the ileum is removed for construction of the reservoir, and the ileum is anastomosed end-to-end. The removed portion is shaped into a W, using absorbable staples. The ureters are attached to the two upper limbs of the W, and the urethra is attached to the bottom of the W. The procedure can be performed quickly, in 12 to 21 minutes.

Wu bunionectomy—a modification of the Mitchell distal metatarsal osteotomy/bunionectomy. Uses a distal transverse first metatarsal osteotomy using Herbert bone screw fixation. Named for Dr. Kent K. Wu.

Wurzburg plating system—titanium craniomaxillofacial plate and screws.

WuScope system—combination laryngoscope and intubation device designed for both awake and anesthetized patient intubation via either the oral or nasal route.

Wylie carotid artery clamp.

Wyse pattern—for reduction mammoplasty.

X, x

Xalatan (latanoprost solution)—used for reduction of intraocular pressure in patients with open-angle glaumoma and ocular hypertension.

Xanar 20 Ambulase CO$_2$ laser—used in dermatologic and gynecologic surgery.

xanthelasma—a flat or slightly raised yellowish tumor, found most frequently on the upper and lower lids, especially near the inner canthus.

xanthogranulomatous cholecystitis—a rare inflammatory condition of the gallbladder associated with marked proliferative fibrosis, which occasionally invades surrounding tissues such as the liver bed and porta hepatis. Unfortunately, this condition so closely mimics gallbladder carcinoma that an intraoperative biopsy is necessary to make a diagnosis. May also be referred to as *ceroid-like histiocytic granuloma* or *fibroxanthogranulomatous inflammation*.

Xatral OD (alfuzosin)—a uroselective alpha-1 blocker for symptomatic treatment of benign prostatic hyperplasia.

X-body—see *Birbeck granule*.

Xcytrin (motexafin gadolinium) **injection**—used for the treatment of cancer patients with brain metastases.

XeCl (xenon, chloride excimer) **laser**.

Xeloda (capecitabine)—new oral treatment for women with breast tumors resistant to treatment with other drugs such as Taxol. Taken by mouth, it is converted by the body into 5FU.

xemilofiban—an oral antiplatelet drug.

Xenical (orlistat) **capsules**—nonsystemic antiobesity medication. It blocks the action of lipases, enabling fat to be absorbed through the intestinal wall. It does not work on the brain to suppress appetite and does not enter the blood stream.

XenoDerm graft—provides a suitable matrix for engraftment of cultured epidermal autografts to generate a reconstituted skin. They are processed porcine dermis, an animal-derived equivalent to LifeCell's patented AlloDerm processed tissue grafts.

xenograft (heterograft)—a term replaced by the phrase *xenotransplantation product*. See *graft*.

Xenomedica prosthetic valve.

xenon arc photocoagulator.

xenon 133 scan (^{133}Xe)—measures cerebral blood flow by isolating the internal carotid artery and injecting xenon 133. The cerebral blood flow is then calculated by automated cerebral blood flow analyzer.

Xenotech prosthetic valve.

xenotransplantation—any procedure that involves the transplantation, implantation, or infusion into a human recipient of either live cells, tissues, or organs from a nonhuman animal source, or human body fluids, cells, tissues, or organs that have had ex vivo contact with nonhuman animal cells, tissues or organs.

xenotransplantation product—live cells, tissues, or organs used in xenotransplantation.

xenotropic donor organisms—organisms originating in nonhuman animal tissue that pose the risk of infectious disease transmission through xenotransplantation.

xenozoonoses—animal diseases that may be transferred through xenotransplantation.

Xerecept (corticotropin-releasing factor)—a synthetic corticosteroid used to treat cerebral edema caused by brain tumors.

Xeroform ("zero-form") **gauze**.

Xillix LIFE-Lung system—GI fluorescence endoscopy imaging system for detection and localization of cancerous and precancerous lesions of the gastrointestinal tract. It is believed to be more effective than conventional white light bronchoscopy alone.

xiphoid ("zi´foid") **process** (Greek, sword-shaped)—the pointed cartilage and bone attached to the lower end of the sternum. Cf. *scyphoid*.

XKnife—software for stereotactic radiation therapy treatment planning. This software is used for the development of radiotherapy treatment plans to treat lesions in the brain, including tumors and vascular malformations.

X-linked familial spastic paraparesis—a disease characterized by spastic gait and increased reflexes without other associated neurologic signs.

X-linked retinoschisis—a splitting of the retina that may be complicated by vitreous hemorrhage and retinal detachment.

X-linked SCID—severe combined immunodeficiency disease of unknown genetic origin.

XMG (x-ray mammogram).

XMMEN-OE5 monoclonal antibody—for patients in shock from a systemic gram-negative infection.

XomaZyme-H65—for children and young adults with acute lymphoblastic leukemia.

Xopenex (levalbuterol HCl) **inhalation solution**—for use with a nebulizer in the treatment or prevention of bronchospasm in adults and adolescents with reversible obstructive airway disease.

Xpeedior 60 catheter—used for removal of clots from dialysis grafts.

XPS Sculpture system—see *liposhaver*.

XPS Straightshot—a micro tissue resector system used in endoscopic sinus surgery.

XQ230 Olympus gastroscope.

x-ray *(not* X-ray)—roentgenogram or roentgen ray.

x-ray tomographic microscope (XTM) —originally invented to analyze ceramic components used in jet engines, this technology is now being used by dental researchers to observe structures in tooth dentin measuring as small as 2 micrometers, about the size of a human cell.

XT cardiac device.

X-TEND-O knee flexer—provides patient-controlled flexion and extension exercises.

XT radiopaque coronary stent—developed by Bard, reportedly more flexible and easier to put in place than other coronary stents.

X-Trode—electrode catheter for intravenous insertion into a cavity of the heart.

xylol pulse indicator.

Xyrem (gamma hydroxybutyrate)—used in treatment of narcolepsy.

Y, y

YAG (yttrium-aluminum-garnet)—see *Nd:YAG laser.*

YagLazr system—used for treatment of a broad range of tattoo colors and epidermal lesions.

Yankauer curette (curet).

Yasargil bayonet scissors.

Yellow IRIS—a workstation that performs blood cell counting in synovial and pericardial fluids and crystal examination in synovial fluid.

Yentl syndrome—refers to the fact that women's cardiac symptoms are often regarded less seriously than men's, with the male-dominated medical profession pursuing a less aggressive management approach to coronary artery disease in women than men, despite greater cardiac disability in women. ("Yentl" is from the story "Yentl, the Yeshiva Boy" by Isaac Bashevis Singer.)

Yeoman uterine biopsy forceps.

Yergason test—used in examining the shoulder to determine if subluxation of the long head of the biceps tendon is present.

Yersinia—genus of gram-negative rods. *Yersinia pestis* is the etiologic agent of plague.

yohimbine—an alkaloid found in the bark of the tree *Pausinstalia yoimbe*. It is used in naturopathic medicine as an aphrodisiac and for treatment of impotence.

Yoon rings—fallopian tube ligation rings.

Yorke-Mason incision.

Young-Dees-Leadbetter bladder-neck reconstructive procedure—to create bladder outlet competence.

Yperwatch gamma control watch—measures exposure to radiation.

YPLL (years of potential life lost)—used in mortality studies.

Y-shaped graft.

Y stenting—an angioplasty technique that utilizes one or more intracoronary stents in an inverted Y configuration.

yttrium-aluminum-garnet (YAG)—see *Nd:YAG laser.*

Yunis-Varon syndrome—extremely rare inherited multisystem disorder

Yunis-Varon *(cont.)*

with defects affecting the skeletal, ectodermal, and cardiorespiratory systems. It is characterized by growth retardation prior to and after birth; defective growth of the bones of the skull along with complete or partial absence of the shoulder blades; characteristic facial features; possible abnormalities of the fingers and/or toes; and, frequently, cardiomyopathy. The syndrome is thought to be inherited as an autosomal recessive genetic trait.

yuppie flu—see *chronic fatigue syndrome*; *myalgic encephalomyelitis*. Also, *postviral fatigue syndrome*.

Z, z

Zacutex (lexipafant)—medication used in the treatment of acute pancreatitis.

Zadaxin (thymalfasin)—a drug used for treatment of AIDS, certain cancers, chronic hepatitis B and C, and hepatocellular carcinoma.

Zaditen (ketotifen)—an oral drug to prevent bronchial asthma attacks.

Zaditor (ketotifen fumarate)—drug that provides temporary relief from itching of the eye due to allergic conjunctivitis.

zafirlukast (Accolate).

Zagam (sparfloxacin)—new-generation fluoroquinolone for respiratory tract infections.

Zahn—see *line of Zahn*.

Zanaflex (tizanidine)—an oral medication treatment for muscle spasticity.

Zancolli clawhand deformity repair.

Zanfel—a topical cream for treatment of poison ivy (urushiol), poison oak, or poison sumac, which is eliminated from the skin in 30 seconds.

Zang Fu differentiations—identifies disease entities and suggests acupuncture treatment by symptoms.

Zantac Efferdose—nonprescription effervescent H_2 antagonist.

Zavanelli maneuver—returns the fetus into the pelvis during cesarean section for failed vaginal breech delivery.

ZD neurosurgical localizing unit—used in stereotactic biopsy and minimally invasive neurosurgery.

ZDV (zidovudine).

Zebeta (bisoprolol).

zebra artifact—see *wrap-around ghosting artifact*.

Zebra exchange guide wire—used with the SoloPass during endoscopic bile duct procedures.

ZEEP (zero end-expiratory pressure).

Zefazone (cefmetazole).

Zeiss—manufacturer of many ophthalmological instruments, cameras, and microscopes.

Zeiss Endolive endoscope.

Zeiss Visulas 690s laser—for activation of Visudyne (verteporfin for injection) therapy to treat wet age-related macular degeneration.

Zelapar (selegiline HCl)—a new formulation of selegiline, an MAO inhibitor, for the treatment of Parkinson's disease.

Zeldox (ziprasidone hydrochloride)—an antipsychotic agent used in the treatment of schizophrenia.

Zelmac (tegaserod)—drug treatment for irritable bowel syndrome in patients whose primary symptom is constipation.

Zelsmyr Cytobrush—used to obtain material from endocervical canal for Pap smear, Chlamydia screen, and other lab tests.

Zenapax (dacliximab)—a humanized monoclonal antibody used in combination with cyclosporin and corticosteroids for prophylaxis of organ transplant rejection in patients receiving kidney transplants.

Zenith AAA endovascular graft system—used for minimally invasive treatment of abdominal aortic aneurysm (AAA). Catheters are guided to the location of the AAA through the femoral arteries; once in position, the self-expanding, fabric-covered, metallic stent/graft is deployed to relieve pressure on the aneurysm.

Zenker's fixative—a mercury-containing solution used to harden and preserve tissue.

Zenotech—a biomaterial for synthetic ligaments.

Zerit (stavudine, d4T)—a fruit-flavored liquid solution of d4T used in the treatment of HIV-infected infants and children.

ZES (Zollinger-Ellison syndrome).

Zest Anchor Advanced Generation (ZAAG) bone anchoring system.

Zestoretic—a combination of the diuretic hydrochlorothiazide and the ACE inhibitor lisinopril. Used to treat hypertension.

Zestril (lisinopril) **tablets**—an ACE inhibitor to be administered within 24 hours of acute myocardial infarction. Used in adjunctive therapy in patients with cardiac failure who do not respond adequately to diuretics and digitalis.

zeugmatography—MRI term.

Zeus—computer- and voice-controlled robotic system that positions and maneuvers instruments in microsurgery, directed by a surgeon working at a Zeus workstation with video monitor.

Zevalin (ibritumomab tiuxetan)—monoclonal antibody linked to the radioisotope yttrium-90.

Ziac (bisoprolol fumarate, hydrochlorothiazide)—a combination drug taken once a day to control mild to moderate hypertension.

Ziagen (abacavir)—a protease inhibitor used in treating AIDS.

Zicam—over-the-counter nasal solution said to significantly reduce the severity of the common cold, including nasal congestion, sneezing, coughing, and sore throat.

ziconotide—analgesic for patients with chronic malignant pain caused by cancer or AIDS.

zidovudine (Aztec)—an antiviral drug for AIDS treatment taken twice daily and reported to cause fewer side effects than Retrovir.

Ziehl-Neelsen stain (Lab)—for acid-fast bacilli.

Zielke curette (curet).

Zielke instrumentation—used to correct thoracolumbar curvatures. It is composed of a threaded rod, bone screws, washers and nuts. Used with

Zielke *(cont.)*
external bracing, it can stabilize a corrected thoracolumber curvature until arthrodesis is considered to be solid.

ZIFT (zygote intrafallopian tube transfer)—used in cases of blocked fallopian tubes, to achieve pregnancy. This is a combination of techniques used in GIFT and IVF. In ZIFT, fertilization takes place in vitro (in a dish), and 18 hours later four of the zygotes that have formed are replaced in the fallopian tubes to work their way into the uterus. See *GIFT, IVF, zygote.*

ZIG vaccine (zoster immune globulin).

Zimmer CPT (collarless polished taper) **hip system**.

Zinecard (dexrazoxane)—used to prevent cardiomyopathy caused by the chemotherapy drug doxorubicin.

Zinnanti Z-clamp.

Zipper Medical—hypoallergenic tracheostomy tube neckband.

zipper scar.

Zipzoc—stocking compression dressing and wrap.

Ziramic femoral head.

Zirconia orthopedic prosthetic heads—made of zirconium oxide ceramic.

Zithromax (azithromycin)—antibiotic drug for treating AIDS patients with MAC infection. Also for strep pharyngitis, chlamydial infections, urethritis, toxoplasmosis, and cryptosporidiosis.

Zixoryn (flumecinol)—for hyperbilirubinemia in newborns.

Z-lengthening of tendons and split tendon transfers.

ZMC (zygomatic-malar complex) **fracture** (of the face).

Z-Med catheter—peripheral, high-pressure balloon catheter, low deflation profile, rapid inflation/deflation time.

ZMS intramedullary fixation system—a Zimmer fixation system that provides easy intramedullary passage over a guide wire through the fracture site without reaming.

Zocor (simvastatin)—lowers levels of LDL in patients with hypercholesterolemia that has not responded to dietary measures. Also raises HDL levels and lowers triglyceride levels.

Zofran, Zofran ODT (orally disintegrating tablets) (ondansetron)—used for postoperative nausea and vomiting. It was previously approved for chemotherapy-induced nausea and vomiting.

Zoladex (goserelin acetate implant)—a once-a-month injection for the treatment of advanced breast cancer in premenopausal and perimenopausal women, as an alternative to surgical removal of the ovaries.

Zoll defibrillator.

Zollinger-Ellison syndrome (ZES)—gastric hypersecretion, peptic ulceration, pancreatic tumor syndrome, ulcerogenic tumor of pancreas syndrome. See *apudoma.*

zolmitriptan (Zomig).

Zoloft (sertraline hydrochloride)—used in treatment of depression, panic disorder, and obsessive-compulsive disorder.

zolpidem tartrate (Ambien)—a sedative/sleeping pill for the short-term treatment of insomnia.

Zomaril (iloperidone)—an antipsychotic agent for the treatment of schizophrenia.

Zometa (zoledronic acid for injection)—for treatment of tumor-induced hypercalcemia, which often occurs

Zometa *(cont.)*
as a complication of bone metastasis in patients with breast cancer, multiple myeloma, and non-small cell lung carcinoma (or cancer).

Zomig (zolmitriptan)—oral drug used for treatment of acute migraine.

zona hamster egg test—used in male infertility to test the ability of spermatozoa to penetrate hamster ova, which approximate human ova.

Zonalon (doxepin hydrochloride cream)—topical antipruritic for eczematous and atopic dermatitis.

zone
electric
Looser's
triangle of doom
triangle of pain

Zonegran (zonisamide)—an antiepilepsy drug used as adjunctive therapy in the treatment of partial (focal) seizures in adults with epilepsy.

zone of partial preservation (ZPP)—in spinal cord injury.

Zone Specific II meniscal repair system—cannulas, needles, and rasps used for inside-out meniscal repair procedures.

zonula occludens—tight junction of endothelial cells.

zonulolysis—dissolution of the ciliary zonule by use of enzymes, to permit surgical removal of the lens.

zoonosis—the transmission of an animal infectious disease to humans, a potential complication of xenotransplantation.

zoonotic retroviruses—retroviruses of animal origin that have the potential to incorporate in the genome of human cells and replicate.

zopiclone—a rapid-acting nonbenzodiazepine hypnotic for the treatment of sleep disorders.

zoster immune globulin vaccine.

Zosyn (piperacillin sodium; tazobactam sodium)—for treatment of intra-abdominal infections. Zosyn is the U.S. product equivalent to European drug Tazocin.

Zovirax (acyclovir)—an antiviral drug for herpes simplex, herpes zoster infections, patients with AIDS, and for treating chickenpox in otherwise healthy children. It is found to cause faster healing of skin lesions with less scar formation.

Z-Pak—packaging form of the antibiotic Zithromax, six capsules.

ZPP (zone of partial preservation).

ZstatFlu—diagnostic test for influenza A and B.

Z stent—a self-expanding stent for bile duct and esophageal stenosis. Its wires are crisscrossed in a Z pattern. Also, *Gianturco prosthesis*.

Z-stitch—used in percutaneous bladder neck stabilization procedure in women with stress urinary incontinence. The stabilization suture is attached at four points on the pubic bone in a Z configuration.

ZTT I and **ZTT II acetabular cups**.

Zucker and Myler cardiac device.

Zuma guiding catheter—used in the coronary or peripheral vascular system to provide a pathway for the introduction of therapeutic devices.

ZUMI uterine manipulator.

Zung Depression Scale.

Zweymuller prosthesis—a cementless hip prosthesis.